MOLECULAR IMMUNOLOGY TECHNIQUES

Prof. Ramesh Chandra and Dr. Heerak Chugh

ALLIED HEALTH PRESS

Molecular Immunology Techniques

Author: **Prof. Ramesh Chandra and Dr. Heerak Chugh**

Allied Health Press
4164 Lakeshore Road
Burlington ON L7L 1A4
Canada
www.alliedhealthpress.com
Email: orders@arclereducation.com

ISBN: 978-1-77956-835-9

ABOUT THE AUTHORS

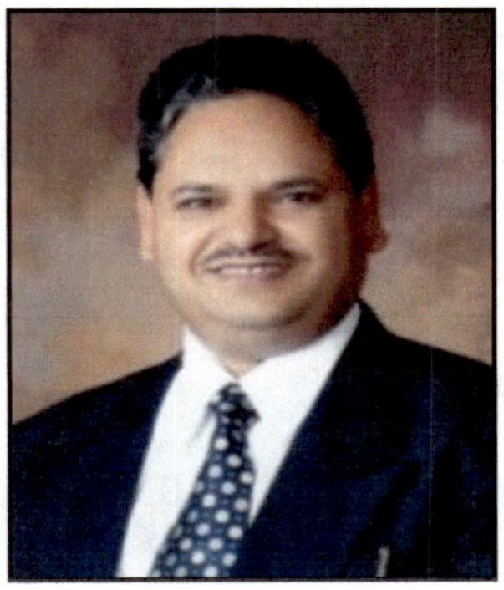

Prof. Ramesh Chandra is a distinguished scientist; Fellow of the Royal Society of Chemistry, London and an outstanding researcher in the field of Biomedical Sciences. Currently, he is the Vice-Chancellor at Maharaja Surajmal Brij University, Bharatpur, Rajasthan, and Founder Director of Dr. B. R. Ambedkar Center for Biomedical Research (ACBR), University of Delhi. He is Official resource person to the Minister and Department of Science and Technology in the kingdom of Lesotho, South Africa.

He started his research career at the University of Delhi, then at The New York Hospital-Cornell University Medical College, and The Rockefeller University, New York; State University of New York at Stonybrook, Harvard University Medical School-Massachusetts General Hospital (MGH) jointly at MIT, Cambridge, USA.

Prof. Chandra has been Vice-Chancellor, Bundelkhand University, Jhansi (1999-2005) as well as President of the Indian Chemical Society, Member, Planning Commission, Government of U.P. India; Secretary - Zaheer Science Foundation, New Delhi and Non-Official Director, Rashtriya Ispat Nigam Ltd, Government of India. He was also Head of the Department of Chemistry, University of Delhi.

He is recipient of several international recognitions: J. William Fulbright Scholarship, The Rockefeller Foundation USA-Biotechnology Career Award, Award of the Highest Honor of Soka University, Tokyo, Japan; Millennium Plaques of Honor (Life Time Achievement Award for contribution in Science & Technology) by the Indian Science Congress Association (ISCA), Lifetime Achievement Award of the Indian Chemical Society (1CS); UGC Research Scientist Award; UGC Career Award; Rajib Goyal Award for Young Scientists and others.

Prof. Chandra shows deep commitment to the cause of higher education & research and possesses in ample measure quality of dynamic leadership, vision required for building academic institutions and excelled in his academic pursuits. To illustrate, he has to his credit several international patents, 9 Books; 28 Book Chapters; and more than 400 original Scientific Research Papers in International journals of repute. He has mentored more than 100 Ph.D. students.

In recognition of his outstanding Scientific Research and Administrative Qualities, Prof Ramesh Chandra has been conferred Capital Foundation Dr A.P.J. Abdul Kalam National Award.

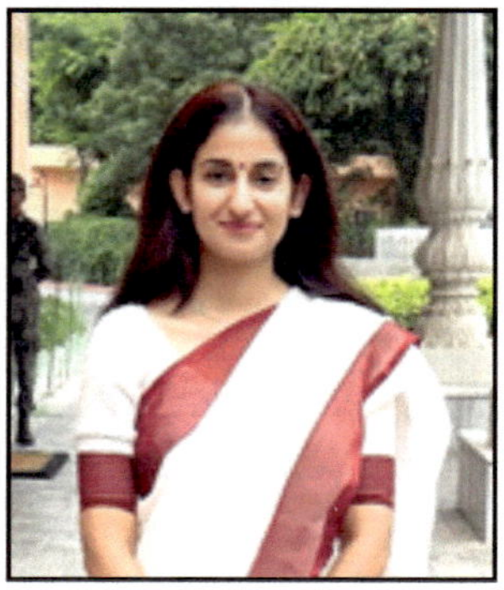

Dr Heerak Chugh is a life scientist who is currently working as a Senior Researcher funded by Indian Council of Medical Research (ICMR) at University of Delhi, Delhi. She is also teaching as an Adjunct Assistant Professor at Maharaja Surajmal Brij University, Rajasthan.

Her Research focusses on advancing our current understanding of cancer and exploring therapeutic interventions to improve treatment (patient) outcomes. She has extensive experience in Cell biology, molecular biology, biochemistry, cancer biology, chemical biology, biophysical chemistry, chemotherapeutics, drug delivery and cancer nanomedicine.

Dr Heerak Chugh completed her graduation and postgraduation in Life Science from Sri Venkateswara, University of Delhi, Delhi and Central University of Punjab, Bathinda, Punjab, respectively.

Dr Heerak Chugh developed her research interest while working as a research intern at CSIR-IGIB where she was working on synthesizing plant-based nanoparticles and cationic nanoparticles as novel anti-microbial agents. To continue her research interests, Dr Heerak Chugh joined a Ph.D. programme in University of Delhi, Drug Discovery and Development Laboratory, Department of Chemistry, University of Delhi wherein she worked on increasing the therapeutic efficacy of Noscapine, an anti-cancer agent.

Dr Chugh was awarded prestigious Prime Minister Fellowship for Doctoral Research by Science and Engineering Research Board (SERB), Government of India and Confederation of Indian Industry (CII); until now, she is the only recipient from University of Delhi. She was also awarded Junior Research Fellowship through National Eligibility Test (All India Rank 60). Further, she was also awarded Senior Research Fellowship by Indian Council of Medical Research.

During her Ph.D., she worked at Department of Biological Sciences, Purdue University, Indiana, USA as Science and Engineering Research Board, Government of India funded Overseas Doctoral Visiting Fellow where she studied HYPE protein and its role in cancer.

She was one of the subject matter experts on Voet's Biochemistry Adapted Edition 2021. She has published over a dozen research articles in various peer-reviewed International Journals, and continues to work and publish actively in the field of cancer biology and cancer therapeutics. She also serves as an invited reviewer for various international journals.

Brief Table of Contents

Detailed Table of Contents

CHAPTER 9

Gene Editing in Immunology 279

CHAPTER 10

High-Throughput Screening in Immunology 315

CHAPTER 13

Immune Profiling and Omics Approaches 421

CHAPTER 14

Immunotherapy and CAR-T Technology 459

CHAPTER 15

Advancements in Vaccine Development Techniques 499

Index 537

LIST OF FIGURES

PREFACE

The immune system, being a finely tuned and intricate protection mechanism, operates through an enormous net of molecular mechanisms that protect the organism from foreign invaders and maintain balance internally. The last decades have witnessed a record growth in the capacity to chart immune processes with precision, thanks to the advances of molecular techniques. These methods allow scientists to investigate immune cell behavior, identify disease biomarkers, and develop targeted therapies with greater assurance. With the increasing convergence of immunology science with molecular biology, new tools and platforms have allowed us to dissect immune responses at the genetic, protein, and single-cell levels.

With the threat of global health issues like emerging infectious diseases, cancer immunotherapy, autoimmune disease, and vaccine research, molecular immunology methodologies have become essential. With their ability to precisely quantify, define, and manipulate immunological components, these methodologies are critical for today's medical science and personalized medicine. From the application of PCR-based immune gene expression detection to CRISPR-mediated genome editing in immune cells, these technologies are defining medical science today and facilitating personalized medicine. Understanding and applying such methods require a well-structured and comprehensive reference that brings together the molecular methods most relevant to immunology.

Molecular Immunology Techniques is designed to be a cohesive, practical, and comprehensive reference for professionals handling the modern methods of molecular immunology. The book consolidates and integrates the fundamental and advanced laboratory procedures used in immunological research with an easy-to-follow explanation of procedures, applications, and interpretations. Every chapter is designed to reflect the modern application and relevance of specific techniques in clinical as well as research settings. Emphasis is placed on experimental design, result interpretation, and assimilation of data from more than one methodology. The content is addressed to beginner students and experienced researchers alike who seek an updated overview of evolving techniques.

Chapter 1 presents an introduction to the basic molecular biology techniques that form the basis of immunological research. It includes nucleic acid extraction, gel electrophoresis, and the polymerase chain reaction (PCR), and their modifications for immune studies.

Chapter 2 discusses immunoassays like ELISA, Western blotting, and radioimmunoassays with a focus on the classical as well as modern modifications for detection as well as quantitation of proteins.

Chapter 3 discusses recombinant DNA technology and applications in designing expression systems for cytokines, antibodies, and immune-modulatory proteins.

Chapter 4 discusses antigen-antibody interactions using tools such as surface plasmon resonance, immunoprecipitation, and microarray formats.

Chapter 5 covers gene expression analysis methods specific to immunology, such as real-time PCR, RNA-Seq, and cytokine and immune marker microarray profiling.

Chapter 6 deals with experimental methods for the study of T-cell and B-cell biology, such as flow cytometry, MHC tetramer staining, and proliferation assays.

Chapter 7 summarizes protein-protein interaction analysis methods, including yeast two-hybrid screening, co-immunoprecipitation, and proximity ligation assays, for immune signaling pathway investigation.

Chapter 8 overviews single-cell analysis methods, including single-cell RNA sequencing, mass cytometry, and microfluidic droplet technologies, for cellular heterogeneity examination in immune responses.

Chapter 9 recapitulates gene editing tools such as CRISPR-Cas9, TALENs, and zinc-finger nucleases with special focus on immune cell engineering for research and therapeutic purposes.

Chapter 10 recapitulates high-throughput screening strategies in immunology, such as small-molecule libraries, peptide arrays, and siRNA screens, allowing for the identification of novel modulators of immune function.

Chapter 11 presents the principal *in vivo* models, i.e., mouse models of autoimmune disease, cancer, and infection, with training in transgenic and knockout technologies.

Chapter 12 presents structural methods such as X-ray crystallography, cryo-electron microscopy, and NMR spectroscopy in gaining insight into the molecular structure of immune complexes.

Chapter 13 presents immune profiling using omics technologies, namely proteomics, metabolomics, and transcriptomics, for the analysis of immune cells and identification of disease biomarkers.

Chapter 14 looks at immunotherapy approaches like CAR-T cell manufacturing, adoptive transfer protocols, and checkpoint blockade studies in preclinical models.

Chapter 15 ends the book with recent innovations in vaccine technology, including mRNA-based platforms, adjuvant engineering, antigen design, and immunogenicity assessment, mirroring the fast pace of vaccinology research.

The book is addressed to a general audience that includes graduate students, postdoctoral fellows, clinical scientists, professorial academics, and laboratory technicians working in immunology, molecular biology, biotechnology, and biomedical sciences. It also serves as a helpful handbook for medical practitioners and drug developers who want to learn more about the application of immune-based technologies in practice.

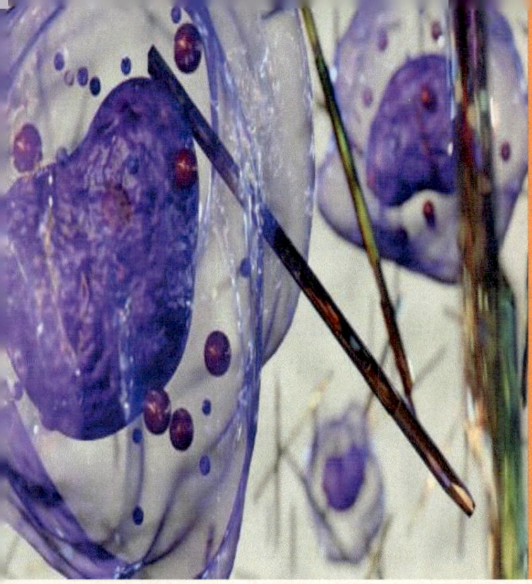

Chapter 1

BASIC MOLECULAR BIOLOGY TECHNIQUES FOR IMMUNOLOGY

Contents

Introduction

Immunology has witnessed spectacular progress over the past decades, and basic molecular biology techniques have been pivotal. They are essential tools by means of which researchers and doctors are able to explore immune phenomena with their intricate mechanisms. By unraveling the molecular and cellular machinery of the immune system, techniques such as polymerase chain reaction (PCR), mass spectrometry, and microscopy have elucidated the pathogen-host defense interaction. Manipulation and characterization of nucleic acids and proteins have propelled immunology to unparalleled heights with novel diagnostics, therapies, and vaccine design in the pipeline. On this account, the integration of molecular biology within immunology has not just elucidated common theories but has also caused the re-evaluation of established views for self and non-self recognition in the immune system. Specifically informative in this regard is research into mycolic acids in mycobacterial analysis, wherein advanced mass spectrometry techniques have been employed for identification. These complex lipids are analyzed to identify species of mycobacteria and thus dictate diagnostic procedures for tuberculosis and other diseases. Highly sensitive and specific procedures for differentiating *Mycobacterium tuberculosis* from non-tuberculous mycobacteria have been established with electrospray ionization tandem mass spectrometry. This technique has proven to demonstrate its worth within clinical settings, surpassing standard diagnosis techniques on both speed and accuracy, underscoring the importance of molecular techniques in the creation of immunological diagnoses (Szewczyk et al., 2013). As we increasingly approach an era of rapid and reliable diagnostics, the marriage of molecular biology and immunology will be imperative in overcoming public health concerns. Furthermore, the philosophical concepts underpinning immunological theory, i.e., the self/non-self model, are being reassessed from a molecular basis. Traditional views established through F.M. Burnet have established a sharp dichotomy between what constitutes the self and non-self entities, yet current experiential data suggest that this model is not entirely representative of the complexity of immune responses. A shift towards conceptualizing immune interactions as continuity and not fixed identity could be a more advanced strategy, in light of recent criticism of metaphysical assumptions in the field (Pradeu & Carosella, 2005). This controversy demonstrates how advances in molecular biology not only advance applied uses but also challenge theory development, with a general appreciation for the complicated dynamics of the immune system.

Definition of Molecular Biology

Molecular biology, essentially, is the study of biological processes at the molecular level, with the overall focus being on the interaction between various cellular systems. Molecular biology entails studying DNA, RNA, proteins, and other macromolecules responsible for carrying out basic functions in cell functioning. Molecular biology presents us with lavish information regarding the process of gene expression, replication, and repair, which are fundamental to learning about cellular functioning and the general biological system. As a preliminary foundation in the broader fields of genetics and biochemistry, molecular biology is a general context for the study of immunological responses. The fusion of the methods of molecular biology with those of immunology both enhances understanding of immunological processes and provides for the creation of new therapeutic and diagnostic techniques. The elucidation of the self/non-self model is perhaps one of the major contributions of molecular biology to immunology. This model, initially proposed by F.M. Burnet, has long been influential in the understanding of how immune systems differentiate between non-self and endogenous material. However, recent criticism suggests that this model may not be capable of explaining all immunological events. For instance, a consideration of immune continuity as opposed to complete differentiation between self and non-self could give more satisfying explanations of immune function. This shift in focus motivates the search for molecular patterns and interactions that regulate immune reactions to lead researchers to develop advanced approaches in immunology in congruence with current biological hypotheses and concepts (Pradeu & Carosella, 2005). Moreover, tools of molecular biology, such as gene editing and protein engineering, play a key role in increasing our comprehension of the immune system's complexity. With the advancing technology in the field of molecular biology, new solutions are on the horizon to address the complex immunological problems. CRISPR-Cas9 gene editing and next-generation sequencing are the finest examples of how the technology is empowering the field of molecular biology to improve our ability to edit and question genetic information. These technologies allow researchers to examine the underlying genetic factors that result in the immune response and thus make interventions in immunotherapy and vaccine development more precise. Besides, cross-disciplinary approaches employing computational biology and synthetic biology are emerging as key in this area. The future second generation of bio-inspired methods reflects growing recognition of the need for the convergence of life sciences and engineering to offer new solutions (Timmis et al., 2005). Such cross-disciplinary merging not only raises technical competence but also leads to a better understanding of biological systems, ultimately driving immunological research and applications (Figure 1.1).

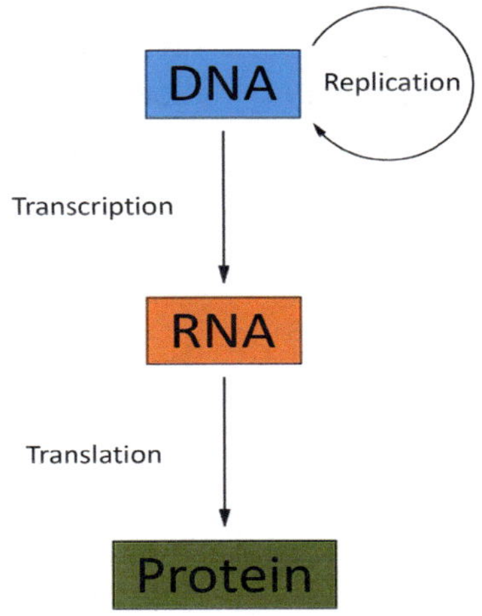

Figure 1.1. The central dogma of molecular biology.

Source: https://thumbs.dreamstime.com/z/central-dogma-molecular-biology-framework-describes-flow-genetic-information-biological-system-297071345.jpg.

Importance of Molecular Biology in Immunology

Molecular biology plays an important role in the study of immunology by providing essential techniques that show the intricate mechanisms of the immune system. With the application of methods such as PCR and gene sequencing, researchers are able to assess immune cell gene expression patterns upon recognition of various antigens. Molecular findings facilitate a better understanding of how self versus non-self is recognized and detected by the immune system, which subsequently accounts for the origin of targeted therapies for autoimmune diseases and infections. As the field of immunology transforms, the function of manipulating and evaluating genetic material becomes increasingly central not only in basic research but also for clinical applications to achieve the aim of increasing immunity and vaccine production. Molecular biology's significance in immunology also encompasses the development of monoclonal antibodies, which have revolutionized therapeutic management for a broad spectrum of disorders. By applying the technology of hybridomas, scientists can generate specific antibodies against corresponding antigens in the immune system and improve diagnostics and therapeutic procedures for ailments such as cancer and chronic inflammatory diseases. As the reliance on such sophisticated methods grows, there is a need to include the rules of molecular biology in the teaching of immunology to prepare the next generation of scientists and healthcare professionals. The ability to comprehend the underlying processes facilitated by these approaches motivates innovation in personalized medicine, indicating the necessity for a sound background in molecular biology. Besides, the collaborative research in marine biotechnology indicates the application of molecular biology in immunology fields. Marine organisms are being utilized by research centers to purify novel compounds with immunomodulatory effects, demonstrating the effectiveness of molecular approaches for the discovery of new therapeutic drugs (Seaman & Whitehouse, 2001). Such interdisciplinarity not only broadens the immunology toolbox but also provokes new research initiatives focused on world health diseases. The commitment of many research and academic institutions to creating such teamwork further underscores the role of molecular biology as a key pillar in improving immunological understanding and interventions, which in turn boosts public health (Asbury et al., 2000).

Overview of Key Techniques

A variety of molecular biology techniques form the essence of immunological investigation, enabling both cellular as well as molecular understanding of immune response. Polymerase chain reaction or PCR, is one of the most significant techniques, as it enables amplification of provided DNA sequences, thereby rendering immune-related genes accessible for analysis. This technique has proven critical in quantifying the levels of gene expression that are required to define the roles of various pathways within the immune system. More advanced versions, such as quantitative PCR (qPCR) and reverse transcription PCR (RT-PCR), provide additional sensitivity and specificity. With researchers further refining and developing such tools, their application in vaccine construction and disease diagnosis grows ever more crucial, filling the lacunae in our comprehension of immune responses and the interactions between pathogens, crucial to health and disease control in human as well as animal populations. In addition to PCR, other key techniques include enzyme-linked immunosorbent assay (ELISA) and Western blotting, which are key to the identification and quantification of proteins associated with immune responses. ELISA takes advantage of the specificity of antibody-antigen complexes to quantify cytokines, antibodies, and other markers of significance in immunology. The technique has enabled high-throughput determination of immune constituents that are involved in roles in infectious and autoimmune diseases. Similarly, Western blotting provides qualitative and quantitative information on protein expression and modification, thereby enabling us to understand the dynamics of immune signal pathways.

Overall, these techniques provide us with a deeper understanding of the fundamental mechanisms of immune function and pathology, forming the basis of more advanced therapeutic interventions and vaccine design. Highlighting the significance of molecular techniques in immunology also encompasses appreciating the expedited advancements offered through the development of technology. Advances in marine biotechnology, for instance, reflect a new frontier that will boost immunological research capability. By merging biological intelligence from numerous aquatic species, researchers can uncover novel immune pathways and potential therapeutic agents unavailable through terrestrial models. This intersection lends to a better understanding of the immune system's evolution and resilience within varying environments, an area being subjected to more research along with technological advancement. Further, the cooperation between the industry and academia, as reflected in studies' surveys like the ones in Seaman & Whitehouse (2001), plays a vital role in encouraging innovation. As immunology increasingly embraces these innovative methods, the information that we gain through these endeavors will be priceless in the prevention and solution of both existing and emerging health issues.

1.1. Polymerase Chain Reaction (PCR)

The PCR is an easy-to-use and widely applied molecular biology method for amplifying segments of DNA, which makes it an essential resource in immunology research. Through cycles of repeated denaturation, annealing, and extension, PCR allows the exponential amplification of desired DNA sequences. This is very useful in immunology, where the detection and quantification of pathogens or immune markers are crucial. For instance, PCR can be employed to detect specific bacterial species linked to periodontitis so that researchers can quantify pathogen load and assess treatment response. In one study, quantitative (real-time) PCR assays were streamlined for simultaneous analysis of multiple periodontal pathogens as a demonstration of PCR's value in enhancing diagnostic precision and informing clinical management (Decat et al., 2012).

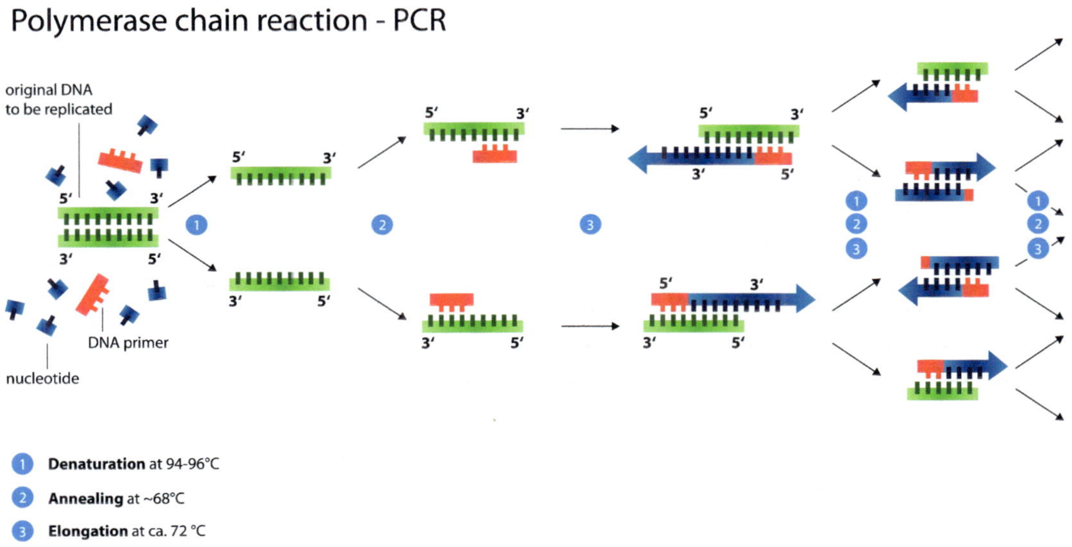

Figure 1.2. Polymerase chain reaction (PCR).

Source: https://microbeonline.com/wp-content/uploads/2016/07/Polymerase_chain_reaction.svg_.png.

The responsiveness and flexibility of PCR are so vital in the diagnosis of infectious diseases, particularly those caused by pathogens with variability in the rates of detection via different methods. For example, in one comparison study of the detection of Leishmania infantum in dogs, PCR displayed a very high sensitivity of 98% in parasite-positive samples. But this sensitivity was observed to be less in post-infection samples, suggesting a mild interaction between the infection timing and the method's efficacy (Quinnell et al., 2001). These observations highlight the necessity to select a suitable molecular technique based on the individual context of the infection as well as the biological targets being considered. PCR's diagnostic capability is compounded when combined with other technologies, such as serological assays, creating a strong framework for immune monitoring and disease regulation. Ultimately, the versatility of PCR extends beyond mere amplification; it is a building block approach to immunological assays utilized for vaccine evaluation, pathogen identification, and immune response measurement. Its specificity and real-time tracking capability allow scientists to distinguish the immunological dynamics of immune responses and interactions of pathogens with host organisms. As illustrated through analysis of periodontal pathogens, PCR-based approaches can be modified to meet various types of applications in immunology, ranging from quantifying disease risk to guiding the selection of therapy (Decat et al., 2012). Also, ongoing advancements in PCR technologies, such as digital PCR and multiplexing technologies, are poised to further enhance its use for comprehensive immunological analysis, providing more efficient diagnostic and therapeutic strategies in the field (Figure 1.2).

1.1.1. Principles of Polymerase Chain Reaction (PCR)

The principles of PCR form the foundation of the majority of molecular biology applications, particularly in immunology. Essentially, PCR is an amplification procedure for specific DNA sequences to enable researchers to make millions of copies of a desired section from an initial small amount. The process is based on the thermal stability of DNA polymerases, which make new strands of DNA through complementary nucleotides added to a template strand. The procedure consists of three main cycles: denaturation, annealing, and extension. Each cycle doubles the quantity of target DNA, exhibiting exponential growth, which is very helpful in the detection and analysis of genetic material of interest to immune response and is of enormous value for the investigation of infectious diseases and autoimmune diseases. Detection and quantification of expression of genes for immune responses is one of the significant roles of PCR in immunology. For instance, IL-21/IL-21R signaling is significant in the majority of inflammation-related conditions because it has been linked to such conditions as rheumatoid arthritis and inflammatory bowel disease. With PCR, researchers have managed to measure the expression level of IL-21R in human tenocytes during tendinopathy, as uncovered in current research. Such an approach not only provides insight into the molecular mechanisms of immune responses but also into the identification of possible therapeutic targets, providing insight into how inflammatory cytokines contribute to the disease pathology (Campbell et al., 2014).

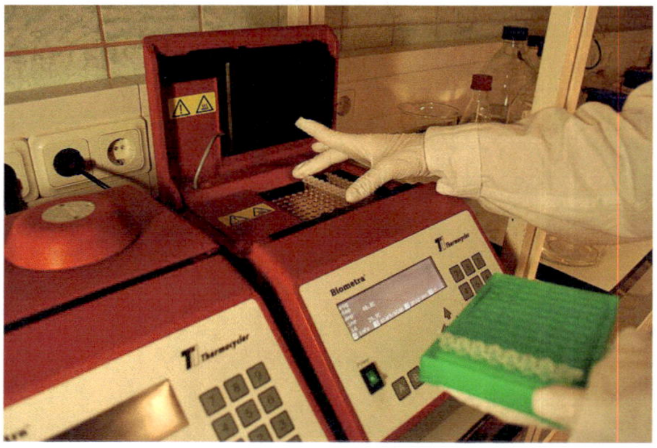

Figure 1.3. Placing a strip of eight polymerase chain reaction (PCR) tubes into a thermal cycler.

Source: https://upload.wikimedia.org/wikipedia/commons/thumb/6/67/PCR_masina_kasutamine.jpg/800px-PCR_masina_kasutamine.jpg.

This perspective accordingly emphasizes the significance of PCR in helping us better understand immunological diseases. Apart from PCR's ease of gene amplification, its application is in its use as a valuable tool in the teaching of immunology. Practical sessions, encompassing demonstrations of hands-on PCR, have shown that students can engage in a range of epistemic practices that support better understanding of abstract concepts. Through the use of PCR in laboratory settings, students can learn how to forecast and analyze outcomes and connect experimental findings with theoretical predictions (de Almeida et al., 2016). These hands-on activities better facilitate an improved understanding of the concepts of immunology and the applicability of molecular techniques to current research. Ultimately, PCR not only progresses the field of immunological research but also improves students' education, readying the scientists of the future within the discipline (Figure 1.3).

1.1.2. Applications of Polymerase Chain Reaction (PCR) in Immunology

PCR has revolutionized the field of immunology by allowing researchers to amplify specific DNA sequences that are crucial to understanding immunity. Low-abundance targets can be detected through this technique, which is particularly convenient when one is working with complex biological samples such as blood or tissue from a patient. For instance, PCR is capable of detecting pathogens or DNA, which helps clinicians diagnose infections that would otherwise not be detected by routine procedures. The sensitive and rapid nature of PCR lowers the time required for diagnosis, thereby enhancing the treatment and management of patients. Additionally, via primer design for unique sequences associated with immune markers, PCR allows for an appreciation of immune mechanisms and regulation understanding, which enhances disease comprehension in the immunological context. For vaccine discovery, PCR is a crucial instrument in evaluating immune responses elicited by vaccines.

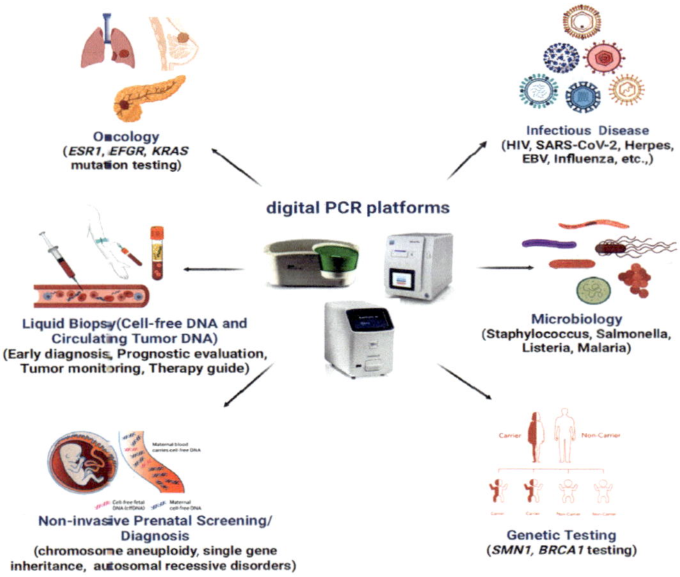

Figure 1.4. An overview of current dPCR applications in clinical laboratories, including infectious disease, microbiology, genetic testing, prenatal testing, liquid biopsy, and oncology.

Source: https://www.researchgate.net/profile/Shivaprasad-Sathyanarayana-2/publication/377150081/figure/fig3/AS:11431281264169072@1722480534377/Applications-of-dPCR-in-clinical-labs-An-overview-of-current-dPCR-applications-in.png.

By identifying unique antibody gene sequences or quantifying T-cell response, researchers can establish the effectiveness of a specific vaccine candidate. The ability to amplify target sequences from immune cells allows it to be possible to profiling the adaptive immune response at a detailed level. For example, PCR has been used extensively to examine the immunogenicity of candidate vaccines against a variety of pathogens, including agents that cause infections such as human immunodeficiency virus

(HIV) and influenza. Further, quantitative PCR (qPCR) methods are enhanced to allow for the precise measurement of genetic expression after vaccination, culminating in better vaccine design and assessment of vaccine efficacy. Such analysis is imperative in achieving immunological insight, but equally in guiding vaccine formulation and deployment strategies most likely to be targeted tightly as needed for public health. Furthermore, PCR's significance extends to the realm of new infectious diseases, which need immediate diagnostic solutions for effective control and containment. As an example, recent outbreaks of new pathogen diseases illustrate the necessity of constructing diagnostics able to detect the genetic makeup of new viruses on time. As highlighted in recent research, PCR not only performs diagnostic purposes but also monitors the real-time evolution of pathogens, hence having a direct bearing on public health interventions. The technique can identify genetic variations impacting pathogenicity or immune evasion mechanisms, as in research addressing the evolution of African trypanosomes with highly complex immune escape mechanisms (Stijlemans et al., 2017). Finally, the variable application of PCR in immunology, from diagnostics to vaccine evaluation, is indicative of its central role in driving both clinical practice and laboratory research in the context of evolving challenges (Figure 1.4).

1.1.3. Limitations and Challenges of Polymerase Chain Reaction (PCR)

PCR has transformed molecular biology, but with great power comes the threat of some limitations and adversity. One of the great ones may be the susceptibility of PCR to contamination. The amplification process is vulnerable to being disturbed by even minute levels of DNA from previous experiments or in the environment. This type of contamination not only leads to false positives but can also skew quantification, rendering the results inaccurate. This is particularly an issue in immunological research, where precise quantitation of target biomarkers is critical. The pervasive use of PCR in the field necessitates observation of these proper uses of the technique, with suggestions that misuses can erode the credibility of findings and ultimately lead to wasted funds in biomedical research (Nour et al., 2014). A second serious limitation of PCR is a function of its specificity, which can limit detection. Its requirement for highly specific primers makes PCR incapable of amplifying all target molecules of interest present in a sample, particularly in the face of pathogen genetic heterogeneity or with complex biological samples. This specificity can exclude low-abundance sequences, leading to analysis incompleteness and potentially misleading immunological research on the basis of comprehensive antigen profile knowledge. Besides, modifications of the PCR technique, for example, qPCR, also have additional complexity in assay design and optimization. This is another challenge since slight variations in conditions can result in varied amplification outcomes, creating challenges for researchers to get reproducible and consistent results (Jorgolli et al., 2019). Other than issues of contamination and specificity, the meaning of PCR result interpretation is a significant challenge for immunology. The quantitative nature of techniques such as qPCR can exaggerate results, particularly when statistical approaches are misused. Misinterpretation can lead to unsubstantiated conclusions about the significance of particular biomarkers or identification of pathogens, which can trigger a link of misinformation in research and even perhaps clinical applications. The demand for robust validation and replication highlights the requirement for critical evaluation of PCR data in immunology studies. Furthermore, with the face of drug discovery evolving and the incorporation of more sophisticated molecular methods, integration of PCR with other approaches is paramount in a bid to avoid its own limitations and enrich findings (Jorgolli et al., 2019).

1.2. Gel Electrophoresis

Gel electrophoresis is a central technique in molecular biology, particularly in research fields such as immunology, where protein and nucleic acid investigation is pivotal. It facilitates the separation of molecules in a sample based on size and charge, which helps identify and characterize elements in a sample. In gel electrophoresis, a current is passed through a matrix of gel, and charged molecules migrate toward their respective electrodes. Smaller molecules travel more quickly than larger molecules in the gel, allowing for efficient separation after electrophoresis. Separation leads to unique band patterns from which scientists can draw conclusions about protein expression and molecular interactions that are critical for understanding immune function as well as disease mechanisms. In immunology, gel electrophoresis is typically paired with other techniques, such as western blotting, which enables the detection of specific proteins involved in immune processes and pathogen interaction.

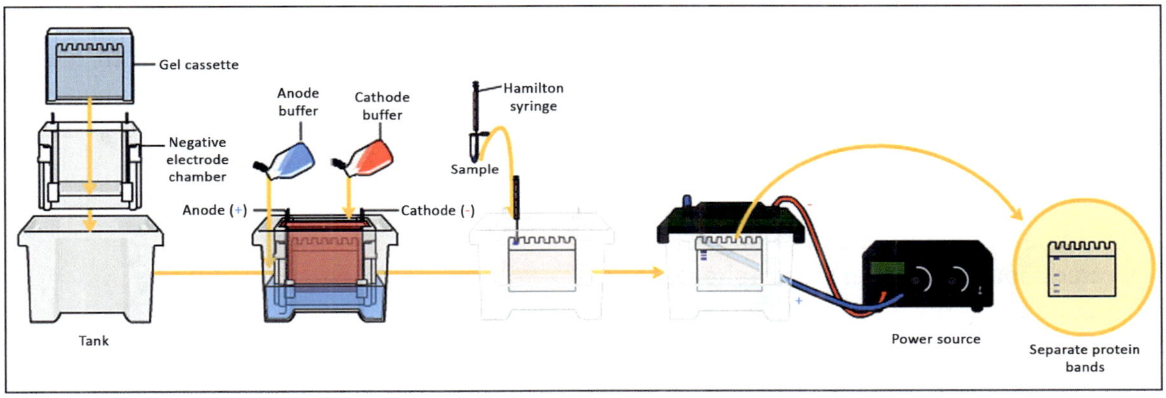

Figure 1.5. Overview of gel electrophoresis.

Source: https://upload.wikimedia.org/wikipedia/commons/4/46/SDS-PAGE_Electrophoresis.png.

Through two-dimensional gel electrophoresis (2-D gel), researchers can concentrate their study of complex mixtures of proteins by fractionating proteins based on isoelectric point and molecular weight. The two-step separation procedure enhances protein spot resolution and allows for closer proteomic investigation. It is particularly critical in disease research into immune modification, as identifying the full set of protein expressions can determine potential biomarkers for diagnostics. This synergy in methodology is critical, particularly in defining pathogens that are responsible for diseases like Primary Amoebic Meningoencephalitis, wherein specific protein markers must be determined quickly to ensure the efficacy of treatment (Park, 2011). Additionally, with improvements in technology in gel electrophoresis, it has become possible to use high-throughput screening and greater sensitivity in the detection of proteins, and hence it is a key tool in biomedical research. With increasing immunological studies, there is a parallel requirement for sophisticated gel electrophoresis methods that enable close examination of protein interactions and post-translational modifications. Marine biotechnology organizations, for example, use gel electrophoresis to examine immunological processes in various species and possibly reveal groundbreaking information about their immunity (Seaman & Whitehouse, 2001). This ongoing research illustrates the usefulness of gel electrophoresis, not just as a single technique but as a foundation technique that supports other molecular biology techniques, thus enhancing our molecular immunology knowledge (Figure 1.5).

1.2.1. Mechanism of Gel Electrophoresis

Gel electrophoresis is a fundamental technique employed in molecular biology that separates macromolecules based on size and charge. This method utilizes an agarose or polyacrylamide gel matrix, which acts as a molecular sieve. When an electric current is applied, negatively charged molecules, such as DNA or RNA, move toward the positive electrode, with the smaller fragments passing faster through the mesh structure of the gel compared to the larger ones.

The separation effect allows researchers to efficiently investigate nucleic acids or proteins, a feature crucial for immunological research. More importantly, the gels' porosity is a variable that can be manipulated by altering the polymer concentration so that separation conditions may be tailored to suit the specific requirements of the analysis being conducted. Visualization of the separated molecules in gel electrophoresis is normally done using the addition of a stain, e.g., ethidium bromide for nucleic acids or Coomassie Brilliant Blue for proteins. Once the electrophoresis run is complete, the gel would typically be exposed to ultraviolet (UV) light or other imaging techniques, enabling the detection and quantification of bands for different fragments or proteins. This aspect of gel electrophoresis not only aids in the confirmation of the presence of specific biomolecules but also aids in estimating their size in comparison with a molecular weight ladder. Therefore, the correct interpretation of these findings can be of great significance, particularly in the area of immunology, where the characterization of antigens and antibodies is critical in the depiction of immune responses and the design of therapeutic modalities. In immunology, gel electrophoresis plays a critical role in many applications, including analyzing the interaction between antibodies and antigens and analyzing the purity of biological samples. For instance, this technique can be employed by scientists to evaluate the efficiency of monoclonal antibodies by ascertaining their specificity and antigen-binding ability to target antigens. Additionally, gel electrophoresis can be employed to analyze EVs, which have been at the center of intercellular communication and immunomodulation in recent times. Gel electrophoresis coupled with other approaches, such as mass spectrometry, enhances the ability for the characterization of intricate biological mixtures to yield a more profound understanding of immunological mechanisms. Through the separation of specific biomolecules and determination of their function and interaction, this technique paves the way for paradigm-shifting advancements in biomarker discovery and therapy for the management of immunological disorders (Huang et al., 2020; Kumar et al., 2024) (Figure 1.6).

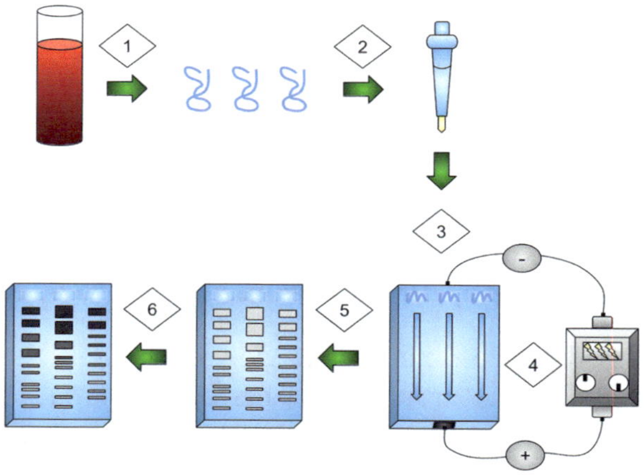

Figure 1.6. Gel electrophoresis is a process where an electric current is applied to DNA samples, creating fragments that can be used for comparison between DNA samples.

Source: https://upload.wikimedia.org/wikipedia/commons/thumb/d/d0/Gel_Electrophoresis_in_DNA_Fingerprinting.svg/800px-Gel_Electrophoresis_in_DNA_Fingerprinting.svg.png.

1.2.2. Role in Analyzing DNA and Proteins

Analysis of DNA and proteins lies at the heart of understanding the mechanisms underlying immunological response. Advanced molecular biology techniques enable researchers to investigate the structure, activities, and interactions of macromolecules, which are critical for the identification of vaccines and therapeutics One application involving liquid chromatography-tandem mass spectrometry (LC-MS/MS) to investigate the complex biomolecules, such as the mycolic acids, serves as an exemplary example. This approach not only aids in describing specific constituents in mycobacterial cell walls but also facilitates the diagnosis of diseases such as tuberculosis. Targeted analysis has the potential to yield various profiles that enable sound differentiation and identification of mycobacterial species, which considerably enhances clinical immunology based on enhanced accuracy and promptness in diagnosis (Szewczyk et al., 2013). Furthermore, the quantification of oxidative stress biomarkers is also a critical element in immunological studies since it is sensitive to disease processes and therapeutic endpoints.

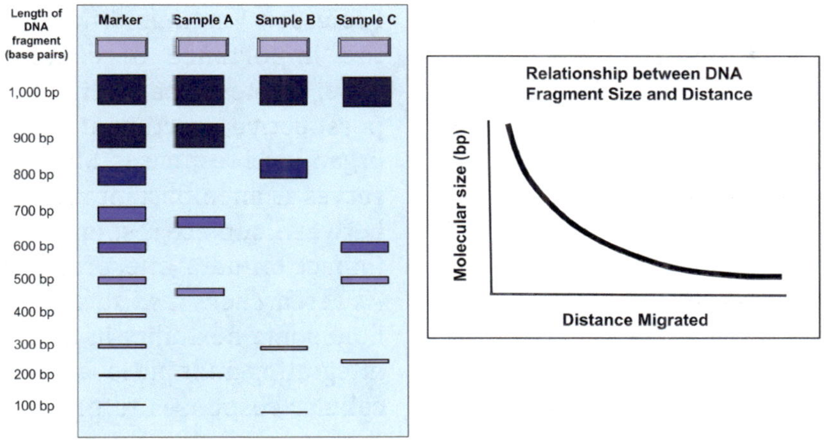

Figure 1.7. The image shows how small DNA fragments will migrate through agarose quickly, but large-sized DNA fragments move more slowly during electrophoresis. The graph to the right shows the nonlinear relationship between the size of the DNA fragment and the distance migrated.

Source: https://upload.wikimedia.org/wikipedia/commons/thumb/7/74/Gel_Electrophoresis.svg/1024px-Gel_Electrophoresis.svg.png.

Reactive oxygen species (ROS) play a crucial role in regulating immune responses, and as such, precise measurement techniques should be employed to quantify their effects on DNA and proteins. Methodological variability, however, poses challenges to quantifying ROS and alterations to biomolecules accurately. For instance, while flow cytometry is largely used for the quantification of ROS in leukocytes, reproducibility and standardization issues can introduce methodological biases. Thus, the generation of global oxidative stress indices by using a combination of multiple markers provides an enhanced representation of oxidative status, of interest in the description of numerous immunological conditions (Marrocco et al., 2017). Combined, these methods and techniques detail the intricate interaction of DNA, proteins, and immune function and highlight their relevance to immunological investigation. The evolution of analytical tools like LC-MS/MS and the necessity for standard methods to evaluate oxidative stress reflect the ever-evolving nature of molecular biology tools. With increasing exploration of the complexities of immune responses at the molecular level, the intersection of such technologies will increasingly define mechanisms of disease, improve diagnostic capability, and ultimately give way to new therapeutic paradigms in immunology. This intricate weave of analysis forms the cornerstone of modern biological science, bridging the divide between molecular mechanism and clinical application (Figure 1.7).

1.2.3. Interpretation of Results

Result interpretation of molecular biology techniques is critical, particularly within immunology, as it is the groundwork for interpreting immune response mechanisms and functions. The effectiveness of these techniques is frequently dependent on precise data interpretation to facilitate the identification of specific biomarkers related to immune responses. For example, advances in mass spectrometry have advanced the identification of mycolic acids in mycobacterial organisms to such a point that scientists can accurately distinguish between types of pathogenic and non-pathogenic strains. The ability to generate unique profiles for the acids demonstrates the diagnostic potential of mass spectrometry as a tool, both in research laboratories and as a clinical tool, for infectious diseases like tuberculosis. Such a strict interpretation helps to enhance the strength of findings, such that conclusions from experiments are drawn using sound analytical protocols. In addition, the relevance of such interpretations extends beyond identification; they serve as indicators for disease occurrence, disease progression, and treatment efficacy. The role of molecular biology tests can be quantifiable in terms of sensitivity and specificity parameters, which are employed in evaluating diagnostic protocols. In diagnosing tuberculosis, studies have shown that the rapid identification protocols using electrospray ionization tandem mass spectrometry yield results that are superior to conventional diagnostic methods. Not only do these results offer quick turnaround time—enabling quicker clinical decision-making—but also improved patient outcomes through timely intervention. By applying such methods to different patient populations and intersecting their responses, researchers can refine the understanding of immune dynamics and hence enable the development of targeted immunotherapies. Additionally, the interpretation of heterogeneous data elucidates the complexity of biological systems, one being forced to account for heterogeneity at more than one level. Investigations by scientists such as Professor Vladimir S. Markhasin demonstrate the importance of comprehending results observed to place within a broader biological perspective, particularly when investigating organ-level responses. Myocardial heterogeneity serves as an important reminder that variability between subject responses necessarily has an impact on data interpretation in immunology. As researchers face such intricacies, they must hold some flexibility in their analysis methods, integrating multiple levels of information—from cellular responses to organismal outcomes. In the end, a general consciousness of outcome interpretation works toward deepening a comprehension of immunological mechanisms, paving the way for innovative solutions to existing health challenges.

1.3. Western Blotting

Western blotting is a fundamental molecular biology method that allows researchers to detect and characterize specific proteins in complex mixtures. Western blotting is a two-step procedure consisting of the separation of proteins according to size by gel electrophoresis and their transfer onto a membrane where they can be attacked by antibodies to target proteins. The key advantage of western blotting is its versatility; western blotting can be employed across a broad field of disciplines, including immunology, for which it is fundamental in its role in identifying mechanisms of disease and potential biomarkers. By the accurate depiction of protein levels of expression, researchers are in a position to make important correlations between protein function and the disease's underlying pathology, thus enhancing the level of diagnosis and treatment possibilities. In addition to its diagnostic use, western blotting plays a unique role in confirming experimental results from other techniques, i.e., ELISA or PCR. In considering the effect of new treatments on protein expression, for instance, western blotting provides a robust means of verifying findings.

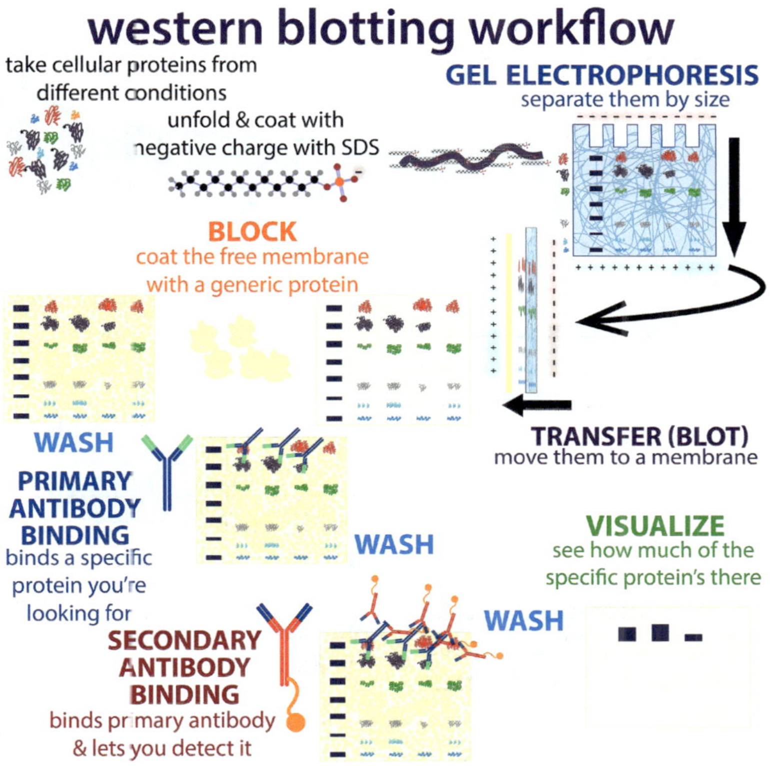

Figure 1.8. Western blot workflow.

Source: https://upload.wikimedia.org/wikipedia/commons/thumb/0/07/Western_blot_workflow.jpg/800px-Western_blot_workflow.jpg.

This cross-validation is not only required to maintain the integrity of scientific research but also to ensure that documented changes in protein quantities are truly representative of biological processes. Recent advances in antibody design and detection methods have further optimized western blotting to provide improved sensitivity and specificity, an important aspect when probing proteins of low abundance or under complex conditions of disease. Consequently, the strategic application of this method can strengthen the immunity of immunological research. The utility of western blotting is not limited to research but also applies to clinical settings, where it can be used to assess inflammatory reactions and disease conditions. As an example, haptoglobin has been found to be an important marker of inflammation, from studies that have demonstrated its determination in various species through techniques like Hp-ELISA that can be complemented with confirmation by western blot analysis. Correct determination of the haptoglobin levels in serum can potentially differentiate normal subjects and inflammatory subjects, illustrating the diagnostic potential of this protein determination method. Also, the versatility of western blotting in the characterization of complex proteins, as noted in comparative studies across species, is a testament to its broad applicability in basic studies and translational medicine (Segawa et al., 2013; Han et al., 2016). Lastly, western blotting is a workhorse technique in the immunologist's toolbox that bridges the gap between basic research and practical clinical application (Figure 1.8).

1.3.1. Process of Western Blotting

The Western blotting technique is an essential molecular biology method through which one can detect and analyze a specific protein in a complicated mixture. Western blotting begins with the separation of proteins using gel electrophoresis, in which proteins migrate based on their size, forming visible bands. Following electrophoresis, proteins are transferred to a membrane, typically nitrocellulose or polyvinylidene fluoride (PVDF). The transfer step is critical as it provides increased access to the proteins at subsequent antibody binding. With the use of a mixture of electric current and careful buffer conditions, researchers can maintain the proteins intact and in proper orientation, such that specific protein characteristics can be properly examined subsequently. The membrane is then incubated with primary antibodies after protein transfer, which bind specifically to the target protein in question. This specific binding is crucial, as it provides the selectivity necessary to be able to distinguish one protein from another in the sample. After leaving enough time for binding, the membrane is washed so as to remove unbound primary antibodies, which minimizes background noise in the results. Following this, a secondary antibody, often enzyme or fluorophore-conjugated, is added. This secondary antibody is attached to the primary antibody, amplifying the signal to allow for sensitive detection. The choice of secondary antibody and detection method contributes considerably to the total efficiency and accuracy of the Western blot result, allowing even low-abundance proteins to be visible.

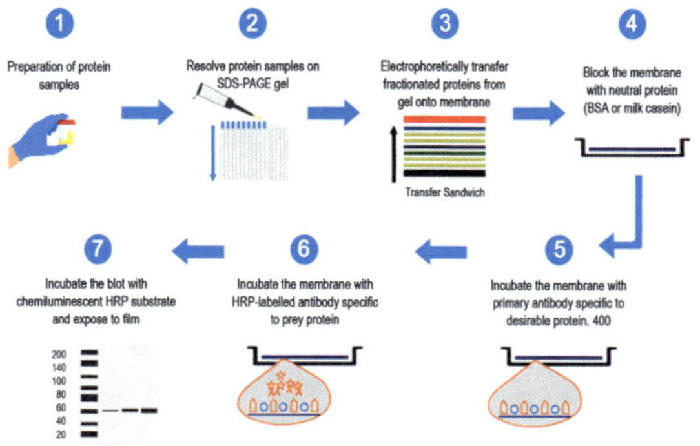

Figure 1.9. Western blot procedure.

Source: https://lh3.googleusercontent.com/fyhWBtaVzOBqvzS4vZDcm-A5CoGRWBIA5LmtW4zgm6qtCsuxPH8A4wvlnuirrtl8KV_rJWWTdqjd0U-fbbPBgcQ1SSPERMwuBj-hoDmura3EmUIrEFBfU4F6XA9KGsqzBTui0vclAzAj3yrEMQ.

Detection of protein-antibody complex is achieved using an array of modalities, such as chemiluminescence or fluorescence. Chemiluminescence relies on a substrate that, when it reacts with the enzyme linked to the secondary antibody, emits light and thus a luminescent signal proportional to the concentration of the target protein. Fluorescence detection, however, employs visualization of the complexes of protein and antibody using specific wavelengths of light. The choice between these detection methods often depends on the requirement for sensitivity and the type of experiment. Notably, technological advancements in the analysis of single cells have greatly improved the optimization and development of Western blotting techniques, enhancing the capability to study heterogeneity of protein expression in different cellular contexts, as discussed in recent literature (Han et al., 2016). Its accuracy and versatility render Western blotting a significant tool in immunological research, where complex biological processes can be elucidated (Figure 1.9).

1.3.2. Significance in Protein Detection

Protein identification is very relevant in immunology, as it provides information on cellular function and disease processes. Techniques such as enzyme-linked immunosorbent assay (ELISA), Western blotting, and mass spectrometry have a crucial role in quantifying and characterizing proteins of interest. By using specific antibodies, researchers can specifically capture target proteins from intricate mixtures for their analysis of function in biological systems. These methods find application beyond basic research; they are pivotal for diagnostic analysis, particularly for the identification of biomarkers for disease. This capability allows immune responses to be followed and pathogen-specific proteins to be determined that can be applied for therapy as well as public health policy. The value of advanced methods for protein detection is seen in aquaculture, where immune response knowledge is key to disease control. With the increasing demand for aquatic protein sources, the dissemination of economically important diseases among shellfish has proven to be a challenge. Sophisticated protein detection techniques enable scientists to grasp mechanisms of immune reactions in crustaceans, thereby forming a foundation for disease control and sustainable production. Recent developments in identifying specific immune pathways and recognition proteins indicate the importance of protein detection in addressing these problems. From the understanding of immune response molecular mechanisms, it is possible to implement controls that minimize the impact of disease as well as increase the tolerance of cultured populations (Hauton, 2012). Protein detection is not only significant for identifying immune mechanisms but also for monitoring the environment. Procedures that accurately quantify protein expression can reveal the impacts of environmental changes on host-pathogen interactions, vital in maintaining biodiversity and ecosystem health. Advances in up-and-coming technologies in protein detection, combined with the collaborative activities of researchers, have the potential to unlock principal knowledge regarding how the environment influences immunity in aquatic organisms. It is essential to the ongoing development of disease prevention and control resources for fisheries. Thus, effective protein detection technologies are a foundation for fundamental research as well as applied sciences in immunology, making them invaluable in the broader context of marine biotechnology and public health programs (Seaman & Whitehouse, 2001).

1.3.3. Common Applications in Immunology

Immunology has employed various molecular biology techniques to dispel the mystique of immune responses, ultimately progressing to the development of research and therapeutic approaches. One of the major techniques used is ELISA, which is used for measuring specific antigens or antibodies in a sample quantitatively. This approach has triggered several milestones in vaccine development and diagnostic testing by offering a sensitive platform for the detection of immune responses to pathogens. In addition, ELISA's versatility is not only limited to that of numerous types of samples, such as serum, plasma, and cell culture supernatants, but also makes it invaluable both in the laboratory and clinical settings. By the power of quantitative analysis of immune markers, ELISA depicts how molecular techniques enhance our understanding of immunological processes and direct the development of new therapeutic strategies. Flow cytometry, excluding ELISA, is another major tool for examining cell populations in immunology. This technique enables researchers to analyze the physical and chemical characteristics of cells as they travel in a stream of liquid within a laser beam. Flow cytometry is particularly valuable in the characterization of immune cell subsets, the detection of the expression of surface markers, and the quantification of cellular activities such as cytokine secretion and apoptosis. Its ability to collect multiparametric data allows researchers to learn about immune system dynamics, which can be used for disease diagnosis and monitoring immunotherapeutic responses. For instance, in cancer immunology, flow cytometry can be used to measure the functionality of T cells in tumor microenvironments and how their activity is related to patient response. Thus, flow cytometry supplements the fundamental molecular biology techniques that enhance the understanding of immune mechanisms. Yet another prime application of molecular techniques in immunology is PCR for DNA or RNA sequence amplification and characterization of specific DNA or RNA sequences. PCR has applications in identifying pathogens and detecting genetic markers of immunity. This efficient tool can detect low-abundance nucleic acids, which are important in the early diagnosis of infectious diseases and the monitoring of chronic illnesses. Additionally, real-time PCR can be used to measure gene expression levels, providing information on the response of different immune genes to external stimuli. As immunological research opens up new avenues of inquiry, methods such as PCR are constantly modified to fit new challenges, including gene therapy and personalized medicine. Therefore, these molecular biology techniques, including PCR, are critical to facilitate advancement in the area of immunology by compelling innovation and unveiling greater understanding of immune-related disease (Asbury et al., 2000; Seaman & Whitehouse, 2001) (Figure 1.10).

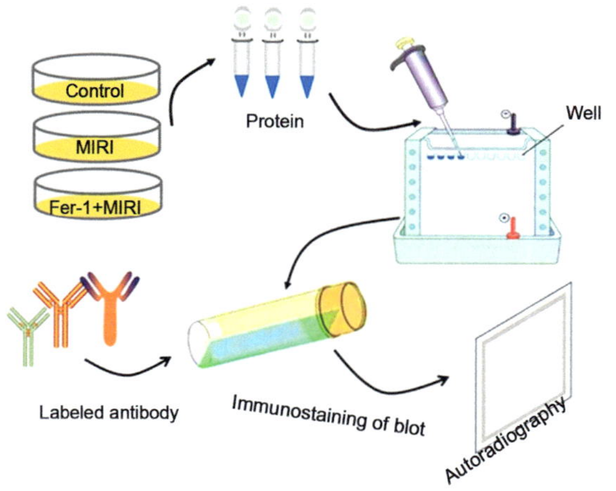

Figure 1.10. Diagram of protein immunoblotting (western blot) to monitor the content of key proteins in normal-treated H9C2 cells (control), hypoxic/re-oxygenation-treated H9C2 cells (MIRI), Fer-1-treated MIRI cells.

Source: https://www.researchgate.net/publication/379146276/figure/fig5/AS:11431281242645973@1715611854249/a-Diagram-of-protein-immunoblotting-western-blot-to-monitor-the-content-of-key.png.

1.4. Flow Cytometry

Flow cytometry is the most important immunology method, offering a powerful analytical tool for the study of the diverse characteristics of isolated cells within complex populations. The method employs fluorescent antibodies to detect and quantify the expression of certain cell surface antigens, allowing researchers to study the immune system more effectively. With the rapid analysis of thousands of cells per second, flow cytometry provides quantitative information regarding cellular activities, state of differentiation, and level of activation. The ability to analyze multiple parameters on each cell in parallel, e.g., size, granularity, and fluorescence level, significantly contributes to our understanding of immune responses under health and disease conditions. This throughput capability not only enhances data acquisition but also allows for the identification of rare cell subsets, which is highly relevant to heterogeneous uses ranging from cancer research to vaccine development. Beyond sheer cell enumeration, the flexibility of flow cytometry also expresses itself in functional assays that measure cell viability, apoptosis, and cytokine secretion. For instance, researchers can utilize flow cytometry to investigate how immune cells are influenced by oxidative stress in terms of ROS measurements. These studies comment on the challenge of harmonizing protocols, as published in the literature, that emphasize the lack of a consensus in validating and reproducing methods applied for measuring oxidative stress in leukocytes and platelets by flow cytometry. This complexity emphasizes the need for a good understanding of various markers associated with oxidative stress, enabling researchers to create elaborate tests that represent true cell conditions. This accuracy in assays is not only important for research but also for applying information to practical use in the clinical environment. In immunology, flow cytometry has played a significant role in the identification of biomarkers associated with diseases. Flow cytometry can be used in the investigation of specific immune responses in autoimmune disease, infections, and malignancies. Through this technique, it is possible to analyze tumor microenvironments by dissecting knowledge on immune cell infiltrates together with their functional status to individualize immunotherapies. This capability is also supplemented by combining flow cytometry with other molecular biology techniques, such as single-cell RNA sequencing, in order to attain a wider characterization of the immune landscape. Nevertheless, the utility of flow cytometry depends on careful experimental design and analysis, as misinterpretation can lead to false conclusions regarding immune mechanisms. Therefore, the integration of flow cytometry with standardized protocols and effective analytical methods is paramount to achieving its utmost potential in immunological investigation (Seaman & Whitehouse, 2001; Marrocco et al., 2017) (Figure 1.11).

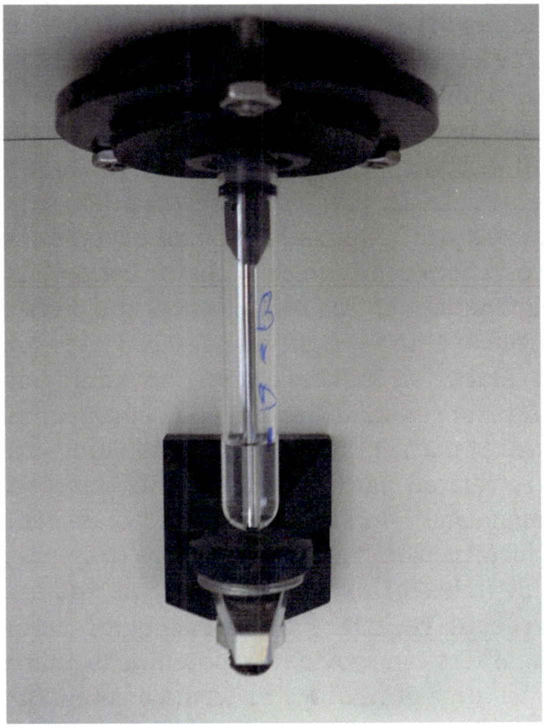

Figure 1.11. Flow cytometer tube with suction straw.

Source: https://upload.wikimedia.org/wikipedia/commons/thumb/d/d1/FACS-buisje.JPG/800px-FACS-buisje.JPG.

1.4.1. Principles of Flow Cytometry

Flow cytometry is a sensitive method widely applied in immunology for the quantitative analysis of various cellular populations. Through the application of laser technology, flow cytometers can quantify several characteristics of single cells as they travel in a stream down the path of the laser beam. This allows them to spot fluorescently labeled antibodies bound to specific cell surface antigens, enabling scientists to count and characterize numerous varieties of immune cells. Collecting information on thousands of cells per second with the power makes the quick acquisition of fine details of information regarding each cell's size, granularity, and expression of given antigens feasible. In addition, developments in flow cytometry technology, for example, the availability of more than one laser and detector, have also improved its use in high-level immunological research where an exact definition of cellular phenotypes is important. With the increasing awareness of oxidative stress in disease pathology, the utilization of flow cytometry in its elucidation has become focal. Researchers utilize flow cytometric methods of measurement of ROS in leukocytes and platelets, thereby gaining insight into the cell's response to oxidative stress challenges. The method does suffer from standardization and reproducibility issues of markers for the estimation of ROS and other related parameters. For this purpose, it is suggested that more rigorous analyses be performed using multiple markers to construct a full index of oxidative status. As indicated by recent research, the merging of various biomarkers can provide the potential to enhance the validity of findings in terms of the clinical relevance of oxidative stress in immunologic diseases (Marrocco et al., 2017).

Moreover, flow cytometry enhances learning processes through practical immunology lessons. By directly engaging students with the technology, the theoretical knowledge is enhanced through its application. Students are provided with the opportunity to make predictions, study data, and grapple with the real-world consequences of their findings. From laboratory experience, students are observed to perform diverse epistemic practices that enhance learning at the deep level, such as explaining experimental steps, making conclusions from data interpretation, and assessing the consistency of their findings (de Almeida et al., 2016). These practices not only reinforce knowledge but also foster a critical thinking approach that is essential for future employment in the field. Therefore, flow cytometry not only turns out to be an instrument of research but also an instrument of great importance for the construction of education in molecular biology and immunology (Figure 1.12).

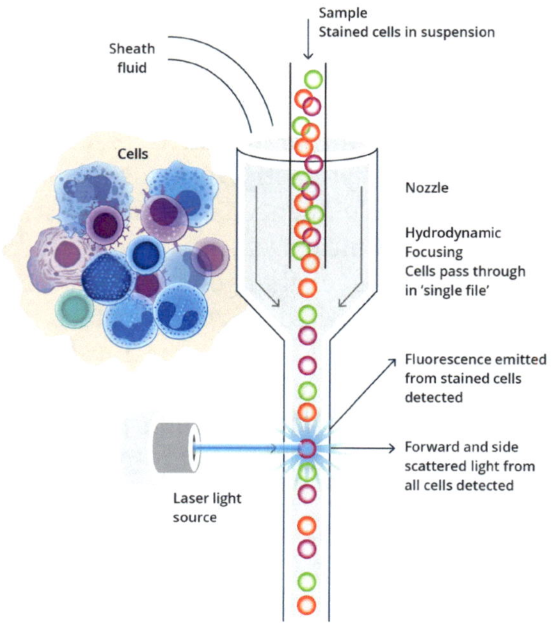

Figure 1.12. Flow cytometry is a powerful technique widely employed in immunology for the quantitative analysis of diverse cellular populations.

Source: https://marvel-b1-cdn.bc0a.com/f00000000288736/www.streck.com/wp-content/uploads/2020/11/flow-cytometry-light-scatter-illustration-1200x1305.jpg.

1.4.2. Use in Cell Analysis and Sorting

Cell analysis and cell sorting are fundamental techniques in the discipline of immunology that provide us with information about cellular dynamics, interaction, and functionality in various biological contexts. One of the predominant technologies in this field, flow cytometry, allows for swift analysis of thousands of cells per second, allowing researchers to study various parameters simultaneously, such as cell size, granularity, and surface marker expression. Using fluorescently marked antibodies to antigens of concern, flow cytometry accurately enumerates and distinguishes multiple cell populations. This has particular utility in immunology, where the identification of defined lymphocyte subsets, e.g., B cells and T cells, is crucial to the study of immune responses, pathologies, and therapeutic targets.

The precision and performance of flow cytometry make it a critical instrument for cell analysis in immune system research. Another significant aspect of cell analysis is the use of extracellular vesicles (EVs), which are increasingly recognized for their role in cell communication and immune regulation. These vesicles, including microvesicles and exosomes, enable proteins and nucleic acids to be exchanged between cells and influence many physiological processes and disease states. It has been reported that EVs could be crucial biomarkers for disease, including metabolic disorders and cardiovascular disease, and hence be useful to provide insight into immune responses at the molecular level. Further, the advancement of sophisticated isolation and characterization techniques has facilitated a comprehensive study of EVs, which has revealed their therapeutic potential due to their ability to deliver targeted miRNAs or peptides to target tissues.

The clarification of EV's role in immunity provides a new therapeutic area for research and a source of biomarkers, ultimately indicating the need for more research in this direction (Lawson et al., 2016). Besides, emerging cell sorting technologies complement traditional analytical methods with the detection of specific cell populations that can be segregated for further analysis. Magnetic-activated cell sorting (MACS) and fluorescence-activated cell sorting (FACS) enhance the recovery of pure immune cell populations, followed by detailed investigation of their attributes and functions.

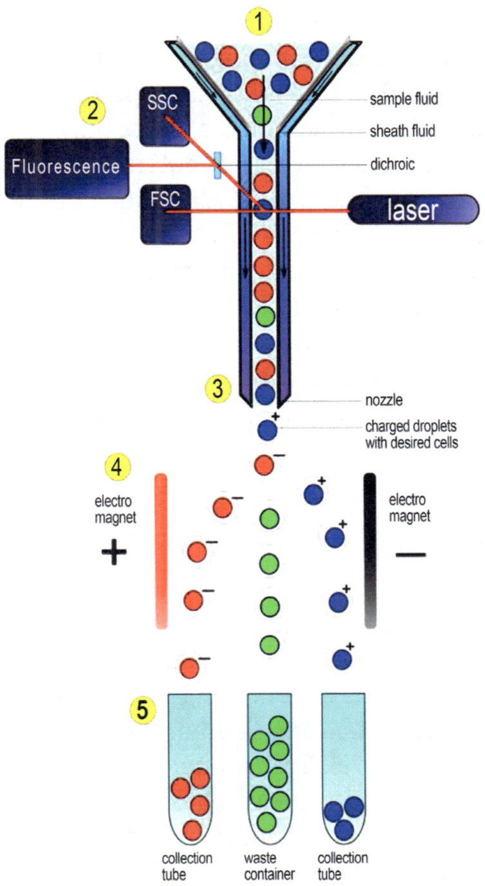

Figure 1.13. Flow cytometry and cell sorting. In the flow cell (1), the single file of cells passes a 622 laser and an array of detectors (2), which measure cell size (FSC), cell granularity/aggregation (SSC) and 623 fluorescence. When the cells exit the flow cell through the nozzle in individual droplets (3), they are 624 either or not given an electrical charge. Droplets with desired cells that possess a charge will be bent 625 out of the downward-going stream by electromagnets (4) into collection tubes on the side (5). The 626 uncharged cells simply drop straight down into a waste collection tank.

Source: https://www.researchgate.net/profile/Robert-Jan-Bleichrodt/publication/326630700/figure/fig2/AS:959467575328768@1605766304020/Flow-cytometry-and-cell-sorting-by-FACS-In-the-flow-cell-1-the-single-file-of-cells.ppm.

The ability to sort and analyze individual types of cells is essential in immunology research, particularly in determining how various immune cells respond to disease or therapeutic reagents. These sorting procedures are not only valuable for basic science but also of potential application to clinics, such as the development of targeted immunotherapy and advanced personalized medicine. With the advancement in technology, integration of sophisticated sorting techniques with cell analysis will definitely yield significant information about immune function as well as disease causation (Seaman & Whitehouse, 2001) (Figure 1.13).

1.4.3. Impact on Immunological Research

The influence of the fundamental molecular biology techniques on immunological research has been dramatic, enabling the enhancement of our understanding of immune responses at a molecular level. Traditional immunology had primarily relied on serological assays and cell culture methods; nonetheless, the addition of molecular biology has brought in capable tools for the investigation of immune mechanisms with unparalleled precision. Techniques such as PCR allow researchers to identify and quantify specific DNA sequences of immune cells, enhancing the ability to follow and examine immune responses in various uses.

This aspect is especially valuable in comprehending immune cell populations' dynamics and functional status during infections, vaccinations, or diseases. These molecular discoveries have paved the way for the creation of targeted vaccines and immunotherapies and, ultimately, the expansion of our knowledge of adaptive and innate immunity. In addition to PCR, additional molecular biology methods have broadened the arsenal at the disposal of the immunologist, such as next-generation sequencing (NGS) and CRISPR-Cas9 gene editing. NGS has transformed our ability to study the complexity of the immune system by making exhaustive immune repertoire profiling and transcriptomic analysis possible. These techniques reveal the specificity and complexity of immune receptors, crucial for defining how the immune system distinguishes between self and non-self antigens. Furthermore, with the advent of CRISPR technology, precise gene modulation makes it possible to study their role in immune response and pathogenesis. These new approaches allow a better understanding of the molecular immune basis of disease, bridging gaps between clinically relevant immunology and molecular biology.

The continued development of these techniques has the potential to unveil novel therapeutic targets and improve vaccine design, emphasizing the importance of the integration of molecular biology with immunology. While these advancements are being made, it is also important to appreciate the biases and pitfalls that molecular approaches bring.

For instance, while PCR and other molecular assays will improve sensitivity, they are inherently dependent upon successful nucleic acid extraction protocols that are not always representative of the microbial or cellular diversity of physiological conditions. Furthermore, oligonucleotide primer bias might result in underrepresentation or overrepresentation of certain immune cell populations and thus skew results. Thus, researchers have to employ a combination of classical and molecular approaches to validate observations and ensure correctness in their studies. As immunology continues to merge with molecular biology, continued discussion of the advantages and disadvantages of these approaches will be important to guide future research areas while advancing their usefulness in acquiring insights into complex immune systems in disease and health (Saunders & Saunders, 1997; Stevenson et al., 2017).

1.5. CRISPR-Cas9 Technology

CRISPR-Cas9 technology represents a groundbreaking evolution of molecular biology, particularly within the field of immunology. Initially discovered in bacteria as a mechanism of adaptive immunity, CRISPR-Cas9 has been repurposed to facilitate high-precision editing of genomic DNA in a wide range of organisms. It acts by using a guide RNA to direct the Cas9 nuclease to a specific genomic site, where it cuts the DNA to create a double-strand break. Such interruption is then corrected by non-homologous end joining or homology-directed repair, and researchers can insert, delete, or modify genes with exquisite accuracy. These capabilities have enormous significance for the study of immune reactions, pathogen interactions, and even therapeutic interventions in disease resulting from aberrant gene expression (Figure 1.14).

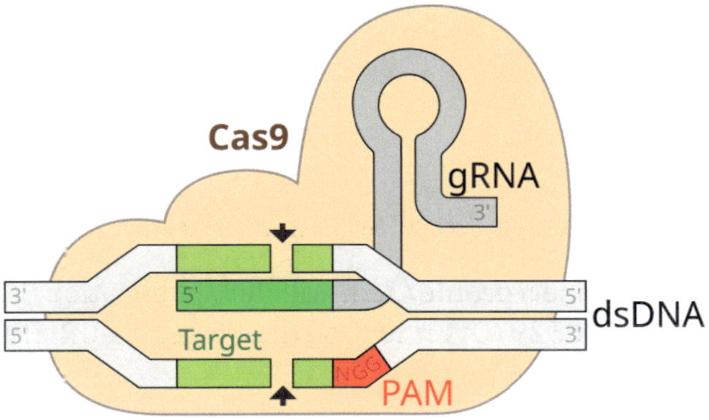

Figure 1.14. Illustration of CRISPR-Cas9.

Source: https://upload.wikimedia.org/wikipedia/commons/thumb/5/57/GRNA-Cas9.svg/800px-GRNA-Cas9.svg.png.

By interrupting or modifying genes associated with immune processes, researchers are able to gain more insights into the roles of such genes under various conditions, including autoimmune diseases and cancers. Also, with CRISPR-Cas9, researchers can develop animal models that closely resemble human immunological diseases, and hence make studies more relevant. They are vital in explaining disease mechanisms as well as in designing therapeutic strategies. For instance, researchers are exploring the use of CRISPR-Cas9 to enhance the efficacy of T cell therapies by gene editing genes that govern T cell function or by checkpoint inhibitor silencing that may impede T cell function. Importantly, the application of CRISPR-Cas9 technology also raises ethical and regulatory concerns, particularly in editing human cells genetically. With the increasing prominence of the technology, addressing potential risks and long-term implications of gene editing is necessary. Unconstrained capability of changing genetic information requires regulation to prevent misuse and ensure the security of engineered biological systems. Considerations of the ethical implications are especially pertinent within the field of immunology, where alterations have the potential to regulate complex immune interactions. These considerations ring true with the necessity of a prudent approach to the application of CRISPR-Cas9, striking a balance between scientific advancement and ethical considerations in order to seek therapeutic breakthroughs in immunology (Gavinho et al., 2019; Robinson et al., 2020) (Figure 1.15).

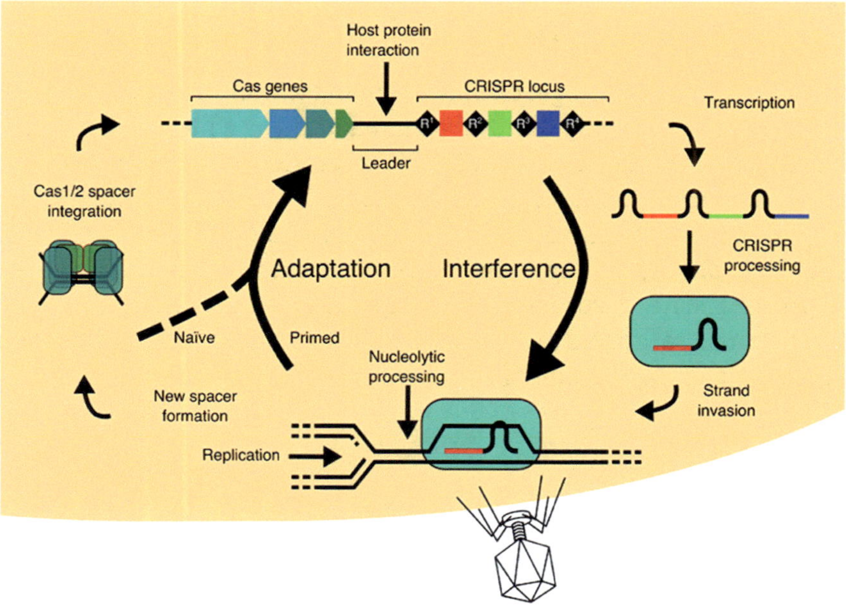

Figure 1.15. Overview of the stages of CRISPR-Cas adaptive immunity.

Source: https://www.researchgate.net/profile/Tom-Killelea/publication/318194437/figure/fig1/AS:530127237124096@1503403590529/Overview-of-the-stages-of-CRISPR-Cas-adaptive-immunity.png.

1.5.1. Mechanism of Clustered Regularly Interspaced Short Palindromic Repeats (CRISPR)-Cas9

The CRISPR-Cas9 system is a novel achievement in the field of molecular biology, more so in immunology, where precise gene editing can lead to the curing of diseases and immune response comprehension. Derived from a bacterial adaptive immune system, CRISPR allows organisms to possess a memory of past infections. The system employs a guide RNA (gRNA) that is complementary to the target DNA sequence such that the Cas9 nuclease can introduce a double-strand break at specific genomic loci. Targeted modification is critical in immunological research, enabling researchers to dissect gene pathways that contribute to immune function and disease susceptibility. Gene editing capability provides, for the first time ever, an opportunity to investigate immune cell behaviors and create novel treatments, particularly for autoimmune diseases and immunodeficiencies. Once the Cas9 creates a double-strand break in the target DNA, the cells' intrinsic repair processes are initiated, primarily by either non-homologous end joining (NHEJ) or homology-directed repair (HDR). NHEJ has a tendency to create insertions or deletions that are damaging to gene function, essentially knocking out target genes. This ability is particularly valuable in the field of immunology, where researchers would like to know the function of individual genes in immunity or pathogen interactions. HDR, on the other hand, can add precise changes with the introduction of a donor DNA template, enabling the fixing of mutations causing immunological disease. The dual capability of NHEJ and HDR emphasizes the versatility of the CRISPR-Cas9 system as a significant reagent in immune system research and manipulation. Beyond mere gene editing, the application of CRISPR-Cas9 extends to enable scientists to study complex interactions between immune system components. For instance, researchers can engineer knockout models using CRISPR-Cas9 to study the effect of a specific immune gene on pathogen susceptibility or the development of autoimmune disease. Moreover, the technology can encompass the analysis of long noncoding RNAs (lncRNAs), which are critical in gene regulation, as evidenced by recent progress in transcriptomic studies. Such an integrated approach not only enhances the understanding of immunological mechanisms but also opens avenues for novel types of innovative therapeutic approaches that could leverage gene editing for the benefit of better patient care (Gavinho et al., 2019; Robinson et al., 2020). As technology continues to advance, its application in unmasking immune responses promises to usher in a new generation of immunological research and therapy.

1.5.2. Applications in Gene Editing for Immunology

The development of gene editing tools, most notably CRISPR/Cas9, has transformed immunology through the possibility of making precise changes to immune cells. This innovation is making it possible for scientists to control genes that play a role in immune responses, hopefully resulting in new therapies for autoimmune disorders and cancer. Scientists can use CRISPR/Cas9 to target genes that suppress immune cell activation, making them better at fighting tumors or infected cells.

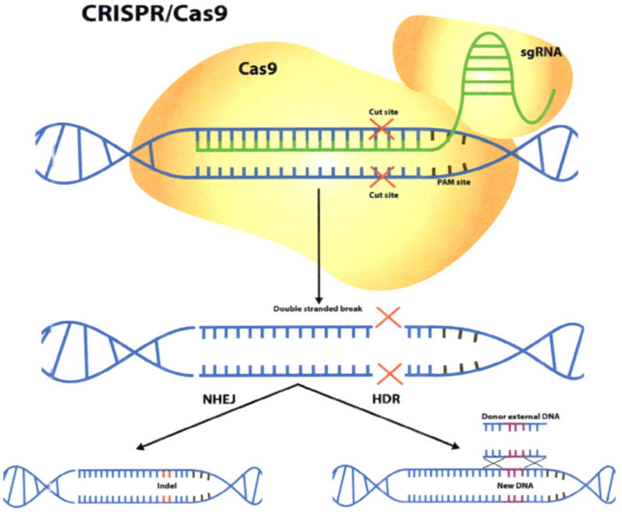

Figure 1.16. CRISPR-Cas9-mediated gene-editing mechanisms. A single guide RNA (sgRNA) recognizes a genomic region followed by a 5'-NGG-3' PAM sequence, which recruits the Cas9 DNA endonuclease. This introduces a double-stranded break that is repaired by (i) non-homologous end joining (NHEJ), an error-prone pathway that can result in the creation of Indels that can disrupt the gene, or by (ii) homology directed repair (HDR) in the presence of a donor construct.

Source: https://www.researchgate.net/profile/Adam-Cribbs/publication/322251194/figure/fig1/AS:579073518256128@1515073293608/CRISPR-Cas9-mediated-gene-editing-mechanisms-A-single-guide-RNA-sgRNA-recognizes-a.png.

This method has not only potential for current therapies but is also paving the way for individualized medicine, where the therapy could be tailored to the specific genetic makeup of each patient. The specificity and the effectiveness of CRISPR/Cas9 render its use in immunological research and clinical applications all the more significant, making it a vital tool in the investigation and treatment of immune-mediated diseases (Powell, 2017). In association with tumor immunotherapy, gene editing plays an important role in developing and optimizing vaccines. With the help of approaches such as CRISPR/Cas9, researchers are able to engineer more effective vaccine candidates by modifying viral genomes or by incorporating adjuvants that can trigger stronger immune responses. For instance, genomic editing allows for the production of live-attenuated vaccines, which stimulate strong immune responses without causing disease. Moreover, gene editing can be employed to enhance the safety and efficacy of mRNA vaccines for targeting the antigenic profiles that more effectively prime the immune system. The versatility of gene editing is not only beneficial in the rapid response to acute infectious disease but also holds potential in developing new vaccines that more effectively guard against chronic pathogens (Seaman & Whitehouse, 2001).

Ethical concerns regarding gene editing within immunology are paramount to its future expansion and application. As CRISPR/Cas9 continues to be developed, concerns regarding off-target effects as well as the consequences of editing germline cells have been identified. These issues necessitate stringent ethical scrutiny, particularly when planning prospective applications within human embryos or heritable change. Policy structures will need to balance the innovation potential of gene editing technology against the requirement not to yield unexpected consequences that will impact generations to come. Collaboration among scientists, ethicists, and policymakers will be essential in establishing guidelines to ensure the appropriate utilization of gene editing in immunology. With continuing advancements in the field, encouraging an educated dialogue of the ethics will be paramount to directing research and application in clinical as well as public health environments (Powell, 2017) (Figure 1.16).

1.5.3. Ethical Considerations and Future Prospects

The addition of basic molecular biology techniques to immunology provokes consideration of ethical concerns underlying such advancements. With scientists expanding into gene manipulation and the development of new treatments, concerns about use and possible abuse of these technologies become paramount. The ethical situation is characterized by consent issues, interpretations of genetic changes, and access to new therapies on an equal basis. Additionally, there are concerns about the dual use of biotechnologies, where research for therapeutic discovery may have applications in harmful purposes. Strong ethics must be built by the scientific community that governs research practice and safeguards responsible innovation. Only with proper supervision can the researchers minimize the risks and maximize the societal payoff potential inherent in the molecular biology techniques employed in immunology. With future opportunities arising in the area of molecular biology and its applications in immunology, ethical guidelines cannot be overstressed. Advances such as CRISPR technology and monoclonal antibody production introduce exciting possibilities for disease prevention and treatment. These advancements do raise some serious ethical questions, however. Gene editing, for instance, poses some challenges as to the ethics of altering human DNA, particularly with regard to germline editing. With a focus on advances in science, there must also be emphasis on the access disparities of these new treatments. Where science and ethical responsibility intersect will ultimately decide the future. Encouraging cross-disciplinary debate between ethicists, scientists, and policy-makers will be necessary to address the challenges of these potent technologies to ensure they are applied in a manner that benefits humanity's common good without compromising ethical standards. The ethical implications of basic molecular biology techniques in immunology will need to keep up with advancing science in the years to come. Anticipatory development of regulations can discourage misuse and foster public trust in biotechnological innovation. For instance, the activity that has been conducted by the Center for Space and Advanced Technology emphasizes the need to obtain an extensive overview of biotechnology's situation and trends to anticipate future ethical dilemmas (Johnston et al., 1988). The information regarding the development of future programs based on ethical responsibility is also accessed through the history presented by previous initiatives (Asbury et al., 2000). Engaging the wider community in these deliberations ensures diverse input, allowing for an open practice of ethical governance. As the stakes are greater, it is increasingly necessary for the scientific community to bridge innovation and integrity and thus set the ground for a future where molecular biology methodologies serve immunology and society as a whole.

SUMMARY

Application of routine molecular biology techniques to immunology has revolutionized our knowledge and management of most diseases. These techniques, which include PCR, ELISA, and NGS, are essential in the diagnosis of diseases and assessment of immune responses. As the science develops, the synergy of these molecular methods enables researchers to identify specific biomarkers and learn more about the mechanisms that are involved with immune function. For example, analysis of mycolic acids (MAs) in mycobacterial isolates with electrospray ionization tandem mass spectrometry demonstrates a significant improvement in the diagnostic capacity in terms of sensitivity and specificity compared with traditional methods (Szewczyk et al., 2013). To boot, the next decade will be marked by the continued evolution of molecular approaches. Improvements in CRISPR tools and single-cell RNA sequencing increasingly enable investigators to disentangle complex immune responses at record specificity. These developments will likely uncover knowledge in the domains of autoimmune disease and vaccine development, ultimately benefiting patients. Moreover, because the field is embracing interdisciplinary concepts, research collaborations among clinicians, biologists, and bioinformaticians will speed up the development of novel therapies. As suggested by observing model programs and initial commitments in favor of them, the future of immunology is in applying these approaches strategically (Asbury et al., 2000). In essence, the application of molecular biology methods to immunology is more than merely a technological breakthrough; it is a paradigm shift in how scientists investigate the immune system. The technologies provide important information that not only advances our scientific understanding but also finds its way into practical applications in healthcare. As the techniques continue to be refined, they will undoubtedly contribute to advancing immunological research and enhancing diagnosis and treatment strategies. In the future, it is essential that scientists and clinicians keep themselves updated with these advancements so that they can maximize the potential of molecular biology in helping to treat nascent immunological problems. The marriage between molecular biology and immunology has the potential to create new avenues of research and development towards a healthier future. Molecular biology techniques are employed in immunology to reveal the complex dynamics between immune cells and pathogens. One of the fundamental methodologies is PCR which allows one to amplify specific DNA sequences and is most helpful in detecting the presence of pathogens or genes concerning immune responses. PCR, apart from amplifying the sensitivity of diagnosis, also facilitates the examination of gene mutations and polymorphisms of interest to immune function. Therefore, it is a critical resource in laboratory and clinical science, aiding the development of targeted therapies and vaccines. The evolution of PCR technology, including quantitative PCR and reverse transcription PCR, has further enhanced its use in immunological research, providing scientists with real-time data on gene expression related to immune responses. Another essential technique is flow cytometry, which is important for the analysis and separation of immune cells. Flow cytometry involves passing cells through a beam of laser light to allow scientists to measure many physical and chemical characteristics, such as cell size, granularity, and surface markers. Flow cytometry enables resolution of the different immune cell populations and their activation status, vastly increasing our understanding of immune dynamics in infection or immunization. Along with fluorescently labeled antibodies, this technique can yield useful information on cellular response, such as cytokine secretion and cell proliferation. The wealth of information that arises from flow cytometry has propelled the development of immunological research and is now a key methodology for exploring the complexity of immune system function and reaction.

Lastly, ELISA is a common technique for measuring protein concentration, namely antibodies, in a sample. This assay has been a staple of much immunology research because it allows for the quantification of immune responses to specific antigens, providing valuable information about host-pathogen interactions. ELISA can be adapted for various targets, such as cytokines, antibodies, and proteins expressed by pathogens, thus offering flexibility in immune monitoring. Its use ranges from clinical immunology diagnostics to research environments, where it allows for the study of vaccine- or therapy-induced immune responses. The data acquired via ELISA also assists in the assessment of human immune responses, as well as informs the development of immune-based medicines, benefitting the general field of immunology by way of its insight into the body's disease defense mechanisms (Asbury et al., 2000; Seaman & Whitehouse, 2001).

A CLOSER LOOK

FUTURE DIRECTIONS IN MOLECULAR BIOLOGY FOR IMMUNOLOGY

Advances in molecular biology will have a dramatic effect on the field of immunology, namely in expanding our understanding of immune responses and disease mechanisms. Future areas of interest will include embracing the connection of genomic, transcriptomic, and proteomic data to characterize complex immune pathways. Utilizing the technologies of high throughput, investigators can characterize new biomarkers and targets for therapy that are critical in enhancing immune responses against pathogens, as well as for vaccine design. This integrated approach will also facilitate the investigation of the strategies of personalized medicine, the tailoring of immunotherapeutic intervention based on individual genetic and proteomic signatures. These advances will not only promote our fundamental understanding of immune mechanisms but also propel disease enhancement in a wide variety of clinical diseases, including autoimmune diseases and cancer (Figure 1.17).

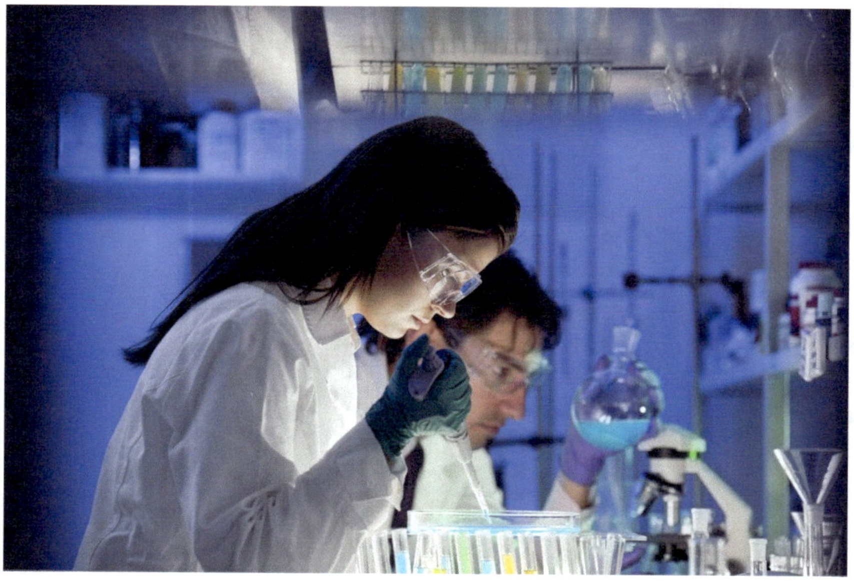

Figure 1.17. Molecular biology techniques applied in immunology research.

Source: https://career-advice.jobs.ac.uk/wp-content/uploads/Molecular-Biology-Jobs-Profile.jpg.optimal.jpg.

Furthermore, the discovery of innate immune responses in invertebrates, e.g., crustaceans, has shown key information that can be applied in the conduct of future immunological studies. The innate immune system of these animals has developed divergent pathways and effector mechanisms that are far from the known characteristics of vertebrates. Knowledge of these distinct systems may provide new avenues for the creation of novel therapies that target specific pathogens. New classes of recognition proteins and immune effectors have been identified in the recent past through research, highlighting how invertebrate immunology can assist in enhancing our knowledge of host-pathogen interactions. Invertebrate immunology can provide unprecedented paradigms for vaccine and treatment design that can be effective in all species, which can ultimately result in the enhanced management of infectious diseases in aquaculture and wild fishery contexts.

Additionally, the evolution of new tools in molecular biology will also redesign the discipline of immunology. New technologies such as CRISPR/Cas9 genome editing and single-cell RNA sequencing have great potential for immunological studies by enabling scientists to manipulate genes in a precise way and analyze cellular responses in real-time. This will provide the key to new therapeutic avenues to engineer the immune system. Coupled with progress in bioinformatics, these technologies enhance our capacity to model immune responses, predict disease outcome, and assess the impact of environmental factors on immune processes. As they advance, these technologies will certainly drive greater insight into immunology, guiding future studies toward more effective prevention and therapy strategies in the context of emerging pathogens and global health concerns.

REFERENCES

1. Abdel Nour, A., Afzal, M., Al-Shahi Salman, R., et al. (2014). The reproducibility of biomedical research: Sleepers awake! https://core.ac.uk/download/77283517.pdf (accessed on 27th June 2025).
2. Abd-Elmagid, M., Adams, M., Adhikari, R., Ali-Shtayeh, M., Altschul, S., Arap, W., Arcate, S., et al. (2016). Diagnostic tests and their application in the management of soil- and water-borne *Oomycete* pathogen species. https://core.ac.uk/download/76977879.pdf (accessed on 27th June 2025).
3. Hauton C. The scope of the crustacean immune system for disease control. *J Invertebr Pathol.* 2012;110(2):251-260. doi:10.1016/j.jip.2012.03.005Marrocco I, Altieri F, Peluso I. Measurement and Clinical Significance of Biomarkers of Oxidative Stress in Humans. *Oxid Med Cell Longev.* 2017;2017:6501046. doi:10.1155/2017/6501046(accessed on 27th June 2025).
4. Stevenson TJ, Alward BA, Ebling FJP, Fernald RD, Kelly A, Ophir AG. The Value of Comparative Animal Research: Krogh's Principle Facilitates Scientific Discoveries. *Policy Insights Behav Brain Sci.* 2018;5(1):118-125. doi:10.1177/2372732217745097(accessed on 27th June 2025).
5. Segawa T, Amatsuji H, Suzuki K, et al. Molecular characterization and validation of commercially available methods for haptoglobin measurement in bottlenose dolphin. *Results Immunol.* 2013;3:57-63. Published 2013 May 25. doi:10.1016/j.rinim.2013.05.003 (accessed on 27th June 2025).
6. Timmis, J., Amos, M., Banzhaf, W., & Tyrrell, A. (2006). Going back to our roots: second generation biocomputing. *International Journal of Unconventional Computing, 2*(4), 349-378. (accessed on 27th June 2025).
7. Arafa, E. (2016). Determining cellular and biochemical function of a novel adhesion molecule in kidneys. https://open.bu.edu/bitstream/2144/16062/1/Arafa_bu_0017N_11077.pdf (accessed on 27th June 2025).
8. Stijlemans B, De Baetselier P, Caljon G, Van Den Abbeele J, Van Ginderachter JA, Magez S. Nanobodies As Tools to Understand, Diagnose, and Treat African Trypanosomiasis. *Front Immunol.* 2017;8:724. Published 2017 Jun 30. doi:10.3389/fimmu.2017.00724(accessed on 27th June 2025).
9. Campbell, A. L., Fazzi, U. G., Kerr, S. C., Leach, R., et al. (2014). IL-21 receptor expression in human tendinopathy. https://core.ac.uk/download/19182571.pdf (accessed on 27th June 2025).
10. Robinson EK, Covarrubias S, Carpenter S. The how and why of lncRNA function: An innate immune perspective. *Biochim Biophys Acta Gene Regul Mech.* 2020;1863(4):194419. doi:10.1016/j.bbagrm.2019.194419(accessed on 27th June 2025).
11. Jorgolli M, Nevill T, Winters A, et al. Nanoscale integration of single cell biologics discovery processes using optofluidic manipulation and monitoring. *Biotechnol Bioeng.* 2019;116(9):2393-2411. doi:10.1002/bit.27024(accessed on 27th June 2025).
12. Asbury, C., Cline, B. L., & Gammino, V. M. (2000). *The Edna McConnell Clark Foundation's Tropical Disease Research Program: A 25-Year Retrospective Review 1976–1999.* https://core.ac.uk/download/71350953.pdf (accessed on 27th June 2025).

13. Decat E, Cosyn J, De Bruyn H, et al. Optimization of quantitative polymerase chain reactions for detection and quantification of eight periodontal bacterial pathogens. *BMC Res Notes.* 2012;5:664. Published 2012 Dec 2. doi:10.1186/1756-0500-5-664 (accessed on 27th June 2025).

14. Quinnell RJ, Courtenay O, Davidson S, et al. Detection of Leishmania infantum by PCR, serology and cellular immune response in a cohort study of Brazilian dogs. *Parasitology.* 2001;122(Pt 3):253-261. doi:10.1017/s0031182001007363(accessed on 27th June 2025).

15. Pradeu, T., Carosella, E.D. The Self Model and the Conception of Biological Identity in Immunology. *Biol Philos* **21**, 235–252 (2006). https://doi.org/10.1007/s10539-005-8621-6(accessed on 27th June 2025).

16. Gavinho, B., Combes, V., Dlugonska, H., Hart, E., Evans-Osses, I., Volpato Rossi, I., Inal, J., et al. (2019). A new landscape of host–protozoa interactions involving the extracellular vesicles world. https://core.ac.uk/download/287580982.pdf (accessed on 27th June 2025).

17. Gorham, K. (2010). Effects of mold exposure on immune cells. https://core.ac.uk/download/56727991.pdf (accessed on 27th June 2025).

18. Han, A., Huebner, A., Mazumder, A., Ribas, A., Sottoriva, A., Ståhlberg, A., Pollen, A. A., et al. (2016). Single-cell analysis tools for drug discovery and development. https://core.ac.uk/download/33125209.pdf (accessed on 27th June 2025).

19. Huang, A., Zheng, H., Wu, Z., Chen, M., & Huang, Y. (2020). Circular RNA-protein interactions: Functions, mechanisms, and identification. *Theragnostic, 10,* 3503–3517. https://doi.org/10.7150/thno.42174 (accessed on 27th June 2025).

20. Szewczyk R, Kowalski K, Janiszewska-Drobinska B, Druszczyńska M. Rapid method for Mycobacterium tuberculosis identification using electrospray ionization tandem mass spectrometry analysis of mycolic acids. *Diagn Microbiol Infect Dis.* 2013;76(3):298-305. doi:10.1016/j.diagmicrobio.2013.03.025(accessed on 27th June 2025).

21. Johnston, R. S., Norton, D. J., & Baldwin, T. H. (1988). *Space and Biotechnology: An Industry Profile.* Contract No. NCC 9-16, Activity IM.5. https://core.ac.uk/download/pdf/42821064.pdf (accessed on 27th June 2025).

22. Katsnelson, L. B., Kohl, P., Panfilov, A., & Solovyova, O., et al. (2016). Mechano-electric heterogeneity of the myocardium as a paradigm of its function. https://core.ac.uk/download/84042819.pdf (accessed on 27th June 2025).

23. Kumar, M. A., Baba, S. K., Sadida, H. Q., Al Marzooqi, S., Jerobin, J., Altemani, F. H., Algehainy, N. A., et al. (2024). Extracellular vesicles as tools and targets in therapy for diseases. *Signal Transduction and Targeted Therapy, 9.* https://doi.org/10.1038/s41392-024-01735-1 (accessed on 27th June 2025).

24. Lawson, C., Yellon, D. M., Gunduz, D., Headland, S., Joop, K., Jorgensen, C., et al. (2016). Microvesicles and exosomes: New players in metabolic and cardiovascular disease. https://core.ac.uk/download/36779172.pdf (accessed on 27th June 2025).

25. Park, H. (2011). *Proteomic Analysis of Two Different States of Naegleria fowleri.* https://core.ac.uk/download/51291040.pdf (accessed on 27th June 2025).

26. Powell, G. E., III. (2017). *Embryos as Patients? Medical Provider Duties in the Age of CRISPR/Cas9.* https://core.ac.uk/download/84098963.pdf (accessed on 27th June 2025).

27. Saeed, A. F. U. H., Wang, R., Wang, S., & Ling, S. (2017). Antibody engineering for pursuing a healthier future. https://core.ac.uk/download/pdf/82883279.pdf (accessed on 27th June 2025).

28. Saunders, J. R., & Saunders, V. A. (1997). The impact of molecular biology on assessment of water quality: Advantages and limitations of current techniques. https://core.ac.uk/download/11020751.pdf (accessed on 27th June 2025).

29. Seaman, W., & Whitehouse, J. H. (2001). *Florida Marine Biotechnology: Research, Development and Training Capabilities to Advance Science and Commerce*. https://core.ac.uk/download/11016354.pdf (accessed on 27th June 2025).

30. Manzoni de Almeida, D., Marzin-Janvier, P., & Frateschi Trivelato, S. L. (2016). Analysis of epistemic practices in reports of higher education students groups in carrying out the inquiry-based activity of immunology. *Investigações Em Ensino De Ciências*, *21*(2), 105-120. https://doi.org/10.22600/1518-8795.ienci2016v21n2p105

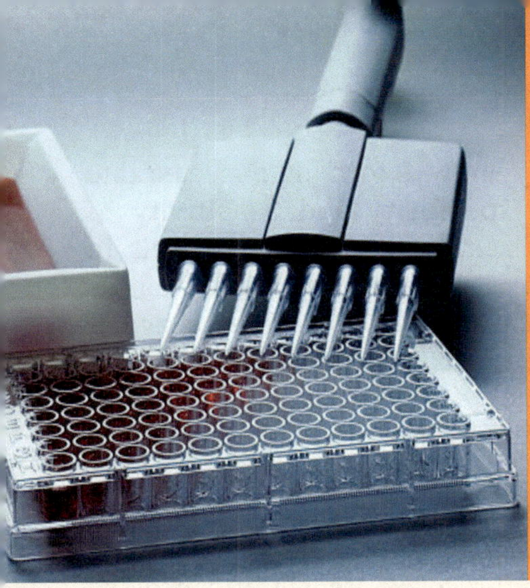

Chapter 2

IMMUNOASSAYS: PRINCIPLES AND APPLICATIONS

Contents

Introduction

Immunoassays are the principal analytical chemistry tools that are known to be sensitive and specific in detecting biomolecules. The assays, underpinned by the principle of antigen-antibody interaction, have gained immense significance in various applications ranging from clinical diagnostics to environmental monitoring. The ability of immunoassays to provide precise results with minimal sample preparation renders them a favorite in laboratory as well as field applications. The versatility of immunoassays allows them to be modified for the analysis of a wide range of analytes, i.e., proteins, hormones, pathogens, and drugs, and hence fulfill different scientific and medical requirements. As a significant advancement in biotechnology, the development of immunoassay methods is a key research area for researchers, influencing healthcare progress and safety practices. Of the different immunoassays, lateral flow immunoassays (LFIAs) have been of special interest for their application in resource-poor environments. LFIAs provide qualitative, semi-quantitative, and in certain instances quantitative information and are thus of great value in the areas of epidemiology, food safety, and veterinary medicine. Ease of operation and rapid turnaround time position LFIAs well in the proximity of situations where expedient judgments are critical, i.e., emergency situations or field operations. However, while the promise of these assays is great, there are nuances in their sensitivity and specificity that need further study. Understanding these limitations as well as their benefits can inform researchers and practitioners about the optimal conditions for applying LFIA technology, ultimately maximizing their effectiveness in real-world applications (Posthuma-Trumpie et al., 2009). Advances in related technologies, such as liquid chromatography tandem mass spectrometry (LC-MS), have also made immunoassays more powerful. LCTMS, to cite one, not only enhances the precision of compound analysis but also increases the range of analyzable compounds beyond traditional methods. The combination of these technologies provides more solid and high-throughput analyses, facilitating new opportunities for clinical laboratory applications that require efficiency and reliability. Besides, a combination of different analyte detection procedures is a sign of the advancing nature of immunoassays, an endeavor that relies on a growing need for deep-level testing alternatives in healthcare and research. As technologies change and the advancing knowledge on immunoassay fundamentals develops, the range of applications of immunoassays keeps on increasing, which yields ongoing discovery and investigation in this evolving field (Vogeser, 2003).

Definition of Immunoassays

Immunoassays are a significant analytical technique applied to detect and quantify specific biomolecules, primarily proteins, through the utilization of antibodies. The method relies on the specificity of antibody-antigen interaction, in which an antibody binds to its complementary antigen, forming a measurable complex. The specificity and sensitivity of immunoassays render them valuable tools in clinical diagnosis, therapeutic monitoring, as well as research. Techniques such as enzyme-linked immunosorbent assays (ELISAs), radioimmunoassays (RIAs), and lateral flow assays all illustrate the diversity of immunoassays, each with its own merits depending on the target analyte and detection conditions required. Immunoassay technology's continued innovation underscores its significance, as it develops to meet the evolving needs for diagnostics and biotechnology. Technological advancements have had significant impacts on the application and efficiency of immunoassays. The application of nanomaterials has been a significant contribution, particularly in the fabrication of electrochemical immunosensors. Graphene quantum dots (GQDs), for example, have exhibited excellent potential according to their superior characteristics like high surface area and higher biocompatibility. These factors enable them to respond more sensitively and at higher rates of detection, making GQD-based immunoassays very effective for clinical analysis. Besides, GQDs can also simulate peroxidase action, thereby making label-free detection processes possible, thus streamlining the diagnostic process. Besides improving performance parameters, this advancement is also an answer to the requirement of cost-effective and rapid diagnostic procedures in developed and developing nations, a great relief for point-of-care testing (POCT) (Mansuriya & Altintas, 2019). Immunoassays are not limited to human disease; they are also finding increasing acceptance in food safety and environmental monitoring. Nanoparticle technology has made it possible to create biosensors that can effectively screen for safety and quality indicators in most foodstuffs. Although the initial focus was on medical applications due to the growing need for accurate point-of-care diagnostics, these technologies have been adapted for the specific needs of food safety testing. For instance, nanosensors detect contaminants at very low levels, which suggests compliance with safety standards as well as consumer protection regulations. However, the fluctuating requirements of the food market may render certain nanoparticle-based sensors commercially unviable, implying the need for specialist strategies suited to this sector (Warriner et al., 2014). As the use of immunoassays widens further, existing research seeks to maximize these technologies for implementation in a wide variety of industries (Figure 2.1).

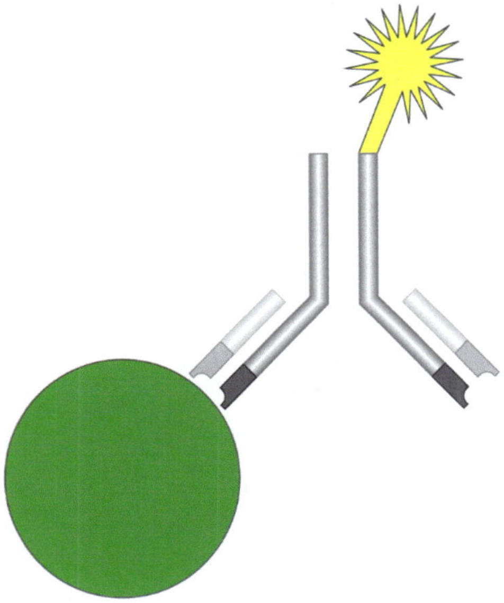

Figure 2.1. Diagram illustrating the basic components of an immunoassay, which includes an analyte (green), an immunglobulin (black), and a detectable label (yellow).

Source: https://upload.wikimedia.org/wikipedia/commons/thumb/3/3c/Immunoassay.svg/800px-Immunoassay.svg.png.

Importance in Biomedical Research

The significance of immunoassays in biomedical research is underscored by their underlying role in diagnostic application. Immunoassays form a firm foundation for the detection of specific biomolecules, for example, proteins, hormones, and antibodies, crucial to the understanding of various disease states. Immunoassays use the specificity of the antigen-antibody interaction to achieve highly sensitive and accurate determination of the analytes and are an indispensable tool in clinical laboratories. In addition to being utilized more than just in routine diagnosis, the assays are also vital in biopharmaceutical development to assess the efficacy of the drug and safety profile during the clinical study. As exemplified in lateral flow (immuno)assays in science, these techniques are at the core of pathogen and prominent biomarker surveillance across a variety of environments, from healthcare to environmental science. In this way, the role of immunoassays in biomedical science cannot be doubted because they are closely linked with therapeutic and diagnostic modalities in progress. Aside from their application in analysis, immunoassays have transformed epidemiological studies through the availability of population-scale screening and surveillance. With infectious disease outbreaks, demand for quick and easy methods of testing has grown manyfold. Immunoassays like ELISAs and point-of-care lateral flow assays provide efficient means for the detection of seroconversion and immune response among populations of different pathogens. This capability is particularly important following global health epidemics since it can monitor disease outbreaks and intervene early. Furthermore, the advantages of lateral flow (immuno)assays, designed for use in resource-limited environments, provide improved access to critical diagnostics (Vogeser, 2003). This democratization of instrumentation for biomedical research ultimately yields improved public health results and parallels the ongoing advancement of immunoassay technologies. Immunoassays also play a significant role in personalized medicine, where information about an individual's unique biological makeup can enable optimal therapy. Immunoassays aid in the identification of biomarkers needed to customize therapeutic strategies for specific patient profiles. In oncology research, for example, immunoassays are employed to measure levels of circulating tumor markers and assess therapy responses so that clinicians can make treatment decisions based on real-time patient data. The use of sophisticated techniques such as LCTMS enhances the quality and efficiency of immunoassays to allow the detection of an increased range of biomolecules in greater throughput and precision than before (Vogeser, 2003). As immunoassays continue to evolve, their role in advancing personalized medicine and improving patient care techniques in biomedical research will become increasingly significant, sealing their vital role in the future of healthcare.

2.1. Historical Background

Historically, immunoassays have their origin in the early 20th century when the field of immunology began gaining pace. Early on, serological methods were employed to identify pathogens and antibodies within clinical samples, laying the ground for the development of more advanced immunoassay technologies.

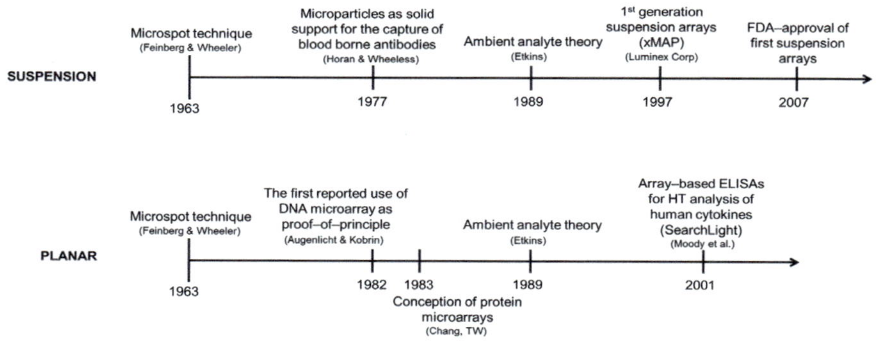

Figure 2.2. Timelines charting the theoretical and practical milestones in the development of multiplex technology for suspension and planar immunoassay formats. The first commercial suspension array was available before the first planar-based array.

Source: https://www.researchgate.net/publication/271335947/figure/fig1/AS:272549087019011@1441992174174/Timelines-charting-the-theoretical-and-practical-milestones-in-the-development-of.png.

Radioimmunoassay (RIA) proved to be a significant advancement in the 1960s with radioactively labeled antibodies to identify antigens in a very sensitive way. The technology revolutionized diagnosis by being capable of measuring hormones and drugs at levels virtually below detection. The widespread application of RIA in clinical laboratories was a milestone when the demand for accurate and rapid disease diagnosis became increasingly prioritized, establishing a standard for future developments in the practice of immunoassay technology. With scientific research developing further, the development of the enzyme-linked immunosorbent assay (ELISA) during the 1970s further enhanced the efficiency of immunoassays. Compared to RIA, ELISA did away with the use of radiation and was thus safer and more convenient for laboratory applications. The development of colorimetric detection methods enabled quantitative analysis of biomarkers and opened their application from research to clinical diagnosis. ELISA's versatility allowed it to be turned into multiplex formats and paved the way for personalized medicine. Nonetheless, despite its advantages, there were challenges, such as how to ensure the specificity and reliability of results for the diverse clinical applications. This advancement is a reflection of the ongoing need for innovation to meet the complexity of biomarker validation and assay standardization, defining the future trajectory of immunoassay technology. The contemporary scene of immunoassays is an expression of innovations both in application and design, most importantly spearheaded by discoveries in nanotechnology and electrochemical strategies. Nanomaterials such as graphene quantum dots (GQDs) have been used more and more to enhance the sensitivity and selectivity of immunoassays to identify disease-associated biomarkers at ultralow levels. The use of these materials not only improved the detection limits but also facilitated miniaturization of diagnostic devices, which is essential in the point-of-care testing platform, particularly in resource-limited settings. In addition, multiplex immunoassays are currently in vogue, offering great advantages over singleplex formats through being more productive and economical (Tighe et al., 2015). Nevertheless, problems such as biomarker validation and assay automation continue to be significant challenges, highlighting research and development for reaping the full potential of immunoassays as clinical diagnostic tools (Tighe et al., 2015) (Figure 2.2).

2.1.1. Development of Immunoassay Techniques

Immunoassay technique development has advanced biomedical diagnostics significantly by providing reproducible means for the detection of single biomolecules in low concentrations. This shift began with the emergence of radioimmunoassay in the 1960s, which utilized radioactive isotopes to measure antigen-antibody interaction. The sensitivity of the techniques created a ground for the later advancements of ELISA and chemiluminescence assays. These techniques utilized the enzymatic nature of enzymes to perform quantifications without using deadly radioactive materials. The trend towards more complex approaches, such as liquid chromatography tandem mass spectrometry (LC-MS), has even further reshaped immunoassay use, adding more robustness and flexibility to clinical labs. LCTMS, with its advanced instrumentation, enables high-throughput analysis, solidifying its place in routine daily diagnostics and our ability to monitor health status optimally (Vogeser, 2003). Nanotechnology has expanded exponentially to advance the complexity of immunoassay techniques, principally through the emergence of electrochemical sensors. The integration of nanomaterials developed highly discriminating and sensitive immunosensors for sensing biomarkers at ultralow concentration levels. For instance, GQDs are becoming an emerging star in electrochemical immunoassays due to their large surface area, excellent biocompatibility, and unique electro-catalytic behavior. These characteristics allow for label-free immunoassay development, reducing costs and simplifying procedures without loss of sensitivity. These advancements have the potential to enhance point-of-care testing (POCT) applications and prove invaluable in resource-limited settings where rapid and efficient disease diagnosis is crucial (Mansuriya & Altintas, 2019). Ongoing studies and applications of these nanomaterials further enhance the field by responding to pressing healthcare needs. The direction of immunoassay techniques in the future is going to adopt even greater synergy with new technologies, with the potential for even more accuracy and efficiency in detection. As methodology improves, the development of microfluidic platforms and hand-held diagnostic units will become more widespread, allowing real-time analysis in diverse environments.

These technological developments not only enhance patient care by allowing for rapid diagnosis but also pave the way toward personalized medicine, whereby therapy may be tailored based on an individual's own unique biomarker signature. In addition, continuing improvements in computational methods for data interpretation will lead to increased precision and quality of immunoassay results. Therefore, the coalescence of these technologies heralds a new era in diagnostics, catalyzing improved disease prevention and management in public health (Mansuriya & Altintas, 2019; Vogeser, 2003) (Figure 2.3).

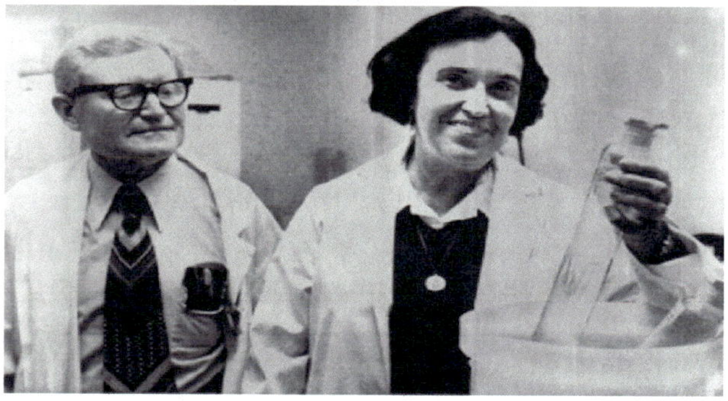

Figure 2.3. Solomon Berson and Rosalyn Yalow first measured PTH via a radioimmunoassay in the early 1960s.

Source:https://www.researchgate.net/profile/Joshua-Bornhorst/publication/311667692/figure/fig1/AS:445924754366464@1483328154656/The-fi-rst-PTH-assay-Solomon-Berson-and-Rosalyn-Yalow-fi-rst-measured-PTH-via-a.png.

2.1.2. Key Milestones in Immunoassay Evolution

The history of immunoassays, which are indispensable biotechnology and clinical diagnostic tools, is characterized by several milestones that have dictated their development. It starts with Paul Ehrlich's suggestion, way back in the early 20th century, that antibodies be utilized in serological analysis, and this formed the foundation for antibody-based diagnostics. This theoretical foundation was built concurrently with advances in serology, leading to technologies such as the RIA of Rosalyn Yalow in the 1960s. The advent of RIAs provided for precise measurement of hormones and drugs at low concentrations, revolutionizing laboratory medicine. As immunoassays gained popularity, their techniques diversified, leading to ELISAs in the 1970s, which were more sensitive and flexible compared to their predecessors and significantly improved their applications in clinical use for disease diagnosis. Advances in immunoassay technology have continued to be fueled by the merger of nanotechnology with other modern developments. Use of nanoparticles in lateral flow immunoassays (LFTs) is a pivotal aspect of such progress, enhancing the detection capacity for biomarkers. LFTs are especially recognized for simplicity, ease of operation, and the ability to provide immediate diagnostic results, thereby supporting personalized medicine principles. The growing demand for low-cost diagnostic equipment to analyze samples in real time is a cry for new testing technologies in medicine. The addition of nanotechnology in LFTs, in addition to the sensitivity improvement, has also expanded the window of the disease to be monitored effectively, a testament to the vast potential of these new immunoassays in the clinical setting (Napione, 2021). Additionally, the rapidly developing field of biomarker identification and validation has opened doors for immunoassays, particularly in complex diseases like Alzheimer's. The construction of *in vivo* diagnostic models using biomarkers such as amyloid-β and tau is another milestone in immunoassay development. These biomarkers contribute significantly to defining accurate diagnostic criteria and improved patient stratification for clinical trials. By monitoring biomarker levels using immunoassays, researchers can better quantify disease progression and thus improve treatment. This immunoadsorption and treatment of neurodegenerative disease illustrates their worth over simple diagnosis, showcasing their role in personalized medicine (Therriault et al., 2024). With the growth of technology, these innovations in immunoassay development will go on to fuel research advancements as well as clinical applications, being integral to better patient outcomes.

2.1.3. Impact of Technology on Immunoassay Advancement

Technological advances have profoundly influenced the practice of immunoassays, and both the level of detail in testing and the quality of testing techniques. The emergence of high-throughput screening technologies has made it possible the simultaneous running of thousands of tests and thus raised productivity and lowered the time for results. This trend towards automation, besides alleviating human error, is further advantaged by addressing the emerging requirement for rapid diagnostic tools in research and clinical settings. Accordingly, these developments have made it possible to apply immunoassays to more conditions, particularly for disease detection at an earlier stage, thus possibly improving patients' outcomes. In addition, the application of sophisticated data analysis computer programs and machine learning methods makes it possible to interpret immunoassay data at a higher level, paving the way for personalized medicine approaches that tailor therapy according to individualized biomarker patterns. The emergence of multiplexing approaches is one of the significant advances of immunoassay technology, which allows multiple analytes to be measured simultaneously from a single sample. This aspect enhances the throughput of immunoassays and assists in conserving valuable biological samples, an important advantage in clinical diagnosis and research applications. Multiplexed immunoassays are capable of allowing full profiling of disease markers, which gives a more holistic view of the biochemical profile of the patient. However, realizing the full potential of multiplexing is no walk in the park, including strict verification of novel biomarkers and maintaining assay sensitivity. The more money organizations invest in developing such complex multiplex assays, the more disease early detection and tailor-made therapeutic strategies become a reality, highlighting the revolutionary potential of technology in this field (Ahsan & Ahmad, 2021). In addition to multiplexing, progress in other fields such as epigenetics and proteomics will revolutionize immunoassay techniques. Leveraging these disciplines can advance immunoassay specificity and sensitivity, alleviating long-standing limitations that have restricted forensic and clinical applications. Research has discovered that epigenetic biomarkers can provide insight into biological sample origin and age estimations and thus enhance contextual data from traditional immunoassays. Similarly, proteomic technologies like mass spectrometry can enable the identification of tissue types and biological fluids without compromising DNA evidence, especially in forensic medicine (Eilerts, 2016). With the advancing maturity of these technologies together, the future for immunoassay applications is expected to expand exponentially, leading to a new era of precision diagnostics and evidence-based therapy interventions.

2.2. Basic Principles of Immunoassays

Immunoassays are laboratory methods that take advantage of the specific binding properties of antibodies to analyze and measure antigens, including proteins, hormones, and microorganisms. Underlying the assays is the antigen-antibody principle, whereby antibodies are designed to bind highly with specific target antigens. Binding generates a signal that can be translated into quantitative data. Immunoassays typically encompass a broad array of formats, including ELISAs, radioimmunoassays, and lateral flow assays, applied to various analytical applications and contexts. Take advantage of the specificity of immune response, the assays have occupied the pivotal position in clinical diagnostics, drug discovery, and environmental monitoring, allowing qualitative and quantitative measurement of a wide range of analytes in complex matrices. Lateral flow immunoassays are a particularly handy format that has gained popularity for on-site use due to the fact that they are so easy and can be rapid in producing results. The assays operate by having a liquid sample travel through a porous membrane, where the sample has access to immobilized antibodies that catch particular antigens. As the sample migrates down the strip, any bound antigen can create a visible signal, typically in the form of a colored line. The technique promotes immediate diagnosis in developing countries, and thus it is a very valuable tool for detecting pathogens and drug screening. In addition to clinical application, the area of application for lateral flow immunoassays also extends to phytosanitary control and environmental monitoring, exemplifying their range of applications in addressing diverse analytical requirements (Posthuma-Trumpie et al., 2009). Advances in technologies such as nanoparticle-based biosensors have further progressed to enhance sensitivity and specificity in immunoassays. Taking advantage of the unique properties of nanoparticles, detection sensitivities can be improved and sample volumes reduced, both of which are important in applications requiring high-throughput screening and point-of-care diagnostics. The use of nanoparticles not only facilitates miniaturization but also provides a means for analyzing multiple targets in parallel, thereby making the analytical process simpler. Despite these advances, there remain problems with realizing the commercial potential of these new sensors, particularly in their uses in ensuring food safety and determining quality, where different requirements may limit their overall application (Warriner et al., 2014) (Figure 2.4).

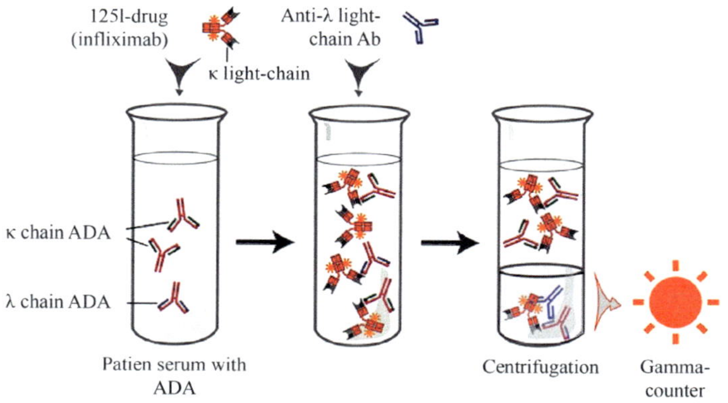

Figure 2.4. Illustration of the principle of radioimmunoassay.

Source: https://www.researchgate.net/profile/Jing-Li-257/publication/346023250/figure/fig4/AS:959615244181510@1605801511279/llustration-of-principle-of-radioimmunoassay-Radioimmunoassay-2020.png.

2.2.1. Antigen-antibody Interactions

Understanding antigen-antibody interactions is core in immunoassay science, where the specificity and affinity of such biological interactions have a direct impact on assay performance. Antigens, which may be proteins, carbohydrates, or nucleic acids, induce an immune response when exposed to a host. Antigens bind to antibodies—Y-shaped proteins excreted from B cells—and allow the formation of antigen-antibody complexes. This can be employed in many assay formats, including ELISAs and lateral flow assays.

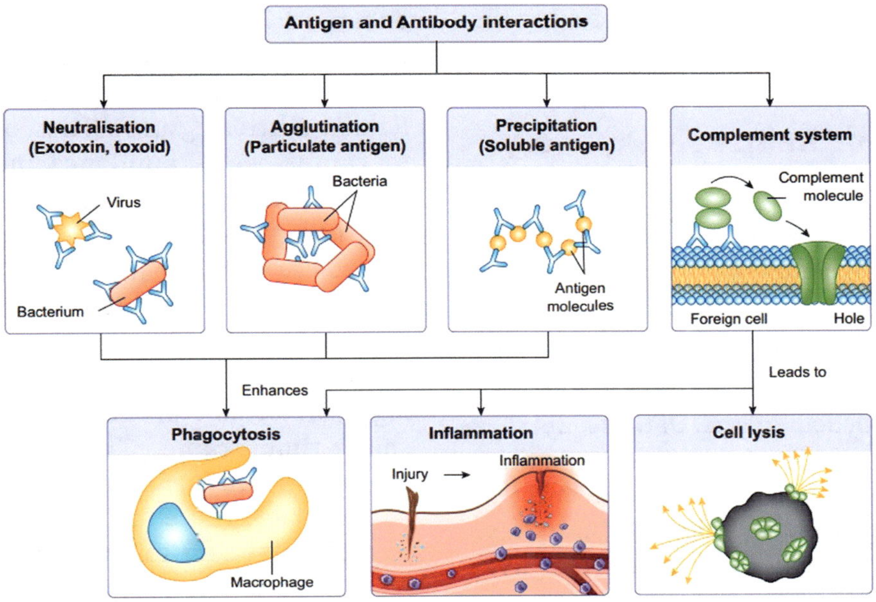

Figure 2.5. Understanding antigen-antibody interactions.

Source: https://img.brainkart.com/imagebk39/8BsYwzt.jpg.

The sensitivity and specificity of these assays are paramount, as they determine the validity of clinical diagnostics. Lastly, the understanding of the dynamics underlying these interactions guides the development of immunoassay methods tailored to the detection of a range of targets, highlighting their essential importance in clinical and research applications. One of the most important applications of antigen-antibody interactions is the development of lateral flow immunoassays, which have become increasingly popular due to their rapid and convenient nature. As Posthuma-Trumpie et al. (2009) explain, such assays provide qualitative or semi-quantitative results in a wide range of environments, from clinical diagnosis through to environmental analysis. By using a specific antigen and antibody, these assays are able to detect a wide range of substances, from pathogens and metabolites. The basis of such assays relies greatly on the specificity and affinity of the antibody-antigen interaction, thus making the test sensitive. While the virtues of lateral flow immunoassays are well known, they also have drawbacks, such as the risk of false positives and false negatives, which demonstrate the need for constant innovation in the method to increase reliability. Additionally, advances in electrochemical sensors have also raised the role of antigen-antibody interactions in biomedicine. The application of nanomaterials, such as GQDs, has revolutionized immunosensor technology with a plethora of advantages in selectivity and sensitivity. As stated by Mansuriya & Altintas (2019), GQDs possess new features, such as a large surface area and biocompatibility, to enable new label-free detection schemes. This integration enables fast identification of biomarkers, which is essential in the early diagnosis and treatment of diseases such as cancer and cardiovascular disease. The establishment of immunosensing methods aided by GQDs confirms the continued relevance of antigen-antibody interactions, as these advances have the potential to bridge gaps in low-cost diagnostics, particularly in resource-poor settings, thereby broadening the applications of immunoassays (Figure 2.5).

2.2.2. Types of Immunoassays (e.g., Enzyme-Linked Immunosorbent Assay [ELISA], Radioimmunoassay [RIA])

Immunoassays are a crucial component of today's diagnostic protocols and yield diverse means toward the identification of antigens or antibodies of a particular type. Of these, ELISA is one of the most prevalent due to its versatility, sensitivity, and ease of use. ELISA is antigen-antibody reaction-based and uses a solid-phase support, ideally a microplate, coated with the to-be-detected antigen. Following sample addition, the addition of antibodies that are enzyme-conjugated leads to the development of a complex that produces a measurable signal following substrate addition. This technique has been applied successfully in numerous applications, from disease testing to biomarker analysis, providing reproducible results that can be applied for clinical decision-making. RIA, however, utilizes radiolabeled antigens to quantify the concentration of a specific antibody within a sample. The technique relies on the principle of competitive inhibition, wherein a sample containing the target antibody competes with a radiolabeled antigen for binding to a specific antibody. Even though RIA is highly sensitive and has heretofore been vital in the measurement of hormones and drugs, its use has declined due to radiation safety concerns, the relatively greater difficulty of manipulating radioactive isotopes, and the availability of safer methods. Nonetheless, the very high accuracy and precision that RIA offers render it a significant research model for the design of newer non-radioactive immunoassays, thus dictating improvements in laboratory diagnosis and therapeutic monitoring. Evolutionary technologies continue to transform the immunoassay discipline, as in the use of surface-enhanced Raman spectroscopy (SERS) in the creation of fast diagnostic tests. This new immunoassay platform exploits the amplified Raman scattering properties of nanoparticles to capture low-abundance biomarkers with high sensitivity. Antibodies are immobilized on gold nanoparticle-containing filter paper in an innovative vertical flow immunoassay design. This allows for the selective capture of target biomarkers, subsequent signal amplification through plasmonic coupling, resulting in a highly detectable product within an extremely short time frame. This demonstrates the dynamic reality of immunoassay technology, with scientists accelerating the development of cost-effective and effective point-of-care tests responsive to the pressing need for the rapid detection of disease in diverse health facilities (Guerra et al., 2016 Amissah, 2024).

2.2.3. Signal Detection Methods

The success of immunoassays largely relies on the effectiveness of signal detection strategies employed. Signal detection strategies form the pillar to quantify the concentration of target antigens or antibodies in a sample. ELISAs, fluorescence-based platforms, and electrochemical sensors are some common detection strategies.

Each technique has unique advantages; ELISAs, for example, are noted for convenience and high throughput, while fluorescence-based methods yield higher sensitivity and specificity. The signal detection technique ultimately decides the LOD and assay robustness, with a direct impact on clinical diagnosis. Developments in signal detection technologies, particularly technologies like LCTMS, are transforming immunoassay technology. For instance, LCTMS is more specific and sensitive than conventional chromatographic techniques and is a highly preferable choice in clinical laboratories (Vogeser, 2003). Recent advances in signal detection tactics have improved immunoassays' diagnostic capability, particularly with the use of nanomaterials. Electrochemical sensors have shown groundbreaking potential in biomedicine through the ability to perform rapid and selective biomarker quantification at trace concentrations. Dominantly, GQDs have emerged as a key component in the fabrication of electrochemical immunosensors. Their inherent properties of extensive surface area and excellent biocompatibility have enabled the enhancement of assay selectivity and sensitivity, which are necessary for accurate disease diagnosis. Moreover, GQDs exhibit peroxidase-mimicking catalysis properties, which enable label-free detection, streamlining the assay process without compromising cost-effectiveness. This evolution in detection methods demonstrates the place of technological innovation in making immunoassays more effective and flexible for use in a wide range of medical contexts (Mansuriya & Altintas, 2019). The addition of new signal detection methods to immunoassays starts a new chapter in clinical diagnostics and holds the potential for applications beyond typical laboratory settings. By utilizing the singular attributes of varying detection technologies, analysts can enhance analytical sensitivity without taking up much time and cost compared to traditional procedures. This paradigm shift revolution is particularly vital in POCT applications since rapid and accurate diagnostics have a crucial bearing on the patient's outcome, particularly in resource-limited settings. The reconfigurability of immunoassays to adopt new-fashioned signal detection mechanisms assures their significance in the ever-evolving domain of medical diagnostics. With constantly evolving methods, the quest to come up with more effective and more affordable diagnosis tools dominates, whose innovations will provide for enhanced disease management requiring early interventions and precision in biomarker detection (Vogeser, 2003; Mansuriya & Altintas, 2019).

2.3. Types of Immunoassays

Immunoassays entail various methods applied to detect and quantify unique antibodies or antigens in a sample. Among the most frequently used are ELISA, RIA, and western blotting techniques. ELISA stands out in its ability to detect proteins, hormones, and antibodies with enzyme-linked antibodies that create measurable signals. It has been invaluable in clinical diagnosis, particularly for infectious diseases and hormone assays. On the other hand, RIA, using radioisotope-labeled antigens or antibodies, finds its primary application in the laboratory, where safety and disposal issues of radioactivity and high sensitivity are acceptable. The sophistication of these methods indicates their particular applications and facility in a large variety of analyses, demonstrating the innovative spirit in immunoassay construction. Immunoassays can be classified based on their detection methods, and hence their usability and performance characteristics. A case in point is the expanding utilization of chemiluminescent immunoassays, which are highly sensitive and fast, and are deemed appropriate for point-of-care testing. In these, a chemiluminescent substrate reacts to yield light, from which quantification is achievable using luminometers. Another new and related area is that of nanoparticle technology immunoassays. These assays employ nanoparticles for signal amplification, which increases sensitivity without greatly enhancing complexity. The incorporation of nanotechnology has also revitalized conventional methods and opened up new diagnostic tools, including rapid lateral flow assays. Combined, these advances underscore the dynamic nature of immunoassay development and its potential to assist in overcoming new challenges in the detection and control of disease, particularly in fields such as oncology and infectious disease control (Heath & Davis, 2008). In addition, there are innovative applications of immunoassays that further demonstrate their multidisciplinary value in research and clinical applications. One such example is the use of immunoassays in identifying autoantibodies in autoimmune diseases such as Type 1 Diabetes Mellitus. Here, tests like the non-radiometric immunoassays to detect insulinoma-associated protein tyrosine phosphatase 2 (IA-2) antibodies demonstrate their feasibility in diagnostic evaluation. Based on the expression of highly pure TrxIA-2ic in *E. coli,* affordable procedures have been developed by scientists to enable sensitive detection of IA-2 autoantibodies in patient samples (Guerra et al., 2016). The development of these individualized immunoassays not only enhances diagnostic accuracy but also enables personalized medicine through the ability to design targeted therapeutic interventions. With the increasing growth of applications, the flexibility and effectiveness of immunoassays will remain at the center of the construction of both clinical diagnostics and biomedical research.

2.3.1. Enzyme-Linked Immunosorbent Assay (ELISA)

ELISA is one of the most frequent immunoassay techniques used in laboratory investigation and diagnosis. ELISA exploits the specificity of antibodies to quantify or detect a variety of proteins, hormones, or antibodies in a sample. ELISA primarily involves an antibody-bound enzyme, which catalyzes a substrate to produce a measurable signal. The sensitivity and flexibility of this assay make it invaluable in clinical practice, such as in the diagnosis of infectious diseases, hormonal disorders, and allergy.

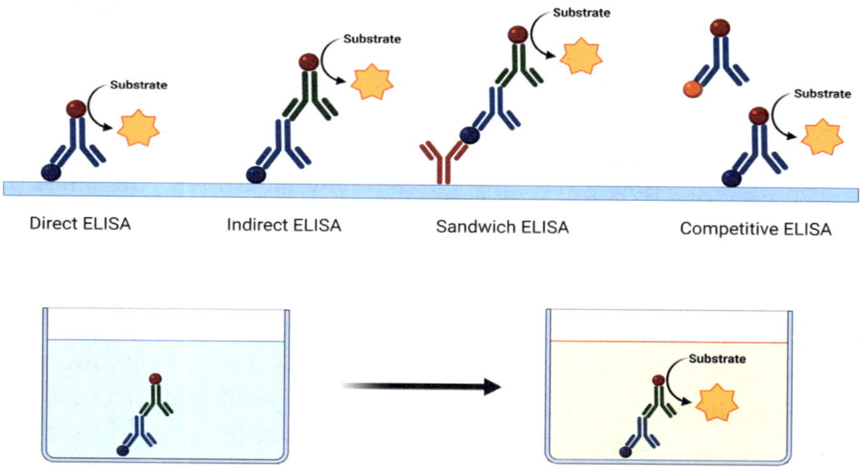

Figure 2.6. Enzyme-linked immunosorbent assay (ELISA) diagram.

Source: https://microbenotes.com/wp-content/uploads/2022/05/ELISA-Diagram.jpeg.

Moreover, developments in ELISA technologies, like modifications that enhance sensitivity and reduce turnaround time, continue to widen its applications, further demonstrating its pivotal role in contemporary biomedical research and diagnostics. ELISA is based on a set of steps that contribute to its success. As the initial step, the target antigen is attached to the solid support, typically a microtiter plate. To this is added a specific antibody in the form of an enzyme conjugate, which reacts with the target antigen and forms a permanent antigen-antibody complex. After removal of free components by washing, an enzyme substrate is added, resulting in a colorimetric or signal response proportional to the amount of target present. The addition of control standards and samples to the assay allows quantitative measurement in order to compare results between samples. This two-step process illustrates how ELISA takes advantage not only of biological specificity but also enhances reproducibility and measurement accuracy. Recent advances in immunoassay technology have contributed to the utility of ELISA, especially in its application to complex diseases. For instance, the ability to develop non-radiometric immunoassays has provided a less harmful and less dangerous alternative for detecting disease markers. Research has come up with new approaches like colorimetric and chemiluminescent detection methods, which not only facilitate easy detection but also increase the sensitivity of the assays several times. The IA-2 study illustrates the efficiency and pragmatic applicability of low-cost ELISA techniques for the quantification of autoantibodies in Type 1 Diabetes Mellitus patients, along with their validity (Guerra et al., 2016). These advances continue to develop ELISA, further establishing its fundamental role in immunodiagnosis and immunoresearch and making possible even broader applications (Figure 2.6).

2.3.2. Radioimmunoassay (RIA)

RIA is a very sensitive technique that makes use of the applications of radioactivity and immunology to quantify antigens within complex biological samples. Developed in the mid-20th century, RIA has revolutionized endocrinology and pharmacology, among others, by offering the ability to quantify hormones, drugs, and metabolites at very low levels. The fundamental principle of RIA is the competition between a nonlabeled and a radiolabeled antigen for limited amounts of specific antibodies. Therefore, the measured radioactivity is inversely proportional to the concentration of the target substance in the sample and can thus be quantified exactly. Its inherent sensitivity and specificity have made this methodology a very valuable reagent in both clinical and research laboratories, particularly where standard analytic methods are not able to meet required detection levels. The effective use of RIA hinges on the planning of a careful assay, comprising several significant elements such as antibody, tracer, and buffer system selection. Most important to the operation of RIA is the affinity of the antibody for the antigen in question, determining the assay's sensitivity and specificity. An optimally optimized assay may offer consistent results for a variety of sample media, ranging from serum to plasma to urine. The tracer, almost always a radioisotope, provides the quantitative aspect required through its quantifiable radioactivity. Though effective, the technique has limitations, i.e., the need for special safety measures to work with radioactive substances and the increased expense of radiolabeled reagents. Thus, alternative non-radioactive immunoassays have been sought by the scientific community, but RIAs remain a benchmark for sensitivity and accuracy for most applications. New developments have led to the design of new non-radioactive alternatives for traditional RIA that continue to enhance assay consistency without increased safety concerns. Assays such as ELISAs and fluorescence immunoassays are gaining popularity because they have better safety characteristics and lower operating costs. But the underlying principles of RIA continue to give useful insights into the construction of these newer assays, especially regarding enhancing antibody specificity and maximizing detection systems. As in the case of several recent studies, such as those on IA-2, new non-radiometric immunoassays have been developed effectively with retention of sensitivity without the use of radioactive materials (Guerra et al., 2016). The evolution of these techniques demonstrates the dynamic and forward-thinking character of immunoassay practice while establishing that RIAs underlying concepts continue to influence modern practices in clinical immunology (Жебентяев et al., 2013) (Figure 2.7).

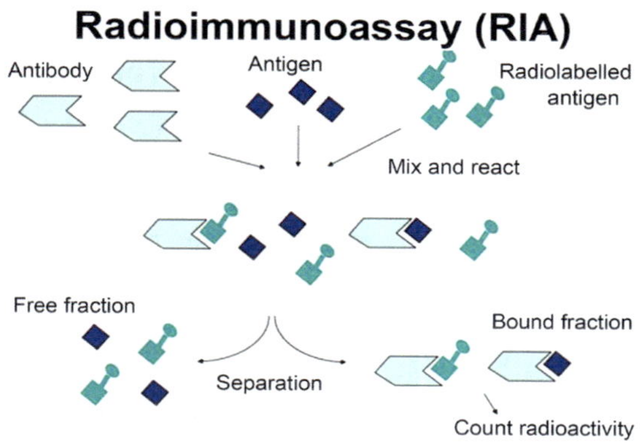

Figure 2.7. Radioimmunoassay (RIA): a highly sensitive technique that exploits the principles of immunology and radioactivity.

Source: https://microscopiaiwm.wordpress.com/wp-content/uploads/2020/11/image-58.png?w=482.

2.3.3. Lateral Flow Assays (LFAs)

LFAs are a significant advancement in the history of immunoassays and yield easy and rapid diagnostics of particular value in low-resource settings. LFAs utilize a simple design based on capillary action to draw liquid along an assay strip, where specific reagents interact and generate a quantifiable signal, usually a colored line. The universal nature of LFAs means that they can be applied to various domains, including biomedical diagnostics, food safety testing, and environmental monitoring. LFAs, for instance, are employed to detect pathogens, drugs, hormones, and metabolites, which means that life-or-death decisions can be made rapidly. The multi-purposefulness captures the primary function of LFAs in global health, particularly in regions where laboratory facilities are scarce (Posthuma-Trumpie et al., 2009). The functionality of LFAs can be tuned by sensitivity, specificity, and the nature of the analyte being analyzed. The design and composition of lateral flow assays are central to their operation in diagnostic applications. Technological advancements, such as the use of paper-based sensors, have significantly boosted the efficacy and accessibility of LFAs. Paper immunoassays, for example, exploit the natural characteristics of cellulose fibers to permit fluid movement while offering a high-quality surface on which biochemical events occur. Advances during the last decade or so have focused on enhancing sensitivity and performance using new materials, including new generations of nanoparticles specifically engineered to maximize signal detection or substitute biological recognition elements with greater specificity towards their objectives. These advances are crucial because they not only increase the quality of the assay results but also expand the range of diseases or conditions detectable, making LFAs a fundamental commodity in diagnostics today (Hristov et al., 2019). Although extremely useful, lateral flow assays are subject to several constraints that must be addressed to achieve full utilization in real-world settings. One such challenge is the inevitable compromise between user-friendliness and precision; while LFAs are designed to be simple to use, this sometimes comes at the expense of reduced sensitivity compared to other, more advanced laboratory techniques. As a further factor, sample quality can be detrimental to the assay's performance, as can environmental conditions. These are countered by ongoing research that develops improved assay formats and the general robustness of LFAs. For example, integrating better signal amplification techniques or designing more sophisticated reader devices could improve quantitative analysis capabilities. Thus, although LFAs are an indispensable part of point-of-care tests, having the knowledge of their limitations is crucial for further progress and wider application in global health policies (Posthuma-Trumpie et al., 2009) (Figure 2.8).

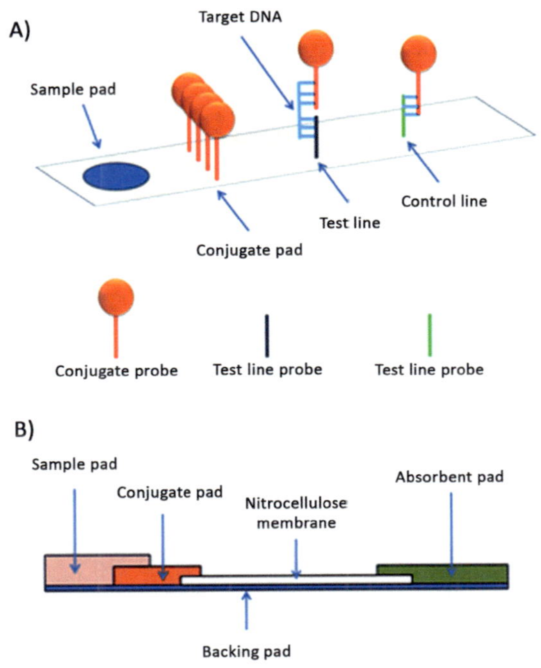

Figure 2.8. Diagram representing the lateral flow assay. This composes of (1) sample pad; the location that the sample is applied, (2) conjugate pad; site of nanogold combined with conjugate probes, (3) Reaction membrane; the main area containing test line-and control line-probes, available for sandwich hybridization of target DNA-nanogold test line probe, and (4) absorbent pad; waste reservoir to draw the sample and collect it.

Source: https://www.researchgate.net/profile/Mongkol-Pongsuchart/publication/271520092/figure/fig1/AS:669950071042070@1536739952816/Diagram-representing-the-lateral-flow-assay-This-composes-of-1-sample-pad-the-location.png.

2.4. Applications in Clinical Diagnostics

Immunoassays have proven to be essential in clinical diagnostics as a result of their ability to perform rapid and sensitive detection of various biomarkers. The assays depend on the specific antigen-antibody interaction, which makes them well-positioned for infectious disease diagnosis, autoimmune diseases, and cancer diagnosis. For instance, the Zika virus epidemic has unleashed unprecedented research in diagnostic testing to effectively detect viral infections among pregnant populations so that appropriate management intervention can be used to prevent public health risks. Specifically, innovative methods such as liposome-based biosensors have been proposed to enhance diagnostic sensitivity through the use of their universal application compared to traditional sensing devices. Accordingly, immunoassays have a central position to occupy in yielding timely and useful diagnostic data that informs public health intervention measures to respond to emergent infectious threats (Shukla et al., 2016). In addition, immunoassays are not only applied in infectious diseases; they have a central place in surveillance for non-infectious diseases such as cardiovascular diseases (CVD). The capacity of these tests to detect specific biomarkers in the blood makes it possible to detect early and prevent adverse health effects. For example, biomarkers such as C-reactive protein (CRP) and cardiac troponins have been extensively studied for their ability to forecast a person's predisposition to cardiovascular events. The growing demand for affordable and portable biosensing instruments to measure these biomarkers highlights the need for alternatives that do not have the drawbacks of laboratory testing. Through the continuous improvement in inventing point-of-care testing, immunoassays pose as the top technique in ensuring fast and precise diagnoses in clinical settings (Qureshi et al., 2012). Finally, the versatility of immunoassays as diagnostic reagents underscores their relevance within clinical laboratories, whether for acute or chronic conditions. Their ability to offer rapid results places them above others within limited-resource settings, particularly in populations with high burdens of infectious diseases like the Zika virus or management of chronic diseases like CVD. Through ongoing research, further refining these assays, innovation through new methodologies and platforms is critical. Future innovation will be poised to improve sensitivity, specificity, and accessibility of immunoassays, ultimately improving patient outcomes. Thus, the continued innovation of immunoassays will be paramount in addressing the challenges laid out in clinical diagnostics and the general efficacy of healthcare delivery (Qureshi et al., 2012; Shukla et al., 2016).

2.4.1. Disease Detection and Monitoring

Practical disease surveillance and detection are integral parts of clinical practice and public health, and immunoassays have emerged as useful tools in this regard. Immunoassays utilize the specificity of antibodies to detect and measure disease-associated biomolecules with great sensitivity, providing clinicians with useful information for management and diagnosis. By detecting specific antigens or antibodies in bodily fluids, immunoassays enable the early identification of pathogens, enabling the use of timely interventions to manage diseases. This is particularly useful in the instance of infectious disease, where early detection can make all the difference to patient management. Immunoassay technologies have seen their use expanded as a result of advancements in them, and they are now suitable for routine laboratory tests and point-of-care testing, thus enhancing their potential in disease surveillance and disease management. The integration of sophisticated technologies such as LCTMS into immunoassay platforms further enhances the capability in detecting disease. LCTMS differs from the traditional methods in its ability to analyze high-throughput data with minimal manual intervention, improving the reliability and efficiency in disease monitoring. LCTMS is more adaptable than the traditional methods with a greater variety of analyzable compounds, which is essential for successful monitoring of multiple diseases.

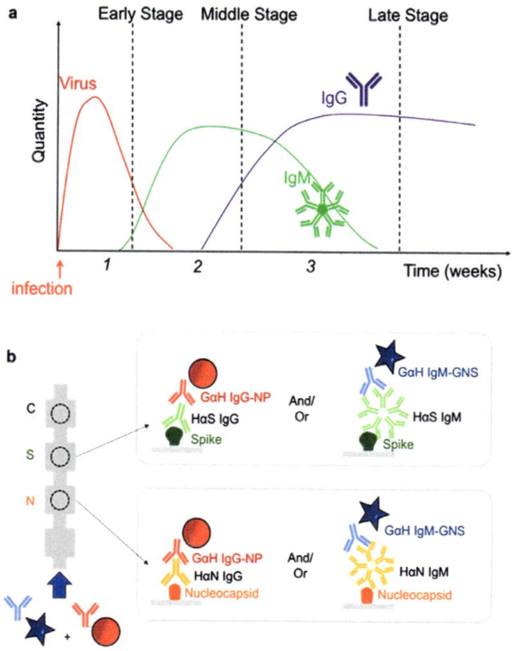

c

Class	αS IgG	αS IgM	αN IgG	αN IgM
Control				
Infected- Early Stage		✓		✓
Infected- Mid Stage	✓	✓	✓	✓
Infected- Late Stage	✓		✓	
Vaccinated- Early Stage		✓		
Vaccinated- Mid Stage	✓	✓		
Vaccinated- Late Stage	✓			
Other- NC IgG			✓	
Other- NC IgM				✓

Figure 2.9. (a) Antibody infection profile. (b) Architecture of the immunoassay. (c) Disease cases investigated.

Source: https://www.researchgate.net/publication/379012590/figure/fig2/AS:11431281236950152@1713442107952/A-Antibody-infection-profile-b-Architecture-of-the-immunoassay-c-Disease-cases.tif.

The LCTMS systems' stability also enables them to be run effectively in clinical labs and meet the demand for quick and accurate diagnosis. This integration of systems with immunoassays is just one of the mechanisms through which new technologies are transforming disease detection, which further leads to improved patient care and outcomes (Vogeser, 2003). In addition, immunoassay development as a high-performance disease diagnostic platform indicates the significance of disease monitoring in chronic disease management as well as infectious disease management. Immunoassays allow real-time disease biomarker monitoring, and this helps clinicians to effectively follow disease progression and treatment response. Real-time monitoring is particularly significant in chronic diseases such as diabetes and autoimmune diseases, where patient management involves ongoing biomarker level monitoring. In addition, immunoassays have made it possible to monitor vaccine responses and provide valuable insights for public health measures. With every emerging disease outbreak, speed and precision of immunoassays will continue to be an essential element in informing public health responses and treatment options, citing their indispensable role in contemporary healthcare (Velghe et al., 2016) (Figure 2.9).

2.4.2. Drug Testing and Therapeutic Drug Monitoring (TDM)

The role of drug testing and TDM plays a vital role in the practice of medication management, particularly in the areas of patient safety and drug efficacy. Immunoassays are commonly employed in such applications, providing sensitive and specific, and rapid detection of therapeutic drugs and their metabolites in biological fluids. These tests aid clinicians in determining if a patient is adherent to prescribed regimens and if drug levels are in therapeutic ranges. Balance between efficacy and toxicity is crucial; hence, appropriate monitoring enables medical professionals to make sufficient adjustments in dosage. This approach, especially with drugs that have narrow therapeutic windows, focuses on putting sensitive immunoassay techniques into practice, maximizing therapeutic outcomes while minimizing adverse reactions that come with incorrect drug levels. Additionally, technology in immunoassays is transforming drug testing and TDM by providing multiplexing capabilities and higher throughput. As emphasized in newer literature, new diagnostic tools are being developed to enable the detection of more than one drug from a single sample at the same time, thus saving time and cost in the clinical environment. These are particularly beneficial for dealing with polypharmacy scenarios where patients are on multiple drugs that require close monitoring to avoid interactions and toxicities. Other attributes, such as increased sensitivity and lowered immunoassay-associated expenses, enable broader use in different healthcare environments. This enhancement in test technologies harmonizes well with the central mission of clinical laboratories to render patient care that is effective as well as efficient, which translates into enhanced management of chronic disorders and complex medication regimens. With the developments in immunoassay technology, the understanding of drug pharmacokinetics and pharmacodynamics enhances the effectiveness of TDM. In-depth understanding of drug absorption, distribution, metabolism, and excretion informs the design and application of immunoassays in real-life clinical circumstances. In addition to ensuring therapeutic effectiveness, monitoring drug levels is also of interest in evaluating the pharmacological effects and potential side effects, and to allow for individualized medicine approaches. For instance, a review revealed that new *in vitro* diagnostic technologies are pivotal in the facilitation of understanding emerging drug activity and their safety profiles, and hence serve as a bridge between laboratory and clinical applications. As pharmacological principles are better understood, their incorporation into immunoassay practice will undoubtedly enhance the position of therapeutic drug monitoring, leading to improved patient outcomes as the fight against disease continues (Figure 2.10).

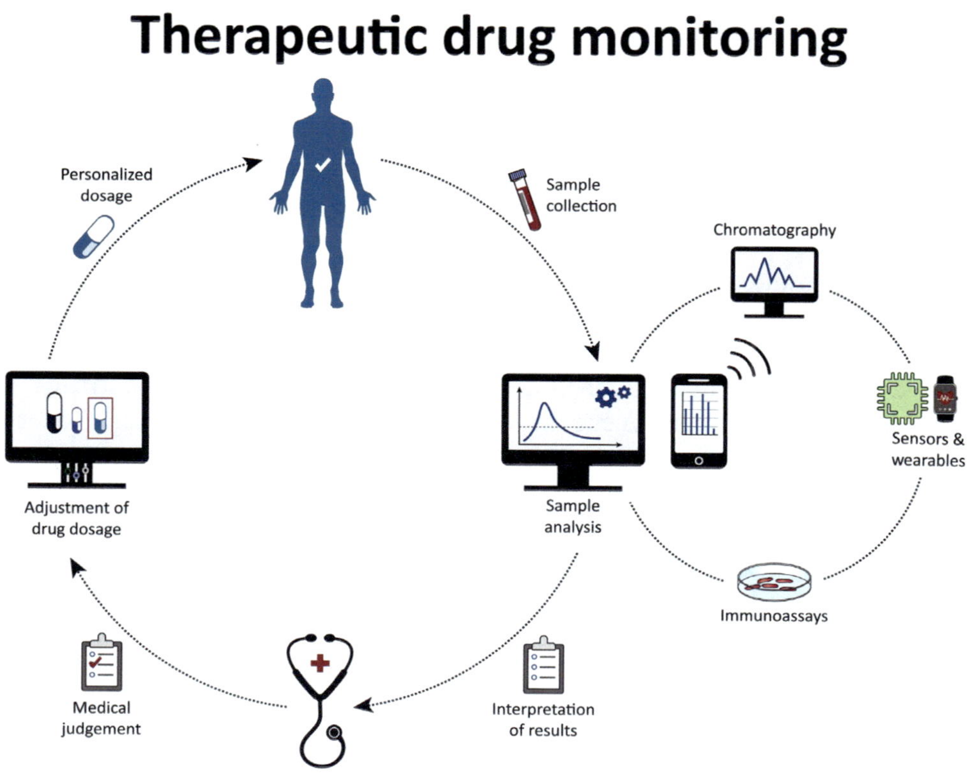

Figure 2.10. TDM should include the active management of free drug concentrations in human body fluids using either chromatographic or immunoassay-based methods or on-site solutions (sensors and wearables) for the optimum benefit of each individual patient.

Source: https://www.researchgate.net/profile/Can-Dincer/publication/340392513/figure/fig2/AS:876030411673602@1585873334987/TDM-should-include-the-active-management-of-free-drug-concentrations-in-human-body-fluids.png.

2.4.3. Infectious Disease Screening

Screening for infectious diseases is an integral part of modern healthcare, providing timely diagnosis and treatment for various pathogens. Immunoassays, particularly multiplexed, have revolutionized this field by allowing for the simultaneous analysis of multiple infectious agents from a single sample. Such efficiency is particularly valuable in the clinical setting, where rapid results can be linked to improved patient outcomes. The intrinsic advantages of multiplex immunoassays over singleplex formats are increased throughput and reduced expense, which provide an environment that is favorable for personalized medicine. However, although such benefits do exist, widespread clinical implementation of multiplex assays for disease diagnosis is hindered by concerns regarding biomarker validation and the requirement for rigorous quality control measures, including calibration and quantitation, that need to be addressed stringently for their efficient use in infectious disease testing (Tighe et al., 2015). Development and application of immunoassays for infectious disease testing have been greatly enhanced by developments in antibody technology. Hybridoma technology provided the means to produce monoclonal antibodies against a multitude of infectious agents, thus increasing diagnostic sensitivity. The challenges of humanizing such antibodies necessitate innovative ways of overcoming defects in specificity and performance. The recent developments in genetic engineering and phage display techniques have led to the development of extremely selective recombinant antibodies that are much better than their conventional counterparts. Besides providing improved immunoprotective responses, these engineered antibodies also allow for the preparation of fusion proteins necessary for successful diagnostics and therapeutic purposes in infectious disease management (Saeed et al., 2017). This antibody design development promises a new day in the quest for more stable and accurate screening. While future immunoassays hold much potential in infectious disease screening, there are still some hurdles to be overcome to allow their useful application in the clinical laboratory. There is a need for standardization of assay protocols so that there is consistent performance in various laboratories and settings. Also, the availability and stability of reagents and cross-reactivity remain critical factors influencing test result reliability. Moreover, automation of assay procedures and the application of validated algorithms for data analysis are critical challenges that, when overcome, would greatly enhance diagnostic competence. With the constantly changing healthcare environment, the addition of new immunoassays to infectious disease screening panels will surely transform patient care through more rapid detection, improved treatment results, and enhanced surveillance against infectious hazards (Tighe et al., 2015) (Figure 2.11).

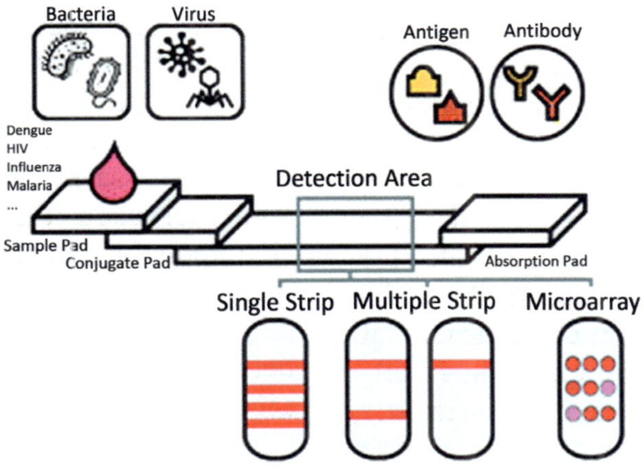

Figure 2.11. A point-of-care test for the diagnosis of infectious diseases based on multiplex lateral flow immunoassays.

Source: https://pubs.rsc.org/en/Image/Get?imageInfo.ImageType=GA&imageInfo.ImageIdentifier.ManuscriptID=C8AN02295J&imageInfo.ImageIdentifier.Year=2019.

2.5. Applications in Research

The use of immunoassays in research has encouraged monumental advances in numerous areas of science, particularly clinical diagnosis and therapeutic monitoring. These immunoassays employ antibodies or antigens to detect specific biomolecular interactions so that diseases, pathogens, and biomarkers can be detected. Immunoassays are versatile and can be utilized in a wide array of areas, including oncology, infectious disease, and autoimmune disease. As scientific techniques of research improve, precise and rapid diagnostic tools have become more crucial; thus, immunoassays are assuming an increasingly pivotal role in experimental designs that enable investigators to yield robust data in studies where high sensitivity and specificity are essential. Actually, the accuracy of immunoassays not only propels scientific research but also contributes to personalized medicine, guaranteeing therapeutic intervention customized by distinctive biomarker profiles. With autoimmune disorders, immunoassays have been extremely useful for research and clinical management. A great case in point is in studies with Type 1 Diabetes Mellitus, where the identification of autoantibodies is of paramount significance for early diagnosis and monitoring of the disease. The IA-2 has emerged as a key autoantigen, providing a target for the development of new immunoassays. Some of the recent advances involve the production of recombinant IA-2 fused with thioredoxin, which results in a stable and highly immunogenic construct that can be made suitable for efficient detection of IA-2 autoantibodies. The process not only makes production easier but also leads to inexpensive and environmentally friendly immunoassays, hence significantly enhancing research activity on autoimmune disorders (Guerra et al., 2016). Moreover, the technological progress in immunoassay methods has introduced new and higher-level techniques such as LCTMS, which provides higher analytical sensitivity and specificity. The combination of chromatographic separation with mass spectrometric detection is reshaping the field of clinical chemistry through the potential for parallel analysis of multiple analytes from a single sample. This high-throughput ability is becoming increasingly necessary as research requirements are expanding for global biomarker profiling. The ruggedness and reliability of LCTMS compared with standard methods bring about a trend for greater flexibility in laboratory testing, culminating in deeper insights into intricate biological systems. With advancements in immunoassays, their applications not only increase knowledge of disease mechanisms but also result in dramatic improvement in patient outcomes and public health in large numbers (Vogeser, 2003).

2.5.1. Biomarker Discovery

Biomarker discovery and validation are key features of modern immunology with significant impacts on diagnostic strategy and therapeutic interventions. Biomarkers such as proteins, nucleic acids, or metabolites serve as indicators for disease states and enable early diagnosis and assessment of therapeutic response. Immunoassays have significantly contributed to the discovery of biomarkers through highly sensitive and specific methods of quantifying the biological markers in various samples. As multiplex immunoassays gain popularity, they present tremendous advantages over classic singleplex assays in terms of enhanced efficiency and increased diagnostic power through simultaneous detection of several biomarkers. Biomarker validation challenges remain, though, major barriers to widespread clinical acceptance before multiplex assays can become universally accepted, as mentioned in the discussion about standardization and control of assay design and conduct (Tighe et al., 2015). In biomarker discovery, the integration of new technological advancements is crucial to enhance the sensitivity and specificity of immunoassays. The emergence of nanotechnology, as exemplified by the development of nanomaterials such as GQDs, has brought new paradigms in biomarker detection. GQDs not only give large surface areas to facilitate efficient biomolecule interaction, but also show unique electro-catalytic properties that can be utilized to elevate traditional detection protocols. These traits enable the production of better performing and cheaper diagnostic immunosensors, which are essential in clinical diagnosis in real-time. The rapid, selective biomarker measurement with such state-of-the-art electrochemical immunosensors illustrates ongoing progress in the technology that provides personalized medicine and disease intervention at an early stage (Mansuriya & Altintas, 2019). Moreover, multiplex immunoassay-based biomarker discovery has a pressing requirement for comprehensive validation frameworks. This is to validate the biomarkers identified by these assays as valid measures of disease. Key validation features involve the evaluation of reagent stability, specificity, and cross-reactivity potential, all of which are imperative to immunoassay integrity. The synergy of these features is imperative for effective crossover from laboratory research to clinical use. By overcoming these challenges effectively, the field can get nearer to its vision of enabling improved diagnostics and therapeutic choices, in turn leading to better patient care and outcomes for a variety of diseases (Tighe et al., 2015) (Figure 2.12).

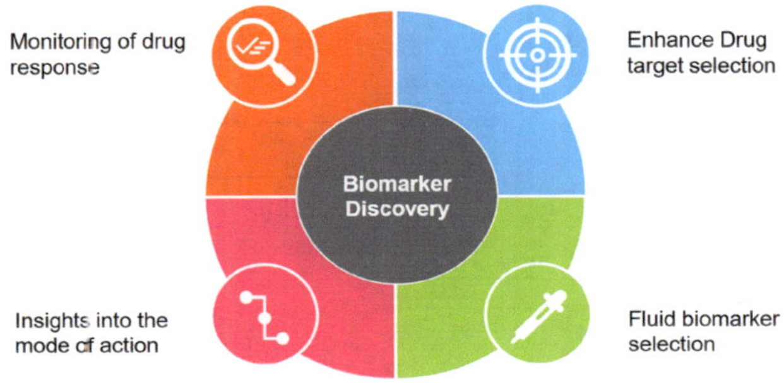

Figure 2.12. Biomarker discovery: Key applications for success.

Source: https://www.svarlifescience.com/hubfs/Discovery%20Biomarker%20key%20applications.svg.

2.5.2. Protein Quantification

Protein quantitation is an elementary requirement of immunoassays, which form the backbone of most clinical applications. By taking advantage of the specificity of antibodies to react with specific proteins, immunoassays present a reliable framework to measure protein levels in different biological matrices. The traditional techniques, e.g., ELISA, have been favored due to their sensitivity and ease of manipulating numerous samples in parallel. These techniques allow researchers and physicians to detect pathological biomarkers, thus facilitating disease diagnosis and monitoring. Improvements in these assays have also led to optimized assay performance that renders them more reliable and precise for clinical use. Technological improvements have also revolutionized protein quantification technologies, which have driven the development of high-throughput methodologies. Techniques like LCTMS offer a very sophisticated technique for protein analysis based on the selectivity of mass spectrometry and the preparatory ability of chromatography. This innovation not only enhances the assays' strength but also extends the range of proteins detectable to more than conventional immunoassays. With LCTMS enabling the quantification of a broader range of proteins in complex mixtures, the clinical laboratory applications are immense. The increased stringency and flexibility of LCTMS make it likely to surpass traditional methods, being a likely weapon for protein quantification in the field (Vogeser, 2003). Technologically, protein microarrays represent another sophisticated avenue for high-throughput protein quantification. The platforms allow the study of numerous proteins simultaneously, significantly increasing analysis efficiency. While earlier microarray technologies were beset with sensitivity and dynamic range challenges, recent advances have overcome these limitations to create digital microarrays with the ability to detect proteins at extremely low concentrations. With new methodologies, such as functionalized gold nanorods as reporters, recent digital microarrays have amazing sensitivity and dynamic range that further extend diagnostic capability. Such advancements confirm the utility of immunoassays in biomolecular studies and clinical diagnostics, marking their irreplaceable role in protein determination (Sevenler et al., 2018) (Figure 2.13).

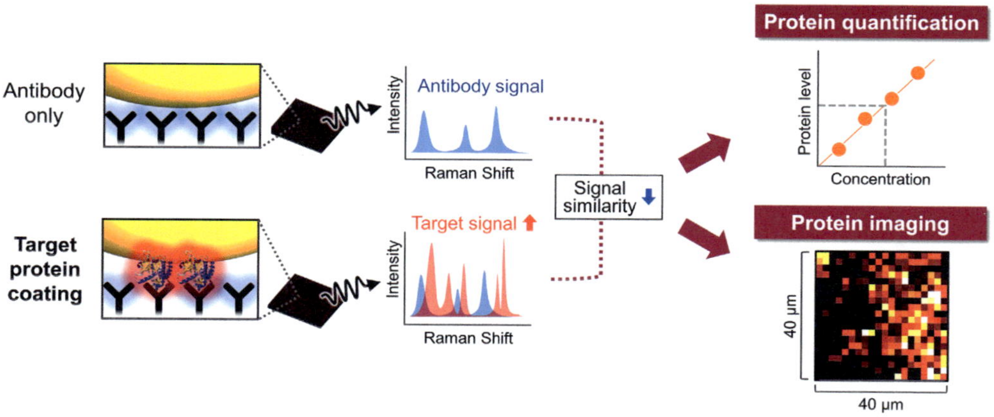

Figure 2.13. Protein quantification and imaging.

Source: https://www.researchgate.net/publication/340688632/figure/fig1/AS:11431281172964502@1688714614055/Protein-quantification-and-imaging-using-the-SERSIA-A-Schematic-overview-of-the.png.

2.5.3. Cell Signaling Studies

The field of cell signaling research has come to be the most important for studying immune response functionality and how it can best be manipulated towards therapeutic effects. Basically, cell signaling is a complex network of molecular interactions that dictate cellular behavior following a multitude of stimuli. This intricate interaction underlies immune responses, particularly T lymphocyte activation and regulation, where signaling pathways orchestrate proliferation and differentiation. Immunoassays are key research tools for demystifying these signaling pathways, such that researchers can quantify various cytokines and signaling molecules involved in mediating immune responses. With continuous reports of new advances in immunoassay technology, the capacity to map such networks of signaling in greater detail is one of the key drivers of immune disease understanding and therapy design (Mohan & Varghese, 2019). There is a fascinating application of immunoassays in cell signaling science, and this is that immunoassays can assist in untangling the mechanisms of specific immune responses. For instance, cloning and expression of porcine IL-2 in recombinant systems have underscored the role of immunoassays in evaluating T cell activation. Analysis of the specificity of antibodies by techniques like Western blotting and ELISA has offered great insights into cytokine-receptor interactions. This not only allows for the immunological description of the immune response in porcine models but also has significance for the description of corresponding mechanisms in humans. The reproducibility of these immunoassays provides an insightful study of cell signaling dynamics, making them invaluable both in basic research and in clinical practice. Improved understanding of these pathways can lead to targeted therapies that boost immune responses in many pathological disorders (Choi & Yoo, 2002). Also, the combination of modern biotech innovations, such as 3D printing and biofabrication, with traditional immunoassays serves to produce new scaffolds in tissue engineering. These scaffolds must interface beneficially with cell signaling pathways in order to facilitate cellular growth and tissue regeneration. By decoding these signaling signals, researchers can optimize the scaffolds in order to more closely mimic the physiological environment required to nurture regenerative activities. Additionally, these novel scaffolds can also be used *in vivo* to monitor real-time signaling events, yet another step towards closing the gap between research into cell signaling and applicable therapeutic intervention. In addition, the intersection of immunoassays and cell signaling studies is a step towards meeting progress in biomedical science, leading to better approaches to immunologically associated diseases and catalyzing tissue regeneration (Mohan & Varghese, 2019).

2.6. Advantages and Limitations

The advantages of immunoassays are numerous, hence making them a necessary component of clinical and research laboratories. Immunoassays are extremely sensitive and specific and enabling the measurement of low analyte concentrations of target analytes such as hormones, drugs, and pathogens, which is quite crucial in diagnosis. For example, immunoassays discriminate effectively between very similar molecules since they take advantage of antigen-antibody binding specificity, thus reducing cross-reactivity. In addition, automation and high-throughput capacity of current immunoassay formats facilitate fast analysis of large numbers of samples, highly beneficial in clinical settings. Also, the versatility of immunoassays makes them flexible regarding assay formats, modes of detection, and binding reagents, and hence makes them extremely usable in numerous fields like pharmaceuticals, environmental monitoring, and food safety (Vogeser, 2003). Despite their advantages, immunoassays have inherent limitations that can affect their validity and reliability. One of the most significant issues is the potential occurrence of false positives or false negatives due to a range of factors, including matrix effects or interfering constituents in the sample. Furthermore, the specificity and complexity of immunoassays require that stringent validation be present to ensure reproducible performance, which can be time-consuming and costly. In addition, the quality and availability of the antibodies could be extremely variable and impact assay performance; suboptimal sensitivity or specificity could be given by poor-quality antibodies, diminishing clinical utility. In light of increasing technological developments in the field, continuous assessment of the current immunoassay technologies is crucial in order to overcome such constraints and maximize their applications (Vogeser, 2003). Advances in technology in immunoassay methods have also introduced new ones aimed at diminishing some of the inherent faults of traditional methods. One such example is the introduction of LCTMS and immunoassays, which enhance sensitivity and versatility through the capacity to analyze multiple analytes from a single sample at once. This technology not only increases the analytical power but also reduces sample preparation time and keeps manual handling to a minimum, promoting high-throughput potential that is paramount to clinical diagnostics. Such advancements mirror the evolving landscape of immunoassays as researchers strive to design more stable formats that can overcome previous limitations. With the potential of innovative immunoassays continuing to expand, research today must focus on making these technologies as good as they can be so that they are reliable and capable of being used in a wide variety of applications in the clinical environment (Matsuda et al., 2015).

2.6.1. Sensitivity and Specificity of Immunoassays

Sensitivity and specificity of immunoassays are determinative criteria that make immunoassays effective and reliable in clinical and research situations. Sensitivity refers to the ability of an immunoassay to correctly identify positive cases and, in the process, avoid false negatives, while specificity refers to the ability of the assay to correctly identify negative cases and avoid false positives. Sensitive assays are useful for detecting disease at the onset, especially in diseases where early treatment can significantly alter outcome, like autoimmune diseases or infectious pathogens. Immunoassays thus must be carefully devised in such a way that they can have high sensitivity and specificity simultaneously, making compromises between the two based on the context of their application.

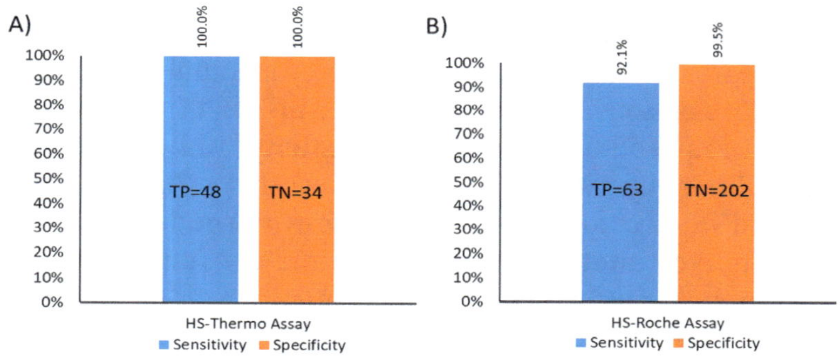

Figure 2.14. Clinical sensitivity and specificity of commercial high-sensitivity benzodiazepine immunoassays. (A) Sensitivity and specificity (Y-axis) of the HS-Thermo benzodiazepine immunoassay in clinical specimens. (B) Sensitivity and specificity (Y-axis) of the HS-Roche benzodiazepine immunoassays in clinical specimens.

Source: https://www.researchgate.net/publication/368899490/figure/fig2/AS:11431281128282346@1679329007072/Clinical-Sensitivity-and-Specificity-of-Commercial-High-Sensitivity-Benzodiazepine.png.

These are indeed important considerations in diagnostic use, where both parameters have direct consequences for clinical decisions and patient management. In designing immunoassays, various aspects can contribute to sensitivity and specificity, for instance, antibody selection, assay format, and the matrix in which the sample is being analyzed. An example is the addition of high-affinity antibodies that would make the assay more sensitive in terms of detecting low levels of target antigens. Additionally, detection strategy selection—colorimetric, chemiluminescence, or mass spectrometry—also contributes to these performance attributes. New advances, which include the merging of advanced technologies such as LCTMS, have proven to improve the ruggedness and specificity of immunoassays. Utilization of rugged methods and diligent optimization results in high-throughput analysis, which is paramount in clinical diagnostics and research (Vogeser, 2003). Additionally, the use of immunoassays transcends the detection of traditional infectious diseases to broader fields, including oncology and autoimmune diseases, the implications of which highlight the importance of sensitivity and specificity to personalized medicine. An example is how the creation of custom immunoassays for the detection of biomarkers such as the IA-2 has been extremely useful for the diagnosis of Type 1 Diabetes Mellitus. The accuracy achieved in autoantibody detection against IA-2, through diligent immunochemical characterization and utilization of recombinant proteins, has greatly enhanced diagnostic sensitivity (Guerra et al., 2016). These advancements demonstrate that high sensitivity and specificity not only help achieve accurate disease diagnosis but also help facilitate an enhanced understanding of disease processes, enabling the development of target-specific therapeutic interventions and improving overall patient outcomes (Figure 2.14).

2.6.2. Cost-Effectiveness and Accessibility

In this era of modern laboratory medicine, the cost-effectiveness of the diagnostic machinery makes a significant difference in its accessibility to a greater population. Immunoassays, which are both very sensitive and specific, are one of the more promising avenues for low-cost diagnostics. Their ability to detect large numbers of biomarkers without extensive and expensive equipment makes them particularly attractive to resource-poor settings. This democratization of health care access is placed within the debates of today for the future of laboratory medicine, with newer technologies and the economic industry being prominent drivers in establishing the efficacy of diagnostic practices, as outlined by the retrospective prediction analysis of trends in laboratory medicine development (Kricka et al., 2015). Therefore, the cost-effectiveness of immunoassays not only renders them practical in clinical settings but also results in improved public health outcomes. Additionally, the application of portable immunoassay technologies is revolutionizing access to diagnostic tests in remote and underserved areas. These innovations make it simpler to use, reduce training needs, and accelerate testing, which is crucial in emergency and low-resource situations. For instance, biomimetic sensor device research illustrates such progress, as a union of efficacy and accessibility. Molecularly imprinted polymers are utilized to utilize these devices within handheld devices capable of sensing analytes with high sensitivity and versatility (Sergeyeva et al., 2010). Through the merging of user-friendly designs with good performance, these innovations are reducing clinical diagnostics entry barriers significantly, and it is now simpler for caregivers to deliver timely interventions in the locations where they are needed most. Altogether, the dual emphasis on cost-effectiveness and access is a transformative shift within the context of immunoassays. As medical systems around the globe grapple to strike a balance between economic constraints and the need for universal diagnostic services, usability and affordability of immunoassays are the watchwords of the day. Future technological developments will not only focus on elevating the sensitivity and specificity of these assays but also on making them accessible at large to a majority of individuals, thereby eliminating the contradiction between high-end diagnostics and actual implementation at the grassroots level. The intersection of novel technologies and affordable solutions ensures that immunoassays will remain a component of improving healthcare outcomes, addressing both the demands of modern diagnostics as well as the underlying imperative towards affordable access to healthcare services (Kricka et al., 2015).

2.6.3. Potential for Cross-Reactivity and False Results

Cross-reactivity risk and false results of immunoassays pose a significant challenge in clinical diagnostics and research applications. Cross-reactivity occurs when a test is developed to quantify a specific analyte and mistakenly identifies and binds with structurally homologous molecules. The spurious reaction creates false-positive results, misdiagnosis, and misdirected therapy. In autoimmune disease screening, for example, antibodies binding to both the target autoantigen and structurally related proteins complicate the interpretation of the result and result in untimely delays in actual diagnosis and initiation of treatment. This issue is particularly relevant for the case of rheumatoid arthritis, in which environmental smoking-induced citrullination of lung tissue proteins is implicated in misleading results arising from increased autoimmune responses, which highlight the complex interplay between the environmental and autoimmune disease states (Lugli et al., 2015). The specificity of reagents applied in assays also directly impinges on the prevalence of cross-reactivity. Variability in the composition and quality of the antibodies used in immunoassays can exacerbate the problem, making it necessary for stringent requirements during manufacturing by the producers. Some cross-reactivity issues might be alleviated by the use of monoclonal antibodies; however, even very well-characterized antibodies are prone to such risk. The phenomenon also emphasizes the need for assiduous assay design, wherein intense testing against a broad panel of possibly cross-reacting agents is conducted to determine specificity. Improvements in assay technologies, such as high-sensitivity multiplex assays, can provide improved specificity but could still struggle with cross-reactivity problems if not properly optimized (Mao et al., 2016). Moreover, resolving cross-reactivity is crucial to the establishment of confidence in routine clinical testing using immunoassays. Understanding the basis of false results can be employed to develop firmer assays for not only minimizing cross-reactivity but also improving sensitivity and specificity. Ongoing dedication to the improvement of assay design, reagent validation, and application of new detection platforms will ultimately translate to improved diagnostic precision of immunoassays. As researchers and clinicians struggle with implications of cross-reactivity, continued dialogue and collaboration between disciplines will be essential in order to further immunodiagnostic potential, moving toward ever more specific and individualized medicine (Lugli et al., 2015; Mao et al., 2016).

SUMMARY

In concluding the discussion of immunoassays, their utility in present diagnostic and research labs should be recognized. Immunoassays are able to exploit the specificity of antigen-antibody interactions in order to quantify a wide range of biological substances, from hormones, proteins to pathogens. This specificity confers immunoassays an unprecedented degree of sensitivity and accuracy, making them suitable for application in a wide array of applications in different fields, including clinical diagnostics, environmental monitoring, and drug development. The development of this technology, from traditional ELISA to newer methods such as LCTMS, is a case in point of how immunoassays advance to meet the demands of high-throughput and intricate analysis. Moreover, as observed in previous studies, the adoption of new methods such as LCTMS is accompanied by increased flexibility and reliability, prompting their widespread application in clinical laboratories (Vogeser, 2003). Furthermore, the ongoing optimization and improvement of immunoassay methods can also improve their performance and broaden their applications. For instance, new findings regarding the regulation of insulin-like growth factor binding proteins (IGFBPs) indicate that immunoassays are also capable of contributing to richer biological information beyond mere quantitation. The proteolytic activity of PAPP-A in modulating IGF availability illustrates the way immunoassays can deconvolute complex biological mechanisms that affect cellular behavior and therapeutic response (D'Elia et al., 2013). This is a reflection of the paradigm shift in the use of immunoassays from simple diagnostic uses to reagents for the enablement of biological research and drug discovery. Eventually, the fate of immunoassays will depend upon their capacity to adapt to evolving scientific queries and technology. Continued development in assay design, sensitivity, and usage of multiplexing capabilities will continue to enhance their utility and reliability exponentially. As clinicians and researchers increasingly desire to learn more about intricate biological systems and maximize patient outcomes, immunoassays will surely be a keystone technology. Their association with emerging fields such as personalized medicine and biotechnology holds out a rosy future, in which immunoassays not only become diagnostic tools but also inspire scientific investigation and innovation to new heights. These trends hold out a rosy future for immunoassays, once again vindicating their usefulness in clinical and research environments.

Immunoassays are valuable analytical tools in clinical and research laboratories, employing the antigen-antibody specificity for detecting and quantifying several substances. They are renowned for their application in diagnosing diseases, monitoring therapeutic responses, and conducting screening tests for other biomarkers. Employing a variety of detection protocols, from colorimetric to luminescent signals, immunoassays can be tailored for specific analytical purposes. This adaptability is also encouraged by advancements in technology, allowing high-throughput screening procedures, efficiency, and volumetric applications in the clinical laboratory. The integration of new technologies, such as LCTMS, illustrates how traditional immunoassay techniques are being modified to further increase sensitivity and specificity, further creating innovations in the field (Vogeser, 2003). In addition to their use in diagnostics, immunoassays play a vital role in monitoring therapeutic intervention, particularly in chronic diseases such as cardiovascular disease and diabetes. For instance, it has been revealed that SGLT2 inhibitors in T2DM have a positive influence on cardiovascular biomarkers. Studies have shown that canagliflozin therapy significantly slows the rise in serum NT-proBNP and high-sensitivity troponin I (hsTnI) over two years compared with placebo. Such information highlights the importance of immunoassays in quantifying treatment efficacy and determining their greater relevance to patient health. By providing crucial information on biomarker levels, immunoassays are indispensable both in therapeutic decision-making and in establishing personalized medicine strategies (Januzzi et al., 2017). Apart from this, ongoing improvement and automation of immunoassay techniques are rendering them increasingly more practical in a clinical environment. Developing stronger methods, such as LCTMS, enables more repeatable and reproducible results, which are essential for high-throughput labs. The complexity and cost of novel technology are often balanced by its improved performance and versatility over existing techniques. As immunoassays evolve, their association with enhanced data analytics and bioinformatics tools will further enhance their value in different biomedical fields, resulting in improved diagnostics and therapies. Immunoassay convergence with next-generation technologies will bring exciting possibilities, remodeling the clinical diagnostics as well as research landscape (Vogeser, 2003).

A CLOSER LOOK

LATERAL FLOW TEST (LFT)

A LFT, also known as a lateral flow immunochromatographic test (ICT) or rapid test, is a simple device that tries to detect the presence of a target analyte in a liquid sample without the need for costly and specialized equipment. LFTs are quickly used in medical diagnostics in the lab, at the point of care, and at home. For instance, the home pregnancy test is an LFT that detects a specific hormone. They are inexpensive and simple to conduct and usually report results within 5–30 minutes. Most laboratory applications render basic LFTs more sensitive by using ancillary purpose-built equipment. Because the target analyte is usually a biological antigen, most lateral flow tests are rapid antigen tests (RAT or ART). LFTs take advantage of the same affinity chromatography that is utilized with ELISA. Basically, these tests allow the liquid sample to travel the surface of a reactive molecule-filled pad with a visible positive or negative result. The pads consist of a series of capillary beds, e.g., pieces of porous paper, microstructured polymer, or sintered polymer. These pads can transport fluid (e.g., urine, blood, saliva) spontaneously (Figure 2.15).

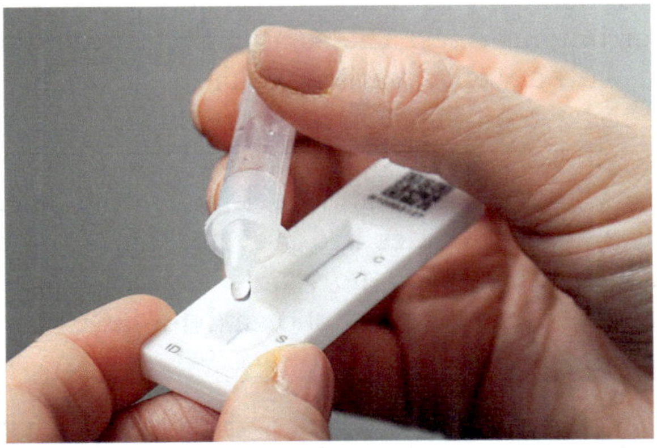

Figure 2.15. Lateral Flow Test (LFT).

Source: https://pharmaceutical-journal.com/wp-content/uploads/2021/05/How-reliable-are-lateral-flow-COVID-19-tests-1.jpg.

The sample pad is a sponge and is in excess of the sample fluid. When it soaks, the fluid flows to the second conjugate pad where the manufacturer has inserted freeze-dried bio-active particles known as conjugates (see below) in a salt–sugar matrix. The conjugate pad contains all the chemicals required for a successful chemical reaction between the target molecule (e.g., an antigen) and its chemical complement (e.g., antibody) immobilized on the surface of the particles. This marks target particles as they travel through the pad and continue over to the test and control lines. The test line shows a signal, typically a color, as in pregnancy tests. The control line contains affinity ligands that tell us whether the sample has passed through and the biomolecules in the conjugate pad are active. The fluid travels from these reaction zones to the final porous material, the wick, which is only a waste holder.

1. **Colored Particles:** Any particle of color can theoretically be used, but latex blue or nanometer-scale gold red particles are most commonly applied. The gold particles are red due to the phenomenon of localized surface plasmon resonance. Fluorescent or magnetic labeled particles can also be used, but require reading using an electronic reader in order to yield the test result.
2. **Sandwich Assays:** Sandwich assays are typically employed for big analytes because they usually possess several binding sites. When the sample travels through the assay, it initially comes in contact with a conjugate, which is an antibody against the target analyte tagged with a visual marker, most often colloidal gold. The antibodies attach to the target analyte in the sample and travel together until they appear at the test line. The test line also has immobilized antibodies of the target analyte that bind to the migrated analyte-bound conjugate molecules. The test line consequently exhibits a visible change due to the concentrated visible tag, thus ensuring the presence of the target molecules. Most sandwich assays also have a control line that will be evident irrespective of the target analyte presence to indicate whether the lateral flow pad is functioning properly. The low-cost, quick sandwich-type assay is used extensively in home pregnancy tests that test for human chorionic gonadotropin (hCG), in pregnant women's urine.
3. **Competitive Assays:** Competitive assays are usually used for small analytes since smaller analytes have fewer binding sites. The sample first encounters antibodies to the target analyte conjugated with a visual marker (colored particles). The test line contains the target analyte immobilized on the surface. If there is no target analyte in the sample, the unbound antibody will react with these immobilized analyte molecules in such a way that a visual marker will be visible. Conversely, when the target analyte is present in the sample, it will bind to the antibodies and prevent them from binding to the immobilized analyte in the test line, and as such, no visible marker will be seen. This contrasts with sandwich assays since, without a band, the analyte must be present.
4. **Quantitative Tests:** Most LFTs are designed on a purely qualitative basis. It is possible, however, to report the strength of the test line to quantify the amount of analyte in the sample. Portable diagnostic testers known as lateral flow readers are used by several companies in order to provide a completely quantitative assay result. Using specific wavelengths of light as illumination along with CCD or CMOS detection technology, the signal-rich image of the actual test lines can be formed. Using image processing algorithms specific to a particular test and medium, line intensities can then be calibrated against analyte concentration levels. One such handheld lateral flow device platform that is good and commercially available is made by Detekt Biomedical L.L.C. Other non-optical techniques are also capable of giving quantitative assay results. A method that falls under the category of such a technique is magnetic immunoassay (MIA) in the LFT also gives ways to achieve a quantified result. Reducing variations in capillary pumping of the sample fluid is another approach to move from qualitative to quantitative results. Recent developments have, for example, demonstrated capillary pumping at a steady rate regardless of the liquid's viscosity and surface energy.

REFERENCES

1. Ahsan, H., & Ahmad, R. (2021). Multiplex Technology for Biomarker Immunoassays. IntechOpen. doi: 10.5772/intechopen.91730(accessed on 27th June 2025).
2. Warriner, K., Reddy, Subrayal M, Namvar, A. and Neethirajan, S. (2014) *Developments in nanoparticles for use in biosensors to assess food safety and quality.* Trends in Food Science and Technology, 40 (2). pp. 183-199.(accessed on 27th June 2025).
3. Mansuriya BD, Altintas Z. Graphene Quantum Dot-Based Electrochemical Immunosensors for Biomedical Applications. *Materials (Basel)*. 2019;13(1):96. Published 2019 Dec 23. doi:10.3390/ma13010096(accessed on 27th June 2025).
4. Amissah, A. A. (2024). Optimization of a SERS-based vertical flow immunoassay utilizing a plasmonic syringe filter for rapid biomarker detection and quantification. https://core.ac.uk/download/621473691.pdf (accessed on 27th June 2025).
5. D'Elia P, Ionta V, Chimenti I, et al. Analysis of pregnancy-associated plasma protein A production in human adult cardiac progenitor cells. *Biomed Res Int.* 2013;2013:190178. doi:10.1155/2013/190178(accessed on 27th June 2025).
6. Therriault J, Schindler SE, Salvadó G, et al. Biomarker-based staging of Alzheimer disease: rationale and clinical applications. *Nat Rev Neurol.* 2024;20(4):232-244. doi:10.1038/s41582-024-00942-2 (accessed on 27th June 2025).
7. Tighe PJ, Ryder RR, Todd I, Fairclough LC. ELISA in the multiplex era: potentials and pitfalls. *Proteomics Clin Appl.* 2015;9(3-4):406-422. doi:10.1002/prca.201400130 (accessed on 27th June 2025).
8. Lugli EB, Correia RE, Fischer R, et al. Expression of citrulline and homocitrulline residues in the lungs of non-smokers and smokers: implications for autoimmunity in rheumatoid arthritis. *Arthritis Res Ther.* 2015;17(1):9. Published 2015 Jan 20. doi:10.1186/s13075-015-0520-x(accessed on 27th June 2025).
9. Sergeyeva TA, Slinchenko OA, Gorbach LA, et al. Catalytic molecularly imprinted polymer membranes: development of the biomimetic sensor for phenols detection. *Anal Chim Acta.* 2010;659(1-2):274-279. doi:10.1016/j.aca.2009.11.065(accessed on 27th June 2025).
10. Januzzi JL Jr, Butler J, Jarolim P, et al. Effects of Canagliflozin on Cardiovascular Biomarkers in Older Adults With Type 2 Diabetes. *J Am Coll Cardiol.* 2017;70(6):704-712. doi:10.1016/j.jacc.2017.06.016(accessed on 27th June 2025).
11. Velghe, S., Capiau, S., & Stove, C. (2016). Opening the toolbox of alternative sampling strategies in clinical routine : a key-role for (LC-)MS/MS. *TRAC-TRENDS IN ANALYTICAL CHEMISTRY, 84*, 61–73. https://doi.org/10.1016/j.trac.2016.01.030(accessed on 27th June 2025).
12. Choi, I., & Yoo, H. (2002). Expression of recombinant porcine interleukin-2 and application of its antibody to immunoassays. *Journal of Veterinary Science, 3*(3), 207–212. https://www.semanticscholar.org/paper/d8bc9d2c35b1771d64b09bbee7994aab1f88e766 (accessed on 27th June 2025).
13. Mao, Y., Shin, KS., Wang, X. *et al.* Semiconductor Electronic Label-Free Assay for Predictive Toxicology. *Sci Rep* **6**, 24982 (2016). https://doi.org/10.1038/srep24982(accessed on 27th June 2025).

14. Sevenler D, Daaboul GG, Ekiz Kanik F, Ünlü NL, Ünlü MS. Digital Microarrays: Single-Molecule Readout with Interferometric Detection of Plasmonic Nanorod Labels. *ACS Nano.* 2018;12(6):5880-5887. doi:10.1021/acsnano.8b02036(accessed on 27th June 2025).

15. Heath JR, Davis ME. Nanotechnology and cancer. *Annu Rev Med.* 2008;59:251-265. doi:10.1146/annurev.med.59.061506.185523 (accessed on 27th June 2025).

16. Eilerts, D. F. (2016). Beyond DNA: Epigenetics and proteomics in forensic science. https://core.ac.uk/download/70427288.pdf (accessed on 27th June 2025).

17. Vogeser M. Liquid chromatography-tandem mass spectrometry--application in the clinical laboratory. *Clin Chem Lab Med.* 2003;41(2):117-126. doi:10.1515/CCLM.2003.020(accessed on 27th June 2025).

18. Kricka LJ, Polsky TG, Park JY, Fortina P. The future of laboratory medicine - a 2014 perspective. *Clin Chim Acta.* 2015;438:284-303. doi:10.1016/j.cca.2014.09.005(accessed on 27th June 2025).

19. Hristov DR, Rodriguez-Quijada C, Gomez-Marquez J, Hamad-Schifferli K. Designing Paper-Based Immunoassays for Biomedical Applications. *Sensors (Basel).* 2019;19(3):554. Published 2019 Jan 29. doi:10.3390/s19030554(accessed on 27th June 2025).

20. Qureshi, A., Gurbuz, Y., Niazi, J. H., et al. (2012). Biosensors for cardiac biomarkers detection: A review. https://core.ac.uk/download/pdf/11743545.pdf (accessed on 27th June 2025).

21. Matsuda R, Rodriguez E, Suresh D, Hage DS. Chromatographic immunoassays: strategies and recent developments in the analysis of drugs and biological agents. *Bioanalysis.* 2015;7(22):2947-2966. doi:10.4155/bio.15.206(accessed on 27th June 2025).

22. Shukla S, Hong SY, Chung SH, Kim M. Rapid Detection Strategies for the Global Threat of Zika Virus: Current State, New Hypotheses, and Limitations. *Front Microbiol.* 2016;7:1685. Published 2016 Oct 24. doi:10.3389/fmicb.2016.01685(accessed on 27th June 2025).

23. Mohan, R., & Varghese, J. (2019). Bio scaffolds in periodontal regeneration. *Journal of Oral Biology and Craniofacial Research, 8*, 428–436. https://www.semanticscholar.org/paper/85d76916a2eb8fccc4646593ffe411cc6e0e70d6 (accessed on 27th June 2025).

24. Napione, L. (2021). Integrated nanomaterials and nanotechnologies in lateral flow tests for personalized medicine applications. https://core.ac.uk/download/524612896.pdf (accessed on 27th June 2025).

25. Saeed, A. F. U. H., Wang, R., Wang, S., & Ling, S. (2017). Antibody engineering for pursuing a healthier future. https://core.ac.uk/download/pdf/82883279.pdf (accessed on 27th June 2025).

26. Guerra LL, Faccinetti NI, Trabucchi A, et al. Novel prokaryotic expression of thioredoxin-fused insulinoma associated protein tyrosine phosphatase 2 (IA-2), its characterization and immunodiagnostic application. *BMC Biotechnol.* 2016;16(1):84. Published 2016 Nov 24. doi:10.1186/s12896-016-0309-2(accessed on 27th June 2025).

27. Posthuma-Trumpie GA, Korf J, van Amerongen A. Lateral flow (immuno)assay: its strengths, weaknesses, opportunities and threats. A literature survey. *Anal Bioanal Chem.* 2009;393(2):569-582. doi:10.1007/s00216-008-2287-2(accessed on 27th June 2025).

28. Жебентяев, А. И., & Каткова, Е. Н. (2013). Современные иммунохимические методы анализа. https://core.ac.uk/download/53875848.pdf (accessed on 27th June 2025).

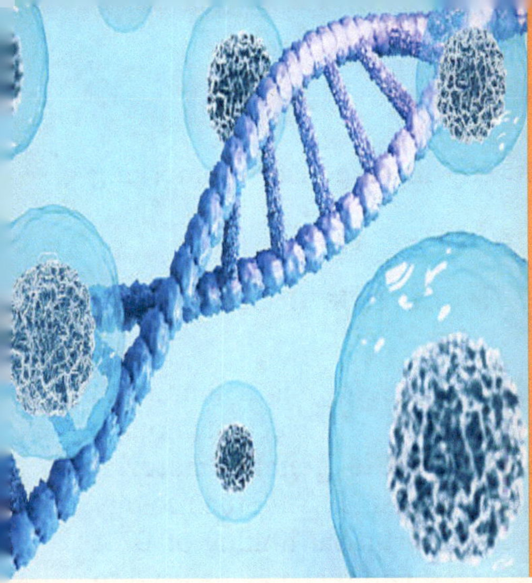

Chapter 3

RECOMBINANT DNA TECHNOLOGY IN IMMUNOLOGY

Contents

Introduction

The advent of recombinant DNA technology has revolutionized immunology to become an exciting discipline with novel and hitherto unimagined opportunities for vaccine design and therapeutic intervention. It allows scientists to, for the first time, manipulate genes and produce vaccines that are capable of inducing potent immune responses without the hazards typically inherent in traditional procedures. This technology allows for the specific introduction of antigen genes, which are then produced in host organisms that are appropriate for this aim, including bacteria, yeast, and plants. The ability to produce specific antigens in quantity not only streamlines vaccine production but also opens doors for manipulating immunological responses to respond effectively to new infectious diseases. These advancements underscore the power of recombinant DNA technology to address world health problems, hence establishing it as the cornerstone of ongoing immunological research and development. In addition, the significance of recombinant DNA technology is more than the simple manufacture of antigens; it is the design of new delivery systems that enhance immunogenicity. Methods like gene agroinfiltration have proved the ability to deliver antigens directly into plants, giving rise to a new generation of plant vaccines. For example, the transient protein expression, e.g., of Staphylococcal enterotoxin B (SEB), in plants is an example of how recombinant DNA technology can be used for quick vaccine development in times of public health crises. The efficacy of these plant-produced vaccines has been established by evidence that intranasal administration of agroinfiltrated plant homogenates can induce protective immune responses in animal models. Such dual utility of antigen synthesis and effective immunogenicity is a reflection of the revolutionary potential of recombinant DNA technology in immunology, which allows for quicker and safer responses to endemic and pandemic threats (Liu et al., 2018). The recombinant DNA technology patent climate highlights the importance of high-tech innovation in creating vaccines, particularly against anticipated rapid mutations of infectious diseases such as influenza.

A thorough analysis of patent documents reveals heightened interest and investment in vaccine technology that triggers immunity to pandemic strains as an active strategy for world health preparedness. The awareness of key stakeholders in this field, including key pharmaceutical companies and government agencies, also calls attention to the cooperative spirit required to ensure vaccine research. This increased focus on recombinant DNA technologies not only plays a part in unraveling the complexity attendant with pathogenic threats but also affects policy strategy formulation. As illustrated in recent epidemics, the ability to innovate quickly through recombinant techniques can play a key role in containing the impact of the next health crises (Cavicchi et al., 2012). Recombinant DNA technology is hence at the forefront of immunology, with an expectation of a future where vaccines are manufactured and distributed instantly in response to emerging health issues.

Definition of Recombinant DNA Technology

Recombinant DNA technology is a landmark innovation in the science of molecular biology to be able to manipulate genetic material across different organisms. The technology basically involves the artificial linking of DNA from different sources, and this may be used to introduce into a host organism to exhibit desired traits or produce specific proteins. The methods utilized include gene isolation, utilization of vectors to transfer the genes into host cells, and subsequent expression of the genetically manipulated gene product. This technology, in addition to enabling scientists to examine gene function, has also enabled them to produce large quantities of proteins for therapeutic reasons. Therefore, recombinant DNA technology is a landmark technology, particularly in the field of immunology, in which it is employed to produce vaccines and monoclonal antibodies vital for disease control and prevention. Furthermore, the application of recombinant DNA technology in immunology is multifaceted and revolutionary. By making certain antigens possible, researchers can come up with vaccines that draw on the body's own immunity to recognize and destroy germs effectively. For instance, through cloning antigens coding genes found in various viruses and bacteria, vaccines can be produced that cause a specific immune response without the disease. Not only is this safer, but it is also more efficient than other vaccine production techniques. As several studies have pointed out, the use of such technologies, or in this case, their development of prophylactic vaccines against new viral strains, highlights the significance of recombinant DNA in solving public health issues. The technology thus has the ability to change the face of the way immunologists respond to disease prevention, showcasing its far-reaching impact on the subject. In addition, the patent landscape for recombinant DNA technology illustrates prominent trends and developments marking its usability in scientific and commercial contexts. Recent patent reviews have indicated an increased rate of innovation for the invention of vaccines, particularly against pandemic threats such as influenza. These patents embrace a variety of methodologies, including the production of recombinant viral antigens and the use of genetic engineering methods to enhance the efficacy of vaccines. Researchers increasingly use recombinant DNA technology to explore platforms ranging from subunit vaccines to vectored virus vaccines, indicating a diversification of approaches towards fighting infectious disease. Also, collaborative research among research institutions and drug companies indicates a mutually shared thrust towards effective utilization of these technologies in immunological interventions. With improving technology, ongoing examination of the patenting scenario continues to reveal further innovations poised to contribute towards world health solutions in the field of recombinant DNA technology (Johnston et al., 1988; Cavicchi et al., 2012) (Figure 3.1).

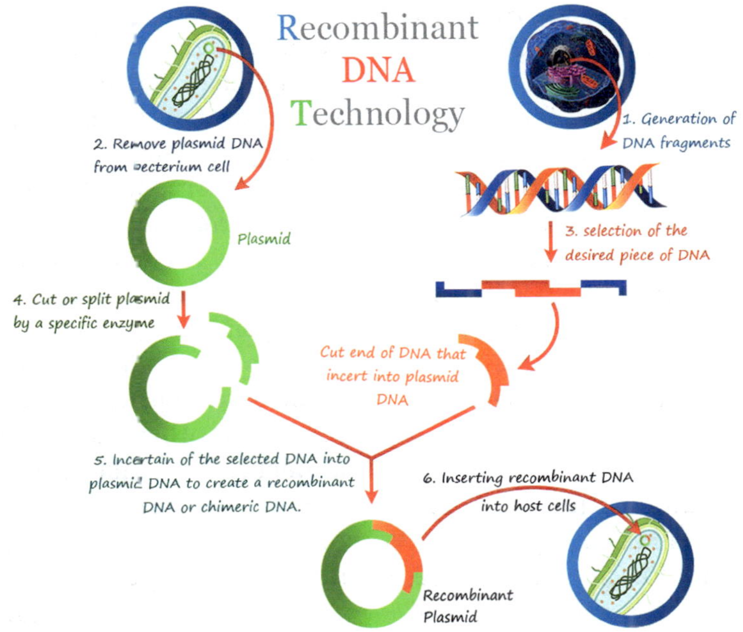

Figure 3.1. Illustration of recombinant DNA technology.

Source: https://www.priyamstudycentre.com/wp-content/uploads/2023/09/Recombinant-DNA-Technology-rDNA-Technology-examples-steps.jpg.

Importance of Immunology in Health And Disease

Immunology plays a vital role in learning about health and disease, especially concerning the development of new technologies to combat infectious diseases and promote improved public health outcomes. The immune system is the body's first defense against microbes, a complex system of cells, tissues, and organs that interact to identify and kill extraneous invaders. This sophisticated mechanism also leads to disease progression when it goes awry, leading to autoimmune conditions or enhanced allergic responses. Therefore, an in-depth knowledge of immune mechanisms informs therapeutic interventions, such as vaccines and monoclonal antibodies, that have revolutionized prevention and treatment paradigms. The impact of immunology on the application of recombinant DNA technology has further enhanced vaccine specificity and efficacy, leading to new therapies that could be tailored to individual immunogenic profiles. Piggybacking on the use of recombinant DNA technology is what, in applied immunology is enabling the manufacture of targeted vaccines against individual pathogens. For instance, work on Clostridium perfringens-type A necrotic enteritis-causing strains in poultry is an excellent example of this potential. Current work emphasizes the requirement for effective vaccination strategies against toxin-secreting bacteria and reflects a general trend wherein immunogenic proteins are being identified for use in vaccines. Studies have proven that although single-protein vaccines can be insufficient, techniques that utilize more than one antigen will result in a stronger immune response, hence the significance of combinatorial techniques in protective immunity. This high level of understanding emphasizes how immunology not only deals with health issues by means of vaccination but also enhances agricultural health, illustrating its multidisciplinary nature. The relevance of immunology extends beyond traditional animal health to encompass essential wildlife conservation science, as exemplified in the investigation of sea turtle viral diseases. Current investigations have employed recombinant DNA techniques to chart out reptilian herpesviruses' immunogenic proteins, providing significant insights into the free-ranging green turtles' immune response to infectious agents. This new area of study outlines the role of immunology in disease processes in wildlife populations and consequently, in the development of conservation. The study, by offering seroepidemiological data and correlating infection, sheds light on the isolation of specific viral infections among marine turtles and leaves space for further immunological investigations. These multidisciplinary activities not only enhance health and disease interaction understanding in other organisms but also help to enhance public education and policy formulation in wildlife and environmental health.

Overview of the Relationship Between Recombinant DNA Technology and Immunology

The convergence of recombinant DNA technology and immunology has stimulated tremendous advancement in both scientific branches, particularly through vaccine development and therapeutic agents. Recombinant DNA techniques, where specific genes are introduced into host organisms, have been employed to generate vaccines that elicit strong and lasting immunity. For instance, in the manufacture of vaccines against infectious diseases, recombinant pathogen proteins, such as bacterial toxins, can elicit immunity to infection but not disease. One of these is the use of toxoided toxins, which have been proven to be efficient immunogenic molecules against Clostridium perfringens in birds. These strategies demonstrate the prowess of recombinant DNA technology in inducing specific immune responses by delivering specific antigens to the immune system, leading to more efficient vaccination regimens in immunology (Mot et al., 2014). Apart from vaccine preparation, recombinant DNA technology has unveiled new approaches to managing chronic ailments induced by immune reactions. This is particularly relevant in the case of autoimmune diseases and allergies, where engineered proteins can assist in modulating immune processes. Through the design of therapeutic agents that act against a particular immune pathway, scientists can come up with treatments that either stimulate or suppress immune activity based on the disease situation. Not only does this technology promise individualized treatment regimens, but it may also have the potential to cure symptoms that are a consequence of aberrant immune responses. Furthermore, the data gleaned from immune mechanisms, for example, between immune cells and disease agents such as trypanosomes, underline the need to understand these systems at the molecular level. For instance, trypanosomes' adaptive immune evasion properties highlight how further sophistications of immunological products might be developed through recombinant technologies, which will improve patient outcomes (Magez et al., 2020). Complementarity of recombinant DNA technology and immunology also applies to how diagnostic devices are improved, disease detection and disease characterization. Traditional diagnostic methods are typically insensitive and nonspecific, but with recombinant technology, one can produce extremely specific antibodies and antigens as diagnostic reagents. Monoclonal antibody production using recombinant means is a prime example, giving rise to improved detection systems for numerous infectious and autoimmune diseases. Furthermore, progress in genetic engineering has enabled the production of biosensors that can identify pathogens using recombinant DNA elements, hence enhancing public health programs. In general, these advancements highlight the ability of recombinant DNA technology to transform immunological diagnostic and treatment strategies, hence increasing our understanding and management of immune-related disorders.

3.1. Historical Background

The development of recombinant DNA technology is a milestone in the history of immunology, filled with scientific inquiry and moral controversy. This new method was conceived in the early 1970s when researchers were able to find out the process of cutting and joining specific segments of DNA and implanting foreign genes in host organisms. The most important of these advances was the pioneering work of Paul Berg, whose lab work, along with that of his colleagues, provided the basis for genetic engineering and molecular cloning. The significance of these discoveries was vast, not only because they enhanced understanding of genetic structures and function, but also because they led to the possibility of vaccine and immunotherapy development. Consequently, the accompanying history of this technology directly shaped the direction of biomedical research, leading to developments that have since transformed immunological practice. As technology for recombinant DNA evolved, it provided a stimulus for research that sought to tap into immune system components as therapeutic agents. Research on various genes related to immune function allowed for the identification of critical genetic markers that underpin conditions such as multiple sclerosis. Research indicated that certain human leukocyte antigen (HLA) alleles could increase or decrease the risk of these conditions, ultimately directing therapeutic interventions. For example, evidence from the HLA-DRB1 locus indicated a multi-factorial association between genetic susceptibility factors and protective alleles in multiple sclerosis (Mamedov et al., 2020). These findings demonstrated how recombinant DNA technology provided potent tools for uncovering the genetic mechanisms of immune-mediated disorders, thereby facilitating more targeted and efficient immunological therapies. Apart from this, the application of recombinant DNA technology in immunology was also not without controversy and raised significant ethical questions regarding genetic manipulation. When researchers began to engineer organisms for therapeutic applications, questions about the results of playing with biological systems were also raised. The resolution of good possibilities against ethical concerns of safety and environmental impact became the focal point of public discourse. This encounter of scientific advancement and public anxiety is epitomized in contemporary debates surrounding the use of genetic modification in medicine and agriculture. The controversy over recombinant DNA continues to have relevance, representing the focal point where ethical consideration occupies in scientific advancement. Thus, understanding this background history is useful to have a proper appreciation not only of the scientific progress in immunology but also of its general impact on society and public policy.

3.1.1. Discovery of DNA Structure and Its Implications

The classic discovery of DNA's double-helix structure by James Watson and Francis Crick revolutionized the discipline of biological sciences and led to numerous technological advancements, especially in the field of immunology. DNA is not only a carrier of genetic information, but it is also the blueprint for protein synthesis, which is necessary for the operation of many physiological processes, including immune defense. This structural architectural characterization of DNA has enabled scientists to manipulate genetic material, such that scientists have been able to investigate and exploit the machinery of gene regulation and expression. In the long term, the characterization of DNA's architecture has far-reaching implications, underpinning the progression of a broad array of disciplines from medicine to biotechnology, shaping the concept and management of disease, most prominently through recombinant DNA technology in immunology. The importance of understanding DNA structure extends to critical uses in recombinant DNA technology, which has had a significant effect on immunology. Through the application of DNA manipulation concepts, scientists can now design recombinant proteins as vaccines or drugs. The manufacture of monoclonal antibodies and the use of recombinant antigens, for example, are now standard practices in vaccine production. These developments not only enhance the specificity and potency of immune interventions but also enhance safety profiles to the point of reduced adverse reactions characteristic of traditional vaccines. Through studies of parasites like trypanosomes in current research, mechanisms of immune evasion have driven target-oriented strategies in vaccine development. Thus, the integration of DNA technology in immunological investigation reflects an important step in the development of potent and efficacious treatments for other infectious diseases (Magez et al., 2020).

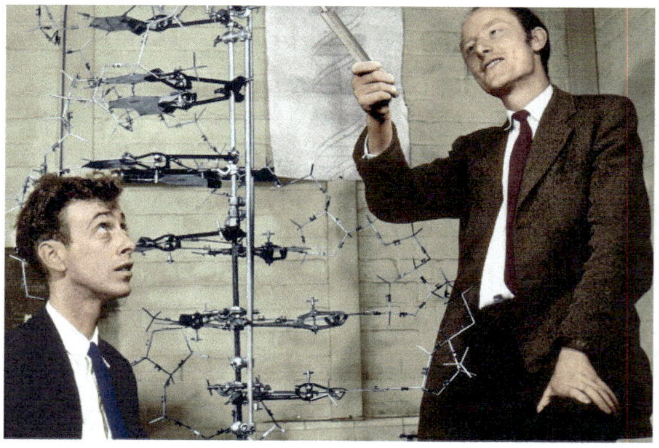

Figure 3.2. James Watson, Francis Crick, and the DNA double helix. Reprinted from Watson JD. The double helix: a personal account of the discovery of the structure of DNA.

Source: https://www.thetimes.com/imageserver/image/%2Fmethode%2Ftimes%2Fprod%2Fweb%2Fbin%2Fee369722-6450-11e8-aeba-dfc3db1a69eb.jpg?crop=4606%2C3071%2C0%2C769.

Besides vaccine development, understanding that has been obtained from studying the structure of DNA has informed significant progress in immune cell regulation and therapeutic manipulation. For instance, selective glucocorticoid receptor modulators, which aim to minimize side effects in the system while maximizing therapeutic effect, are a product of the evolution of recombinant DNA technology. Such modulators can be crafted to act selectively on immune responses, thus maximizing the treatment of chronic inflammatory diseases without side effects. By relating the molecular underpinnings of DNA directly to real-world immunological treatments, scientists can now engineer improved therapies for dysregulated immune process ailments. As scientific study continues to progress, further advancements in DNA-based technologies could further revolutionize immunology procedures, leading to new ways to combat complex diseases (Chirumamilla et al., 2017) (Figure 3.2).

3.1.2. Recombinant DNA Technology

The search for new recombinant DNA techniques has further developed immunology, particularly in making vaccines and therapeutic compounds. First conceived during the 1970s, these techniques allow scientists to manipulate genes of various species.

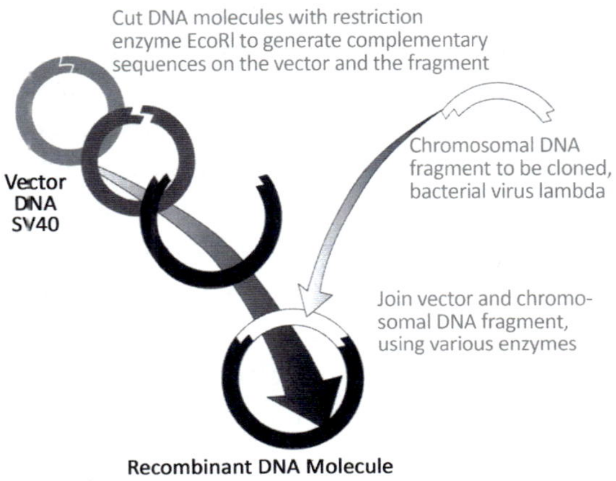

Figure 3.3. The process of making recombinant DNA, as pioneered by Paul Berg.

Source: https://www.sciencehistory.org/wp-content/uploads/2025/06/berg_recombinant-dna-molecule.jpeg.

By utilizing restriction endonucleases and ligases, scientists can combine DNA fragments to form recombinant molecules. This forms the foundation for the production of pathogen-like proteins that can be recognized by the immune system to combat and detect diseases without exposure to live pathogens. Agroinfiltration is one such example, which presents a novel method of vaccine antigen expression in plants and evading traditional purification methods and transgene dissemination risk, something of topical interest with respect to vaccine manufacture biosecurity (Liu et al., 2018). In immunology, recombinant DNA techniques enhance the promise of vaccine efficacy with specific antigen targeting. Targeted antigen inclusion in vaccine products enhances immune response, as in recombinant subunit vaccine trials for such pathogens as Neospora caninum. Use of adjuvants like immunostimulating complexes (iscoms) for hydrophilic proteins enhances immunogenicity, as traditionally hydrophilic proteins have trouble eliciting strong immune responses. The innovative application of biotin-streptavidin interactions for immobilization of recombinant proteins onto iscom matrices demonstrates the creativity in vaccine development in today's era. These methods not only enhance the efficacy of vaccines but also provide a strategic move towards controlling infectious diseases that have no useful means of prevention, such as neosporosis in livestock (Pinitkiatisakul et al., 2007). In the end, the ongoing development of recombinant DNA techniques is more a revolution in public health than a scientific endeavor. As technology becomes better, these techniques promise increased understanding of antigen presentation and interaction with the immune system. For instance, the ability to create targeted antibodies to designer antigens significantly improves vaccine design, ensuring a tailored immune response that can adapt to newly evolving pathogens. The research on recombinant technology, as illustrated through its application in immunogenicity research, proves its ability to address global health challenges. Scientists continue to identify and advance these techniques, paving the way for the development of vaccines that seek to enhance immunological immunity against all manners of infectious diseases (Figure 3.3).

3.1.3. Immunological Milestones Influenced by Recombinant DNA

Recombinant DNA technology has provided monumental immunological milestones, particularly in vaccine development and therapy. The earliest breakthroughs were the generation of recombinant insulin and recombinant human growth hormone, in particular demonstrating the capability of making biologically active proteins. These pioneering achievements led to more sophisticated immunological applications, such as the creation of recombinant vaccines. As opposed to traditional methods that often relied on live attenuated or inactivated pathogens of disease, recombinant vaccines enable the use of defined antigens, which are safe and effective as well as reducing risk. The transformation has had a radical effect on how infectious diseases are dealt with, where scientists can weigh immunogenicity against safety. These innovations established a precedent that has become central in developing modern vaccines, particularly for complicated diseases like malaria, where traditional methods are faced with serious challenges (Johansen et al., 2024). A milestone worth noting in the position of recombinant DNAs in immunology is the invention of monoclonal antibodies (mAbs), which revolutionized diagnostics and treatment options. With the use of hybridoma technology, scientists can generate antibodies of high specificity against targeted antigens that facilitate therapeutic targeting. Such specificity has profound implications in oncology and autoimmune disease therapy, where dysregulated immune response leads to compromised patient health. Success with mAbs has not just transformed cancer therapies with targeted therapy but has also facilitated more accurate and dependable diagnostic testing. By the specific targeting of pathogens or infected cells, mAbs provide better patient outcomes and fewer side effects. The ongoing optimization of such technology is a testament to the promise that recombinant DNA brings, with research continually advancing therapeutic methods (Tandel et al., 2020). Along with advancements in monoclonal antibodies, recombinant DNA technology has played a key role in the development of gene therapies, particularly in the control of immunological disorders. Genetic components are manipulated to allow corrective therapy in genetic immunodeficiency patients. For example, the application of CRISPR and other gene-editing tools has opened avenues for the repair of faulty genes that lead to diseases like Severe Combined Immunodeficiency (SCID). The patient management implications are deep, converting previously fatal diseases into treatable illnesses by restoring normal immunity. These advances in gene therapy represent a milestone in immunology, illustrating the capability of recombinant DNA technology for reshaping our perception of disease. As the science evolves, the integration of genetics and immunology may usher in future developments that transform the understanding and management of many immune-mediated conditions (Johansen et al., 2024).

3.2. Mechanisms of Recombinant DNA Technology

The mechanisms of recombinant DNA technology form the basis of using it in immunology, through the creation of new vaccines and therapeutic substances. The mechanism involved in this technology is in the cloning of genes, whereby specific pieces of DNA are isolated and inserted into vectors—such as plasmids or viruses—that can be replicated within host cells. This procedure usually utilizes restriction enzymes that cut the DNA at particular sequences so that there is a precise insertion of foreign genes.

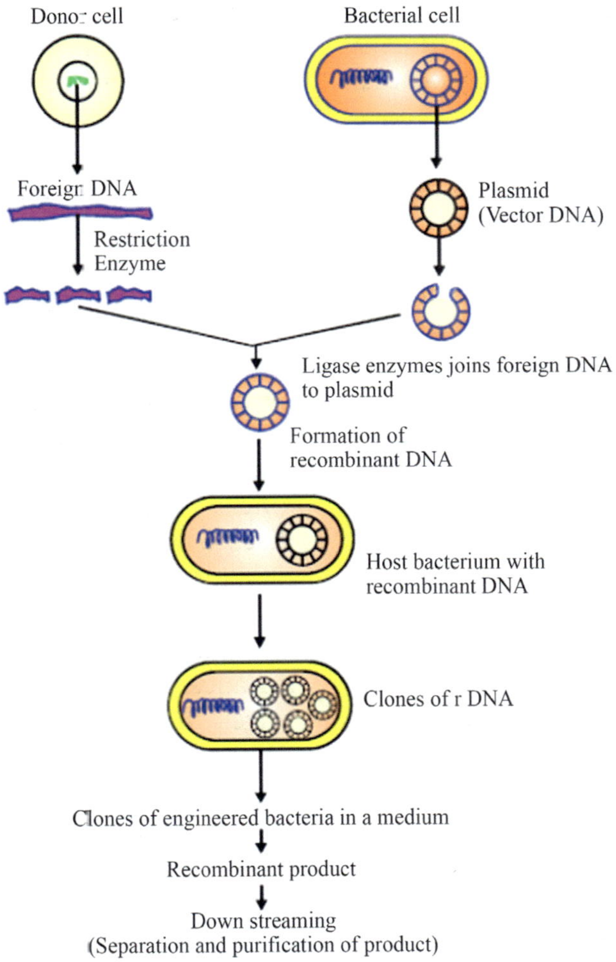

Figure 3.4. Recombinant DNA technology general process.

Source: https://www.google.com/url?sa=i&url=https%3A%2F%2Fwww.ozguryayinlari.com%2Fsite%2Fcatalog%2Fdownload%2F124%2F869%2F2061&psig=AOvVaw0qA25hihs2CeD704TCiMai&ust=1750482195098000&source=images&cd=vfe&opi=89978449&ved=0CBcQjhxqFwoTCIi0pcSc_40DFQAAAAAdAAAAABAE.

This method allows one to produce large amounts of an antigen, which can be used to trigger the immune response. In immunology, the ability to produce high levels of immunogenic proteins, such as those found in pathogens and used as antigens, plays a crucial role in developing effective vaccines that might provide immunity against disease. Agroinfiltration is a new use of recombinant DNA technology nicely illustrated through the revolutionary approach taken with plant-based vaccines. By directly transforming genes encoding for antigens, such as those associated with Staphylococcal enterotoxin B (SEB), into non-reproductive plant tissue, researchers can gain transient antigen expression *in vivo*. Not only is this an enhanced safety feature through the decrease of introgression risk of the gene, but it also allows for the co-expression of multiple antigens within one leaf of a plant. Demonstrated in radish plants, the efficacy of such an approach was confirmed through research wherein ICR mice were immunized intranasally with transgenic leaves, resulting in high antibody yields and immune protection against SEB-induced immune responses. Such breakthroughs demonstrate the promise of quicker vaccine production, which proves helpful specifically in the context of emergent infectious diseases (Liu et al., 2018). Another of the major mechanisms that exists in recombinant DNA technology includes the engineering of glucocorticoid receptor (GR) ligands, which advance the therapeutic intervention in immunology. Synthesis of selective glucocorticoid receptor agonists (SEGRAs) is a top-down strategy that seeks to modulate inflammation with fewer side effects than conventional corticosteroids. By creating analogs such as GSK866 that covalently bind to the GR, scientists can extend therapeutic effects, thereby needing smaller doses to be effective and lowering systemic side effects. The in-depth investigation of these covalent-binding ligands has revealed strong anti-inflammatory activity, as well as simultaneously elucidating GR activity using biochemical assays. Cumulatively, these advances reflect the enormous synergy of recombinant DNA technology with drug discovery innovation towards more and safer therapeutic options for inflammatory diseases (Chirumamilla et al., 2017) (Figure 3.4).

3.2.1. Gene Cloning and Its Applications

Gene cloning is a pillar of modern biotechnology, offering enormous advancement in the area of immunology. Through the selective isolation and replication of a specific DNA sequence, researchers can engineer organisms to synthesize targeted proteins, such as antibodies and cytokines, that are central to the immune response. This is particularly groundbreaking for vaccine development in that cloned genes encoding immunogenic proteins can be used to add vectors in an attempt to induce robust immunologic responses without the risk posed by live pathogens. Consequently, gene cloning enables the production of recombinant proteins that can be employed to enhance vaccine efficacy, hence proving its pivotal relevance in disease protection and treatment regimens in immunology. Gene cloning is not just confined to vaccine production; it also entails research on immune cell signaling and function. For instance, focused cloning of cytokine genes has solved the complexities of immune responses. Research has confirmed the functional abilities of various cytokines in birds and mammals, and their homology despite varying structural forms. Advances in gene cloning techniques have allowed the identification of key avian cytokines, such as interferon-gamma (IFN-γ) and interleukins, that were not properly studied due to the difficulties of their identification. This innovation advances enhanced knowledge of immune functions in various species, uncovering information on evolutionary mechanisms and possible applications in poultry medicine and immunization regimes (Staeheli et al., 2001). In addition, implications for cloning of genes for therapeutic applications in immunology are considerable. Investigation confirms the effectiveness of recombinant cytokines, including chicken interferon-γ (rChIFN-γ), in immunomodulation of activities. It has been demonstrated through scientific research that rChIFN-γ can enhance the phagocytic activity of heterophils in poultry, thereby stimulating the innate immunity against pathogenic bacteria such as *Salmonella enteritidis*. The modulation of cytokines primes immune cells and thereby enhances their capability to respond strongly to subsequent infections. Such findings highlight the potential of employing cloned cytokines as immunotherapeutic medications, not merely for veterinary medicine but also for human health improvement through more effective therapeutic intervention in infections and immune diseases (Kogut et al., 2001). The continuous improvement in gene cloning techniques thus promises more future achievements in the intersection of recombinant DNA technology with immunology (Figure 3.5).

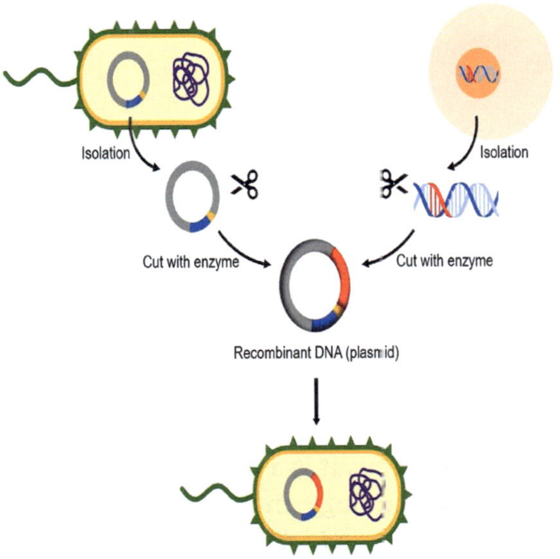

Figure 3.5. The basic steps of gene cloning.

Source: https://www.antibody-creativebiolabs.com/img/1-6-1-1-gene-cloning-1-1.jpg.

3.2.2. Use of Plasmids in Gene Expression

Plasmids play an important role in gene expression, particularly in the field of immunology. Plasmids as extrachromosomal DNA can be engineered to carry genes of interest. By utilizing their ability to replicate independently within host organisms, researchers can introduce foreign DNA into organisms purposely. This has enormous potential for investigating immune mechanisms as well as the development of new vaccines. For instance, the production of genes encoding the pathogen antigens can be done with the use of plasmids, such that the host immune system can identify the antigens and respond. The versatility of plasmid-based platforms enables a platform for high-throughput rapid prototyping of various immunological constructs to be tested for protective immunity elicitation or the modulation of immunological processes, a key endpoint for translational immunology. Besides their role of displaying antigens, plasmids have been utilized to examine immune modulation. As an example, to examine how certain parasites are able to escape host immune responses, it is possible to express molecules with immunomodulatory functions via plasmids. By utilizing DNA plasmids that display functionally inactive forms of such molecules, scientists can examine the intricate interactions between pathogens and the immune system of the host. In experiments on Litomosoides sigmodontis filarial nematodes, plasmid expression of mutant proteins was shown to increase cytokine and antibody responses significantly, effectively thwarting the immunosuppressive tactics of the parasite. These developments not only deepen our knowledge of parasitic infections but also highlight the potential of plasmid-directed expression as a methodology for enhancing immunity to chronic infections, exemplifying the dual utility of plasmids in both medicine and research. Plasmids can also serve as indispensable instruments in constructing more effective immunotherapeutics. Through the utilization of plasmids that stimulate immune processes, researchers can strategically improve the efficacy of vaccines and treatments. This is particularly prevalent in studies where plasmids are co-administered with cytokine-encoding sequences in order to facilitate particular immune pathways. The combined approach has seen elevated immune responses, such as those seen with research indicating the high similarity of the elicited responses to protective antibody production. This method has important implications in vaccine development against various diseases, such as those caused by challenging organisms that have evolved sophisticated mechanisms for evading immune recognition. The use of plasmids in gene expression systems is thus paramount in propelling immunological research, providing new avenues for effective vaccine strategies and therapeutic intervention of infectious diseases, thus reinforcing their importance within the perspective of recombinant DNA technology in immunology (Figure 3.6).

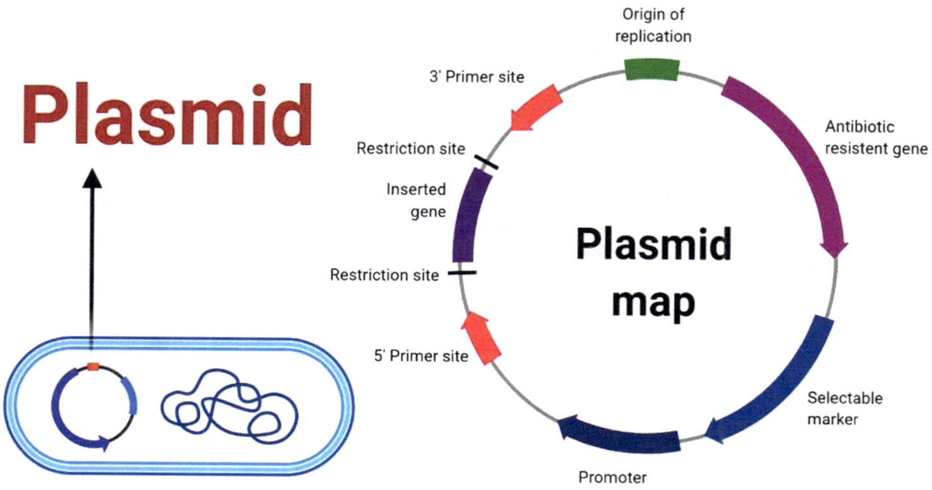

Figure 3.6. Plasmids.

Source: https://microbenotes.com/wp-content/uploads/2022/03/Plasmids-1024x537.jpeg.

3.2.3. Techniques for Gene Editing, Including Clustered Regularly Interspaced Short Palindromic Repeats (CRISPR)

Gene editing tools, particularly CRISPR and CRISPR-associated proteins (Cas), have revolutionized the world of molecular biology and immunology. The targetability of the CRISPR/Cas9 system allows scientists to introduce site-specific gene modifications, and thus it is a useful tool to develop therapies intended for the treatment of genetic diseases. This technology enables the elimination, addition, or change of genes with high accuracy. Specifically, in the field of immunology, CRISPR technology enables immune cells to be engineered so as to enhance their action against cancer or pathogens. For example, through the reprogramming of T cells into CAR-positive cells, the immune system can be enhanced against cancer cells, showing the great potential of CRISPR technology to be applied to therapy. Apart from its use in clinical settings, CRISPR technology is pivotal in the production of therapeutic proteins such as mAbs. mAbs are critical in treating many diseases, including autoimmune diseases and cancers. With the promising market growth of mAbs, such that the growth has increased from USD 60 billion in 2014 to potentially hit USD 300 billion in 2025, production is still a challenge. Advances in gene editing, particularly through CRISPR/Cas9, offer ways to maximize the productivity of cell lines like Chinese Hamster Ovary cells utilized predominantly for mAb production. Gene modifications, such as the deletion of the C12orf35 gene, have been shown to increase output, demonstrating how CRISPR can make production processes more efficient in biotech (Barentine, 2022). The moral concerns related to gene editing technologies cannot be ignored, and particularly how they are applied in the field of immunology. The ability to edit or delete certain genes raises significant questions about the extent and limits of doing so. For instance, while gene mutations lead to fatal diseases like cystic fibrosis and sickle cell anemia, editing genes associated with less severe traits is questionable (Mullen 2020). Debates regarding the acceptability of gene editing for non-lethal diseases, or the capacity to engineer genes, underline the need for a prudent ethical strategy. Coordination among scientists, ethicists, and policy-makers is essential to address the complexities of gene editing so that advances are for the good of all without trespassing on the domain of ethics (Figure 3.7).

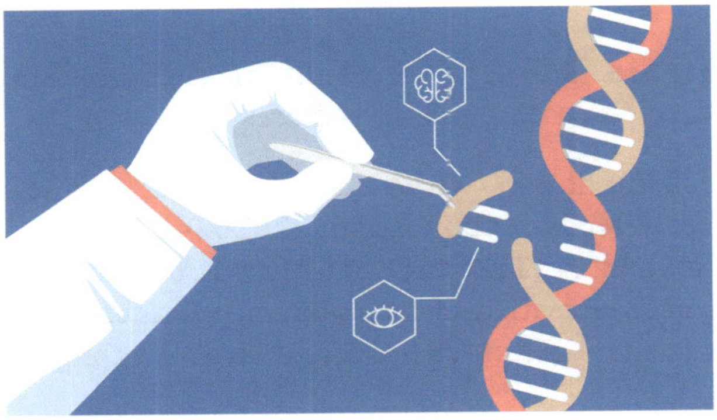

Figure 3.7. Illustration of gene editing.

Source: https://static.scientificamerican.com/sciam/cache/file/18015641-8D4B-4F1B-ADEC0DEA56DDB8FC_source.jpg?w=1200.

3.3. Applications in Vaccine Development

Applications of recombinant DNA technology in vaccine development are a revolutionary breakthrough in immunology that enables vaccines to be designed to induce powerful immune responses that are specifically targeted. With the ability of genetic engineering, researchers can now introduce certain genes from disease-causing organisms into vectors that subsequently express antigens that trigger immunity without the risk of inducing actual disease. This is particularly observed in plant vaccine development, where agroinfiltration techniques facilitate the introduction of transgenes into non-reproductive plant tissues, minimizing the risk of transgene introgression. For instance, studies have indicated that SEB genes can be agroinfiltrated into radishes with great efficiency to permit transient expression of SEB and subsequent immunization in animal models, thereby suggesting a promising path to rapid vaccine production in the case of an outbreak (Liu et al., 2018). Recombinant DNA technology has unveiled a diverse array of potential vaccine platforms, particularly in managing emerging pandemics. The recent patent landscape reviews of vaccine technologies against influenza viruses highlight the technology-driven innovations. The analyses point toward robust advancement in several vaccine formulations and production methods, including subunit vaccines and novel viral vectors that enhance the efficiency of immune responses. Additionally, the steep rise in recent years of influenza vaccine patent filings and research results reflects a global effort to increase vaccine preparedness in the face of recurring outbreaks, as instigated by H5N1 and H1N1 viruses (Cavicchi et al., 2012). This reflects a concerted effort by industry and academia to utilize recombinant DNA technology in developing effective prophylactic strategies against rapidly mutating viral incursions.

Moreover, the use of recombinant DNA technology in vaccine development provides a model for producing vaccines that are not only effective but can also be produced in bulk to immunize large numbers of individuals. The possibility of producing genetically modified plants and other novel expression systems allows for the rapid production of vaccine antigens under conditions of public health crises. With the incidence of infectious diseases escalating, public health concerns are also increasing, and hence, the adoption of these new approaches is sure to make the vaccine programs globally much better. Further, with the patent landscapes, collaborative arrangements among the pharmaceutical sector, government agencies, and research institutes also reflect a shared purpose of creating vaccine technology. These developments together constitute an important milestone towards improving international health security through more efficient and effective vaccination strategies (Cavicchi et al., 2012).

3.3.1. Creation of Recombinant Vaccines

The recombinant vaccine development is an important milestone in the field of immunology, constituting a more targeted mode of action compared to traditional vaccines. The process generally involves placing pathogen genes within a vector, typically a virus or plasmid, that produces specific antigens evoking an immune response without exposing the entire pathogen. This procedure not only reduces the threat of side effects typically associated with live attenuated or killed pathogens but also allows for better control of the immune response. The ability to rapidly design and produce recombinant vaccines for novel emerging infectious diseases has drawn increased attention, particularly after the pandemics triggered by H1N1 and, more recently, by global health issues posed by other viral epidemics, highlighting the requirement for new vaccine technologies as critical public health tools. An understanding of the terrain of patent filings and technological advancements in the case of recombinant vaccines is crucial to their creation. There have been reports of a sudden spike in patent applications for recombinant vaccine technology, particularly for flu vaccines, which have seen greater focus following viral pandemics and emerging strain threats.

Analysis of the patent documents and mapping of various technologies addressed has revealed a broad spectrum of methodologies, from reverse genetics to the use of altered cell lines for manufacturing viruses.

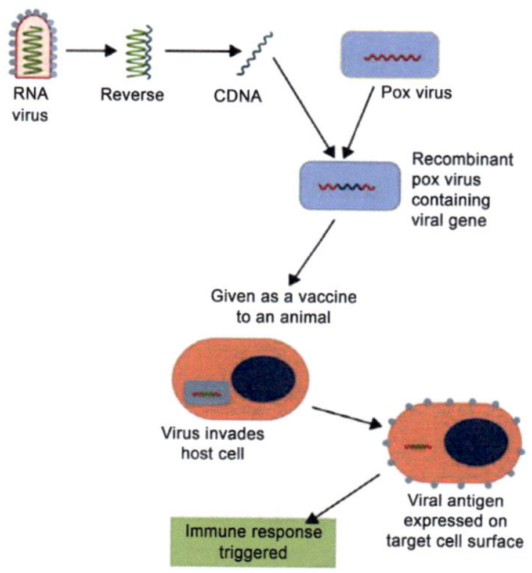

Figure 3.8. The creation of recombinant vaccines with vaccinia vectors.

Source: https://www.researchgate.net/profile/Tesfa-Mossie/publication/370267442/figure/fig4/AS:11431281153615912@1682510681439/The-creation-of-recombinant-vaccines-with-vaccinia-vectors-The-vaccinia-virus-was.png.

Recording such observations facilitates the stakeholders in guiding the intricacies of vaccine development toward meeting research agendas aligned with the current requirements in vaccine efficacy as well as producibility in scale, which are essential to address the needs of pandemics

(Cavicchi et al., 2012). Further, the relationships between biotechnology sectors and space exploration emphasize the versatile applications of recombinant technologies. The Center for Space and Advanced Technology illustrates in research the growing interest of the biotechnology industry in space biotechnology, investigating how space conditions can generate novel approaches to biological research and vaccine development. Researchers are also increasingly investigating the potential impact of microgravity on cellular functions, with the hope of advancing vaccine effectiveness or novel production methods. This cross-pollination highlights the necessity for a multi-disciplinary strategy for the creation of next-generation vaccines, and that advancements in one area can have a major effect on international health efforts. These perspectives legitimize an adaptive response in vaccine production to guarantee immunological responses are tailored not only to earth pathogens but to emerging threats in different settings (Johnston et al., 1988) (Figure 3.8).

3.3.2. Examples of Successful Recombinant Vaccines

Recombinant vaccine development has been a game-changer in immunology, particularly in the combat of infectious diseases.

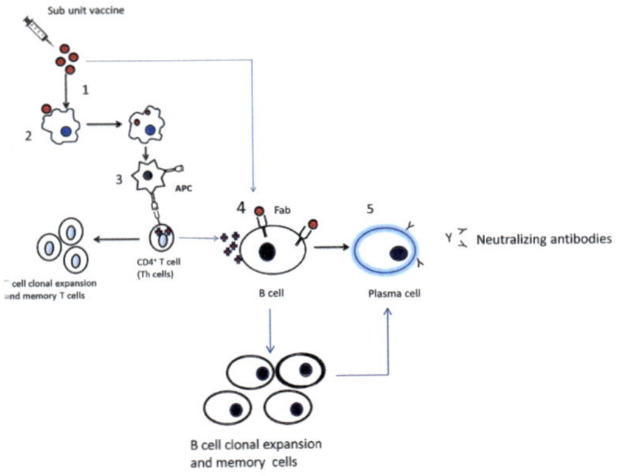

Figure 3.9. Schematic representation of the mechanism of action of HBV vaccine 1. The injected HBV vaccine containing HBsAg proteins are engulfed and processed by the antigen-presenting cells. 2. The antigen-presenting cells process the antigen and attach the same to the surface of the antigen-presenting cells. 3. The antigen-presenting cells present the antigen to the T helper cells, leading to clonal expansion of the T cells as well as production of memory T cells. 4. The antigen can be recognized directly by B cells, producing a weak immune response, with binding of the antigen to the Fab region on the B cell receptor and secondary signaling from cytokines released by T-helper cells; B cells begin somatic hypermutation at the Fab region, which further increases the corresponding fit between the Fab region and the antigen. 5. The B cells mature to plasma cells to produce neutralizing antibodies.

Source: https://www.researchgate.net/publication/333612380/figure/fig1/AS:11431281276381917@1725629372485/Schematic-representation-of-the-mechanism-of-action-of-HBV-vaccine-1-The-injected-HBV.tif.

One of the most prominent players is the uses of recombinant DNA technology to develop the hepatitis B vaccine. Isolation of the surface antigens of the hepatitis B virus (HBV) and expression in yeast cells enabled researchers to produce a vaccine that can induce immunity without infecting anyone. This innovation was not only safer than earlier approaches, but it also made mass production possible, enabling vaccination to be extended to various parts of the globe. Such outcomes bear witness to the potency of recombinant methodology in the creation of efficient immunity against viral infections and to the public health benefits of biotechnological advances (Figure 3.9). Another such compelling example of a successful recombinant vaccine is the outer membrane vesicle (OMV) meningococcal vaccine produced against *Neisseria meningitidis* serogroup B. The vaccine utilizes OMV for encapsulation and display of bacterial antigens, thus creating an artificial infection, which enhances the immune response. Cuba's Finlay Institute has succeeded in streamlining the Good Manufacturing Practice (GMP) processes for the production of OMV from different strains, including those of serogroups A, W, and X. Immunogenicity trials have shown that these vaccines are able to elicit specific antibodies, thereby establishing their protective potential. Here, OMV vaccines are a model of the flexibility of recombinant technology in immunization approaches, underscoring the importance of continued research and development in vaccine innovation and use in various populations (Acevedo et al., 2014). In the landscape of recombinant vaccines, much progress has occurred in the field of influenza vaccine technology. Recent advancements have focused on applying recombinant DNA technology for developing vaccines against pandemic virus strains of the influenza virus. This includes recombinant subunit vaccines that are formulated from purified viral proteins aimed at eliciting adequate immune responses. Additionally, the analysis of patents presents growing interest in employing reverse genetics, enabling the generation of recombinant influenza viruses towards more consistent vaccines. As has been observed in recent studies, an increasing number of patent applications involving influenza vaccine technologies indicates an undeniable trend in the field. The direction reflects the urgency and necessity to develop effective vaccines against looming attacks and marks the likely impact of recombinant DNA technology on global health policies (Cavicchi et al., 2012) (Figure 3.10).

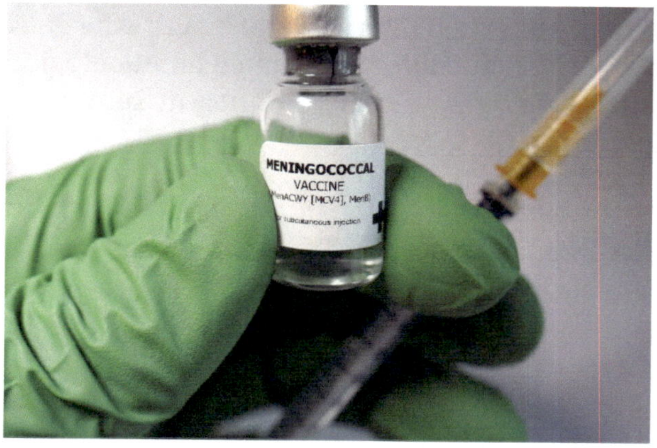

Figure 3.10. Illustration of the meningococcal vaccine.

Source: https://www.sakethospital.in/wp-content/uploads/2025/02/Meningococcal-Vaccine-1.jpg.

3.3.3. Advantages Over Traditional Vaccine Methods

The discovery of recombinant DNA technology has drastically altered the landscape of immunology, particularly vaccine production. Compared to traditional vaccine approaches, which at times rely on live-attenuated or inactivated pathogens, recombinant DNA vaccines offer a more accurate approach using specific antigenic components. The specificity reduces the possibility of causing disease; thus the recombinant vaccines are safer, especially for immunocompromised patients. By isolating and employing only the required proteins from a pathogen, such vaccines can elicit considerable immune responses without the potential dangers of encountering the entire pathogen. It is particularly beneficial in the case of infectious diseases, where safety is still always a primary concern when it comes to vaccine delivery. Moreover, the ability to trigger specific immunity also has the potential to make vaccination against more complex diseases more effective, with the advantage of recombinant methods over traditional methods standing out. Improved capability for rapid production and alteration is also another major advantage of recombinant DNA technology. Traditional vaccine manufacture typically involves lengthy processes, including culturing pathogens in test tubes and passing through lengthy trial phases that can take decades, without necessarily leading to any breakthrough (Pöri, 2018). Recombinant vaccines, however, can be rapidly constructed and manufactured as soon as the genetic composition of an infectious pathogen is determined. This rapid response is crucial in disease outbreaks, such as the recent COVID-19 pandemic, in which the ability to produce useful vaccines at short notice can save lives and halt the spread of infection. The technology of recombinant DNA is also easy to use for altering vaccine constructions so that scientists can react to mutating pathogens or even combine antigens from multiple strains to immunize against a large variety of infections. This flexibility provides an inherent strength in preserving public health against impending health crises. Last but not least, recombinant DNA vaccines spearhead in reducing side effects that are usually associated with traditional vaccination processes. Side effects of traditional vaccines range from mild effects to unwanted immune responses, which are a cause of concern during vaccination campaigns (Pöri, 2018). By comparison, recombinant vaccines have a decreased side effect profile as they lack live pathogens or their toxic byproducts. Because they utilize engineered proteins, these vaccines can evoke an effective immune response with fewer bad effects and thus maximize public acceptance and immunization program participation. In addition, adjuvants specifically designed to enhance immune responses may also be included in the recombinant constructs so that their efficacy is enhanced without diminishing safety. Consequently, the technology is not only enhancing immunological strategies but also playing a crucial role in supporting public trust in vaccination, which is an integral part of the global fight against infectious diseases.

3.4. Role in Monoclonal Antibody (mAb) Production

The advent of recombinant DNA technology has changed the situation of producing mAbs and now makes it possible to have more efficient therapeutic and diagnostic applications in immunology. Previously, mAb production was achieved by fusing immunized mice spleen cells with myeloma cells to get hybridomas that secrete one clone of antibodies. But with the advent of recombinant DNA techniques, scientists are now able to construct individual antibody genes and express them in various host cells. This process not only enhances the specificity and affinity of the produced antibodies but also allows the incorporation of human immunoglobulin frameworks, thus reducing the immunogenicity for therapeutic use. Furthermore, the application of genetic engineering in the production of monoclonal antibodies brings with it the promise of new antigen discovery and modes of vaccination. For instance, some of the latest technology improvements in recombinant protein expression, for instance, antigens, can facilitate rapid vaccine development. Technologies such as agroinfiltration have been promising in the context of transient expression of multiple antigens from plant systems, which are then harvestable for immunogenic evaluation. This is just one instance of the new field of recombinant DNA-vaccine technology convergence that requires the application of methods like those utilized to produce NcSRS2-iscoms, enabling powerful design of immunization against single pathogens, demonstrating the versatility of recombinant techniques in modern immunology (Pinitkiatisakul et al., 2007). Apart from expanding the yield and selectivity of monoclonal antibodies, recombinant DNA technology has a more general contribution to making more heterogeneous and productive antibody libraries. Phage display and other selection methods permit researchers to screen vast libraries of designed antibodies for high-affinity binders against antigens of interest. This capacity is highly critical while working with difficult-to-treat diseases like emerging infectious diseases and cancer. The creation of such varied pools of antibodies enhances the chances of isolating good candidates for therapeutic use, especially if combined with new tactics like antigen gene fusion expressing Staphylococcal enterotoxin B in plant tissue. This combined method of monoclonal antibody preparation emphasizes the crucial role of recombinant DNA technology in speeding up immunological research and therapy development (Liu et al., 2018).

3.4.1. Process of Generating Monoclonal Antibodies (mAbs)

mAb generation is a milestone technological advancement in immunology and therapy development. The procedure begins with the immunization of a suitable host, typically a mouse, against a specific antigen.

The host immune response initiates antibody-secreting B lymphocytes against the antigen. Later, B cells are isolated and fused with myeloma cells, which are immortal and can be cultured an infinite number of times. Such formed hybrid cells are termed hybridomas and possess the ability to produce antibodies as well as divide indefinitely. This new technique revolutionized antibody production to allow scientists to develop monoclonal antibodies with high specificity and affinity towards their antigens of interest, hence allowing their use in diagnostics and therapy. The hybridomas are screened for the desired antibody production following the fusion of the B cells and the myeloma cells. This involves the selection of the hybrids producing the desired mAbs for the antigen of interest. The selection is initially performed via a series of assays to identify successfully fused cells producing target antibodies. Once identified, the hybridomas are cloned so that the resulting mAbs are homogeneous. A single one of the cloned hybridomas can be cultured, paving the way for bulk production of the specific antibody. Specificity and efficacy achieved through this procedure have rendered mAbs beneficial in numerous fields, such as cancer treatment, wherein they can be designed to target a specific tumor marker, and vaccine development, which underscores the significance of their production procedure in modern medicine.

Advances in genetic engineering and antibody engineering techniques in recent times have also enhanced the monoclonal antibody production procedure. Techniques such as phage display allow for the high-specificity, high-affinity selection of particular antibodies against target molecules, avoiding the issue typically encountered with the use of standard hybridoma methods. Recombinant DNA technology also enables genetic engineering to develop chimeric or humanized antibodies that are more therapeutic in nature but less immunogenic in human patients.

These engineered antibodies could potentially engage with immune systems or serve as drug carriers. This breakthrough in antibody production techniques highlights the ongoing innovation in the science of immunology, which will further contribute to more effective treatments and a better understanding of immune interactions in disease and health, as observed in studies on antibody development and immunization practices (Saeed et al., 2017; Liu et al., 2018) (Figure 3.11).

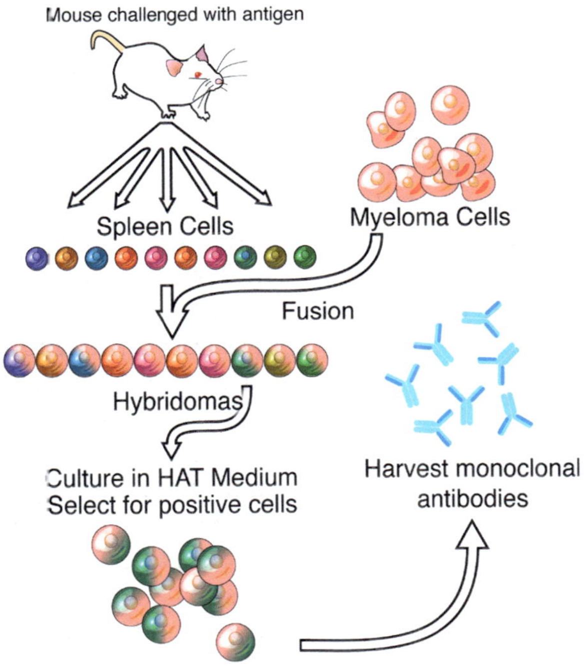

Figure 3.11. A general representation of the method used to produce monoclonal antibodies.

Source: https://upload.wikimedia.org/wikipedia/commons/thumb/9/9a/Monoclonals.png/330px-Monoclonals.png.

3.4.2. Therapeutic Applications of Monoclonal Antibodies (mAbs)

Monoclonal antibodies have emerged as key reagents in therapeutic applications, significantly enhancing the treatment protocol of most diseases, including cancers and autoimmune disorders. Target-specific antibodies are synthesized in the laboratory to selectively bind target antigens, providing highly selective and potent therapeutic action. The emergence of hybridoma technology, which allows for the production of cloned cell lines secreting antibodies, was a landmark achievement in the area of immunotherapy because it became a reality to produce specific antibodies to disease antigens on a large scale. The technology led to the development of humanized and chimeric antibodies with limitations in specificity and function, but laid the ground for newer generations of antibody engineering and therapeutics. The long-term objective is to stimulate immune cells with effectors in a manner that would be able to treat those diseases that were previously difficult to control effectively, thereby improving patient care. Recent advances in recombinant DNA technology have revolutionized the manufacture of monoclonal antibodies by creating techniques that enhance their efficiency and potency. New technologies such as phage display and genetic alteration of antibody fragments have enabled the production of highly selective antibodies with improved affinity. The engineered antibodies can bind to conserved epitopes, and they are of benefit in cases where traditional treatments do not work as well. Moreover, with antibody engineering thrown into the mix, it is now possible to generate fusion proteins wherein the targeting function of antibodies can be married with the therapeutic function of other biologic molecules. The research of new antibody engineering approaches is imperative as it not only allows the construction of more effective therapeutics but also provides the possibility of studying complex effects on immune modulation and disease treatment strategies, widening the field of immunotherapy applications. Applications of monoclonal antibodies are not restricted to oncology but extend to infectious diseases and autoimmune diseases, attesting to their diversity in modern medicine.

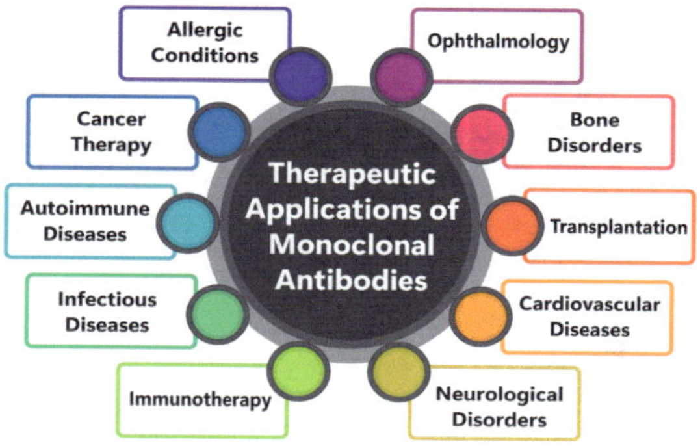

Figure 3.12. Illustration of therapeutic applications of monoclonal antibodies.

Source: https://encrypted-tbn0.gstatic.com/images?q=tbn:ANd9GcTh108Y9FP6zky5Gzz-MxoN9wNRWJe7zbsmBw&s.

For example, the capability of encapsulating antigens in plant tissue, such as in the use of agroinfiltration based on SEB genes, demonstrates a new approach to rapid vaccine development (Liu et al., 2018). They demonstrate how useful monoclonal antibodies are in facilitating not only treatment but also prophylaxis against a wide range of pathogens. With more and more such new modalities being developed, utilization of engineered antibodies for preventing and treating disease will further escalate, holding the promise of improved prevention and therapy strategies. The effort to incorporate such new methodologies into the therapeutic regimen is testimony to the complementarity between recombinant DNA technology and immunology as a quantum leap in the development of effective and targeted immunotherapeutics (Saeed et al., 2017) (Figure 3.12).

3.4.3. Impact on Treatment of Diseases Such as Cancer

The invention of recombinant DNA technology has brought a revolution in the treatment of diseases, especially cancer, by increasing the accuracy and effectiveness of immunotherapeutic strategies. This technology allows for the design of genetic manipulation to create targeted therapies, such as monoclonal antibodies and gene therapy, against known cancer cell antigens. These rationally designed agents exploit the intrinsic activity of the immune system and lead to more efficient killing of malignant cells without causing damage to normal tissues. Through the production of highly specific drugs, recombinant DNA technology not only improves patient care but also reduces the severity of side effects normally associated with conventional cancer treatment modalities such as radiation and chemotherapy. Therefore, the creation of such cutting-edge therapies within clinics demonstrates the power of genetic engineering in changing paradigms of cancer therapy, paving the way to more tailored therapy. In recent years, the role of dendritic cells (DCs), the key antigen-presenting cells, has attracted significant attention in the context of cancer immunotherapy. Traditional therapy is unable to provoke a sufficient immune response, but the use of recombinant DNA technology enables one to enhance the activity of DCs, key elements in the induction of naïve T cells. By utilizing tumor-derived microvesicles (MVs) to modulate DC antigen processing, researchers have demonstrated that these microvesicles modify the phagosomal microenvironment of DCs, enhancing ROS levels and alkalinization. These modifications are capable of significantly augmenting the immunogenicity of such tumor antigens as MUC1, facilitating the presentation of the antigens to T cells. The ability of DCs to prime antigen-specific CD8+ T cells effectively is crucial in the induction of long-lasting anti-tumor immunity, and thus DC-targeted therapy is a promising candidate in recombinant DNA-based cancer therapy (Battisti et al., 2017). Recombinant DNA technology has found its way into collaborative studies within the biotechnology sector, as evidenced by findings from research led by the Center for Space and Advanced Technology (CSAT) on behalf of NASA-JSC. This research highlights the industry's engagement with the biotechnology domain in space biotechnology to explore new environments that enable biotechnological innovation. Captains from the industry insights offer a reflection of the dominant trends and issues that influence the biotechnology sector, which are likely to have a far-reaching influence on cancer treatment development. Inter-pollination of ideas between unlike disciplines offers an affluent matrix for cancer therapeutics innovations, illustrating the potential of inter-disciplinary approaches to propel novel solutions. By merging the experience gained from the space projects with the premises of the recombinant DNA technology, the available treatment options for cancer can be potentially enlarged in a remarkable fusion of science and technology (Johnston et al., 1988) (Figure 3.13).

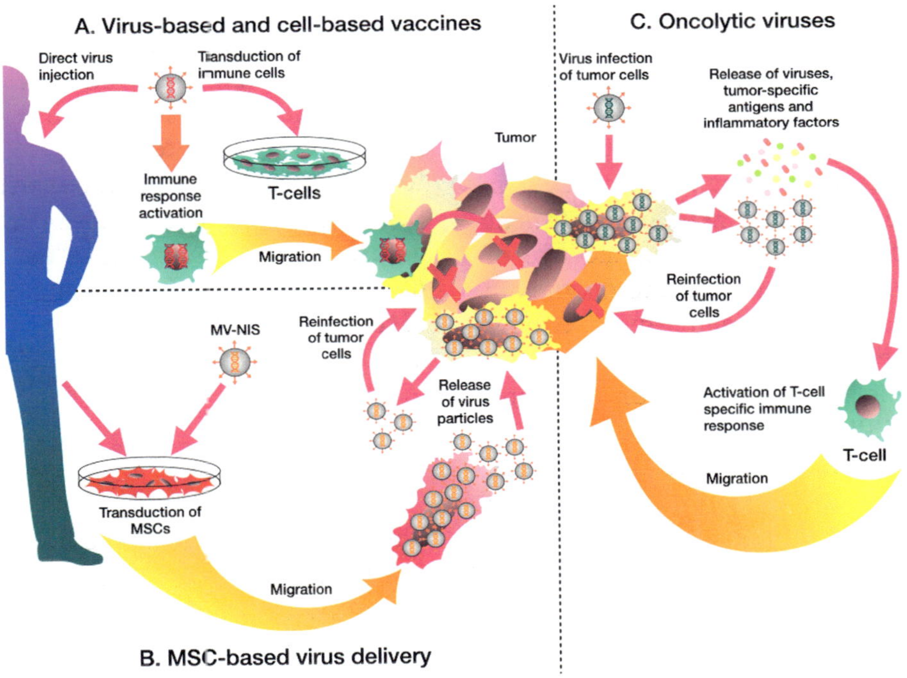

Figure 3.13. Recombinant virus-based treatment of cancer. (A) Antitumor therapeutic vaccines, which are based on viruses encoding tumor-specific antigens, boost anti-cancer immune responses by enhancing presentation of the tumor antigens to immune cells. (B) Therapeutic viruses, for example, MV-NIS (the Edmonston strain of measles virus), can also be delivered to the tumor with mesenchymal stem cells (MSCs), which have a natural tropism toward tumor niches. (C) Oncolytic viruses preferentially infect tumor cells and induce tumor cell death.

Source: https://www.mdpi.com/biomedicines/biomedicines-06-00094/article_deploy/html/images/biomedicines-06-00094-g001.png.

3.5. Enhancements in Diagnostic Tools

The evolution of immunology's diagnostic tools has been significantly influenced by advances in recombinant DNA technology. These technologies have enabled extremely specific and sensitive assays that provide the capability for identifying infectious agents at an unprecedented level. For instance, monoclonal antibody production, a product of recombinant DNA technology, has enhanced diagnostic examination to the extent that efficient identification of pathogens such as viruses and bacteria is achievable. Apart from enhancing the accuracy of tests, specificity decreases the likelihood of cross-reactivity, which has been a problem with conventional immunoassays. Thus, clinicians can make more precise judgments as a result of the exact diagnostic outcomes, leading to improved management and treatment regimens for patients. In general, the use of these technological advances in the diagnostic models has made the introduction of a new era of immunological testing possible, a step forward from less accurate older methods (Asbury et al., 2000). Other than monoclonal antibodies, recombinant DNA technology has also enabled the production of rapid diagnostic tests with little time and capital outlays. This is particularly significant in emergency clinical conditions where rapid diagnosis can significantly impact patient outcomes. For example, the production of polymerase chain reaction (PCR) tests for disease diagnosis is a strong illustration of speed and accuracy achievable with recombinant DNA technology. PCR enables the amplification of target DNA sequences from a sample, enabling the detection of low levels of pathogens in a rapid and efficient manner. These improvements not only enable early intervention for infectious diseases but also assist in tracking disease outbreaks and the efficacy of vaccine strategies. The ability to deploy rapid diagnostics in a variety of settings is the revolutionary impact of recombinant DNA technology on global health paradigms (Krattiger et al., 2006). In addition, the potential for global availability of these new diagnostic tools poses problems and opportunities that are unique. While recombinant DNA technology has created new opportunities for the development of precise diagnostic tests, intellectual property (IP) and access issues frequently prevent their use in resource-poor settings. For instance, the complexity of patent environments for diagnostic tests can restrict the technologies needed from being made available to developing countries. According to estimates, although options like patent pools are theoretically possible, they are typically plagued by legal and functional complexities, and thus cooperation is called for in terms of improved access. Eliminating these hindrances is a priority in order to provide diagnostic technological achievements to all groups, especially those with the greatest health burdens. Equilibrating innovation with accessibility is important to the future success of immunological diagnostic reagents from recombinant DNA technology (Asbury et al., 2000).

3.5.1. Development of Recombinant Antigens for Diagnostics

The development of recombinant antigens for diagnostics has fundamentally altered the climate of immunology, enhancing the specificity and sensitivity of detection assays. With the use of recombinant DNA technology, researchers can produce tailored antigens that closely mimic those present in causative organisms. This is achieved by translating the relevant genes participating in the antigen synthesis in suitable host systems and thereby producing pure, scalable antigen proteins. Significantly, the recombinant antigens allow the development of diagnostic assays that are able to distinguish between very related pathogens, thus yielding vital information for successful disease management and prevention measures. In the quest for successful vaccines and diagnostics, plant-based systems have come forth as promising platforms for the generation of recombinant antigens. For example, recent studies illustrate agroinfiltration of SEB genes into radishes, resulting in the transient presentation of this antigen in plant tissue. Such novel approaches do not just make vaccine production easier but also yield high-throughput capability that is useful in times of public health emergencies. By expressing the antigen using non-reproductive plant parts, the method decreases the possibility of transgene introgression and is thus an environmentally friendly approach towards diagnostics and vaccine production (Liu et al., 2018). The association of immunological assays and recombinant antigens has also opened doors to novel ways of studying host-pathogen interactions. Investigations on marine turtles, such as the identification of CTLV and FPHV herpesviruses, depict recombinant antigen technology utilization in the diagnosis of wildlife viral diseases. Here, the purified antigenic proteins from these viruses are breakthrough finds, as they are the first of their type to be expressed and characterized for host species immunogenic activity. This finding not only supports the presence of these viral diseases in free-ranging populations but also emphasizes the potential of recombinant antigens to direct conservation methods and disease control measures (Klein & Jacobson, 2001) (Figure 3.14).

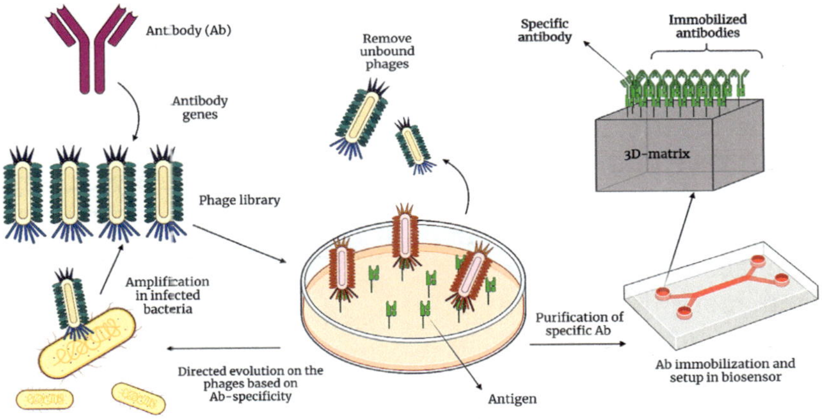

Figure 3.14. Development of recombinant antigens for diagnostics.

Source: https://www.researchgate.net/publication/359801951/figure/fig4/AS:11431281210574506@1702053302761/Production-of-recombinant-antibodies-using-phage-display-technology-First-a-recombinant.tif.

3.5.2. Use of Recombinant DNA in Serological Tests

The application of recombinant DNA technology in serological tests is a significant advance in immunological diagnostics. Through this new technology, very specific antigens can be generated, which are needed for the proper identification of antibodies associated with infectious and autoimmune diseases. By cloning DNA sequences encoding known proteins, it is possible to generate vast quantities of such antigens, rendering serological tests more sensitive and specific. Besides augmenting the diagnostic insight, it is also possible to construct tests with the ability to differentiate between closely related diseases, an essential feature in clinical practice wherein early and precise diagnosis can greatly impact patient management and treatment schedules. Recombinant antigens usage indicates a significant step towards precision medicine, where personalized diagnostics lead to enhanced patient care and the proper use of healthcare resources within healthcare systems. Besides, the use of recombinant DNA technology in serological assays has led to the standardization of diagnostic protocols across laboratories. Serological assays have traditionally employed natural antigens, whose quality and composition turned out to be variable in most instances. Application of recombinant antigens provides a more stable product that can be produced consistently, thereby improving consistency of test results in various research and clinical settings. Researchers have noted that standardized tests not only improve comparability of results in several different laboratories but also minimize regulatory processes for test validation and approval.

This shift contributes to the overall diagnostic effectiveness of procedures and contributes to greater trust among clinicians and patients regarding test outcomes. Additionally, this replicability helps collaboration between the scientific world, and more development of immunology studies and their uses is thereby aided. In addition to the improvement of accuracy and standardization of serological analysis, recombinant DNA technology has facilitated the development of multiplex assays. These diagnostic tests enable the identification of more than a single pathogen or antibody in a single sample, which enhances efficiency in diagnosis. Through the use of recombinant antigens for diseases, physicians are in a position to promptly measure a patient's immune response to these infections within a short time frame. This is particularly valuable in public health scenarios, such as epidemics and pandemics, where the incidence of multiple pathogens is required to engage effective control of the disease. The modularity of recombinant DNA technology thereby not only improves the quality of care for individual patients but also improves public health interventions by facilitating multidimensional surveillance and timely intervention. Therefore, recombinant DNA application in serology continues to revolutionize immunology, proof of its central role in contemporary medical diagnostics.

3.5.3. Innovations in Rapid Diagnostic Tests

Recombinant DNA technology has greatly revolutionized immunology, particularly through rapid diagnostic test advances. These advances enable the faster and more accurate detection of pathogens, thereby improving patient outcomes. These traditional methods of diagnosis were typically time-consuming and required large amounts of laboratory equipment, thereby sacrificing timely decision-making in the clinical setting. Rapid diagnostic tests, on the other hand, employ recombinant DNA technology to identify specific antigens or nucleic acids with high sensitivity and specificity. This not only accelerates the diagnostic process but also helps facilitate better infectious disease control, especially in resource-limited settings. As the health care environment keeps improving, the integration of such innovative test technology is essential to enhancing disease surveillance and outbreak response capacity. The prospects for scalability and availability of recombinant DNA technology-based rapid diagnostic tests are also impressive. As has been noted by recent reviews, evolution in laboratory medicine is not so much about the development of technology as it involves understanding economic and social forces that can drive such innovation. Rapid tests most often use transportable devices, and it is more convenient to use them in remote or underdeveloped areas where laboratory facilities may be limited. This democratization of medical diagnosis helps broader public health objectives through the delivery of important testing to those populations that would otherwise lack access. Through ongoing research and development, it is hoped that these advances will increasingly make healthcare access expand, delivering early and precise diagnosis to more individuals globally. In addition to diagnostic functional enhancements, recombinant DNA technology also has lucrative avenues to enhance the performance and consistency of rapid tests. Trends suggest that the intersection of synthetic biology and bioinformatics with diagnostic test design will further define the future of test development. Interdisciplinary approaches can enable tests to have the ability to simultaneously detect multiple pathogens, presenting an instantaneous snapshot of infectious disease patterns. Furthermore, the modular character of these tests allows for rapid responsiveness to newly arising and re-emerging pathogens, something that is absolutely critical in the presence of pandemics worldwide. In the future, the integration of recombinant DNA technology with new diagnostics has promise not only for present-day clinical use but also for planning for the future management of infectious disease epidemics. This interplay between public health and technology puts rapid diagnostic tests at the forefront of immunology's evolving context (Asbury et al., 2000; Kricka et al., 2015) (Figure 3.15).

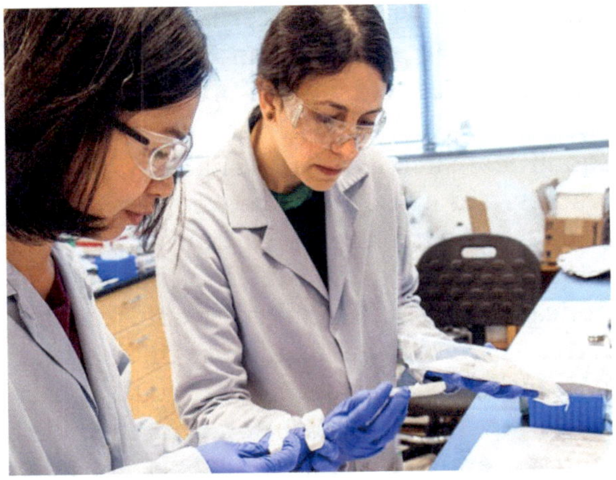

Figure 3.15. A team of scientists focuses on advancing high-impact diagnostic technologies.

Source: https://media.path.org/images/Hero_Image.max-1440x960.jpg.

3.6. Ethical Considerations

The addition of recombinant DNA technology to immunology brings with it a myriad of ethical concerns that must be addressed to ensure responsible scientific advancement. One of the most significant ethical concerns is the potential danger of genetic manipulation, particularly when dealing with human subjects. The unknown nature of genetic changes raises concerns over long-term implications for health and the unintended effects on individuals who undergo gene therapy. As scientists explore the potential of recombinant DNA technology, they have to make sure that there is informed consent from their subjects, such that individuals have a full grasp of the potential risks involved. Consent here is not a process but an ethical requirement that respects the right of freedom and decision-making capacity of persons in the scientific process, thus building trust in biomedical applications and research. Fair access to therapies generated through recombinant DNA technology is a second critical ethical dimension. Advances in biotechnology have historically been largely reserved for wealthy communities, generating concerns associated with health disparities. The promise of this technology, particularly in the creation of personalized vaccines or gene therapies, risks exacerbating existing inequalities if access is limited by socioeconomic class. The absence of equity in this technology contravenes the ethical precept of justice, and there ought to be policies guaranteeing fair distribution of the biotechnological gains. Assuring these new treatments for all, irrespective of socio-economic position, not only fulfills an ethical requirement but also does the greatest good for the greatest number by ensuring the highest possible overall impact of public health measures, guaranteeing more benefit to society from science. In addition, the environmental implications of recombinant DNA technology are worthy of close ethical scrutiny.

Genetic changes that enhance the virulence or resistance of pathogens can inadvertently create organisms with broader extensible transmission and unforeseen ecological impacts. Such risks necessitate robust regulatory frameworks governing the manipulation and release of genetically modified organisms into the environment. Ethical stewardship for the biotechnology industry must entail meticulous risk assessment, as well as ongoing monitoring to prevent potential adverse outcomes. Besides, public engagement on these issues is crucial; open dialogue between scientists, policymakers, and the public will ensure that community values guide development within the field. As envisioned in the prevalence of contemporary biotechnological reviews, there must be a constant reminder to maintain ethical issues at the forefront of research activities, as with progress in pharmaceutical sciences and education from the narrative development of the industry (Johnston et al., 1988; Stoimenova et al., 2011).

3.6.1. Concerns Regarding Genetic Manipulation

The advent of recombinant DNA technology has certainly altered the complexion of immunology, but it has also ushered in a plethora of problems with genetic manipulation. The foremost among them is the moral problem of the potential for designer organisms or the deliberate alteration of genetic information within human and animal populations. Critics argue that those manipulations would have unforetold consequences such as ecological imbalances and loss of biodiversity. For instance, releasing genetically modified organisms (GMOs) into the environment could cause the displacement of native species, disturbance of food webs and ecosystems irreversibly. The unintended interactions between genetically modified and naturally occurring organisms produced by the resulting create legitimate fear about the consequences of long-term genetic manipulation on environmental sustainability and conservation of biodiversity, necessitating extensive studies prior to the large-scale application of such technologies. In addition, the health risks to humans caused by genetic manipulation cannot be overlooked. The randomness of genetic alteration raises questions of possible allergenic impacts or other adverse health effects when such genetically modified organisms find their way into the food chain. These involve biotechnologies in medicine, where genetically modified vaccines and medicines may elicit unpredictable side reactions in human patients. Based on these possible risks, regulatory frameworks governing genetic alteration have assumed greater significance. The use of strict testing protocols and transparent labeling of genetically altered foods can guarantee the protection of public health and facilitate informed consumer choice. In the view of the Center for Space and Advanced Technology, the rapid advances in the biotechnology sector necessitate consistent monitoring to prevent health hazards from animal and human genetic interventions (Johnston et al., 1988). Besides, the moral and social concerns of genetic manipulation create severe challenges to its acceptance. Public concern is normally a product of fear of the technology and what it will introduce. Individuals are worried that genetic manipulation will further exacerbate inequalities, such as the availability of new therapies, and cause a gap between those who can pay for such therapies and those who cannot. Questions of consent and the rights of genetically altered beings further obfuscate the picture. As we struggle to address these issues, it is clear that there must be an interdisciplinary solution—a participatory solution involving scientists, ethicists, and society as a whole. Resolving issues about the ownership of genetic materials and the ethics of manipulating organisms that have been modified will be crucial to guaranteeing that recombinant DNA technology in immunology is ethically promoted

(Stroud et al., 2016). It is only through honest debate and moral reflection that we may hope to guide the complex landscape of genetic manipulation responsibly.

3.6.2. Regulatory Frameworks Governing Recombinant DNA Technology

Legal regimes governing recombinant DNA technology must provide security, ethical behavior, and scientific honor in biotechnological innovations, particularly in immunology. These regulations are established by various international and national organizations, which aim to monitor the use and impact of recombinant DNA techniques. In the United States, the National Institutes of Health (NIH) oversees the guidelines on recombinant DNA by implementing the NIH Guidelines for Research Involving Recombinant or Synthetic Nucleic Acid Molecules. This guideline offers a complete series of safety measures intended to restrict risks to the environment and researchers while promoting responsible use of genetic engineering. It is crucial to comprehend and adhere to these guidelines since they aim at curbing potential unintended effects that may arise due to unregulated manipulation of genetic material in immunological studies. At a global level, organizations such as the World Health Organization (WHO) and the Organisation for Economic Co-operation and Development (OECD) take the lead in harmonizing regulatory needs for recombinant DNA technology. The organizations create guidelines that transcend national borders, fostering cooperation and technology transfer and protecting safety and ethical needs. The WHO, for instance, is dedicated to biosecurity and biosafety during genetic research such that unintended consequences are prevented from modified organisms. Through setting uniform regulations, the agencies foster an environment of research friendliness in which immunologists can research new solutions without risking public confidence in scientific advances. The global regulatory system for systems thus not only enhances scientific progress but also addresses public concern about the safety of recombinant DNA technology. Regulation is important to researchers who are handling recombinant DNA technology because it poses very serious implications if violated, from canceled research, legal penalties, to grant withdrawal.

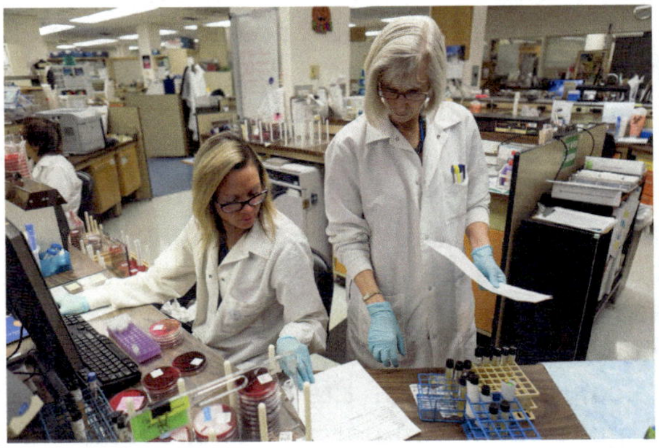

Figure 3.16. The National Institutes of Health (NIH) oversees the guidelines for recombinant DNA research.

Source: https://www.actfornih.org/wp-content/uploads/2020/03/28756947676_ebeaf4fe36_o.jpg.

Institutions are typically required to establish new Institutional Biosafety Committees (IBCs) that review proposed projects to the level of adequacy as per regulations before implementation. Although such double-layered control not only focuses on the experimental methodology, but also includes an additional layer of ethical reflection, there exists the problem of revising the regulations with ongoing advances in biotechnology that necessitate constant communication between scientists, regulators, and policy-makers. With the evolution of technologies, regulatory frameworks must be adaptive to adapt and accommodate new scientific realities. This adaptability ensures the benefits of recombinant DNA technology, particularly in immunology, can be maximized while any potential hazard to society and the environment is minimized to the barest level, thereby facilitating sustainable scientific activity (Figure 3.16).

3.6.3. Public Perception and Societal Implications

Societal opinion regarding scientific advancements is partly determined by public opinion about such advancements, as in the instance of recombinant DNA technology in immunology. The greater the level of exposure of the general population to discourse on genetic engineering, the more sophisticated the public opinion is. While some people recognize the potential benefits of recombinant DNA technology as a vehicle for creating vaccines and drugs against disease, there is also the concomitant fear of the ethical implications of genetic manipulation. These fears are normally served by coverage in the media and sensationalist reports, which can distort facts and cause fear among the public. Thus, the quiet perspectives of individuals and groups come to the forefront to aid informed conversation regarding this technology and any myths that may propagate. Implications for society stemming from recombinant DNA technology development extend beyond health and safety threats as well. As genetic modification becomes more integrated into existing immunological protocols, questions of justice, access, and consent emerge. Certain populations, particularly those from historically marginalized groups, may become disproportionately affected by the effects of genetic technologies. This raises with it the pressing question of who benefits from these technologies and who gets left behind. As emphasized in arguments regarding directed evolution and biotechnology's future, deeply society-generating change might become inevitable if protecting that the progress is made for the public good, rather than creating further inequalities, is to become an objective (Annas et al., 2003). Therefore, fair policies and stakeholder involvement must be at the forefront of the agenda when the future of biotechnology is being discussed. In addressing the long-term consequences of recombinant DNA technology, one must include consideration of the role of public attitudes in driving regulatory forces and ethical values. The interplay between societal values and scientific advancement is what can make or break biotechnological development and applications. For instance, if popular opinion leans heavily towards fear and suspicion, regulatory bodies will consequently have strict controls that would unwittingly stifle innovation. Conversely, where there is an educated and interested public to take up these technologies, then regulators will be less inhibited in permitting their development and application (Annas et al., 2003). Lastly, achieving a balance between technology and the public good demands collaborative deliberation among scientists, ethicists, legislators, and the public. In this manner, society can move through the oppositions of recombinant DNA technology with a considered strategy for advancement.

SUMMARY

Recombinant DNA technology has advanced the field of immunology enormously and hence changed our understanding and capability in combating numerous infectious and malignant diseases. With genetic manipulation, the new technology has taken the opportunity to develop custom-made therapies and vaccines and bypassed the limitations of the old treatment protocols. For example, in the case of oral canine malignant melanoma (CMM), scientists have employed plasmid DNA vaccines coding for human tyrosinase, demonstrating the potential of these technologies in veterinary medicine and human medicine too (Atherton et al., 2016). The interactive dynamics between the immune system and genetic engineering open up new horizons for personalized therapies, indicating the importance of the role of recombinant DNA technology in enhancing therapeutic options. Furthermore, techniques of antibody engineering are a demonstration of the capability of recombinant DNA technology for generating precise and effective immunotherapeutics. The identification of hybridoma technology revolutionized the manufacturing of antibodies; however, the complexities of classical technology prompted one to look for new methods. Existing advancements, particularly phage display and genetic engineering, allow the construction of high-affinity recombinant antibodies with enhanced properties (Saeed et al., 2017). Not only do the engineered antibodies improve therapeutically, but they also broaden application prospects in immunology towards groundbreaking diagnostics and treatments. Therefore, the union of recombinant DNA technology and antibody engineering is a pioneering effort to realize improved health outcomes. Finally, the applicability of recombinant DNA technology to immunology is not only evident in short-term therapeutic applications but also in establishing the groundwork for research and development in the field. As scientists decipher the immunological enigma, the ability to control genetic components will further shed light on autoimmunity, cancer, and infectious diseases. Recombinant DNA technology enables targeting with greater precision for a selected antigen, enabling treatments to be more efficient while generating fewer side effects. Through embracing this technology, the scientific community is well-positioned to tackle existing challenges and identify new therapies that improve patient care and clinical outcomes. Overall, the integration of recombinant DNA technology into immunology is a paradigm shift milestone that guarantees a healthier future through new therapeutic strategies and enhanced scientific inquiry. The exploration of recombinant DNA technology within immunology illustrates a revolutionized role in vaccine and therapeutic development. Significant advancements have been made towards the recombinant design of vaccines that leverage genetic engineering to enhance immunogenicity with reduced risk for pathogenic response. Through the application of recombinant DNA technology, researchers are able to position selected antigens into expression systems in order to produce proteins that mimic natural pathogens, a technique that significantly maximizes immune response without the risks presented by traditional vaccines. Overall, this approach provides a streamlined pathway to vaccine development, which leads to public and personal protection on a larger scale. Indeed, the utilization of these technologies has led to landmark developments in disease prevention and control, underscoring the need for further research in the field of immunology.

Another significant aspect noted in the context of recombinant DNA technology is its utilization in the manufacture of monoclonal antibodies. These antibodies are now vital for therapeutic treatment as well as diagnostic use of a multitude of diseases, ranging from cancers to autoimmune diseases. The method involves the fusion of myeloma cells and spleen cells of immunized mice to form hybrid cells that secrete one type of antibody. The targeted therapy becomes more specific and less immunogenic than the conventional therapies. The clinical use of monoclonal antibodies underlines the demand for continuous innovation in recombinant DNA technology to develop such products as trastuzumab and rituximab, whose impact has greatly improved patient outcomes in cancer and immunology. The argument over the use of new eukaryotic systems, such as *Leishmania tarentolae*, also addresses the versatility of recombinant DNA technology in application to immunology. The protozoan parasite constitutes an amenable host for recombinant protein expression, offering specialized attributes in glycoprotein expression important for effective immunotherapies. According to recent reviews, *L. tarentolae* expression of mammalian recombinant proteins not only increases the promise for vaccine production but also raises issues of biosafety since infectivity in mammals exists in some strains. The similarity between its harmless expression capability and the specificity towards any range of hosts will be discussed tarentolae and pathogenic Leishmania species pointing out the significance of careful safety examinations in biotechnological applications. In general, these arguments lean towards a promising future with recombinant DNA technology at the helm for future innovations in immunological research and drug discovery (Asbury et al., 2000; Klatt et al., 2019).

A CLOSER LOOK

GENE CLONING

Gene cloning, otherwise known as molecular cloning, is a basic technique in immunology and molecular biology that is utilized to create multiple copies of a specific gene or DNA segment. It is a pivotal technique in isolating, growing, and analyzing genes, including those that are employed in immune responses and disease (Figure 3.17).

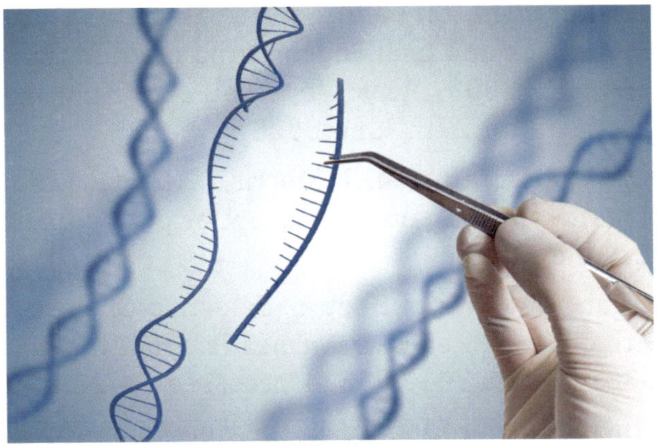

Figure 3.17. Genetic engineering on humans.

Source: https://biokimicroki.com/wp-content/uploads/2021/01/1-11-2018-genetic-engineering-on-humans-1024x683-1.jpg.

1. **Importance of Gene Cloning in Immunology:**

   a. **Immune System Component Analysis:** Gene cloning enables researchers to purify and examine genes encoding various components of the immune system, i.e., antibodies, cytokines, and receptors.

   b. **Immune Response Analysis:** It helps one understand how the components are involved in healthy immune responses and in diseases like autoimmune diseases and immunodeficiencies.

   c. **Immunological Tool Development:** Gene cloning is necessary to produce vast quantities of proteins for research, diagnostics, and therapy, like recombinant antibodies or vaccines.

2. Key Steps in Gene Cloning:

   a. **Gene Isolation:** The target gene is isolated from the DNA of the source organism.

   b. **Vector Preparation:** A suitable cloning vector (e.g., a plasmid) is chosen and made ready for gene insertion.

   c. **Recombination:** The isolated gene and the prepared vector are joined together using enzymes like restriction enzymes and DNA ligase.

   d. **Transformation:** The recombinant DNA is introduced into a host organism (e.g., bacteria).

REFERENCES

1. Acevedo, R., Acosta, A., Campa, C., Cardoso, F., et al. (2014). Bacterial outer membrane vesicles and vaccine applications. https://core.ac.uk/download/19767454.pdf (accessed on 27th June 2025).
2. Stoimenova, A., Savova, A., Manova, M., Angelovska, B., & Petrova, G. (2011). Pharmaceutical Biotechnology in Pharmacy Education: USA Pharmacy Schools. *Biotechnology & Biotechnological Equipment*, *25*(3), 2533–2537. https://doi.org/10.5504/BBEQ.2011.0074(accessed on 27th June 2025).
3. Annas, G., Berwick, R., Campbell, D., Cantor, N., et al. (2003). The future of human nature: A symposium on the promises and challenges of the revolutions in genomics and computer science, April 10, 11, and 12, 2003. https://open.bu.edu/bitstream/2144/22887/1/Conf03-Human-Nature.pdf (accessed on 27th June 2025).
4. Atherton, M. J., Lichty, B. D., McDermott, M. R., Morris, D. G., et al. (2016). Cancer immunology and canine malignant melanoma: A comparative review. https://core.ac.uk/download/42370176.pdf (accessed on 27th June 2025).
5. Chirumamilla CS, Palagani A, Kamaraj B, et al. Selective Glucocorticoid Receptor Properties of GSK866 Analogs with Cysteine Reactive Warheads. *Front Immunol.* 2017;8:1324. Published 2017 Nov 1. doi:10.3389/fimmu.2017.01324(accessed on 27th June 2025).
6. Barentine, C. (2022). Increasing production of therapeutic mAbs in CHO cells through genetic engineering. https://core.ac.uk/download/533934333.pdf (accessed on 27th June 2025).
7. Stroud C, Dmitriev I, Kashentseva E, et al. A One Health overview, facilitating advances in comparative medicine and translational research. *Clin Transl Med.* 2016;5(Suppl 1):26. doi:10.1186/s40169-016-0107-4(accessed on 27th June 2025).
8. Jon R. Cavicchi, Stanley P. Kowalski, et al, "Patent Landscape of Influenza A Virus Prophylactic Vaccines and Related Technologies" (2012). The Franklin Pierce Center for Intellectual Property, University of New Hampshire School of Law International Technology Transfer Institute, Concord, NH, USA (accessed on 27th June 2025).
9. Mamedov A, Vorobyeva N, Filimonova I, et al. Protective Allele for Multiple Sclerosis HLA-DRB1*01:01 Provides Kinetic Discrimination of Myelin and Exogenous Antigenic Peptides. *Front Immunol.* 2020;10:3088. Published 2020 Jan 17. doi:10.3389/fimmu.2019.03088(accessed on 27th June 2025).
10. Asbury, C., Cline, B. L., & Gammino, V. M. (2000). *The Edna McConnell Clark Foundation's Tropical Disease Research Program: A 25-year retrospective review 1976–1999.* https://core.ac.uk/download/71350953.pdf (accessed on 27th June 2025).
11. Tandel N, Trivedi D, Mohan Krishnan A, Kumar Dalai S. Application of Radiation Technology: A Novel Vaccine Approach to Induce Protective Immunity against Malaria Infection [Internet]. Ionizing and Non-ionizing Radiation. IntechOpen; 2020. Available from: http://dx.doi.org/10.5772/intechopen.85491(accessed on 27th June 2025).
12. Mot D, Timbermont L, Haesebrouck F, Ducatelle R, Van Immerseel F. Progress and problems in vaccination against necrotic enteritis in broiler chickens. *Avian Pathol.* 2014;43(4):290-300. doi:10.1080/03079457.2014.939942(accessed on 27th June 2025).

13. Anatole Krattiger, Stanley P. Kowalski, Robert Eiss & Anthony Taubman. "Intellectual Property Management Strategies to Accelerate the Development and Access of Vaccines and Diagnostics: Case Studies on Pandemic Influenza, Malaria and SARS." 2 Innovation Strategy Today 2 (2006). (accessed on 27th June 2025).

14. Kricka LJ, Polsky TG, Park JY, Fortina P. The future of laboratory medicine - a 2014 perspective. *Clin Chim Acta.* 2015;438:284-303. doi:10.1016/j.cca.2014.09.005(accessed on 27th June 2025).

15. Fredriksen, A. B., Pedersen, A. B., O'Connell, A. E., Schwab, A. E., de Andres, B., Manoury, B., Makepeace, B. L., et al. (2012). Deletion of parasite immune modulatory sequences combined with immune activating signals enhances vaccine mediated protection against filarial nematodes. https://core.ac.uk/download/16458801.pdf (accessed on 27th June 2025).

16. Liu PF, Wang Y, Ulrich RG, et al. Leaf-Encapsulated Vaccines: Agroinfiltration and Transient Expression of the Antigen *Staphylococcal Endotoxin* B in Radish Leaves. *J Immunol Res.* 2018;2018:3710961. Published 2018 Feb 7. doi:10.1155/2018/3710961 (accessed on 27th June 2025).

17. Generalov, I. I., Sencovich, S. A., & Zheleznyak, N. V. (2014). Instructions for laboratory training in general microbiology & immunology. Ministry of Health Care, Republic of Belarus Vitebsk State Medical University Department of Clinical Microbiology. https://core.ac.uk/download/80150439.pdf (accessed on 27th June 2025).

18. Staeheli P, Puehler F, Schneider K, Göbel TW, s B. Cytokines of birds: conserved functions--a largely different look. *J Interferon Cytokine Res.* 2001;21(12):993-1010. doi:10.1089/107999001317205123(accessed on 27th June 2025).

19. Hood, L., Korber, B., & Stroynowski, I. (1987). Regulation of murine class I genes by interferons is controlled by regions located both 5′ and 3′ to the transcription initiation site. https://core.ac.uk/download/4873444.pdf (accessed on 27th June 2025).

20. Klein, P. A. & Jacobson, E. (2001). Sero epidemiological studies of herpesvirus-associated diseases of marine turtles: Fibro papillomatosis and lung-eye-trachea disease. Florida Cooperative Fish and Wildlife Research Unit , University of Florida. https://core.ac.uk/download/11017006.pdf (accessed on 27th June 2025).

21. (2024). State of the art of synthetic biology–Literature review. https://core.ac.uk/download/653697438.pdf (accessed on 27th June 2025).

22. Johnston, R. S., Norton, D. J., & Baldwin, T. H. (1988). *Space and Biotechnology: An Industry Profile.* Contract No. NCC 9-16, Activity IM.5. https://core.ac.uk/download/pdf/42821064.pdf (accessed on 27th June 2025).

23. Kogut MH, Pishko EJ, Kaspers B, Weining KC. Modulation of functional activities of chicken heterophils by recombinant chicken IFN-gamma. *J Interferon Cytokine Res.* 2001;21(2):85-92. doi:10.1089/107999001750069944(accessed on 27th June 2025).

24. Klatt S, Simpson L, Maslov DA, Konthur Z. Leishmania tarentolae: Taxonomic classification and its application as a promising biotechnological expression host. *PLoS Negl Trop Dis.* 2019;13(7):e0007424. Published 2019 Jul 25. doi:10.1371/journal.pntd.0007424Magez, S., Obishakin, E. T., Pinto Torres, J. E., Radwanska, M., et al. (2020). Infections with extracellular trypanosomes require control by efficient innate immune mechanisms and can result in the destruction of the mammalian humoral immune system. https://core.ac.uk/

download/288817508.pdf (accessed on 27th June 2025).

25. Mullen, B. (2020). The (ab)uses of CRISPR-mediated human genome editing. https://core.ac.uk/download/327110863.pdf (accessed on 27th June 2025).

26. Pinitkiatisakul, S. (2007). Recombinant subunit vaccines against *Neospora caninum*. https://core.ac.uk/download/11695141.pdf (accessed on 27th June 2025).

27. Pöri, P. (2018). Development of vaccines. https://core.ac.uk/download/161424545.pdf (accessed on 27th June 2025).

28. Battisti F, Napoletano C, Rahimi Koshkaki H, et al. Tumor-Derived Microvesicles Modulate Antigen Cross-Processing *via* Reactive Oxygen Species-Mediated Alkalinization of Phagosomal Compartment in Dendritic Cells. *Front Immunol.* 2017;8:1179. Published 2017 Sep 25. doi:10.3389/fimmu.2017.01179(accessed on 27th June 2025).

29. Saeed, A. F. U. H., Wang, R., Wang, S., & Ling, S. (2017). Antibody engineering for pursuing a healthier future. https://core.ac.uk/download/pdf/82883279.pdf (accessed on 27th June 2025).

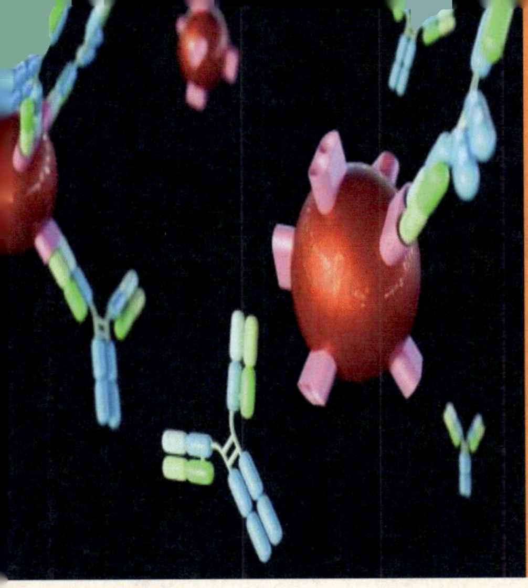

Chapter 4

ANTIGEN-ANTIBODY INTERACTIONS: MOLECULAR TECHNIQUES

Contents

Introduction

The study of antigen-antibody interactions is the signature of immunological research and of great importance in diagnostic and therapeutic sciences. Understanding such interactions at the molecular level enables researchers to design highly specific probes that are capable of detecting various biomarkers crucial in the detection and monitoring of diseases. The advent of proteomic analyses has intensified the need for engineered antibodies, which have long been preferred due to their specificity and affinity for single targets. Issues such as directional immobilization and specificity loss are significant hurdles. Such issues point towards innovative strategies since researchers seek to engineer antibody formats capable of overcoming such limitations and maintaining their functional integrity. Recent developments in protein engineering have enabled the introduction of novel antibody development methods into concise formats like Fab fragments and single-domain antibodies. These miniaturized forms not only retain the major features of traditional antibodies but also enhance the ease of assay assembly by minimizing steric hindrance and improving biosensor stability. In this case, the selection of immobilization strategies and solid supports plays a leading role as it comes as a great way to control antibody-based assay performance. The ongoing efforts to optimize these parameters are poised to further enhance biosensing strategies and their adaptability in diverse fields ranging from clinical diagnostics to environmental monitoring. This state-of-the-art research environment is a milestone for antibody technology and future research avenues and applications. Furthermore, breakthroughs in computer methods, particularly in silico epitope prediction, have revolutionized our understanding of antigen-antibody interactions. Predictive models enable the identification of the respective epitopes that the antibodies need to target, which is crucial in designing effective immunoassays and vaccines. By using molecular mechanics for epitope categorization and valuation, researchers are capable of improving the accuracy of prediction and streamlining the development process. Such a new method complements traditional experimental techniques, enabling a more systematic exploration of the antigen structure and the resulting antibodies. With predictive algorithms getting better and better, incorporating such methods in the greater framework of antigen-antibody interaction research has the potential to unlock new information and enhance the efficiency of molecular techniques for biosensing and therapeutic applications (Reitmaier, 2007; Saerens et al., 2008).

Definition of Antigens and Antibodies

The terms antigen and antibody are fundamental constituents of the immune system, both of which are vital in the defense of the body against foreign substances. An antigen is typically defined as any molecule or molecular aggregate that is capable of provoking an immune response; among these are an enormous number of things, such as proteins, polysaccharides, and even nucleic acids. Antigens are recognized by immune cells, particularly lymphocytes, which call for an attack of defensive responses. Antibodies, or immunoglobulins, are dedicated proteins produced by B cells that bind specifically to antigens. Binding results in neutralization of microorganisms or tagging them for removal by other immune components. Antigen specificity of the antibody is a highly significant property of both immunological memory and vaccine preparation, exhibiting the intricate synergy between the two factors in the induction of a robust immune response. Antigen-antibody interaction is regulated by intricate molecular mechanisms, and therefore, it is a significant topic of study within the discipline of immunology. These interactions are often described by the lock and key model, in which an antibody (the key) binds preferentially to an antigen (the lock). This is a gross oversimplification of what occurs, as work published recently has established that there are many factors that contribute to the specificity and affinity of such interactions. For instance, prediction of B-cell epitopes has been enhanced by advances in in-silico tools and molecular mechanics that allow the classification, evaluation, and prediction of epitopes—that is, the exact regions on antigens recognized by antibodies. As described in the literature, these tools represent a significant advancement in knowledge of antigen-antibody interactions and are required to develop targeted vaccines and immunotherapies (Reitmaier, 2007). Yet, once such a pivotal role has been played by antibodies, their validity for experimental purposes has come into question. Issues of the specificity and quality of the commercially produced antibodies have been among the biggest headaches for scientists handling the tools in different assays. Proper localization of antigens by techniques like immunocytochemistry requires that such antibodies employed be not only extremely specific but also reproducible in binding modes. The richness of the discovery of real specificity goes beyond binding upfront, demanding strict experimental proof. As outlined in recent reviews, it has increasingly become apparent that many off-the-shelf commercial antibodies are below the high standards for scientific relevance. Good practices for the selection of antibodies and antibody testing are essential, particularly since quantitative electron microscopy methods can provide further information about reproducible labeling patterns, leading to the robust interpretation of experimental results (Griffiths & Lucocq, 2014) (Figure 4.1).

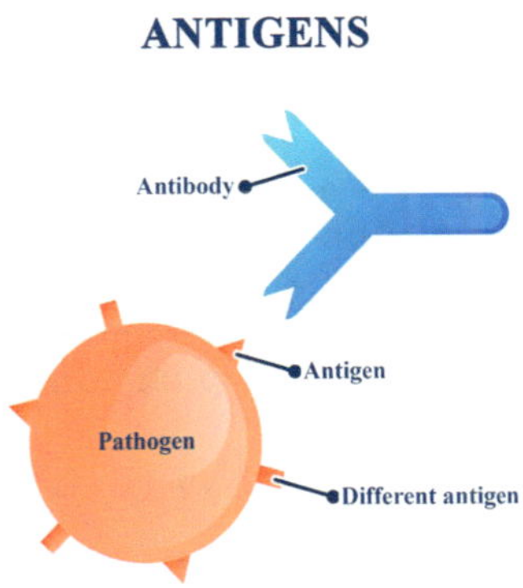

Figure 4.1. Antigens.

Source: https://media.istockphoto.com/id/1220171709/vector/antigens-vector-illustration-labeled-antibody-pathogen-educational-scheme.jpg?s=612x612&w=0&k=20&c=q6la9jQc8_yxCUgEehrDSlsS5VkzHUh2hZYdOgV6xpQ=.

Importance of Antigen-Antibody Interactions in Immunology

Antigen-antibody reactions form the basis of the science of immunology and are the mechanism through which the immune system can recognize and block pathogens. Such interactions are characterized by high specificity, whereby antibodies can recognize specific epitopes presented by antigens. This specificity, apart from facilitating effective targeting of pathogenic microbes, is essential in vaccine development. Through the use of specific antigens in vaccines, scientists are able to elicit a robust immune response, allowing them to establish memory cells that are responsible for long-term immunity. Hence, understanding mechanisms of antigen-antibody interactions is significant in driving forward therapeutic strategies, especially in vaccine design, where antigen-antibody interactions are utilized to provide long-term immunity against infection. Antigen-antibody interactions are also important beyond the recognition of pathogens, as they are vital in therapeutic interventions in cancer and autoimmune diseases. For instance, monoclonal antibodies may be engineered to bind specifically to cancer cells, marking them for destruction by effector immune cells or delivering cytotoxic substances directly to neoplastic tissues. Targeting avoids normal cells from being harmed by collateral effects, maximizing the efficiency of treatment and minimizing side effects. In addition, the ability to determine the antigenic features of tumor cells through the interaction of antibodies allows physicians to tailor immunotherapies according to each patient's unique profile of tumors. All these advancements highlight the two-way nature of antigen-antibody interactions to both diagnose and treat disease, further solidifying their roles in today's immunology research and clinical applications. Moreover, new molecular technologies, such as adaptive immune receptor repertoire sequencing (AIRR-seq), have transformed our understanding of the complexity inherent in antigen-antibody interactions. AIRR-seq enables end-to-end immunoprofiling of immune repertoires at the genomic level, explaining the complex antibody and T-cell receptor landscape engaged in adaptive immunity. This high-dimensional strategy allows investigators to probe the evolution of immune responses to many stimuli, from infections to cancers. Through the correlation of computational analysis with AIRR-seq data, scientists are capable of detecting diversity and specificity patterns in immune responses, which impart insights that are used to develop new immunotherapeutics and diagnostics. In the process, molecular breakthroughs enhance our knowledge of antigen-antibody interactions, cementing their central place in both basic immunological studies and functional clinical use (Tan et al., 2015; Miho et al., 2018) (Figure 4.2).

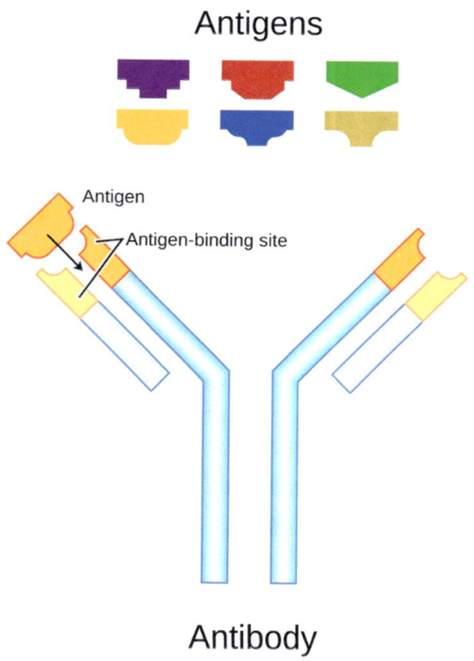

Figure 4.2. An illustration that shows how antigens induce the immune system response by interacting with an antibody that matches the molecular structure of an antigen.

Source: https://upload.wikimedia.org/wikipedia/commons/thumb/2/2d/Antibody.svg/800px-Antibody.svg.png.

Overview of Molecular Techniques Used to Study These Interactions

Antigen-antibody interactions are facilitated a great deal through an array of molecular techniques by which scientists can study the intricacies of immune responses. Of all these techniques, molecular docking simulations have received much attention as they can predict how antibodies and antigens will behave at the atomic level. Through simulations that use algorithms to define the spatial relationship of molecules, researchers can compute the optimal binding positions and affinities, hence accelerating the drug discovery process. For example, the F2 Dock protocol is representative of such advancements by including improved scoring and ranking parameters that consider shape complementarity and electrostatic interactions, which help towards more accurate predictions of docking poses. This approach not only enhances the identification of drug candidate ability but also generates information regarding the pathways involved in immune responses, thus simplifying the development of therapeutics against certain antigen-antibody interactions (Chowdhury et al., 2013). Another essential approach to investigating such interactions involves the use of recombinant proteins, particularly when evaluating the performance of diagnostic assays. For instance, surface antigens like Apical Membrane Antigen 1 (AMA-1) of pathogenic *Babesia bigemina* have been expressed and purified to measure antibody response in cattle. Production of the protein allows the development of enzyme-linked immunosorbent assays (ELISA) for the specific detection of some antibodies. By correlating the presence of some antibodies with disease status, scientists can obtain a better understanding of the immunological status in infected populations. This also reinforces the importance of specificity in immunological analysis, as exemplified by the ability of AMA-1 to discriminate between *B. bigemina* infections and infections by other diseases and thus illustrate how molecular technology can enhance diagnostic specificity (Torina et al., 2016). In addition to recombinant protein techniques, high-throughput sequencing and bioinformatics have now emerged as useful tools for identification and antibody repertoire characterization. These methods allow for comprehensive analysis of B-cell diversity and characterization of antibody specificity upon exposure to varied antigens. With next-generation sequencing (NGS), researchers are able to identify broad ranges of immunoglobulin sequences, allowing for the investigation of clonal expansion and affinity maturation. These data not only illustrate the dynamic nature of immune responses but also allow for correlations of the exposure to specific antigens and the generation of antibodies. Taken altogether, these molecular approaches form a firm basis for comprehension of the complex antigen-antibody relationships and further elucidation of their role in disease, health, and the development of immunotherapies.

4.1. The Basics of Antigen-Antibody Interactions

Appreciation of the fundamental principles of antigen-antibody interactions is essential to the comprehension of the immune response. Antigens, in general, foreign molecules such as proteins or polysaccharides found on pathogens, trigger the immune system's response upon recognition. When such foreign substances enter the body, B cells recognize and bind to specific epitopes of the antigen via their respective antibodies. Strong specificity is facilitated through non-covalent forces like hydrogen bonds, ionic interactions, and Van der Waals forces. The resulting antigen-antibody complexes play a significant role in neutralizing pathogens or tagging them for immune component elimination. Therefore, the subtlety of this interaction highlights the acumen and sophistication of the adaptive immune response, providing an important basis for further investigation of molecular approaches that utilize these dynamics to optimal benefit in scientific and clinical applications. Antibody diversity contributes to antigen recognition specificity. There are five principal classes of antibodies (IgA, IgD, IgE, IgG, and IgM) that are all designed to perform distinct functions in the immune system. For instance, IgG is renowned to cross the placenta and provide passive immunity to the fetus, whereas IgA predominates the mucosal surfaces, protecting against incoming pathogens by respiratory and gut routes. The structural variations among such classes also affect their affinity for binding and functional potential. Moreover, the formation of an antigen-antibody complex is required for the initiation of complement cascades, phagocytosis, and antigen presentation to T cells, thereby enhancing the immune response. These interactions facilitate the easy flow of therapeutic interventions, i.e., in the development of monoclonal antibodies to targeted therapy against infections and cancer. Improvements in molecular techniques identify the potential of antigen-antibody interaction manipulation for therapeutic use. The single-domain antibody, or Nanobody as it is widely known, is a good example of such progress since its initial discovery in the 1990s. VHHs possess traits like unparalleled solubility, stability, and smaller size compared to regular antibodies, which have revolutionized the use of affinity reagents across various disciplines. Their modular nature predisposes them to fusion with other modules of molecules, which has been found incredibly useful in designing strategies for combating viral diseases, e.g., those caused by HIV-1 and influenza viruses. The usability and effectiveness of VHHs not only lead to affinity and immune response but also reduce the potential for viral escape, marking a revolutionary change in therapeutic design. The ongoing research into these molecular techniques portends a rosy future for antiviral approaches targeted, being spurred by the intimate understanding of how antigens and antibodies interrelate.

4.1.1. Mechanisms of Binding Between Antigens and Antibodies

Understanding the mechanisms of antigen-antibody binding is at the heart of immunology and biochemistry. Antigen-antibody binding is generally described in terms of non-covalent forces such as hydrogen bonds, van der Waals forces, ionic interactions, and hydrophobic effects. The specificity of these antigen-antibody interactions is, in large part, determined by the unique structures of both the antibody and antigen. Every antibody has a variable region that is suited to recognize specific antigens on the basis of their three-dimensional shape.

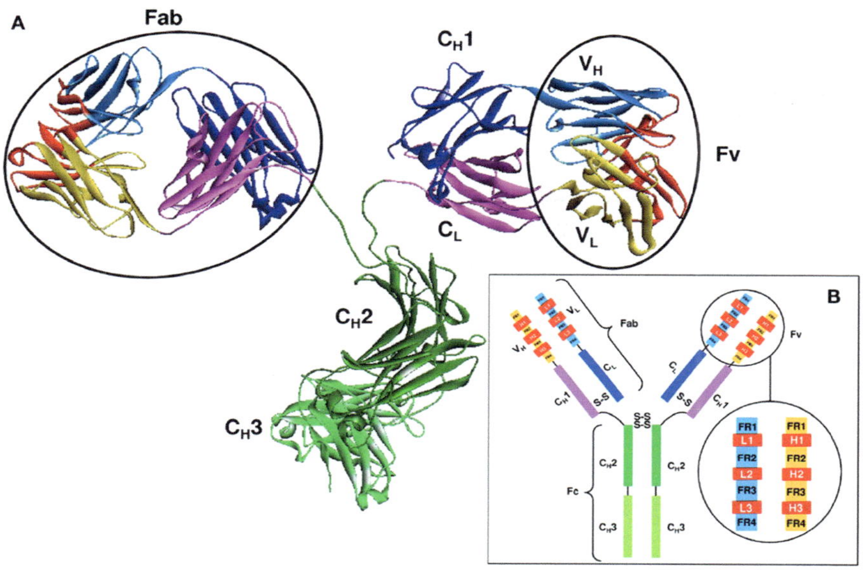

Figure 4.3. Structural model of an antibody molecule. Rounded portions indicate antigen binding sites.

Source: https://upload.wikimedia.org/wikipedia/commons/thumb/6/62/Structure_of_antibody_molecule.jpg/800px-Structure_of_antibody_molecule.jpg.

Consequently, by extrapolation, it has been proven through research that HLA antibodies can lead to acute and chronic antibody-mediated rejection of transplanted organs and thus affect graft survival. As described by current studies, while donor-specific antibodies have been most in the limelight, evidence implicating non-HLA-specific antibodies continues to grow, and their detection is being implicated with allograft damage. Despite the development of novel technology like single antigen bead assays, more research is required to define the characteristics of these antibodies that are implicated in AMR pathophysiology. This sustained research into antibody characteristics and graft rejection affirmations indicates the significant role that understanding antigen-antibody reactions plays in transplant immunology as well as individualized medicine (Januzzi et al., 2017) (Figure 4.3).

This specificity serves as the foundation of numerous therapeutic and diagnostic applications, as the specificity of antibodies for binding to antigens can serve to target causative disease agents. Additionally, the binding affinity, depending on concentration and environmental conditions, is a determinant in the efficiency of immune response as well as other molecular mechanisms of antigen-antibody interaction. Deeper still, the antigen-antibody binding process can be questioned through molecular approaches, which unveil the dynamic nature of such interactions. More advanced developments put more focus on the application of in-silico methods for B-cell epitope prediction in order for researchers to be able to predict which regions of an antigen should react immunologically. Such application of molecular mechanics not only contributes to advancing knowledge but also assists in vaccine and immunotherapy development by giving insight into potential targets for antibody production. These approaches represent a considerable step forward in the field, providing robust instruments to optimize epitope classification and evaluation. Furthermore, these methods allow for an ordered approach to exploring the functional consequences of antibody binding, leading to an enhanced appreciation of antibody-mediated immunity and its manipulation in the clinic (Reitmaier, 2007). Furthermore, the antigen-antibody binding reactions are not mere theory; they play a role in clinical transplants and immunemediated disease.

4.1.2. Types of Antibodies and Their Specificities

The immune system utilizes a variety of antibodies with specificities that enhance its capacity for recognizing and neutralizing various antigens. The five principal classes of antibodies—IgG, IgA, IgM, IgE, and IgD—possess variant functional characteristics and structural properties. For instance, IgG is the most dense antibody in serum and plays a role in opsonization and neutralization, while IgA is dense primarily in mucosal locations such as the gut and respiratory tract to create a first line of defense against infection. IgM, on the other hand, is an early immune response, present in large pentameric formations that agglutinate antigens very effectively. These structural diversities among antibody classes then result in a powerful immune response, fitting the body's defenses to specific dangers. Antibody specificity is largely regulated by its unique variable regions, which can fine-tune so as to recognize specific epitopes on antigens. Each antibody's ability to bind to these epitopes by non-covalent interactions—i.e., hydrogen bonding, van der Waals forces, and electrostatic interactions—enhances the precision of the immune system in targeting pathogens. Following the advancements in molecular techniques, researchers developed high-complexity techniques for B-cell epitope prediction and annotation. As explained in Reitmaier (2007), new computational algorithms have emerged, utilizing molecular mechanics for epitope evaluation, enhancing accuracy in the design of antibodies. This has deep implications for therapeutic progress, enabling monoclonal antibodies to be developed that can selectively bind to disease-related antigens, e.g., of cancer or autoimmune diseases. Advances in biosensor technology in recent times have made it possible to study antibody specificities for diagnostic applications even more. Silicon nanochannel field-effect transistor (FET) biosensors are a good example, with a superb sensitivity to identify specific antibodies at the molecular level. These systems not only allow detection of individual molecules but also provide a platform for multiplexed analysis, expanding the list of diagnostic applications. According to Mohanty et al. (2012), such FET biosensors take advantage of conventional semiconductor technology, resulting in high-performance, low-cost, and sensitive biosensors capable of real-time monitoring of biomarkers. The coming together of these technologies with antibody specificity research further enhances the promise of early cancer diagnosis, allowing for the crucial information on disease presence and disease progression based on antigen-antibody interaction in biological samples (Figure 4.4).

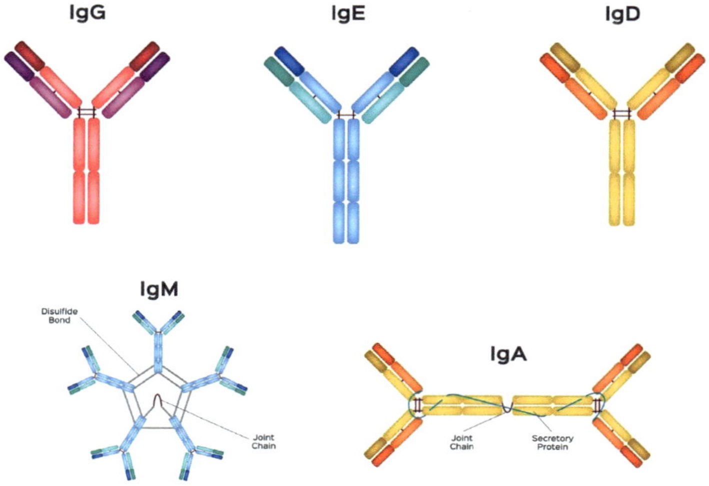

Figure 4.4. Antibody types.

Source: https://www.news-medical.net/images/Article_Images/ImageForArticle_16427_17386092428414821.jpg.

4.1.3. Role of Epitopes in Antigen Recognition

Epitopes play a pivotal role to play in antigen recognition, which is a fundamental process in the immune response. These structurally dissimilar antigen regions are recognized by antibodies to enable the immune system to distinguish between non-self and self. The binding specificity depends largely on the unique three-dimensional conformation of the epitopes and their ability to bind to the paratopes on antibodies. It is important to understand epitopes in vaccine and therapeutic antibody design because the correct choice of proper epitopes can be employed for enhancing immune responses. The efficiency of epitope-based vaccines also relies on their ability to allow a strong and extended immune memory, which further underlines the importance of epitope characterization in immunology. Technological advancements in molecular methods have greatly enhanced epitope prediction and analysis, as well as epitope-antibody understanding. For example, novel in-silico tools are being created to predict B-cell epitopes from structural and sequence information. Studies indicate that using molecular mechanics to classify, assess, and predict epitopes has high potential to improve epitope discovery processes (Reitmaier, 2007). These predictive tools facilitate researchers to rapidly predict possible epitopes, thus making it possible to develop more specific immunotherapeutics. These developments also enhance the ability of vaccines to be designed to a particular population or pathogen and hence offer better protection against pathogens through precise targeting of the immune system. In addition, computational modeling, as introduced in the software package SIMMUNE, enables researchers to analyze immune system activity at a microscopic level, with particular focus on immune agent interaction (Meier-Schellersheim & Mack, 1999).

By simulating immune system components responding to various epitopes, researchers can investigate the antigen recognition dynamics in a simulated environment. Such a method not only allows for the prediction of optimal epitope presentations but also explains the immune system interactions with minimal assumptions. Consequently, such epitope predictions and molecular simulations pave the way for improved vaccine design concepts and the development of novel immunotherapies, significantly advancing our overall understanding of antigen-antibody interactions (Figure 4.5).

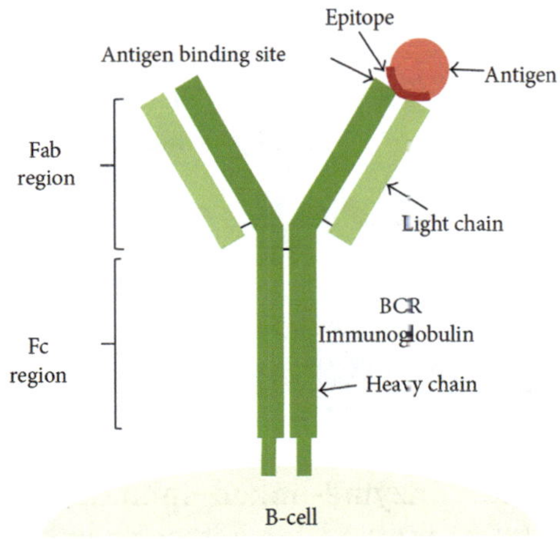

Figure 4.5. B-cell epitope recognition. B-cell epitopes are solvent-exposed portions of the antigen that bind to secreted and cell-bound immunoglobulins. (a) B-cell receptors encompass cell-bound immunoglobulins, consisting of two heavy chains and two light chains. The different chains and regions are annotated. (b) Molecular representation of the interaction between an antibody and the antigen. Antibodies are secreted immunoglobulins of known specificity.

Source: https://www.researchgate.net/publication/322128738/figure/fig1/AS:1086490968895495@1636051041596/B-cell-epitope-recognition-B-cell-epitopes-are-solvent-exposed-portions-of-the-antigen.jpg.

4.2. Techniques for Detecting Antigen-Antibody Interactions

The identification of antigen-antibody interactions is of the essence in numerous biological and clinical applications, and so advanced techniques need to be developed. One of the leading methods is through the application of biosensors, which are instruments that translate biological interactions into measurable signals. Antibodies are used as highly selective probes within these biosensors because they can bind specifically to target antigens. However, traditional antibody-based assays are often plagued with issues such as steric hindrance and direction-based immobilization problems that limit their performance. In an effort to reverse these drawbacks, novel protein engineering techniques have been employed in designing smaller antibody formats such as single-domain antibodies and Fab fragments. In addition to size reduction, these engineered antibody fragments enhance their stability, thus enhancing more efficient biosensor designs for biomarker detection (Saerens et al., 2008). Yet another promising technique consists of silicon nanochannel FET biosensors, which have been demonstrated to be very effective in quantifying antigen-antibody interactions. These advanced devices benefit from the high surface-to-volume ratios found in silicon nanochannels, and single molecules can be detected with high sensitivity. The electrical character of FETs also allows for label-free detection, which evades possible pitfalls of fluorescent labeling in traditional assays. In addition, the use of Complementary Metal Oxide Semiconductor (CMOS) technology aids in the fabrication of highly multiplexed sensor arrays, which enhance the throughput and versatility of these biosensing platforms. These advancements are a quantum leap towards low-cost, high-speed diagnostics for applications like cancer diagnosis, where precise and efficient identification of biomolecules is of utmost significance (Mohanty et al., 2012). The application of more than one detection method is a growing trend towards multi-modal sensing in biosensing, which increases assay robustness and specificity. Techniques such as surface plasmon resonance (SPR) and electrochemical impedance spectroscopy (EIS) complement antibody-based detection by monitoring antigen-antibody interactions in real time. These methods can be used in conjunction with engineered antibodies to benefit from their high affinity, resulting in highly amplified signal amplification and the ability to detect low-abundance targets. Furthermore, microfluidic developments allow the miniaturization of these approaches, cutting down on sample handling and volume demand for sensitive detection. As the biosensing environment continues to evolve, the merging of these diverse methodologies will progressively become more efficient at measuring and detecting antigen-antibody interactions, transforming diagnostic progress and improving therapeutic intervention.

4.2.1. Enzyme-Linked Immunosorbent Assay (ELISA)

ELISA is a prominent technique in the study of immunology, which primarily harnesses the capability of antigen-antibody reactions to quantify specific proteins and other biomolecules. The method involves coating a microplate with an antigen so that it can bind with antibodies that are attached specifically to the plate. When the target analyte-containing sample (e.g., a protein or a microorganism) is presented, it is trapped by antibodies specific to the analyte, leading to the formation of an immune complex. The technique not only facilitates the detection of low-abundance targets but also enhances the sensitivity of assays, which is desirable in clinical diagnostics as well as research laboratories. The built-in flexibility of ELISA allows it to be adapted into various forms, including direct, indirect, sandwich, and competitive assays, each of which is tailored to meet a specific experimental need. ELISA's flexibility is again confirmed by its applications in a large number of areas beyond the traditional clinical diagnostic uses, extending into research and therapeutic monitoring. For instance, in a study on the conjugation of a novel aldobiouronic acid to methylated bovine serum albumin (BSA), antibodies were generated and subsequently characterized by ELISA to demonstrate specificity towards wood cell wall polysaccharides.

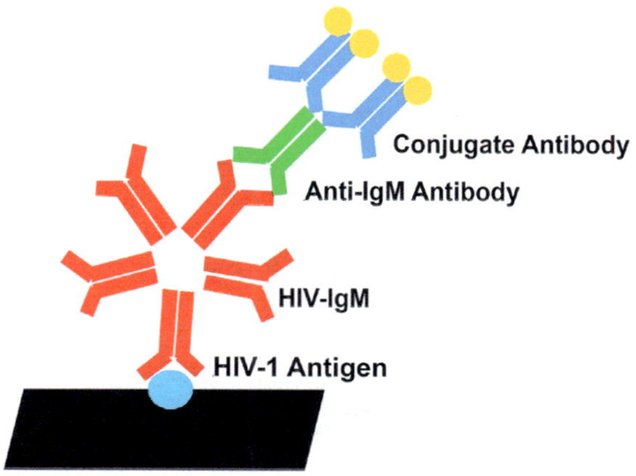

Figure 4.6. Enzyme-linked immunosorbent assay (ELISA) method for detecting anti-HIV-1 IgM antibody captured by membrane-bound recombinant gp41.

Source: https://www.researchgate.net/publication/281340996/figure/fig7/AS:669650295734279@1536668480363/Enzyme-linked-immunosorbent-assay-ELISA-method-for-detecting-anti-HIV1-IgM-antibody.jpg.

The obtained antiserum displayed specific binding towards some sugar-protein conjugates, a demonstration of ELISAs utility in the exploration of complex biological interactions and interrogating target specificities (Sumiya & Takahashi, 1990). This ability to not just provide quantitative data, but also qualitative findings serves to further demonstrate ELISA's utility as a molecular tool that can be applied in various research contexts, continuing to build our understanding of antigen-antibody interactions. Perhaps more importantly, the role of ELISA in diagnostic medicine cannot be stressed enough. The technique has revolutionized the process of detecting disease, particularly infectious pathogens. Its high throughput and reproducibility make it an important tool in epidemiological research and vaccine development, allowing clinicians and researchers to assess immune responses cost-effectively. For example, novel applications of ELISA in gene therapy research illustrate its application for the measurement of immune responses against therapeutics (Khan et al., 2013). In such contexts, the measurable outcomes derived from ELISA are of significant value in the comprehensive assessment of immune system function. As an approach paradigm in immunodiagnostics, ELISA is still evolving, paving the way for future directions in the quest to comprehend health and disease through the antigen-antibody interaction paradigm (Figure 4.6).

4.2.2. Western Blotting

Western blotting is now a central technique in biochemistry and molecular biology used to detect and study specific proteins in complex biological samples. On the principle of antigen-antibody reactions, the technique works by separating the proteins via gel electrophoresis prior to transferring them onto a membrane. The immobilized proteins are then probed with antibodies that bind specifically to the antigens for qualitative and semi-quantitative analysis. The ability to see them in a visual form renders Western blotting an indispensable piece of equipment for a broad spectrum of applications, including protein expression profile characterization, the identification of post-translational modifications, and the validation of other assays. Its versatility is yet to uncover new applications in researchers from various disciplines, ranging from basic science research to diagnostic research, rendering it an essential instrument in the characterization of protein biology. The efficacy of Western blotting is prone to various factors, e.g., purity of the antibodies used and the conditions for the assay.

One such critical factor is the selection of a suitable buffer during transfer, which can potentially affect the integrity and availability of target proteins on the membrane. In addition, sample preparation options, such as the inclusion of denaturing agents like sodium dodecyl sulfate (SDS), can also affect outcomes. New advances in methods have introduced new strategies to detection abilities, such as the use of benzophenone-functionalized hydrogels, which allow for the covalent immobilization of proteins for multiplex detection. However, with these advancements, there is increased analysis depth but also raises the issue of possible signal loss during reprobing and stripping steps, which compromises the assay's reliability (Gopal & Herr, 2019).

Additionally, Western blotting plays a critical role in the identification of protein dynamics during pathological conditions, such as myocardial infarction. By using this technique in conjunction with other methods, i.e., laser confocal microscopy, researchers can not only detect but also locate the expression of inflammatory proteins in tissue samples. The use of Western blotting in conjunction with new imaging methods provides greater information regarding inflammatory response and protein expression kinetics over time, allowing a more extensive exploration of the mechanisms of disease onset (Cantatore et al., 2015). This cross-disciplinary approach allows for meticulous investigation of how single proteins operate in biological processes and thus allows for a greater knowledge of their functions within disease and health contexts. As more is learned about antigen-antibody interactions, the value of Western blotting in both basic research and clinical application will grow (Figure 4.7).

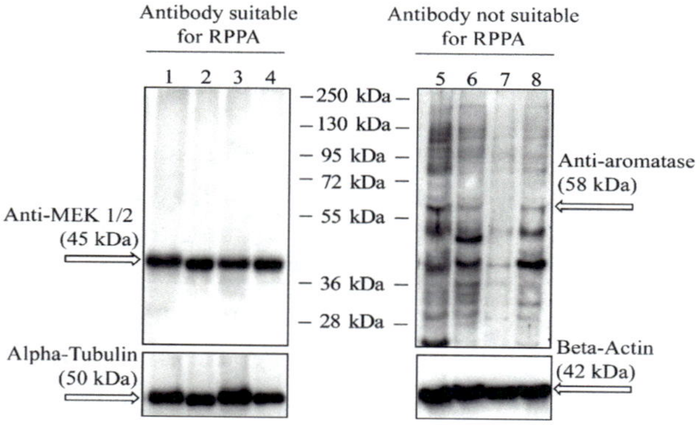

Figure 4.7. Antibody validation by Western Blot using different cell lines. The left panel shows an antibody that is suitable for RPPA analysis as it detects a single protein band at the expected molecular weight. The antibody used for the right panel should not be used for RPPA studies, as there are numerous bands besides the proposed " specific " band. 1–4: lysates from breast cancer FFPE-tissue; 5–8: lysates from different cell lines; arrows indicate the expected molecular weight.

Source: https://www.researchgate.net/publication/277574328/figure/fig2/AS:391297983631375@1470304117795/Antibody-validation-by-Western-Blot-using-different-cell-lines-The-left-panel-shows-an.png.

4.2.3. Immunofluorescence Microscopy

Immunofluorescence microscopy is a critical method of studying antigen-antibody interactions, as it allows for the visualization of specific proteins or antigens in cell environments. Immunofluorescence microscopy employs fluorochrome-labeled antibodies, which are used to bind to target antigens such that they can be detected with fluorescence microscopy. With the use of different wavelengths of light, researchers can observe the spatial localization and distribution of proteins in cells and tissues and have in-depth information about cellular functions and interactions. The technique has now come to be recognized in greater terms as it is capable of providing qualitative as well as quantitative data, enabling us to better understand biological processes and disease states. Notwithstanding that, there are still issues, like those of antibody specificity and the threat of nonspecific binding, which can complicate the interpretation of the data, demanding tight validation protocols to ensure the reliability of targets identified (Griffiths & Lucocq, 2014). The complexity of antigen-antibody interactions can strongly influence the efficiency of immunofluorescence microscopy. It should be noted, however, that while the lock-and-key model presents a crude picture of such interactions, it is a much more complicated affair in reality. Antibody affinity, cross-reactivity, and sample preparation protocol can affect binding specificity, and as such, scientists must conduct thorough analyses of their antibodies. Current evidence also suggests that the majority of commercially available antibodies do not meet the reproducibility standard necessary for reproducible immunolabeling, hence questioning the effectiveness of their utility in experiments (Griffiths & Lucocq, 2014). It is thus crucial to have a standard antibody validation protocol, inclusive of specificity assays and control experiments, to avoid misinterpretation and obtain valid data on antigen localization of interest. Immunofluorescence microscopy has been very instrumental in the observation of complex cellular structures, such as sensory hair cell tip links. Identification of related antigens in these structures has opened new avenues for study, particularly in auditory and visual systems. By the use of monoclonal antibodies that target these antigens, researchers can study their mechanisms in mechanotransduction and sensory signal processing. For instance, the discovery of the tip-link antigen has demonstrated its occurrence in both photoreceptors and hair bundles and therefore demonstrated its functional relevance in different sensory modalities. This intersection between immunofluorescence and molecular biology underlines the importance of ascertaining antigen localization and function. Subsequent studies employing this technique have the potential to uncover sophisticated disease mechanisms and sensory perception, illustrating the significant contribution of immunofluorescence to the broader field of molecular techniques (Figure 4.8).

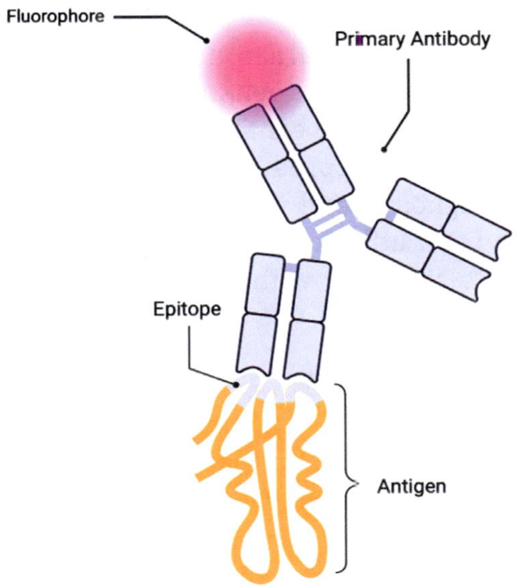

Figure 4.8. Basic concept of Primary Immunofluorescence: An antibody with a conjugated fluorophore that is specifically bound to an epitope on the target molecule.

Source: https://upload.wikimedia.org/wikipedia/commons/4/43/Primary_Immunofluorescence.png.

4.3. Molecular Cloning and Antibody Production

The process of molecular cloning serves as a foundation for the generation of antibodies and assumes a pivotal position in generating monoclonal antibodies. The process involves the manipulation of DNA to generate copies of specific gene sequences, which can be employed to express desired proteins, including antibodies, in host cells. One of the key benefits of molecular cloning is the ability to get enormous quantities of antibodies specific to particular antigens, which is of utmost importance for many applications in diagnostics and therapeutics. Cloning is usually achieved by the insertion of the antibody gene into a plasmid vector before transformation into suitable host cells, e.g., bacteria or mammalian cells. The correct expression of these antibodies then permits their subsequent purification and characterization and paves the way for application in a wide range of fields, from cancer treatment to disease control in infectious diseases. Defining specificity and binding affinities for antibodies produced is essential to their effective use, especially where therapeutic use is contemplated. Techniques such as glycan microarray screening are employed in high-throughput assays to determine antibody binding properties against carbohydrates and other substances. For instance, the production of monoclonal antibodies such as TKH2 for targeting the tumor-associated carbohydrate antigen sialyl-Tn (STn) highlights the significance of precise characterization procedures. Through quantitative analysis to evaluate apparent affinity constants (KD values), researchers are able to comprehend the antigen-binding interactions between the target antigen and antibody. Furthermore, advanced techniques such as saturation transfer difference NMR enhance the understanding of the interaction of glycan antigens, allowing for rational design and optimizing the antibodies against specific antigens and thereby affording higher therapeutic benefit (Amon et al., 2018). Physiological relevance and multifaceted functional role of molecularly cloned antibodies entail more than a simple binding interaction, shaping the entire field of immunology. Insight into the molecular environment under which antibodies are produced is essential to such advancements.

The soluble adenylyl cyclase (sAC) enzyme, for example, has been identified as a key player in various cellular processes, prompting further research into methods of antibody production. As sAC occurs in many organisms, knowledge of learning about its functional dynamics helps to inform the design of antibodies and can assist one to learn about how these antibodies might function in different biological contexts. The variability of sAC variants and their varying physiological roles underscores the importance of personalized approaches in antibody manufacturing and application, indicating the interactive game between molecular mechanisms and antibody-mediated responses in living organisms (Tresguerres & Salmerón, 2018).

4.3.1. Overview of Monoclonal vs. Polyclonal Antibodies

The distinction between monoclonal and polyclonal antibodies is paramount in immunology, particularly in the utilization of monoclonal vs. polyclonal antibodies in antigen-antibody interaction. Monoclonal antibodies are derived from one clone of B cells and hence exhibit uniform specificity for one particular antigen epitope. This uniformity leads to very reproducible results, and that is why they are found to be of immense benefit in the diagnostic and therapeutic applications. For example, the specificity of monoclonal antibodies has been utilized to great success in target therapies and particular diagnostic tests with very low cross-reactivity with non-target molecules.

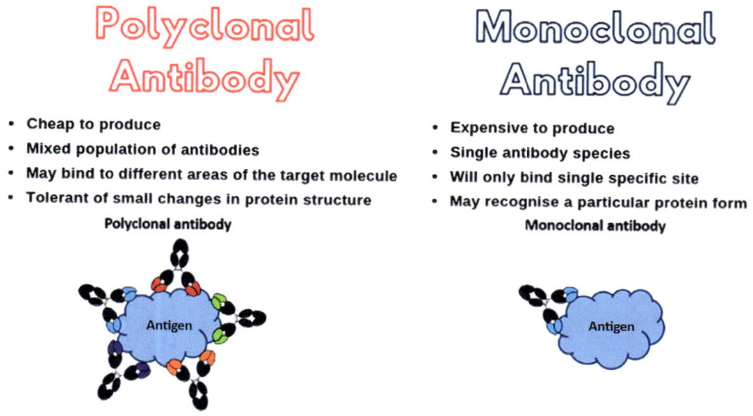

Figure 4.9. Monoclonal vs. polyclonal antibody.

Source: https://www.labclinics.com/wp-content/uploads/2018/09/Polyclonal_vs_Monoclonal.png.

On the other hand, polyclonal antibodies are a mixture of various antibodies from different B cell clones in response to an antigen that can bind to more than one epitope on the same protein. This will enhance sensitivity in assays, particularly in immunoassays where binding to multiple sites maximizes detection. Despite their advantages, each of these types of antibodies has its own setbacks. Monoclonal antibodies, though specific, could be expensive and time-consuming to produce, thereby making them unavailable for common use. Also, the development of a hybridoma cell line for monoclonal antibody production is extremely labor-intensive and requiring in terms of skill and material. Polyclonal antibodies, though simpler and less expensive to produce, are a source of heterogeneity and inconsistency between batches, thereby posing problems regarding their consistency in experimental use. As well documented in current literature, proper controls are required in working with polyclonal antibodies, as specificity and cross-reactivity issues may be present, which might lead to erroneous conclusions in research studies (Griffiths & Lucocq, 2014). Therefore, choosing between monoclonal and polyclonal antibodies must weigh factors such as specificity, sensitivity, cost, and complexity of experiment design. In practice, the selection of an appropriate type of antibody depends on the purposes and situations of experiments. Monoclonal antibodies typically find applications in those requiring high specificity and quantitative detection, such as flow cytometry or Western blotting. Conversely, polyclonal antibodies find applications in those requiring high sensitivity, for instance, immunohistochemistry, where one can label antigens effectively, utilizing them in many tissues. For instance, polyclonal antibody studies against GMP-140 showed impressive enhancement in the delineation of protein localization upon activation of platelets, highlighting their utilization for strong profiling (Stenberg et al., 1985). Establishing specificity and correct utilization of either class of antibody enhances the credibility of the outcome, valuing the understanding of their inherent differences in the general framework of antigen-antibody interaction in molecular techniques (Figure 4.9).

4.3.2. Techniques for Generating Monoclonal Antibodies (mAbs)

Production of monoclonal antibodies is founded on sophisticated procedures that enhance specificity and yield. One of the typical methods begins with the immunization of suitable host animals, typically mice, with the target antigen. Following immunization, the animal spleen cells secreting multifarious antibodies against the antigen are harvested. They are subsequently fused with myeloma cells to create hybridomas that are engineered to proliferate indefinitely while still possessing the capability for secreting the target antibody. This fusion process is crucial because it allows for the selection of hybridomas secreting antibodies with high target antigen affinity. The produced mAbs can be cloned and amplified, leading to the production of a homogeneous population of antibodies, which is beneficial for many uses in research, diagnostics, and therapeutics. The production of hybridomas is the most critical once they are generated, and that is selecting the clones secreting the desired antibody. This is normally done by using ELISA to screen for secreted antibodies against the target antigen. Optimization of culture conditions, like nutrient composition and temperature regulation, is needed to be able to produce high concentrations of monoclonal antibodies. According to recent advances, high-concentration formulation issues also apply to monoclonal antibodies to be used in antibody-drug conjugates (ADCs), to need tailored formulations to provide the stability and activity of the antibodies under various conditions (Alves, 2019). Optimal selection and amplification of hybridoma cells are the key to ensuring that the resulting antibody product possesses the necessary specificity and functionality for its intended application. Furthermore, novel protein engineering techniques are expanding the horizons of monoclonal antibody production. As the demand for customized probes in biomarker research grows, the application of various antibody formats like Fab fragments, single-chain variable fragments (scFvs), and small nanobodies is rapidly gaining prominence. These smaller antibody formats offer enhanced tissue penetration and reduced steric hindrance, which can be bothersome for larger antibodies (Saerens et al., 2008). Such engineering not only fills the gaps in conventional mAbs but also enables the generation of more generalized reagents for diagnostic and therapeutic use. As the science continues to advance, such approaches are sure to optimize the efficacy and availability of monoclonal antibody-based technologies, highlighting their significance in molecular techniques and antigen-antibody interactions (Figure 4.10).

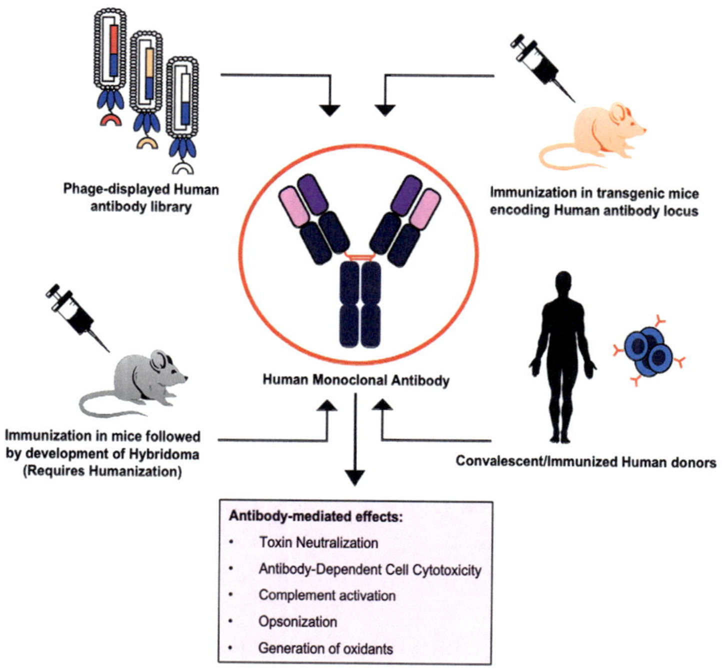

Figure 4.10. Strategies available for the development of human monoclonal antibodies (mAbs).

Source: https://www.researchgate.net/profile/Vaishali-Verma/publication/365860634/figure/fig1/AS:11431281103757409@1669812814762/Strategies-available-for-the-development-of-human-monoclonal-antibodies.png.

4.3.3. Applications of Recombinant Antibodies in Research

Applications of recombinant antibodies in research have transformed various industries, particularly diagnostic and drug research. Recombinant antibodies are very specific and exhibit strong affinity to antigens, and thus they make it simple for scientists to analyze complex biological systems. Their use is realized in the creation of biosensors, where recombinant antibodies serve as molecular elements of recognition that can detect biomarkers associated with various diseases. But the traditional antibodies possess some limitations, for instance, instability and loss of specificity when immobilized to sensor surfaces. Protein engineering is what has given rise to smaller antibody fragments like single-chain variable fragments (scFvs) and nanobodies, which shun these pitfalls. These improvements drastically enhance the performance of assays, offering researchers more sensitivity and accuracy in biomarker measurement, which is essential for detecting disease at an early stage and monitoring (Saerens et al., 2008). In addition, recombinant antibodies are at the center of revolutionizing drug discovery methods by their application in antibody engineering and bioassay development. As the knowledge about biological systems enhances and new technologies are being exploited, engineered antibodies allow for high-throughput screening of potential therapeutics against many diseases. New phage display and hybridoma technologies have speeded up the discovery of suitable antibodies with the desired characteristics, thus enhancing biologics development. Furthermore, the integration of lab-on-a-chip technologies has fueled these processes, allowing scientists to reduce complex experiments and amplify throughput. These innovations not only conserve time and costs in the drug discovery pipeline but also improve the overall efficacy and safety of therapeutic antibodies, marking a significant advancement in biopharmaceutical science and clinical translational uses (Jorgolli et al., 2019). The use of recombinant antibodies in several molecular techniques underscores their versatility and unequivocal role within a broad spectrum of research environments. Their use in personalized medicine is an example; recombinant antibodies can be engineered to bind to specific antigens associated with the disease profile of an individual. This individualized setting holds considerable utility in treating diseases like cancer, where specific tumor markers can be targeted easily. By employing recombinant antibodies, researchers can design targeted therapy with fewer off-target effects and enhanced treatment efficacy. The prospect of future study has more promise for recombinant antibodies to establish answers to erstwhile intractable questions in immunotherapy, vaccine development, and diagnostics, once again foreshadowing their fundamental significance in scientific research and clinical progress (Saerens et al., 2008; Jorgolli et al., 2019).

4.4. Advanced Techniques in Antigen-Antibody Interaction Studies

A comprehension and examination of antigen-antibody interactions has been greatly improved with the ability created by high-level molecular techniques. The techniques are important to the examination of specificity and binding affinity at the molecular level, an importance of considerable importance in applications to vaccine development, diagnostics, and therapy design. One of the promising avenues is the use of in-silico methods towards the prediction of B-cell epitopes, which has been shown to be more accurate and effective at identifying possible epitopes that are capable of eliciting strong immune responses. By the use of molecular mechanics, researchers have better described and ranked epitopes, thus paving the way for novel approaches to designing and manufacturing antibodies (Reitmaier, 2007). This shift towards computational methods not only offers increased prediction accuracy but also reduces the time and resources typically required in more traditional laboratory conditions. Furthermore, the integration of three-dimensional quantitative structure-activity relationship (3D-QSAR) models and experimental methodology is revolutionizing study of antigen-antibody interaction. Of special interest was a study that employed comparative molecular field analysis (CoMFA) to derive a 3D-QSAR model for monoclonal antibody (MabSMR) binding sulfonamide analogs. The interdisciplinary work combined fluorescence polarization immunoassay (FPIA) and CoMFA to measure binding affinity, with high r2 values indicating good predictive ability. This new strategy not only facilitates the assessment of interactions but also provides a powerful tool for designing novel antibodies and haptens with optimized properties, contributing immensely to the field of immunochemistry (Wu et al., 2008). These advances underscore the power of cooperative research in science, with advances that can result in groundbreaking therapeutic advances. Lastly, the achievements in antigen-antibody interaction studies are further evidenced by the use of high-throughput screening strategies, which permit the simultaneous analysis of vast libraries of antibodies. This method enables the identification of low-abundance antibodies with desirable binding characteristics, thereby accelerating the development process for certain immunological applications. Augmented by recent breakthroughs in gene editing tools such as CRISPR, researchers can now efficiently design and screen engineered variants of antibodies with tailored specificities. By integrating these high-throughput methods with computational predictive models, researchers not only can identify good antibody leads but also can refine their characteristics to achieve optimal efficacy while reducing off-target activities. Together, these advanced techniques collectively facilitate greater understanding of antigen-antibody interactions, which in turn facilitate the development of more effective diagnostic tools and therapeutic reagents within the biomedical field.

4.4.1. Surface Plasmon Resonance (SPR)

SPR has also emerged as a major technique in the study of antigen-antibody interactions, with a label-free, real-time approach to monitor binding events. This optical sensor exploits the unique properties of surface plasmons—coherent free electron oscillations at the metal-dielectric interface—whose coherence is sensitive to the refractive index. SPR's appeal lies in the fact that binding kinetics, i.e., association and dissociation rates, which are essential in understanding molecular interactions giving rise to immune responses, can be measured. By monitoring the movement of the resonance wavelength or intensity, researchers can examine such interactions with sensitivity and specificity, providing insights into the biolayer formation, binding affinities, and molecular recognition dynamics in applications ranging from drug discovery to clinical diagnosis.

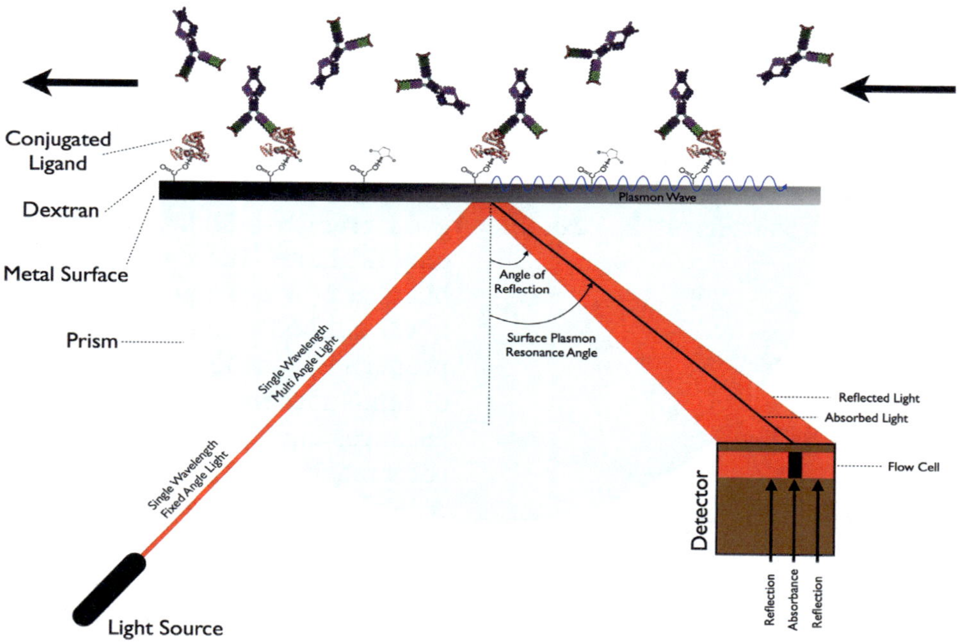

Figure 4.11. Illustration of surface plasmon resonance (SPR).

Source: https://upload.wikimedia.org/wikipedia/commons/thumb/d/d5/Surface_Plasmon_Resonance_%28SPR%29.jpg/800px-Surface_Plasmon_Resonance_%28SPR%29.jpg.

SPR technology is facilitated by flexibility in a broad range of biological environments, including application in immunoassays for disease biomarker detection. As highlighted in recent literature, an enormous advancement has been observed in the use of optical sensors like SPR for developing quick and sensitive diagnostics for clinical applications. SPR-based devices can detect low concentrations of target proteins, such as cardiac troponin, necessary in the diagnosis of acute myocardial infarction. This ability to detect particular antigens within complex biological matrices such as blood or serum places SPR at the forefront of leading-edge diagnostic methods. The simplicity of real-time analysis label-free makes SPR a valuable resource for facilitating speed and accuracy in clinical assessments, particularly in the detection of disease at an early stage and monitoring therapeutic response, as explored in a number of reviews of optical sensors (Pirzada & Altintas, 2020). Furthermore, the marriage of SPR with advanced multiplexing even expands its application in clinical diagnostics. By allowing simultaneous detection of a greater than one antigen, SPR enhances its utility as a personalized medicine tool. This is particularly relevant in the context of the growing need for whole biomarkers that can guide treatment decisions, particularly for the individual patient. The ability to define several interaction profiles also allows for further understanding of disease processes through defining the complex interplay between various antigens and antibodies. With researchers making leaps in this direction, the evolution of SPR technology promises big things to radically improve the development of effective and efficient diagnostic devices. The ongoing investment in such molecular techniques not only enhances our diagnostic potential but also stimulates future forays into biomolecular interactions and therapeutics (Abdolrahim et al., 2015) (Figure 4.11).

4.4.2. Bio-Layer Interferometry (BLI)

BLI is a prominent breakthrough among biomolecular interaction analysis methods, particularly applicable to studies on antigen-antibody interactions. BLI is an optical biosensing approach allowing researchers to monitor the process of binding in real time, providing valuable information on kinetics and affinity without labeling the participating biomolecules. BLI operates on the principle of sensing the changes in interference patterns caused by molecules binding to a biosensor surface. Through this non-destructive technique, BLI can generate fine interaction profiles, thereby significantly enhancing our knowledge of the binding processes of antigen-antibody interactions. Therefore, BLI has been a versatile tool not only for standard research but also for drug discovery and diagnostic applications, and it is vital in molecular techniques dealing with immunology. One of the key strengths of BLI is that it is capable of detecting label-free, as this eliminates potential artifacts created through labeling methods. This feature yields more accurate measurements for real-time interactions under physiological conditions. For example, the bio-layer on the sensor surface can be functionalized with diverse capture agents, including antibodies or protein receptors, and thus be suitable for use in multiple types of assays. New breakthroughs have also broadened the applications of BLI by introducing new immobilization strategies. Methods like polyethylene imine (PEI)-based immobilization of antibodies have been proven to increase the sensitivity and reproducibility of binding in assays. Specifically this method leveraged the deposition of a hyperbranched layer of PEI through which antibodies could be immobilized effectively and, ultimately, a label-free assay of target proteins such as C-Reactive Protein (CRP) (Kurunczi et al., 2013). These advances represent the pivotal role of BLI in serving as an enrichment of experimental setups that investigate antigen-antibody interactions. Moreover, the use of bio-layer interferometry with molecularly imprinted polymers (MIPs) is a promising prospect for enhancing sensor performance in biosensing. MIPs are artificially made polymers with specific binding sites for target molecules, which are similar to natural antibodies. When incorporated with BLI, these kinds of polymers can potentially enhance selectivity and sensitivity to analytes like proteins. For example, research demonstrated that polyacrylamide-based MIP efficiently created a specific layer over BLI sensors for precise measuring of bovine hemoglobin interactions. The results identified that with the presence of an imprint, the sensor efficiently captured the target molecule with low cross-reactivity toward other proteins and displayed the enhancement of the detection parameters (Reddyy et al., 2012). This BLI-MIP synergy represents the changing landscape in molecular methodology, as both enable strong analysis of antigen-antibody interactions that have therapeutic and diagnostic development potential (Figure 4.12).

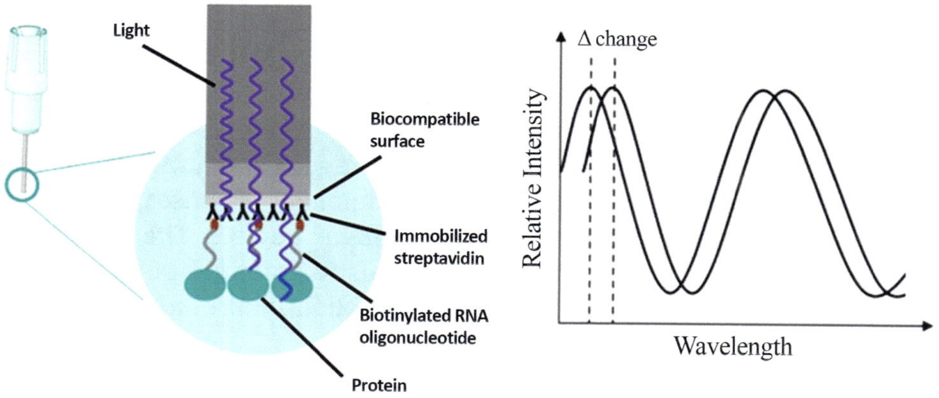

Figure 4.12. Schematic representation of the principle of the bio-layer interferometry (BLI) system.

Source: https://www.profacgen.com/wp-content/themes/profacgen/img/Bio-layer-Interferometry-BLI-Service.jpg.

4.4.3. Mass Spectrometry for Interaction Analysis

Mass spectrometry is a highly effective analytical tool for interaction analysis in antigen-antibody interactions. This approach capitalizes on the ability to measure the mass-to-charge ratio of ions, which can be used to characterize biomolecules in a very sensitive and specific way. With mass spectrometry, researchers can study the subtleties of antigen-antibody interactions at the molecular level. The ability to monitor and quantify binding affinities and kinetic processes provides a thorough comprehension of how antibodies bind antigens. Consequently, mass spectrometry enhances the process of designing therapeutic antibodies and developing more efficient diagnostic tools, making it a critical technique for encouraging molecular immunology. Furthermore, the diversity of mass spectrometry is also usable in structural biology since it provides data regarding antibody-antigen binding conformational changes. By studying the resultant fragmentation patterns of complexed molecules, researchers learn about the structural dynamics and regions that are involved in the interaction. Such information is relevant in designing monoclonal antibodies, for which small differences in binding sites can influence efficacy and specificity significantly. Furthermore, the integration of mass spectrometry with other techniques, such as surface plasmon resonance and high-resolution imaging, facilitates a complete investigation of antigen-antibody interactions. Synergistically, this increases both the information derived from mass spectrometry and the accuracy of interaction analysis in practical circumstances. Mass spectrometry is certainly very useful in resolving antigen-antibody interactions. Nevertheless, it also has some weaknesses to which scientists must address their attention. For instance, a need for complex sample preparation and the potential for ion suppression in matrices can make analysis more difficult. Moreover, because applications of immunology will often involve large proteins or glycoproteins, the mass spectrometric analysis may require advanced techniques or adjustments to facilitate accurate outcomes. Addressing difficulties of this sort is crucial to the development of mass spectrometry-based approaches that are not only robust but also readily applicable on a large scale to immunological study. As highlighted by recent studies, the integration of mass spectrometry into routine analytical protocols for antibody-drug conjugates demonstrates the ongoing development and potential of this technology in the field of molecular techniques (Hulme et al., 2017; sAlves, 2019) (Figure 4.13).

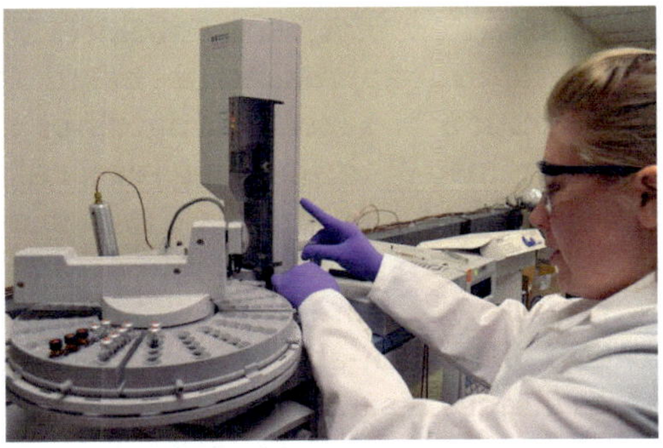

Figure 4.13. Mass spectrometry is a powerful analytical tool for antigen-antibody interactions analysis.

Source: https://img.mlo-online.com/files/base/ebm/mlo/image/2021/10/Mass_spec_courtesy_of_CDC.616744449f166.png?auto=format,compress&fit=max&q=45&w=640&width=640.

4.5. Applications in Disease Diagnosis

The role of antigen-antibody interactions in disease diagnosis has gained more importance in the wake of increasing development in biosensor technology. One of the most important developments that have been made here is the silicon nanochannel FET biosensor, which offers a very sensitive and label-free means of identifying certain biomarkers specific to numerous varied diseases, such as cancers. These sensors exploit silicon nanochannels' particular electrical properties, including their ability to detect single molecules due to their high surface-to-volume ratios. Therefore, FET biosensors can detect disease-related antigens at high speed and accuracy, thus paving the way towards early detection and apt monitoring of diseases such as breast cancer. The ability for the manufacture of highly multiplexed sensor arrays by top-down manufacturing strategies also enhances the utility of these biosensors in clinics and presents a paradigm shift in modern diagnostics (Mohanty et al., 2012). Besides biosensors, systems biology integration into disease diagnosis has entirely revolutionized the appreciation of various pathologies. The paradigm is shifting from purely phenomenological models to very sophisticated network models explaining the molecular origins of cancer and other diseases. This integrated approach tries to bring biological data together with clinical diagnostics and thereby significantly enhance our ability to predict disease progression and modulate therapy on this basis. Emerging technologies, such as nanotechnology and microfluidics, are at the forefront, holding the promise of cheap and precise high-throughput diagnostic measurements. Through the integration of antigen-antibody interactions with these platforms, clinicians will be able to deliver stratified diagnostics tailored to individual patient profiles, thus avoiding one-size-fits-all treatment and diagnosis (Heath & Davis, 2008). The application also extends to the field of therapy with the development of nanoscale-based therapies. Not only do these illustrate the magnitude of antigen-antibody interactions as a diagnostic tool, but also their implication in therapy, since nanoparticles can be tailored to deliver drugs directly to the site of cancer cells. By bridging the gap between therapy and diagnostics, these novel strategies aim to maximize therapeutic efficacy with minimal risk of the common side effects of chemotherapy. With growing research, diagnostic strategies grounded on advanced molecular interactions increasingly appear as a necessity. Such innovations not only have the potential to enhance early detection but also to play a pivotal role in the ongoing battle against multifactorial diseases, ultimately improving their patients' longevity and quality of life (Heath & Davis, 2008).

4.5.1. Role of Antigen-Antibody Interactions in Infectious Disease Detection

The intricate interaction between antigens and antibodies plays a vital role in the realm of infectious disease detection. Antigens, i.e., substances that cause an immune response, are either of pathogenic origin, e.g., from bacteria, viruses, or fungi. When the immune system recognizes such foreign material, antibodies specific to the respective antigens are produced. The antigen-antibody reaction is a fundamental concept of diagnostic tests, permitting the detection of infectious agents. Techniques like ELISA and western blotting are used most frequently to detect these interactions. Sensitivity and specificity of the tests become a matter of utmost significance, given the rapidly evolving infectious disease scenario, where correct and timely diagnosis can prove to be a game-changer for patients. New advances in molecular techniques further enhance the role played by antigen-antibody interactions in the detection of disease. Techniques such as polymerase chain reaction (PCR) have improved the detection of recognized pathogens by targeting their genetic material. For example, in studies on enteric disease in pigs, PCR-based diagnostic tests have provided reliable detection of pathogenic microorganisms such as *Lawsonia intracellularis* and reduced the time needed for diagnosis (Jacobson, 2003). These molecular approaches not only increase the sensitivity of detection but also make it possible to identify pathogens in complex biological samples, where traditional methods may not be successful. Therefore, antigen-antibody binding combined with molecular approaches is a promising field in infectious disease diagnostics, with the potential for more specific and quicker identification of infectious pathogens. Besides, the increased prevalence of drug-resistant infections highlights the importance of advanced detection methods that are not only able to detect the presence of pathogens but also the drug susceptibility of the pathogens. The issue posed by opportunistic infections, such as those caused by resistant yeast species, stresses the importance of rapid and accurate detection methods in healthcare centers (Consortium OPATHY & Gabaldón, 2019). Present therapeutic approaches are based on the early recognition of specific antigens of these resistant strains. With ongoing research, the combination of high-throughput technologies, such as next-generation sequencing and proteomics, may potentially revolutionize the application of antigen-antibody interactions to infectious disease diagnosis. These technologies hold promise for accelerating and refining diagnostics, ultimately leading to improved infection control and patient care in the face of emerging pathogenic threats.

4.5.2. Use in Autoimmune Disease Diagnostics

Antigen-antibody interactions have also received serious consideration in autoimmune disease diagnosis due to the ability to improve early diagnosis and therapy response. Autoimmune diseases are diseases in which the immune system attacks the body's own tissues rather than pathogens, and they are difficult to diagnose due to the variety of clinical manifestations as well as overlapping symptoms. Traditional diagnosis traditionally relies on indirect markers of autoimmune activity through clinical presentation, radiologic evaluation, or tissue biopsy. New advances in molecular technology, particularly in biomarker identification, can allow the detection of specific autoantibodies that can serve as good markers for autoimmune disease. Through the application of techniques such as ELISAs or western blotting to detect these autoantibodies, clinical laboratories are able to achieve an earlier and more specific diagnosis, allowing timely intervention and treatment regimen in autoimmune disease patients.

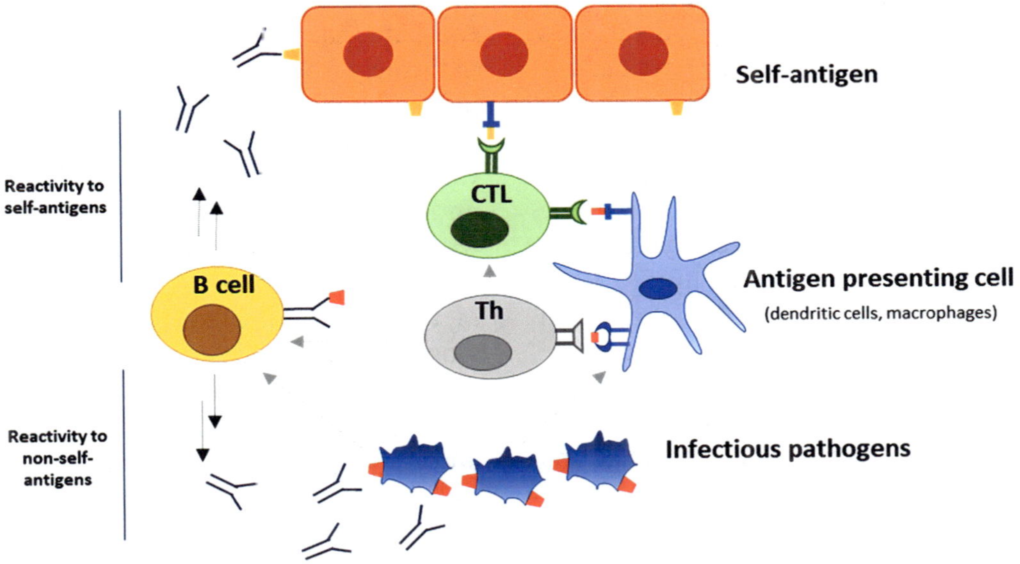

Figure 4.14. Schematic illustration of molecular mimicry associated with autoimmunity. Infectious pathogens express non-self-antigens (red box) that are similar in amino acid sequence or structure to self-antigens (yellow box). The immune response directed toward the infectious pathogens may cross-react with self-antigens, resulting in tissue damage, among others, by antibody effector functions stimulating complement activation along with antibody-dependent cytotoxicity, and cytotoxic T cells (CTL) inflicting cytotoxic tissue damage.

Source: https://www.mdpi.com/ijms/ijms-24-13609/article_deploy/html/images/ijms-24-13609-g002.png.

To be specific, taking advantage of the specificity of antibodies to autoantigens is a paradigm shift to personalized medicine in autoimmune diagnosis. Autoantibodies vary significantly from one person to another and thus reflect the unique autoimmune profile of any patient. This variation has prompted scientists to discover different biomarkers corresponding to various autoimmune diseases. For instance, anti-nuclear antibodies (ANAs) have been used routinely as a screening test for systemic lupus erythematosus, while rheumatoid factor and anti-citrullinated protein antibodies are essential for rheumatoid arthritis. As hybridoma technology and recombinant antibody production advance, the development of more sensitive and specific assays for the detection of these autoantibodies becomes increasingly possible. These newer technologies hold out the promise of enabling healthcare professionals to diagnose autoimmune diseases more efficiently, possibly even before massive tissue damage can occur, validating the utility of biomarker detection techniques in contemporary diagnostics (Saeed et al., 2017). In addition, newer molecular techniques have increased the diagnostic horizons for autoimmune diseases even more. Advanced technologies, such as phage display technology, enable scientists to identify rare and specific autoantibodies, giving a better insight into the immune status of an individual. Using genetically engineered antibodies, scientists are now able to construct assays that are not only more sensitive but also more specific and targeted towards relevant autoantigens. This is particularly valuable in that it reduces the possibility of false positives associated with serological analysis. In addition, utilization of multiplex assays enables simultaneous measurement of multiple autoantibodies, providing a more comprehensive picture of a patient's autoimmune profile. With these diagnostic tools advancing, they hold great potential to revolutionize the clinical environment for the treatment of autoimmune disease, enhancing patient outcomes by precision-directed therapeutic interventions (Jamal, 2017) (Figure 4.14).

4.5.3. Applications in Cancer Biomarker Identification

Verification and identification of cancer biomarkers are necessary in the creation of diagnostic and therapeutic methods. A few molecular techniques have been formulated, employing antigen-antibody interactions to enhance sensitivity and specificity in biomarker detection. Through the use of advanced immunoassays such as ELISA, scientists can measure biomarkers present in body fluids, thus facilitating early cancer detection. Also, the application of optical sensors has been reported to improve the performance of these assays considerably, with the capability to generate rapid and reproducible results. Recent studies illustrate how optical sensors are applied to detect proteins and disease biomarkers in various sample types and how they can be applied to real-time clinical applications, especially in point-of-care testing environments (Pirzada & Altintas, 2020). Successful biomarker discovery ultimately facilitates personalized medicine approaches, which improve patient outcomes through targeted therapy that is specially designed to match individual molecular signatures. In cancer biomarker discovery, the value of specific and stable recognition moieties cannot be overemphasized. The employment of antibodies has been a venerable norm for the detection of biomarkers because they are extremely specific and possess high binding affinities for target antigens. However, there are issues such as steric hindrance and instability that call for the development of more advanced antibody formats to ensure efficient analysis (Saerens et al., 2008). Techniques such as protein engineering have enabled the manipulation of antibodies into smaller versions such as single-chain variable fragments (scFv) and nanobodies, which maintain the efficiency of binding while preventing issues related to size and stability. These new forms find the greatest utility in complex biological samples, where they can navigate dense environments more effectively. The structural design optimization of binding probes is therefore at the forefront of enhancing the accuracy and reliability of cancer biomarker detection. The dynamic nature of cancer biomarkers means constant innovation in detection technologies. Leveraging the strength of antigen-antibody interaction through molecular technology advancements is essential to addressing this challenge. For instance, multiplex assays are now capable of detecting an array of biomarkers in a single analysis, providing an overall perspective on tumor development and behavior. In addition to the multiparameter approach aiding diagnosis, it also allows therapeutic decision-making by determining biomarker expression in specific cancer phenotypes. With the capability of newer biosensor technologies, scientists can now make use of more advanced assays that enhance the accuracy of diagnosis and prognostic potential. Application of molecular methods in the study of antigen-antibody interactions has been of tremendous potential in revolutionizing cancer detection through treatment, an area that underscores the critical junction of antigen-antibody interactions and molecular approaches in cancerology.

4.6. Challenges and Limitations

Studying antigen-antibody interactions with molecular approaches is confronted with various challenges and limitations that must be overcome by researchers. One of the fundamental issues lies with the precision and uniformity of current diagnostic testing. For instance, routine assays are usually preceded by preliminary culturing of the specimen, leading to delays in diagnosis and treatment. The sensitivity and specificity of these assays may also be less than optimal, leading to false positives or false negatives. This flaw is particularly crucial in clinical settings where timely intervention is imperative. As noted in Gwinner et al. (2016), the occurrence of opportunistic infections necessitates rapid and accurate identification, indicating a primary need for better techniques in detecting antigens and their respective antibodies. The biological variation inherent in samples is another urgent issue and complicates antigen-antibody interaction interpretation. Interindividual variability in immune response generates heterogeneity in the production and affinity of antibodies, which becomes a challenge in replicating results across populations. Moreover, external factors and comorbidities tend to skew the immune response, hence making standardization of assays challenging. Such heterogeneity might be particularly important in transplant patients, whereby rejection, as herein defined in Gwinner et al. (2016), is determined by numerous dynamic variables. This ultimately leads to the requirement of individualized strategies based on patient profiles, making it more complex to adopt molecular strategies into clinical practice. Moreover, the application of new technology in reality is itself difficult. Although innovations such as proteomics and high-throughput sequencing have the capacity to enhance diagnostic potential, they also require significant investment in terms of infrastructure and resources. The transition from laboratory research to clinical application normally encounters challenges as far as scaling and technology compatibility are concerned. On top of this, stringent testing of these approaches in different clinical conditions cannot be overemphasized, as in existing research efforts discussed in Consortium OPATHY & Gabaldón (2019). As these emerging methodologies continue to advance, addressing the deficits will be crucial to effective implementation in the diagnosis and treatment of antigen-antibody interaction with accuracy.

4.6.1. Specificity and Cross-Reactivity Issues

The specificity of antigen-antibody is paramount to an accurate diagnosis and cure of diseases. Antibodies are designed to bind specifically to their antigens with great specificity, like a lock and key; however, this is an oversimplification of a very complex reality. As discussed in most literature, the achievement and validation of antibody specificity involve overcoming serious issues. Various studies have established that the majority of commercially available antibodies do not possess the quality required for effective applications, and they have high cross-reaction rates. This has been aggravated when antibodies react to common epitopes among many proteins, and this can lead to false experimental results where non-target proteins are falsely labeled as positive, rendering the immunocytochemistry and other techniques null and void (Griffiths & Lucocq, 2014). Cross-reactivity is a big impediment to the successful application of antibodies in research and clinical settings. Not only does it compromise the integrity of experimental results, but it also results in misdiagnosis when used in diagnostic screens.

This intrinsic obstacle demands rigorous validation processes for antibody specificity, wherein scientists are being asked ever more frequently to screen their antibodies against a series of related antigens. Also, cross-reactivity could be the consequence of conformational changes within the antigen or the cross-reactive epitopes, which underscore the necessity of applying molecular approaches that interrogate these interactions at a high degree of detail. The necessity of generating antibodies that possess a minimum degree of cross-reactivity further complicates the situation since it requires an awareness of both the structural and functional characteristics of the involved antibodies (Yazdani et al., 2015).

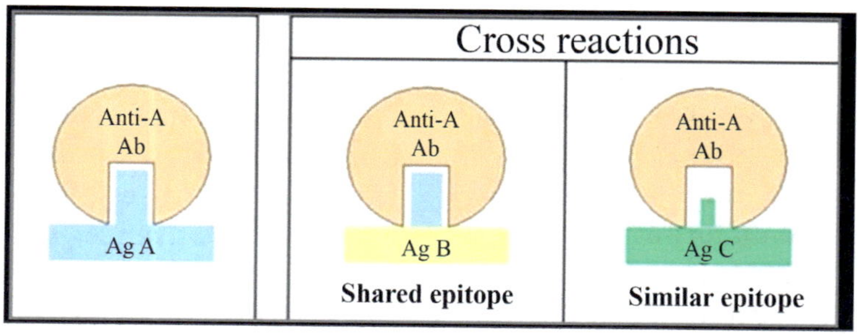

Figure 4.15. Showing cross cross-reactive interaction between antigen and antibody.

Source: https://www.researchgate.net/profile/Manzoor-Mir/publication/348555653/figure/fig29/AS:981897345765388@1611113978298/Showing-Cross-reactive-interaction-between-antigen-and-antibody-Source.jpg.

Most applicable here is the role additives play in stabilizing antibodies so that they become more specific and functionally reliable. Recent advances have indicated that while antibodies are precious reagents, their performance can be significantly affected by environmental factors and formulation strategies. Addition of stabilizing excipients such as sucrose and trehalose has been shown to play a major role in maintaining the structural integrity of antibody binding sites. Research has indicated these additives inhibit aggregation and degradation, and thus maintain the relative reactivity of antibodies throughout critical procedures, such as ELISA (Yazdani et al., 2015). This is to highlight one of the novel solutions to specificity as well as cross-reactivity issues, suggesting that correct formulation strategies might unlock the formula to maximize the clinical use of antibody-based assays, leading to improved diagnostic results (Figure 4.15).

4.6.2. Limitations of Current Detection Techniques

Current detection procedures for antigen-antibody interactions, while being vital to molecular diagnostics, face daunting limitations that can hinder their usability and efficiency. Traditional methods, such as ELISAs and Western blotting, involve multiple steps and are thus labor-consuming and prone to human errors. Moreover, these approaches are not very sensitive in determining low-abundance biomarkers in complicated matrices that might be particularly valuable in cancer diagnosis. Missing such subtle changes can lead to false negatives that mask important changes that can be employed in the direction of treatment. Hence, the issue is not only to develop more sensitive assays but also to ensure that these processes can be used efficiently in clinical settings, particularly in situations where fast results have to be provided for timely medical treatment. Moreover, the currently employed methods of detection often lack specificity, which can lead to cross-reactivity with non-target antigens. This issue is particularly severe in multiplex assays that attempt to measure multiple biomarkers in parallel, leading to trouble in interpreting the results. As a result, the overall performance of such assays can be compromised, which is highly undesirable in critical applications like cancer diagnosis, where precise biomarker identification is critical in establishing targeted therapies. Efforts toward the exploitation of novel biosensing technologies aim to bridge these limitations. For instance, silicon nanochannel FET biosensors promise to provide greater sensitivity and specificity and therefore represent a robust alternative to conventional detection techniques (Mohanty et al., 2012). Such advancements are critical to the development of reliable diagnostics, particularly in very complex biological systems. Novel approaches, such as single-cell analysis, bring with them promising improvements but present their own challenges. While techniques like electrowetting nanopipette sensing are able to probe cellular dynamics at unprecedented resolution, they often require very sophisticated equipment and technical proficiency that is not readily accessible to most researchers (Bulbul et al., 2018). Moreover, issues of sample preparation, contamination, and the need for functionalized probes can complicate the process. As researchers continue to integrate such advanced technologies into practical applications, reproducibility of results and scalability are also important features to consider. Overcoming the limitations in current detection strategies for antigen-antibody interactions is fundamental to unlocking the full potential of molecular diagnostics in an effort to enhance patient outcomes through more and earlier detection strategies.

4.6.3. Ethical Considerations in Antibody Production

In the context of monoclonal antibody production, ethics emerges as a critical element that impacts research protocols as well as therapeutic use. The conventional production of monoclonal antibodies involves the use of living animals, which is a threat to the welfare of animals and the ethical issues related to utilizing living animals for science. While researchers work to reconcile the demands for practical diagnostic reagents and treatments with ethical responsibilities to minimize animal distress, alternative techniques become increasingly important. The research on synthetic antibodies, which might bypass a variety of traditional production problems, is only one instance of an expanding initiative to bring scientific advancement into consonance with moral responsibility. Such an identification is not only seminal in establishing public confidence but also key to ensuring the integrity of scientific research within the broader context of medicine and biotechnology. While the pursuit of synthetic antibodies presents a viable alternative, questions still linger regarding the ethical standards that control their creation and application. For instance, the new approach to the addition of unnatural amino acids into peptide sequences raises questions about safety and regulatory clearance. Though engineered peptides, made to mimic monoclonal antibodies, hold promise as therapies against certain diseases, their long-term effects are not yet fully understood. Ethical consideration needs to be conducted to ensure that such biomolecules made by synthesis do not cause unforeseen injury to patients or the environment. Alongside, the regulatory framework also needs to be calibrated to address such nuances of novel drugs so that ethical practice never undermines either patient safety or scientific integrity. The endeavor towards innovation must therefore go hand in hand with a will to ensure ethical integrity in the process. The introduction of engineered peptide biomolecules is not only accompanied by a shift in production methods but also by the need to challenge existing ethical frameworks in the study of antibodies. The use of computational design for peptide modification towards target specificity is a significant technological advancement, but it raises very profound intellectual property and commercialization questions. With scholarly studies increasingly aligning with commercial interests, the risk of ethical conflict in profit-generating goals needs a cautious approach to ensure equal access to innovations. Furthermore, commercial dynamics may drive the quality of ethics toward compromises, leading to potential exploitation by clinical trials of vulnerable populations. As the field progresses, an intense framework that incorporates ethical considerations will be important to guide decision-making so that developments in antigen-antibody interactions are inclusive, accessible, and devoted to the welfare of all concerned stakeholders.

SUMMARY

The study of antigen-antibody interactions by molecular techniques has significantly enhanced our understanding of immunological activity and its implications. The advances in biotechnology, particularly epitope prediction and characterization, have led the way to more targeted therapeutic interventions. For instance, the advent of new methodologies such as those that employ molecular mechanics for epitope categorization underscores the dynamic nature of research in this area. With the development of current techniques and new ones, scientists can advance the specificity and efficacy of antibody-based therapies to ultimately result in more efficient interventions in diseases like cancer and autoimmune disorders (Reitmaier, 2007). This emerging fact implies that a thorough knowledge of antigen-antibody interactions will continue to be at the heart of both fundamental research as well as clinical application. Furthermore, the synergy of interdisciplinary approaches has been key in shaping the science of antigen-antibody interactions. Recent studies involving genetic engineering combined with structural biology techniques such as X-ray crystallography have enabled investigators to determine the structure and affinity of various ligand-receptor systems at unprecedented levels of accuracy. These developments are further supported by developments in computing power and simulation techniques, which allow for intensive investigation of macromolecular interactions at the molecular and cellular levels. These developments not only enriched our theoretical knowledge but also introduced immediate experimental data to the dynamics of single ligand-receptor bonds, thus enriching our knowledge on the kinetic and mechanical nature of these interactions (Bongrand, 1999). Therefore, the convergence of several disciplines is an impetus for immunological innovation and treatment. Finally, given the enormous number of techniques developed to investigate antigen-antibody interactions, it is obvious that in the future there will be many more discoveries to follow. Ongoing invention of experimental techniques, such as atomic force microscopy and biomembrane probes, is a testament to the importance of observing in real time in order to unravel biological interactions. With the scientific world becoming more and more advanced in instruments and techniques, the possibilities of discovering new targets of therapy and improving existing treatment modalities will be enhanced manifold. This relentless pursuit of information, coupled with the enhanced understanding of the principles of antigen-antibody interactions, makes scientists more capable of dealing with complex health problems. Ultimately, the passion to advance molecular techniques within this field is a process of change that will revolutionize the future of immunotherapy in the coming years. Research into antigen-antibody interactions through the use of molecular techniques signals the complexity that resides within these fundamental biological interactions. Points noted emphasize the reliance on standardized antibodies within many applications, such as immunocytochemistry. While these reagents are in widespread use, the binding of antibodies to their respective antigens is more subtle than suggested by the classical "lock and key" model. Maintaining antibody specificity remains an open problem, since large numbers of commercially acquired antibodies fail to meet the stringent levels of quality required for reproducible experimental outcomes. This highlights an important point of antibody research: the need for rigorous validation and testing of the specificity of antibodies, particularly in immunolabeling procedures in light and electron microscopy (Griffiths & Lucocq, 2014).

Apart from antibody specificity, the physiology of neural crest cell interaction with laminin are valuable lessons in the dynamic nature of cell adhesion. The data indicate that the extent of attachment by the neural crest cells is proportional to the laminin concentrations. The interactions are mediated by β_(1-)integrins, as demonstrated by cell adhesion blockage by the CSAT antibody, which specifically binds to the chick β1 subunit of integrin. Additionally, the differential functionalities of integrins for cellular adhesion at varying laminin concentrations suggest that the neural crest cells utilize various mechanisms for interaction with extracellular matrices. Such a difference serves to underscore the importance of antibodies towards illuminating the structural and functional interactions underlying cell attachment processes and presents a future direction of research into cellular behavior and migration (Lallier & Bronner-Fraser, 1991).

The antigen-antibody interaction debate also encompasses methods to test and validate antibodies utilized in various assays. The increasingly recognized limitations of commercially sourced antibodies necessitate strict guidelines to ensure the acquisition of high-quality reagents. Quantitative methods, such as electron microscopy, need to be adopted by researchers in order to ascertain antibody labeling reproducibility. By adopting stringent testing regimens, molecular biology's precious resources can be made even more reliable and specific through the collective efforts of the research community. In conclusion, the incorporation of these watershed points illumines not just the intricacies and intricaments of antigen-antibody studies but also the necessity of stringent verification in broadening our understanding of molecular interactions as well as easing the efficacy of research protocols (Griffiths & Lucocq, 2014).

A CLOSER LOOK

ANTIBODY-MEDIATED REJECTION (AMR)

AMR is a clinical complication of organ transplantation, particularly kidney transplantation, where it is among the most common causes of late graft loss. AMR occurs when the immune system of the host produces antibodies that attack the transplanted organ, triggering inflammation and injury. It's critical to know the mechanisms, diagnosis, and treatment of AMR in an effort to improve long-term transplant outcomes (Figure 4.16).

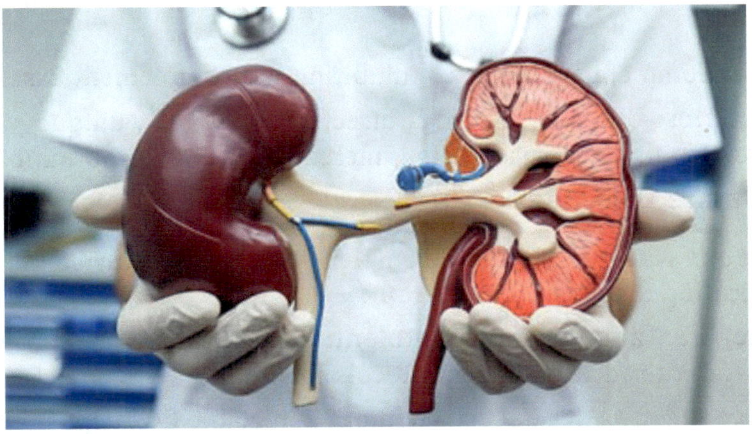

Figure 4.16. Kidney transplantation.

Source: https://images.onlymyhealth.com/imported/images/2024/September/23_Sep_2024/tmb-kidney-transplant.jpg.

1. Mechanisms of AMR:

a. **Donor-Specific Antibodies (DSAs):** The presence of DSAs, that is, antibodies directed against donor organ antigens, is typical of AMR. These may be pre-formed or newly formed de novo after the transplant.

b. **Complement Activation:** Complement proteins are activated by binding of DSAs to donor cells and initiate a cascade process that amplifies the inflammation and leads to tissue damage.

c. **Endothelial Damage:** AMR first targets the endothelium of the blood vessels of the graft and induces inflammation, microvascular injury, and eventually fibrosis.

d. **Histological Alterations:** Biopsy, in AMR, shows microvascular inflammation, C4d deposition (marker for complement activation), and signs of damage to the endothelium.

2. Diagnosis of AMR:

a. **Detection by DSA:** Detection of DSAs in recipient serum is an important diagnostic maneuver.

b. **Allograft Biopsy:** C4d staining, microvascular inflammation, and endothelial injury on biopsy support the diagnosis of AMR.

c. **Grading:** AMR diagnosis is typically graded by the intensity of DSA and biopsy findings, e.g., "possible," "probable," and "definite."

3. **Management of AMR:**

a. **Plasmapheresis:** Removes circulating DSAs from the recipient's blood.

b. **Intravenous Immunoglobulin (IVIg):** Can suppress antibody production and modulate immune response.

c. **Rituximab:** Monoclonal antibody directed against B cells, reducing antibody production.

d. **Bortezomib:** Proteasome inhibitor directed against plasma cells, reducing antibody production.

e. **Eculizumab:** Complement inhibitor inhibiting the complement cascade.

f. **Other Therapies:** Other novel drugs directed against the unique pathways responsible for AMR are also under consideration, including interleukin-6 inhibitors.

4. **Challenges and Future Directions:**

a. **Heterogeneous Nature:** AMR is a complex process with varied clinical manifestations, thus complicating diagnosis and therapy.

b. **Insufficiency of Standardized Treatment:** A need exists for more robust clinical trials to create standardized treatment protocols for AMR.

c. **C4d-Negative AMR:** AMR can occur without detectable C4d deposition, leading to further research on non-C4d diagnostic markers and treatment strategies.

d. **Prevention of New Pathways:** Ongoing research still attempts to discover new targets and treatments with which to prevent and treat AMR.

e. **Improving Organ Allocation:** Donor-recipient matching based on HLA typing or epitope matching could reduce the risk of AMR.

REFERENCES

1. Abdolrahim, M., Alhosseini, S. N., Rabiee, M., Tahriri, M., et al. (2015). Development of optical biosensor technologies for cardiac troponin recognition. https://core.ac.uk/download/213059311.pdf (accessed on 27th June 2025).
2. Tresguerres M, Salmerón C. Molecular, Enzymatic, and Cellular Characterization of Soluble Adenylyl Cyclase From Aquatic Animals. *Methods Enzymol.* 2018;605:525-549. doi:10.1016/bs.mie.2018.02.022(accessed on 27th June 2025).
3. Miho E, Yermanos A, Weber CR, Berger CT, Reddy ST, Greiff V. Computational Strategies for Dissecting the High-Dimensional Complexity of Adaptive Immune Repertoires. *Front Immunol.* 2018;9:224. Published 2018 Feb 21. doi:10.3389/fimmu.2018.00224 (accessed on 27th June 2025).
4. Pierre Bongrand. LIGAND-RECEPTOR INTERACTIONS. Reports on Progress in Physics, 1999, 62, pp.921-968. ffhal-00320498 (accessed on 27th June 2025).
5. Reddy, Subrayal M, Hawkins, DM, Phan, QT, Stevenson, D and Warriner, K (2012) Protein detection using hydrogel-based molecularly imprinted polymers integrated with dual polarisation interferometry. Sensors and Actuators, B: Chemical, 176 (Januar). 190 - 197. (accessed on 27th June 2025).
6. Pirzada M, Altintas Z. Recent Progress in Optical Sensors for Biomedical Diagnostics. *Micromachines (Basel).* 2020;11(4):356. Published 2020 Mar 30. doi:10.3390/mi11040356(accessed on 27th June 2025).
7. Alves, N. J. (2019). Antibody conjugation and formulation. https://core.ac.uk/download/189104594.pdf (accessed on 27th June 2025).
8. Amon, R., Chen, X., Fleishman, S. J., Glushka, J., et al. (2018). A combined computational-experimental approach to define the structural origin of antibody recognition of sialyl-Tn, a tumor-associated carbohydrate antigen. https://core.ac.uk/download/323068873.pdf (accessed on 27th June 2025).
9. Consortium OPATHY, Gabaldón T. Recent trends in molecular diagnostics of yeast infections: from PCR to NGS. *FEMS Microbiol Rev.* 2019;43(5):517-547. doi:10.1093/femsre/fuz015(accessed on 27th June 2025).
10. Stenberg PE, McEver RP, Shuman MA, Jacques YV, Bainton DF. A platelet alpha-granule membrane protein (GMP-140) is expressed on the plasma membrane after activation. *J Cell Biol.* 1985;101(3):880-886. doi:10.1083/jcb.101.3.880(accessed on 27th June 2025).
11. Chowdhury R, Rasheed M, Keidel D, et al. Protein-protein docking with F(2)Dock 2.0 and GB-rerank. *PLoS One.* 2013;8(3):e51307. doi:10.1371/journal.pone.0051307(accessed on 27th June 2025).
12. Batiuk, E., Kiyohara, C., & Nguyen, T. (2017). Engineering synthetic antibody by expanded genetic code. https://core.ac.uk/download/84118620.pdf (accessed on 27th June 2025).
13. Torina A, Cordaro A, Blanda V, et al. A promising new ELISA diagnostic test for cattle babesiosis based on Babesia bigemina Apical Membrane Antigen-1. *Vet Ital.* 2016;52(1):63-69. doi:10.12834/VetIt.74.237.2(accessed on 27th June 2025).

14. Saerens D, Huang L, Bonroy K, Muyldermans S. Antibody Fragments as Probe in Biosensor Development. *Sensors (Basel)*. 2008;8(8):4669-4686. Published 2008 Aug 8. doi:10.3390/s8084669(accessed on 27th June 2025).

15. Lallier, T., & Bronner-Fraser, M. (1991). Avian neural crest cell attachment to laminin: involvement of divalent cation dependent and independent integrins. *Development (Cambridge, England)*, *113*(4), 1069–1084. https://doi.org/10.1242/dev.113.4.1069(accessed on 27th June 2025).

16. Khan, G., E., S., Denniss, F., Sigurdardottir, D., & Gui, B. (2013). Identification and Validation of Targets for Cancer Immunotherapy: From the Bench-to-Bedside. InTech. doi: 10.5772/54698(accessed on 27th June 2025).

17. Bulbul, G., Chaves, G., Olivier, J., Joseph, A., Ozel, T., et al. (2018). Nanopipettes as monitoring probes for the single living cell: State of the art and future directions in molecular biology. https://core.ac.uk/download/323063966.pdf (accessed on 27th June 2025).

18. Januzzi JL Jr, Butler J, Jarolim P, et al. Effects of Canagliflozin on Cardiovascular Biomarkers in Older Adults With Type 2 Diabetes. *J Am Coll Cardiol*. 2017;70(6):704-712. doi:10.1016/j.jacc.2017.06.016(accessed on 27th June 2025).

19. Cantatore, S., De Carlo, D., Fineschi, V., Fiore, A., et al. (2015). Confocal laser scanning microscope, Raman microscopy and western blotting to evaluate inflammatory response after myocardial infarction. https://core.ac.uk/download/54248088.pdf (accessed on 27th June 2025).

20. Mohanty, P., Chen, Y., Erramilli, S., Hong, M. K., et al. (2012). Field effect transistor nano sensor for breast cancer diagnostics. Invited Review in Biosensors and Molecular Technologies for Cancer Diagnostics, edited by K. H. Herold and A. Rasooly (CRC Press, 2012) https://open.bu.edu/bitstream/2144/28273/1/1401.1168v1.pdf (accessed on 27th June 2025).

21. Jorgolli M, Nevill T, Winters A, et al. Nanoscale integration of single cell biologics discovery processes using optofluidic manipulation and monitoring. *Biotechnol Bioeng*. 2019;116(9):2393-2411. doi:10.1002/bit.27024

22. Heath JR, Davis ME. Nanotechnology and cancer. *Annu Rev Med*. 2008;59:251-265. doi:10.1146/annurev.med.59.061506.185523(accessed on 27th June 2025).

23. Evans, T., & Therriault, J. H. (2016). Computational design of synthetic antibodies for consumer diagnostic tests. https://core.ac.uk/download/72852881.pdf (accessed on 27th June 2025).

24. Goodyear, R. J., & Richardson, G. P. (2003). A novel antigen sensitive to calcium chelation that is associated with the tip links and kinocilial links of sensory hair bundles. https://core.ac.uk/download/2721964.pdf (accessed on 27th June 2025).

25. Gopal, A., & Herr, A. E. (2019). Multiplexed in-gel microfluidic immunoassays: Characterizing protein target loss during reproving of benzophenone-modified hydrogels. https://core.ac.uk/download/286362232.pdf (accessed on 27th June 2025).

26. Griffiths, G., & Lucocq, J. M. (2014). Antibodies for immunolabeling by light and electron microscopy: Not for the faint hearted. https://core.ac.uk/download/30318334.pdf (accessed on 27th June 2025).

27. Tan HR, Gross J, Uhlhaas PJ. MEG-measured auditory steady-state oscillations show high test-retest reliability: A sensor and source-space analysis. *Neuroimage*. 2015;122:417-426. doi:10.1016/j.neuroimage.2015.07.055(accessed on 27th June 2025).

28. Gwinner, W., Husi, H., Marx, D., Metzger, J., et al. (2016). Proteomics for rejection diagnosis in renal transplant patients: Where are we now? https://core.ac.uk/download/46559952.pdf (accessed on 27th June 2025).

29. S. Kurunczi a , A. Hainard b , K. Juhász a, D. Patkó a, N. Orgován a, N. Turck b , J.C. Sanchez b , R. Horvath(2013). Polyethylene imine-based receptor immobilization for label free bioassays. Sensors and Actuators B 181 (2013) 71-76. https://core.ac.uk/download/11856936.pdf (accessed on 27th June 2025).

30. Jacobson, M. (2003). Enteric diseases in pigs from weaning to slaughter. https://core.ac.uk/download/11694636.pdf (accessed on 27th June 2025).

31. Jamal, T. (2017). Cancer biomarkers, and novel techniques for detection. https://open.bu.edu/bitstream/2144/26755/5/Jamal_bu_0017N_13232.pdf (accessed on 27th June 2025).

32. Meier-Schellersheim, M. & Mack, G. (1999). SIMMUNE, a tool for simulating and analyzing immune system behavior. e-Print: cs/9903017 [cs]. http://arxiv.org/abs/cs/9903017 (accessed on 27th June 2025).

33. Yazdani Y, Mohammadi S, Yousefi M, Shokri F. Preliminary Assessment of Various Additives on the Specific Reactivity of Anti- rHBsAg Monoclonal Antibodies. *Avicenna J Med Biotechnol.* 2015;7(4):145-150.(accessed on 27th June 2025).

34. Hulme HE, Meikle LM, Wessel H, et al. Mass spectrometry imaging identifies palmitoylcarnitine as an immunological mediator during Salmonella Typhimurium infection. *Sci Rep.* 2017;7(1):2786. Published 2017 Jun 5. doi:10.1038/s41598-017-03100-5(accessed on 27th June 2025).

35. Reitmaier, R. (2007). Review of immunoinformatic approaches to *in-silico* B-cell epitope prediction. https://core.ac.uk/download/pdf/287415.pdf (accessed on 27th June 2025).

36. Saeed, A. F. U. H., Wang, R., Wang, S., & Ling, S. (2017). Antibody engineering for pursuing a healthier future. https://core.ac.uk/download/pdf/82883279.pdf (accessed on 27th June 2025).

37. Sumiya, K., & Takahashi, N. (1990). Preparation and characterization of the antibody against the aldobiouronic acid unit of Xylan. Wood research: bulletin of the Wood Research Institute Kyoto University. 1990, 77: 8-17. https://core.ac.uk/download/39187464.pdf (accessed on 27th June 2025).

38. Wu, C., Jiang, H., Shen, J., Cheng, L., Beier, R. C., Cao, X., Yang, X., et al. (2008). Three-dimensional quantitative structure-activity relationships of sulfonamides binding monoclonal antibody by comparative molecular field analysis. https://core.ac.uk/download/pdf/288200.pdf (accessed on 27th June 2025).

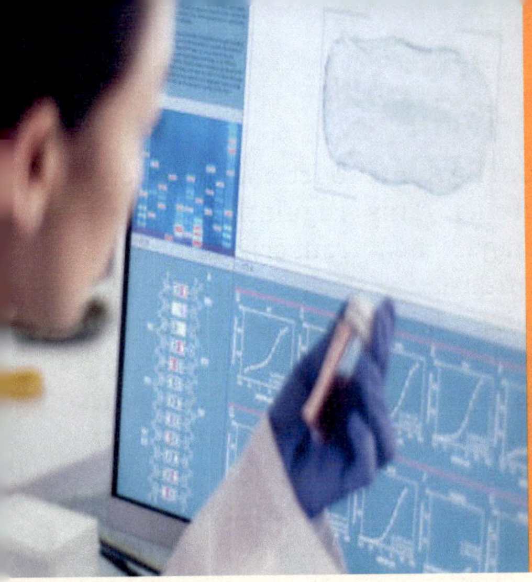

Chapter 5

GENE EXPRESSION ANALYSIS IN IMMUNOLOGY

Contents

Introduction

Gene expression is a fundamental concept that serves as the foundation of studying biological functions, particularly in immunology. Gene expression refers to the process whereby genetic information encoded in DNA is translated into mRNA and further into proteins. These proteins frequently have key functions in immune responses, including the ability to recognize pathogens and coordinate the elimination of foreign entities. With advances in molecular biology and bioinformatics, it is now possible to deconstruct the gene expression profiles of immune cells during different immune challenges, allowing us to better appreciate how gene regulation is involved in the establishment of immunity. By examining differential gene expression during infections, scientists are able to explain the mechanisms that control immune cell activation and differentiation, which may result in the development of more effective therapeutic strategies in immunological diseases and infections. In recent years, focus on gene expression analysis has been expedited in immunology because of a boom in technological advances such as high-throughput RNA sequencing and microarray analysis. Such methods provide never-before-possible data on immune activation and resolution of inflammation dynamics at the gene activity level. Through comparison of gene expression patterns in different immune cells and under different conditions, researchers have found novel biomarkers that represent immune status and function. Such studies are of great importance, particularly in terms of recognizing how some genes, such as RELM-β, are involved in maintaining gut barrier integrity and overall immune function. RELM-β, which has been studied in a number of research works, is an important biomarker of the immune response during gastrointestinal infection, depicting how expression of the genes can track the body's adaptive as well as physiological status in eliminating pathogens (Ahmed et al., 2019). The integration of gene expression analysis into immunology not only identifies cellular processes in immune responses but also highlights the issue that scientists face in translocating these into clinical applications. The relative paucity of genomic resources for certain species, particularly those relevant to aquaculture and marine biology, has been discussed in some recent reviews. The decapod crustacean immunology is the prime example of this issue; while our understanding of their innate immunity has come a long way, the lack of immortal cell lines and genomic information constrains current research (Hauton, 2012). Hence, it is essential to invest in genomic resources and innovative technologies that enhance our capacity to follow and regulate gene expression in immunology. By continuous research and collaboration, the utility of gene expression analysis can be expanded, eventually leading to improved disease control in wildlife and farmed populations.

Definition of Gene Expression

Gene expression is a fundamental biological process that defines the translation of genetic information from DNA into functional products, primarily proteins. This regulation occurs at different stages, i.e., transcription, RNA processing, and translation, each of which plays a crucial role in determining the quantity and type of proteins synthesized in a cell. In immunology, gene expression is particularly critical because it regulates the functioning and differentiation of immune cells. For example, immune responses are greatly dependent on the expression of certain genes encoding cytokines, receptors, and other effector molecules necessary for immune function and cell communication. Hence, knowledge regarding gene expression patterns is very important in providing insights into how immune cells react to pathogens and how homeostasis is established within the body. Gene expression can be controlled by numerous internal and external cues, illustrating the complexity of cell response. In the immune system, environmental stimuli through cytokines or pathogens can heavily alter gene expression profiles among immune cell subsets. For example, innate lymphoid cells (ILCs) are plastic in their gene expression because they can adapt and respond to different inflammatory signals. Specifically, ILC3s can convert to a type 1 response phenotype under the influence of specific cytokine conditions, representing a dynamic interplay between gene regulation and cell fate determination. As shown in recent studies, the presence of IL-23 can trigger specific transcription factors like STAT4 and T-BET that regulate the expression of critical effector molecules like IL-22 and IFN-γ, showing how precisely balanced gene expression is required for normal immune responses (Mikami et al., 2018). Moreover, the concept of gene expression is not just mere transcriptional events; it encompasses intricate processes of post-transcriptional modifications and epigenetic control. In macrophages, for example, autophagy-related signaling pathways might tune gene expression for genes that are involved in polarization, emphasizing the role of cellular milieus of expression. CD5L, an essential glycoprotein, controls macrophage polarization through the regulation of inflammation and the process of repair-related gene expression. Evidence indicates that CD5L-induced autophagy enhances gene expression for genes regulated by the ID3 transcription factor and, correspondingly, dictates macrophage reactions to inflammatory stimuli (Sanjurjo et al., 2018). This illustrates the interconnectedness of gene expression mechanisms and immunological impact, evincing the necessity of gene expression analysis in its entirety for understanding immune reactions and designing therapeutic interventions (Figure 5.1).

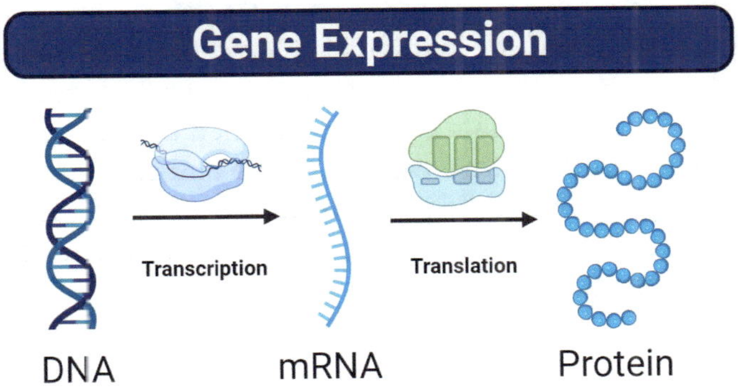

Figure 5.1. Illustration of gene expression.

Source: https://microbenotes.com/wp-content/uploads/2023/10/Gene-Expression.jpeg.

Importance in Biological Processes

The intricacies of gene expression are significant controls over biological function and the basis for cellular and organismal response to stimuli. In immunology, the control of gene expression is crucial to immune cell development and function. In invasion by pathogens, specific genes become activated to initiate a protective response, leading to the production of proteins that facilitate immune recognition and tissue repair. As an illustration, the process of activation of cytokine-related genes is at the core of determining the resolution of immune reactions, including inflammation and immune tolerance. Therefore, understanding the nuances of gene expression not only streamlines our grasp of immune mechanisms but also reveals the potential of therapeutic interventions to modulate these genetic processes to combat disease efficiently. In addition, advances in gene expression analysis have significantly enhanced our capacity to examine the complexity of immunological processes. Through techniques such as quantitative PCR and RNA sequencing, researchers are able to quantify variation in gene expression levels among various immune cell types under varied conditions. Such specificity is essential for defining the immune landscape during health and disease and the discovery of prospective biomarkers and therapeutic targets. The addition of bioinformatics tools further supports such activities by promoting the interpretation of vast quantities of data acquired during the process of gene expression studies. Such methods are a demonstration of the role played by gene expression in biology, especially as it relates to achieving the dynamicity of immune responses and the implication in diseases like autoimmunity and cancer. With the deluge of information from biomedical research, the requirement for formal frameworks of data interpretation has been apparent for a long time. The sheer quantity of articles and findings could obscure valuable insight and consequently hinder full knowledge of gene function and regulation in immunology. Work towards establishing minimum information standards and controlled vocabularies is most critical in overcoming this barrier. Through creating systematic, machine-readable frameworks for the representation of data, researchers can enhance the availability of data and facilitate collaborative analysis. This systematic approach not only facilitates the extraction of gene expression data but also allows researchers to connect, thus expanding the knowledge base of the research community regarding gene expression and its function in immunological phenomena (Seaman & Whitehouse, 2001; Scheuermann et al., 2009;).

Overview of Gene Expression Analysis Techniques

The landscape of gene expression analysis methods is incredibly wide-ranging, mirroring advances in technology and methodology. High-throughput sequencing, or RNA-seq, is a significant technique applied to the capture of transcriptomic data of unprecedented depth and accuracy. The method can estimate gene expression levels in the entire transcriptome and can show how genes are regulated in various states of physiology. In immunology, RNA-seq has allowed researchers to identify novel biomarkers linked to immune responses, allowing scientists to dissect the complex dynamics of immune cell-pathogen interactions.

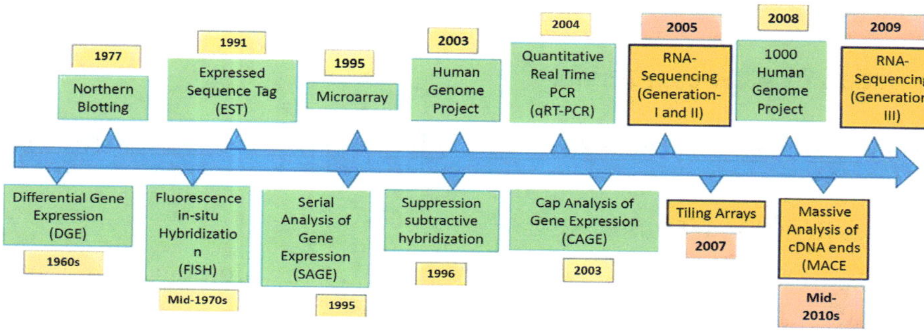

Figure 5.2. Historic timeline of technologies involved in gene expression analysis.

Source: https://www.intechopen.com/chapters/83046.

Such specificity was previously inaccessible with microarray-based technology, which was frequently hindered by limitations in sensitivity and specificity. In accordance, while microarrays still remain in use for diagnostic purposes, RNA-seq is a step beyond revolutionary in gene expression analysis that is particularly suited to immunological research. Quantitative PCR (qPCR), except for gene expression analysis, is still the rock on which one can rely because of its precision and reliability. This technique offers the possibility for discrete amplification and quantitation of specific RNA molecules, enabling scientists to validate findings from general measurements such as RNA-seq. qPCR is particularly valuable in immunology in order to investigate gene expression for genes having a central function in immune cell function and activation. The ability to quantify levels of single cytokines or immune receptors at various stages of immune responses significantly improves our understanding of disease pathologies and therapeutic opportunities. Furthermore, integration with other omics approaches is becoming more common, where it provides a supplementary layer of information that can confirm high-throughput data. This convergence is largely to blame for driving the field of immunology, particularly the comprehension of complex host-pathogen interactions. Another track worth pursuing is the integration of computational and statistical models aimed at better gene expression data interpretation. As gene expression research generates extensive datasets, the use of advanced bioinformatics tools is now indispensable to transform raw data into interpretative biological information. Computational approaches, including network analysis and machine learning, are able to reveal intricate patterns of gene regulation and expression within the immune system. These approaches are capable of identifying potential therapeutic targets and biomarkers by correlating disease phenotypes with expression profiles. For example, through the use of network-based approaches to analyze gene expression after infection, one might be able to discern important pathways used in immune response and thereby track gut barrier integrity and immune responses non-invasively, as has recently been demonstrated through the use of new techniques that pair fecal analysis with measurements of gene expression (Ahmed et al., 2019). Furthermore, these computational advancements enhance the use of translational medicine, particularly by establishing stable biomarker systems for clinical applications (Wang & Sarwal, 2015) (Figure 5.2).

5.1. Basics of Immunology

In order to comprehend how gene expression influences immune responses, the fundamentals of immunology must be grasped. The immune system is an intricate network composed of various cells and proteins that coordinate synergistically to defend against pathogens. Immune cells at the center of the network include lymphocytes, macrophages, and dendritic cells. The cells are central in the perception and response to foreign antigens. Additionally, every cell type has distinct gene expression patterns that dictate its function. For instance, activation of T-cells involves a signaling cascade leading to precise gene expression alterations, which will give rise to cytokine production and cell growth. This dynamic immune cell behavior supports the necessity for the analysis of gene expression in order to dissect the processes underlying immunity and disease pathology. Gene expression analysis offers insights into the regulation of the immune response from the identification of genes being activated throughout various immunological events. Pathogen recognition by pattern recognition receptors (PRRs) activates cascades of signals leading to transcriptional changes in immune cells. These changes are typically evident in the expression of cytokines, chemokines, and receptors that promote adaptive immunity. For instance, studies on non-coding RNAs (ncRNAs) have enhanced our understanding of immune cell gene control. As noted in ongoing studies, ncRNA characterization is significant, but the field is hindered by semantic annotation problems in the data due to its lack of standard ontologies. The development of the Non-Coding RNA Ontology (NCRO) fills this gap and, therefore, facilitates data exchange as well as our insight into immune function-related gene expression (Huang et al., 2016). The interaction between hematopoietic stem cells (HSCs) and their microenvironment exerts considerable influence on gene expression and, therefore, immune behavior. Fresh evidence demonstrates that transcription factors such as Ebf1 play a crucial role in controlling the structure and MSC function, as well as controlling HSCs. Changes to MSC gene expression patterns can potentially impose long-term implications on HSC functionality and the ability to sustain the immune system. Specifically, the Ebf1 knockout in MSCs has been shown to regulate stem cell adhesion, reducing quiescence and subsequently impacting myeloid lineage production. Such long-term functional impacts are key to understanding how genetic and environmental factors are able to mold the immune landscape, emphasizing the value of studying gene expression within an immunological context (Derecka et al., 2020).

5.1.1. Key Components of the Immune System

The immune system is a network of multiple components that work synergistically, working cellular and molecular components conferring defense on the body against pathogens. Innate immune cells, such as macrophages and dendritic cells, constitute a key component of the first line of defense. Macrophages are heterogeneous in function and, as such, are able to react to a wide variety of environmental stimuli and signals. Current research has shown the utility of gene expression profiling to clarify the natural strain-to-strain variability in populations of macrophages at baseline levels indicative of their readiness to act against infection. This is paramount and important in immunology since gene expression variations between states of being unstimulated and stimulated for these cells can inform and predict therapy and responses to disease, thus uncovering the active nature of macrophages in the immune context (Breda et al., 2022). Moreover, lymphocytes, including T and B cells, constitute the second very important component of the adaptive immune response.

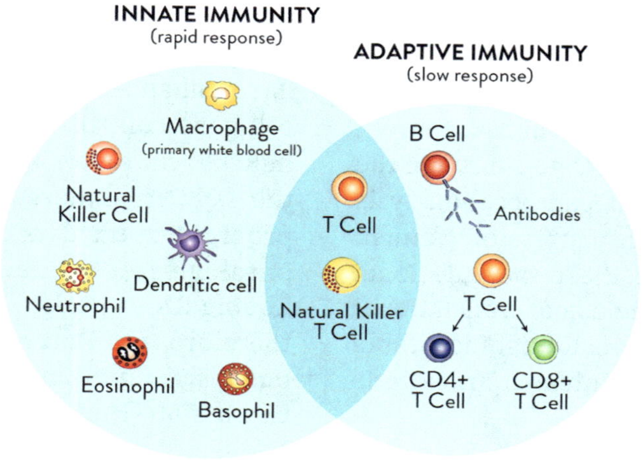

Figure 5.3. Components of the immune system of the body.

Source: https://www.researchgate.net/profile/Preeti-Dubey/publication/325767063/figure/fig3/AS:671943455936512@1537215212174/Components-of-immune-system-of-the-body.png.

These cells are characterized by their specificity in recognizing pathogens through specific receptors generated through somatic recombination. Gene expression analysis may give us information about lymphocyte activation, differentiation, and memory generation, which are important in long-lasting immunity. T cells, for instance, have significant alterations in their gene expression pattern on activation against antigens so that they can proliferate and execute effector functions effectively. These events are recognized through insights, which can allow researchers to interpret disparities among different strains, such as enhanced polarization of macrophages in C57BL/6 mice compared to BALB/c counterparts, that can enhance resistance to pathogens (Breda et al., 2022). This shows the key connection between gene expression patterns and immune cell function in the immune system. Finally, immune cell components like cytokines and other signal molecules play key functions in enabling communication between immune cells. Cytokines are important signaling molecules responsible for coordinating immunity by triggering inflammation and guiding immune cell differentiation and activity. Gene expression analysis breakthroughs have made available more knowledge of how various immune cells respond to these signals, so that particular regulatory pathways and networks can be recognized. For example, comparing immune challenges and their variations at the gene expression level can not only reveal mechanisms for good immunity but also the probable possibility of maladaptive immune responses resulting in autoimmunity or chronic inflammation. By characterizing these changes, researchers are able to generate targeted therapies based on the power of the immune system with fewer side effects, which makes gene expression analysis key to immunology (Figure 5.3).

5.1.2. Role of Genes in Immune Response

The interplay between genes and the immune response is a central tenet of immunology that defines how genetic expression defines immune response efficacy. Genes play a critical role in encoding proteins that regulate many of the immune response's functions, including antibody production, activation of immune cells, and regulation of inflammation processes. For instance, immune checkpoint gene expression may determine whether T cells are inhibited or stimulated and may influence the body's ability to combat infection and cancer. Gene function becomes involved, particularly in the case of cancer, where mutation can have a very significant effect on the immune environment, creating a microenvironment to suppress or enhance immune activity. Understanding these genetic factors can lead to improved immunotherapy methods, particularly in cancer treatment, so as to render the immune system more effective against cancer cells. Recent studies have highlighted the strong influence some gene expression profiles have on the immune system, particularly in cancer. Research has indicated that genes that are implicated in nitrogen metabolism significantly impact immune cell infiltration and patient outcomes in cancers such as hepatocellular carcinoma (HCC) (Duan et al., 2024). By creating predictive models based on gene expression, researchers have been able to forecast patients into risk groups, with their findings indicating that patients with certain genetic signatures possess increased immune infiltration and, consequently, superior responses to immunotherapy. These observations highlight the promise of using gene expression analysis as a biomarker for therapeutic response prediction, marking a move toward personalized medicine. This drift underscores the need for stringent genetic investigations to determine mechanisms underlying immune response differences between individuals. Additionally, the interaction between genetic mutations and the immune microenvironment can be pivotal to determining the outcome of therapies like immune checkpoint blockade (ICB). It has been elucidated by research that the immune microenvironment of the tumor is modulated by mutations affecting DNA damage repair pathways, which direct gene expression in terms of innate immune responses (Vaninov et al., 2023). For example, DDR-deficient tumors exhibit distinct immune profiles characterized by heterogeneous chemokine secretion and infiltration of immune cells. These findings not only provide deeper insights into tumor biology but also guide the design of specific immunotherapeutic approaches. Gene expression in this context can thus reveal key mechanisms that either enable or hinder effective immune activation, to new treatments that leverage the potential of the immune system against cancer.

5.1.3. Interaction Between Genes and Environmental Factors

Genes and environmental factors is significant as far as the factor of gene expression is concerned, particularly under the framework of immunology. Environmental stimuli such as pathogens, toxins, and the availability of food can regulate gene expression, thereby changing immunity. Research has shown that various immune-related genes exhibit differential expression when exposed to specific environmental stresses. For instance, in crustaceans, environmental stress triggers special immune signaling pathways that are not available in vertebrates. This highlights the resilience of the immune system to fluctuating environmental pressures, offering an example of how innate immunity adjusts over time in reaction to ecological stress. The information is significant in providing us with an understanding of how environmental factors may increase disease susceptibility and resistance and therefore has implications for aquaculture practices and wildlife conservation policies, as discussed in Hauton (2012). In addition, the interaction between environment and genetics can have significant implications for infectious disease epidemiology, specifically for vector-borne infections such as malaria. For mosquito interactions with the Plasmodium parasite, ecological immunology has become an area of interest where gene-environment interactions are highlighted to determine immune responses. Insecticide resistance among mosquito populations has been shown to impact susceptibility to infection, and therefore dynamics of malaria transmission could also be affected by environmental conditions. Understanding such interactions would help researchers better enhance vector control and disease management programs because innate immunity responses in mosquitoes are subtle and context-dependent, worthy of further investigation exploring population-level mechanisms in natural conditions. The importance of studying such interactions *in situ* compared to laboratory conditions is brought forth in Tripet (2009). Finally, it must be mentioned that genetic predispositions and environmental factors cooperate to affect immune responses throughout an organism's life. The resultant effect of these forces is observed in most species, whereby genetic evolution follows adaptations to some pressures of the environment, and genetic variation may dictate the range of reactions to changing environments. For example, immune genes can be increased or decreased by pathogens, but the magnitude of this increase or decrease typically depends on the genetic makeup of the organism and the environmental context. This interaction exhibits the complexity involved in immune system functioning and demands an integrative approach in immunology research. Through the study of coordination between genetic and environmental aspects, scientists are able to determine sophisticated intelligence regarding immune system dynamics, enabling effective interventions in health and disease circumstances, as shown in Tripet (2009) and Hauton (2012) (Figure 5.4).

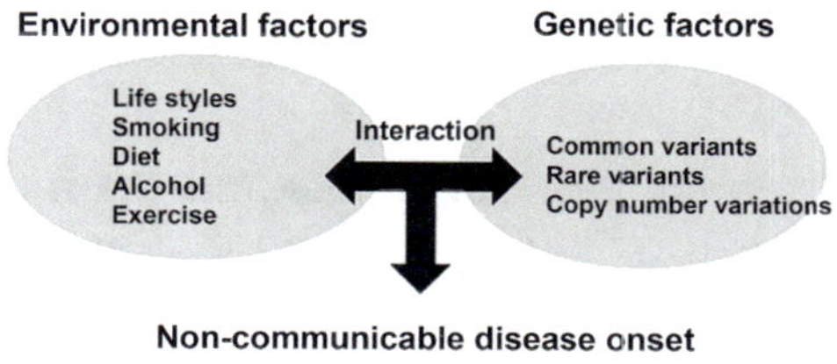

Figure 5.4. Interaction between genes and environmental factors.

Source: https://pub.mdpi-res.com/ijms/ijms-18-00302/article_deploy/html/images/ijms-18-00302-ag.png?1488444865.

5.2. Techniques for Gene Expression Analysis

The intricate processes of gene expression analysis form the core of immunological investigation as they enable scientists to value the dynamism of the immune response under various conditions. From the wide variety of approaches available, quantitative polymerase chain reaction (qPCR) stands out due to its sensitivity and specificity in measuring the levels of gene expression. Through the amplification of particular sequences, qPCR allows researchers to quantify the levels of certain mRNA transcripts following stimulation through infection or vaccination. The technique is particularly enlightening in immunology because it can provide insight into the expression of genes implicated in immune function, such as cytokines and activation markers of immune cells. The ability to quantify changes in gene expression accurately is important for understanding how immune cells respond to pathogens and how such changes might be used for therapeutic benefit. In addition to qPCR, high-throughput gene expression profiling technologies such as NGS have revolutionized immunology by offering incredibly powerful tools for the analysis of transcriptomes. NGS allows for the quantification of thousands of genes simultaneously, providing a complete view of gene expression profiles upon immune reactions. The technique can be of great use, particularly in the case of complex diseases that involve more than one gene. For instance, NGS can detect alterations in the expression of immune-associated genes in autoimmune diseases or infection. Furthermore, the integration of bioinformatics tools allows for the interpretation of the vast data generated by NGS, which allows researchers to identify new biomarkers or drug targets that can enhance clinical outcomes. Application of such sophisticated technology underscores the evolving field of gene expression analysis in immunology. Also, novel non-invasive techniques of expression analysis are under development, expanding the potential for the exploration of immune responses in real time without having subjects undergo invasive methods. An illustration of this is the development of techniques that quantify alterations in gut barrier function by assaying exfoliated epithelial cells found in fecal matter. This approach not only allows one to track immunity against gastrointestinal infections but also underscores the function of the gut in keeping the body overall immune. Employing markers such as RELM-β to quantify the integrity of the gut barrier and the associated immunity, researchers can now make observations previously difficult to make without being invasive. This novel method is a great example of how novel approaches can enhance the comprehension of complex immunological interactions and broaden the applicability of gene expression analysis in immunology (Ahmed et al., 2019). Further development in this area may reveal unprecedented progress in both diagnostics and therapeutics, bridging the gap between basic research and clinical applicability in immunology (Wang & Sarwal, 2015).

5.2.1. Quantitative PCR (qPCR)

qPCR in immunology, is a milestone technique for investigating gene expression. Based on qPCR, researchers can quantify the amount of specific RNA transcripts in an example sample, which can tell them about the operational state of immune cells under various conditions. From the measurement of gene expression levels, researchers can make inferences about correlations between the immune system function and the effect of extrinsic factors, i.e., infections or diseases. For instance, qPCR has been used to explore immune responses within populations of different organisms, where significant differences in immune gene expression profiles according to environment have been shown, for example, using the threespine stickleback fish as a model species (Mathieu et al., 2010). Such findings underscore the utility of qPCR as a precious tool in the exploration of the intricacies of gene control within immunological responses. The power of qPCR lies in its ability to provide highly specific and sensitive determinations of gene expression. By the use of procedures such as reverse transcription, this method allows cDNA generated from RNA to be amplified and detected even low-abundance transcripts. This feature is particularly vital when quantifying levels of expression of gene markers that may be involved in immune modulation. For example, cancer/testis antigens like HAGE exhibit a differential expression pattern in cancer and normal tissues. Experiments with qPCR have revealed differences in the levels of mRNA and protein expression and are an indication of the need for cross-validation of results using various means, including immunohistochemistry.

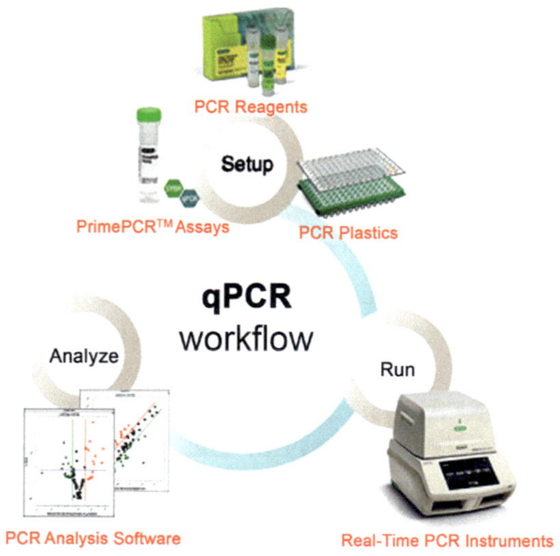

Figure 5.5. Quantitative PCR (qPCR) workflow.

Source: https://www.bio-rad.com/webroot/web/images/lsr/solutions/technologies/gene_expression/qPCR_real-time_PCR/technology_detail/real-time-qpcr-workflow.jpg.

These differences highlight the finely tuned control of gene expression and how it has implications for the creation of targeted immunotherapies, as explored in cancer research into HAGE as a vaccine target (Mathieu et al., 2010). Furthermore, the application of qPCR goes beyond mere quantification; it also offers a system by which to comprehend how gene expression is related to various physiological parameters. Within immune response research, condition, reproductive status, and pathogen load have been shown to play an important role in influencing immune gene expression profiles. Employing qPCR, researchers can analyze the relationships of these variables in a population and understand the adaptive basis of immune responses. For instance, the threespine stickleback study above demonstrated how differences in environmental conditions were able to modulate immune function and presented the complexity of immune regulation (Robertson et al., 2016). It is this versatility of qPCR to augment our understanding of immunological processes that paves the way for innovative therapeutic strategies and enhances our understanding of immune system dynamics overall (Figure 5.5).

5.2.2. RNA Sequencing (RNA-seq)

RNA-seq has revolutionized gene expression analysis, particularly in immunology. By providing a comprehensive and unbiased estimate of RNA transcripts, RNA-seq allows researchers to investigate dynamic transcriptomic changes that occur with immune responses. Unlike traditional microarray technologies, RNA-seq can detect an extended repertoire of transcripts, including novel and low-abundance genes, and thus improves understanding of immune functions. This function is crucial in the differentiation of the complex process of gene regulation to differentiate immune cells and for their activation, giving an understanding of how heterogeneous immune responses can be tailored to combat various pathogens. Apart from that, RNA-seq application in immunology studies has significantly enhanced the determination of how diseases such as tuberculosis operate, in support of the identification of several differentially expressed genes and pathways within immune response, as seen in the recent study of *M. bovis*-infected cattle (McLoughlin et al., 2014). In addition, RNA-seq also offers the potential to investigate genetic interactions, as well as regulatory mechanisms within immune cells. With single-cell RNA-seq platforms, researchers are able to dissect immune cell population heterogeneity and unearth the complex cellular interactions driving immune responses. This resolution is crucial for learning how many variables, such as cytokine signaling and intercellular communication, influence patterns of gene expression during immune activation. In studies using mesenchymal stromal cells (MSCs) and HSCs, for instance, RNA-seq has illuminated how modulation of transcription in MSCs can have long-term consequences for the functional features of HSCs, again underscoring the extracellular niche's control over immune dynamics (Derecka et al., 2020). These findings are the promise of RNA-seq in uncovering the sophisticated molecular dialogues that characterize our immune landscape. The uses of RNA-seq extend beyond research; they are also highly promising for clinical applications in immunology. By virtue of its ability to identify characteristic gene expression signatures for specific immune responses or disease pathologies, RNA-seq can assist in the development of novel diagnostic and therapeutic approaches. For example, with an understanding of the transcriptomic profiles of immune cells under disease conditions, personalized medicine approaches can be developed, allowing targeted interventions based on individual genetic profiles. Apart from this, RNA-seq can also strengthen vaccine development by unveiling the gene expression changes linked with effective immune responses. While researchers continue to apply RNA-seq technologies, what is learned is certain to advance our understanding of immunological complications, paving the way for novel solutions toward immune-related disease and disorder eradication (Figure 5.6).

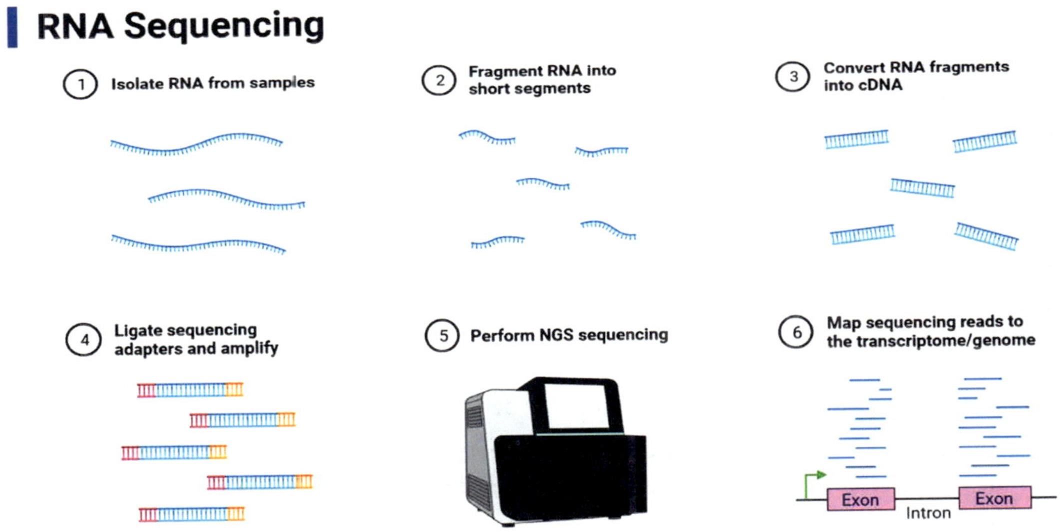

Figure 5.6. Illustration of RNA sequencing (RNA-seq).

Source: https://microbenotes.com/wp-content/uploads/2022/07/RNA-Sequencing.jpg.

5.2.3. Microarray Technology

Microarray technology has enabled the transformation of gene expression analysis, particularly in the field of immunology. Microarrays can enable researchers to compare, simultaneously, the level of expression of thousands of genes, and thus empower researchers to explore complex biological processes such as immune response. Microarray technology is based on hybridization, where fluorescent-labeled cDNA samples hybridize to complementary DNA probes bound to a solid substrate. As a result, the differences in gene expression can be quantified and provide data on how genes are up- or down-regulated upon immune stimulation. Such functions play a key role in immunology, with nuances in gene expression contributing to enhanced vaccine design and therapies for various immune disorders. In the background of recent breakthroughs, researchers have used BioMicroarrays to analyze the intricate transcriptomic reactions of immune cells in response to various stimulations. For instance, researchers have identified a large number of differently expressed genes (DEGs) in some immune cells upon challenge with Toll-like receptor (TLR) ligands, enhancing our understanding of their functional importance. A single study showed variations in 530 DEGs in porcine intramuscular mature adipocytes upon TLR ligand stimulation. Immune response and lipid metabolism pathways were found to be significant in this study, with CXCR4 and PPARA being major genes targeted in the immunometabolic profile (Igata et al., 2019). Such evidence points out the effectiveness of microarray technology's ability to account for gene interactions and pathways at the core of immune system functionality. Moreover, bioinformatics resources, together with microarray data, facilitate the analysis of gene networks on a broad scale, thereby facilitating the discovery of immunological research biomarkers. Functional characterization of the DEGs and their interaction within networks can illuminate the role of different genes in immune regulation as well as metabolic processes. Findings of major regulatory genes, as in this study above, unveil therapeutic potential in designing target-modulating immune responses for clinical benefit (Igata et al., 2019). Significantly, continued research and funding within this specialism, supported by the offer of grants like those offered by the BBSRC, are important in increasing our understanding of gene expression in immunology and the development of new treatments (Figure 5.7).

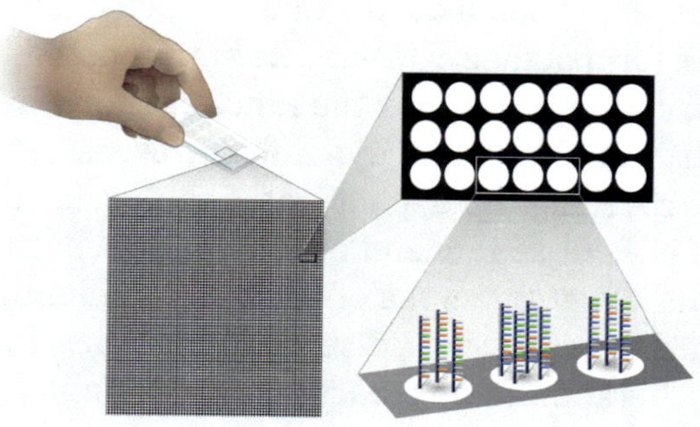

Figure 5.7. Microarray technology has revolutionized the field of gene expression analysis.

Source: https://www.genome.gov/sites/default/files/media/images/2022-05/Microarray-technology.jpg.

5.3. Applications of Gene Expression Analysis in Immunology

Immunology has made significant applications of gene expression analysis, particularly in explaining complex immune responses. By analyzing gene expression in distinct immune cells, scientists can identify pathways that are induced by exposure to specific immune challenges, such as infections or inflammatory conditions. By analyzing this kind of information, it is now possible to separate cellular responses that are normally masked when conducting bulk tissue analysis. For instance, single-cell RNA sequencing can reveal transcriptional heterogeneity among immune cells and hence identify rare cell populations that may be of vital significance for immune pathology or regulation. Not only do such findings shed greater insight into immune mechanisms, but they also promise avenues for the creation of targeted therapies with the ability to modulate immune responses well. Throughout the last decade, advances in gene expression analysis technologies have led to breakthroughs in biomarker discovery for immunological diseases. The combination of high-throughput sequencing tools and advanced computational algorithms allowed researchers to identify specific gene expression signatures corresponding to conditions like autoimmune diseases or transplant rejection. For example, careful analysis of peripheral blood mononuclear cells can uncover unique expression profiles linked to disease activity or treatment response. The potential for their application to clinical diagnostics is significant since such biomarkers have the potential to direct customized medicine approaches, with the ability to provide insights into the prognosis of disease as well as modifying therapeutic interventions in accordance with an individual patient's immune landscape. This paradigm shift brings with it a revolutionary age for immunology as precision medicine is dictated by real-time gene expression data. Gene expression analysis has uses beyond diagnosis and therapeutic monitoring and opens avenues to research into the very fundamental mechanisms of the immune system. Exploring immune cells' transcriptional responses to different conditions further improves our understanding of immune tolerance and cellular interaction dynamics in the immune microenvironment. Examining how gene expression profiles change upon encountering stimuli, such as pathogens or treatment drugs, offers critical details regarding the mechanisms of immunity and inflammation. Scientists are also increasingly using gene expression analysis to explore these dynamics and illuminate how changes in gene regulation lead to such afflictions as chronic inflammation or tumor immunology. This more detailed knowledge then eventually seeks to inform the development of novel immunotherapies, transforming the landscape of existing options for treatment for immune-related afflictions (Wang & Sarwal, 2015; Chirumamilla et al., 2017).

5.3.1. Understanding Autoimmune Diseases

A critical analysis of autoimmune diseases reveals the complexity of their etiology and pathogenesis. Autoimmune diseases arise when the immune system responds to healthy cells by mistake, producing many symptoms that affect multiple organ systems. Among the causes of this abnormal immune response are genetic predispositions, environmental triggers, and hormonal influences. Recent data show that autoimmune disorders inordinately occur in females, perhaps due to the hormonal and genetic characteristics of the X chromosome. It is worthwhile knowing about such sex-dependent variations, as it may help explain why some microRNAs, which are of the utmost significance in gene expression regulation and modulation of immune responses, are differentially regulated between males and females. These facts can result in the establishment of more targeted treatments that take into account the unique biological characteristics of each sex (Sharma & Eghbali, 2014). One of the most known autoimmune diseases is vitiligo, a disease that presents depigmented patches on the skin as a consequence of melanocyte cell killing by autoreactive cytotoxic T cells. This autoimmune response not only causes cosmetic concerns but also significantly impacts the quality of life of the patients, which very often leads to psychological distress. The association of vitiligo with other autoimmune disorders, such as Hashimoto's thyroiditis, also makes it difficult to comprehend its pathophysiology. The most frequent autoimmune hypothesis is that dysregulation of the immune system, possibly mediated by environmental and genetic factors, is the key determinant in the onset of vitiligo. Further, the presence of melanocytes within other organs, including the auditory and nervous systems, also provides a possibility of extension of autoimmune mechanisms outside the skin, with presentation of a broader clinical picture of implications and associated risks for the patient with vitiligo (Baldini et al., 2017). Gene expression analysis in immunology has become a central element in the investigation of the intricacies of autoimmune disease. Through an examination of gene expression changes in autoimmune disease, researchers can mark disease severity and response to treatment through identified biomarkers. This is particularly significant for disease conditions like vitiligo, wherein the intricate relationship between genetic expression and immune pathways can lend insight into disease mechanisms. Further, the examination of microRNAs as regulatory elements brings new evidence on what pathways are employed in autoimmune processes. With continued research on unraveling the genetics of autoimmune disease, it is increasingly becoming evident that sex-specific and individualized treatments can significantly enhance therapeutic efficiency. Hence, the addition of gene expression analysis provides a promising avenue to increase our understanding of autoimmune disorders and improve patient care in immunology (Sharma & Eghbali, 2014) (Figure 5.8).

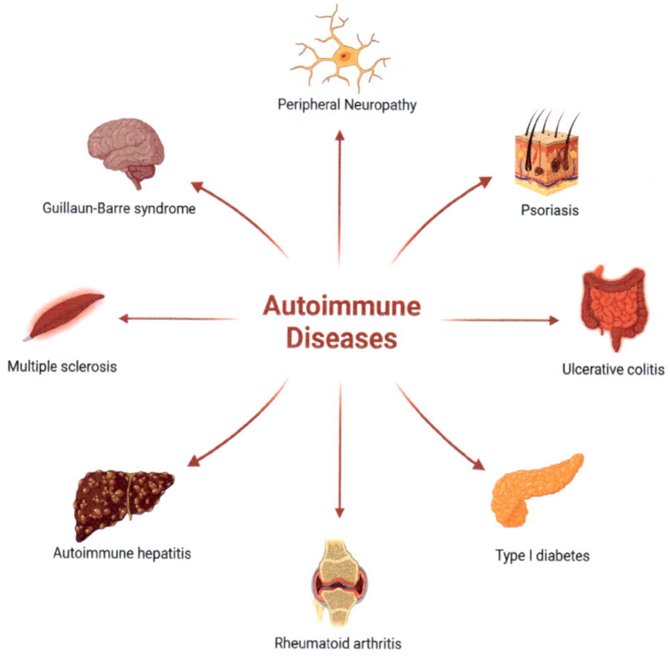

Figure 5.8. Common autoimmune diseases.

Source: https://biotech.ucdavis.edu/sites/g/files/dgvnsk2696/files/media/images/Figure%201_Why%20women.png.

5.3.2. Vaccine Development and Efficacy

The vaccine development process has historically relied on a deep understanding of the immune response, namely, in how gene expression profiles direct the body's response to pathogens. Vaccines aim to immunize the immune system so that it will identify and efficiently combat infectious diseases or cancer cells. The key to this process is the detection of distinct tumor-associated antigens (TAAs) capable of eliciting a robust immune response. Various methods have been established, including the use of dendritic cell (DC)-based vaccines, which hold the potential for generating antitumor immunity. These vaccines can utilize many TAAs to induce cytotoxic T cell responses that are critical for effective tumor killing. However, while laboratory findings are promising, several clinical trials have encountered challenges in surmounting obstacles that make the successful translation of these outcomes into widespread clinical effectiveness difficult. The problem remains how to optimize vaccine formulations that can traverse the tumor microenvironment and generate effective immune responses against resistance mechanisms within tumors (Koido et al., 2010).

A major hindrance to the success of cancer vaccines is the complex structure of solid tumors and their detailed microenvironment. Solid tumors consist not only of malignant cells but also of various non-malignant cells that contribute significantly to tumor behavior. Tumor antigens have a tendency to provoke tolerance to the immune system rather than active immunity. The tumor stroma in the vicinity, especially the vascular architecture, has a crucial function in regulating immune responses by modifying the tumor microenvironment, restricting immune effector cell access. Studies emphasize that disorganized and permeable tumor vasculature is one of the reasons current immunotherapies are not effective, calling for novel vaccine approaches targeting not only the tumor cells but also the supportive cells within the tumor microenvironment. This strategy of integration could prove to enhance the activation of T cells cytotoxic to TAAs against tumor evasive moves (Sabins & Storkus, 2013). Genetically engineered vaccines provide a powerful tool to overcome these hurdles in vaccine design. These vaccines can deliver specific genes associated with pro-inflammatory responses or encode antigens of interest within tumor cells. In this manner, they can optimize the delivery of TAAs to the immune system and induce more efficient adaptive and innate immunity. Additionally, patterns of gene expression induced by the vaccines can be traced to assess the efficacy of the immune activation. Knowing how the genetic elements interact within the immune system is not only critical to vaccine construction but also to the prediction of their success in clinics. By this filter of analysis, researchers are able to infer optimal dosing regimens and immunization schedules specific to the nuances of an individual patient's response and ultimately improve therapeutic prospects in oncology (Koido et al., 2010; Sabins & Storkus, 2013) (Figure 5.9).

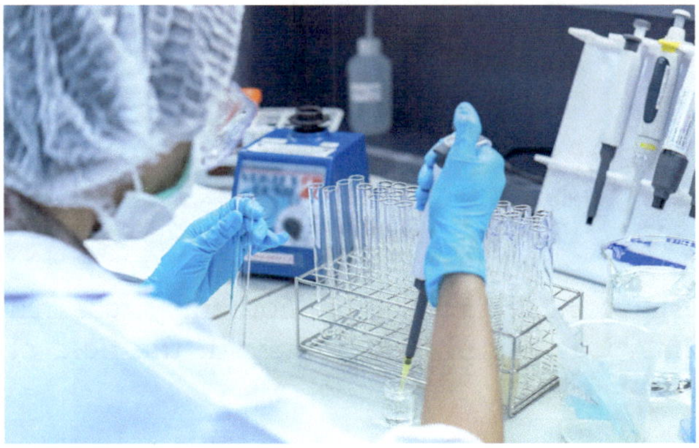

Figure 5.9. The development of vaccines relied on a deep understanding of the immune response.

Source: https://static.cepi.net/images/3840x2160/2024-01/shutterstock_1921538018-scaled.webp.

5.3.3. Cancer Immunotherapy Research

Cancer immunotherapy has emerged as the key oncology frontier, focusing on using the body's immune system to fight against cancer cells more effectively than current treatments. Gene expression analysis has now enabled us to decode the molecular events involved in the immune microenvironment of tumors. This analysis forms the foundation to discover future biomarkers, which may assist in prognostication and treatment decisions, finally leading to more tailored therapy plans. For instance, single-cell RNA sequencing technologies uncover details regarding tumor-infiltrating lymphocyte heterogeneity and their engagement with cancer cells. By identifying the gene expression patterns of various subsets of immune cells, researchers can simplify immunotherapeutic methods and enhance their efficacy in various cancers, especially for cancers that are resistant to traditional treatments.

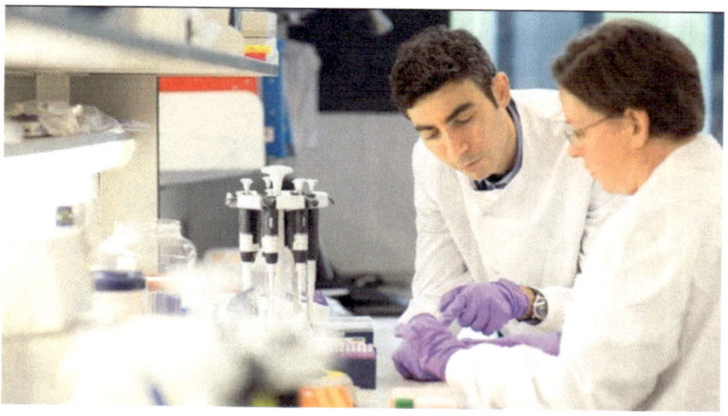

Figure 5.10. Cancer immunotherapy research emerged as a pivotal frontier in the field of oncology.

Source: https://news.cancerresearchuk.org/wp-content/uploads/2021/05/science-5-16.webp.

Current studies highlight the central role played by certain genes in making immunotherapy more effective, particularly in the case of hepatocellular carcinoma, a cancer notorious for its poor prognosis. Cancer stem cells have been involved in tumor growth and therapy resistance and therefore make the best target for treatment. The integration of advanced machine learning approaches with gene expression profiling is able to dissect key stem cell-associated genes with prognostic value and therapeutic targets for liver cancer. S100A10 has been identified as a very useful gene by research that highly correlates with patient prognosis and with responses to immunotherapies. These findings underscore the importance of gaining more information about stem cell gene expression, which could be utilized to tailor immunotherapeutic approaches for enhancing therapeutic responses in liver cancer patients and potentially other tumor types as well (Huang & Tu, 2025). While exploring the entire category of immunotherapy, researchers have also shifted their focus to novel immune checkpoint targets that could enhance therapeutic responses. Siglec-15 has also emerged as a strong candidate since it's highly expressed in the tumor microenvironment and lowly expressed in normal tissues. Interestingly, studies of Siglec-15 co-expression patterns with classical immune checkpoint molecules such as PD-L1 show complex interactions that can be exploited for the optimization of combination therapies. The varying expression levels of these checkpoints in different tumors reflect the need for specific immunotherapeutic strategies. For instance, the synergistic interaction of Siglec-15 and PD-L1 expression in different cancers indicates the combined effects when both signaling pathways are targeted, hence opening up new avenues for the development of cancer treatment protocols. These findings by gene expression profiling not only present a finer view of tumor immunology but also open up novel combinations in cancer therapy (Watkins et al., 2024) (Figure 5.10).

5.4. Case Studies in Gene Expression and Immunology

Gene expression is progressively becoming pivotal to understanding various immunological diseases, particularly when it comes to cancer. A famous case study involving papillary thyroid carcinoma (PTC) and anaplastic thyroid carcinoma (ATC) is important in terms of insight into mechanisms of immune evasion. By examining the mRNA expression levels of PD-1 ligands (PD-L1 and PD-L2) and CTLA-4 ligands (CD80 and CD86) in 94 PTC and 11 ATC patients, researchers uncovered dysregulation patterns that correlate with clinicopathological features.

The findings indicate that both carcinomas had down-regulation of CD80, particularly in ATC. In addition, the amplified PD-L1 expression was correlated with classical histological variants and certain genetic mutations, demonstrating the intricate relationship between gene expression and tumor development. These case studies describe how gene expression analysis can guide possible treatment interventions in cancer immunology (Tuccilli et al., 2018). Another relevant case study is that of interactions between MSCs and HSCs, which play an essential role in maintaining hematopoietic homeostasis. The research focused on transcriptional regulation of bone marrow MSCs and their long-term consequences on HSC function. Using single-cell analysis, researchers uncovered that specific transcription factor genes, such as Ebf1, were expressed consistently but crucial to maintain HSC niches. Conditional deletion of Ebf1 led to alterations of cellular composition and adhesive properties within the MSC niche, resulting in decreased quiescence and impaired myeloid lineage production by HSCs. This disturbance had a cascading effect on HSCs to demonstrate the manner in which alterations in the bone marrow niche hold enormous significance for immunological well-being. Thus, this case study explains the function of gene expression to describe the dynamics of stem cell interactions within the immune system (Derecka et al., 2020). Synthesis of findings across various case studies in gene expression and immunology demonstrates the intricate interaction between genetic control and immune reactions. They identify the potential of gene expression profiling not only for the diagnosis of disease but also for disease outcome prognostication. As these studies delineate immune evasion in cancer and stem cell homeostasis, they set the stage for directed therapies that may regulate these pathways to optimize immune reactions. Interjection of such knowledge into the clinic would have the potential to revolutionize personalized medicine. Thus, a systematic strategy in gene expression analysis is essential in designing successful immunotherapeutic interventions and research in the area is a must for future advancements in immunology. The immune-related disease scenario is complex; however, the understanding of the underlying current of gene expression will enable further therapeutic advancement (Tuccilli et al., 2018; Derecka et al., 2020).

5.4.1. Gene Expression Profiles in HIV Research

The intersection of gene expression profiles and HIV research is a field of urgent research within the broader framework of immunology. Clarification of how HIV exploits host cellular processes is not merely crucial to understanding the viruses virulence but also therapeutically in terms of proposing treatment avenues. Research conducted on gene expression dynamics following vaccination in recent years has shown that transcriptional signatures are accurate predictors of immunity. For instance, specific patterns of gene activation of DEGs were established within blood samples of subjects that had been administered an HIV-1 envelope glycoprotein subunit vaccine and found that certain gene activation tracks quite closely with good antibody production. The findings indicate that gene expression signatures can serve as a vaccine efficacy biomarker, thus placing relevance to their use in the development of new immunotherapeutic strategies against HIV (Anderson et al., 2018). Further, growing RNA interference (RNAi) technologies in HIV research underscore the significance of gene expression manipulation in clinical applications. By targeting specific genes such as chemokine (C-C motif) receptor 5 (CCR5), researchers have been able to manipulate immune cell reactions to HIV. The sustained expression of RNAi molecules in primates has led to recurrent down-regulation of CCR5 and thereby rendered increased resistance to SIV infection. These advances not only highlight the potential of gene expression modulation as a mode of therapy but also define the intricate interaction between host genetics and susceptibility to virulent infection. This new approach can pave the way to creating long-term therapies that take advantage of gene expression machinery for the treatment of HIV-1 and other blood-borne pathogens (An et al., 2007). Furthermore, transcriptomic research on HIV reveals critical information on the landscape of immunity during infection and therapy. These analyses of gene expression facilitate dissecting immune cell interactions and pathways invoked by viral replication. For example, the discovery of blood transcription modules (BTMs) associated with different immune cell types illuminates the activation mechanisms of the immune system against HIV. By comparing these profiles at different stages of infection or treatment, scientists can gain further insight into the immune evasion mechanisms of HIV. Additionally, the definition of these gene expression changes aids in the identification of new targets for therapy and vaccine candidates, further underscoring the significance of gene expression analysis in today's fight against HIV (Anderson et al., 2018) (Figure 5.11).

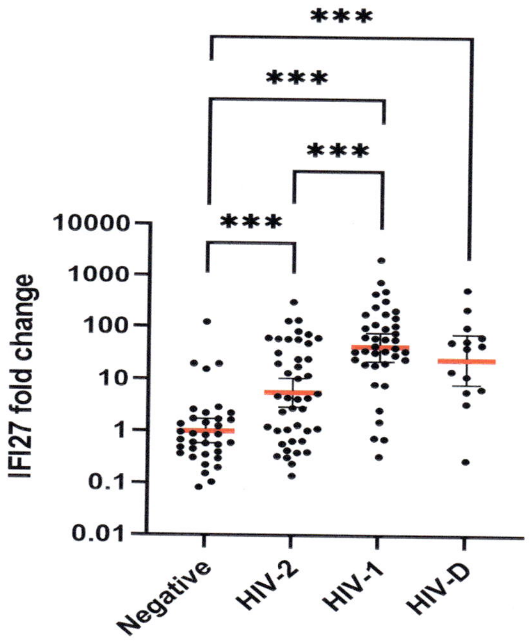

Figure 5.11. IFI27 gene expression by HIV infection status.

Source: https://www.researchgate.net/publication/361266163/figure/fig1/AS:116666842012876 9@1655166835200/IFI27-gene-expression-by-HIV-infection-status-The-relative-IFI27-fold-change-gene.png.

5.4.2. Analysis of Cytokine Gene Expression in Allergies

Cytokine gene expression analysis is a key technique for understanding the immunological mechanisms of allergies. Cytokines, as components of the immune response, control the activity of many immune cells, and their production determines both the development and extent of allergic reactions. Overexpression of inflammatory cytokines is characteristic of allergic diseases such as asthma and atopic dermatitis, leading to activation of pathological processes. For instance, in research, it has been unveiled that higher levels of interleukin (IL)-4, IL-5, and IL-13 have been linked to the exacerbation of allergic reactions. With gene expression profiling techniques such as quantitative PCR and microarray, scientists are capable of determining the specific cytokine patterns in allergic subjects, which provides prospects of therapeutic interventions being made patient-parameter-specific. Cytokine gene expression characterization is hence critical in the development of personalized medicine in the management of allergy.

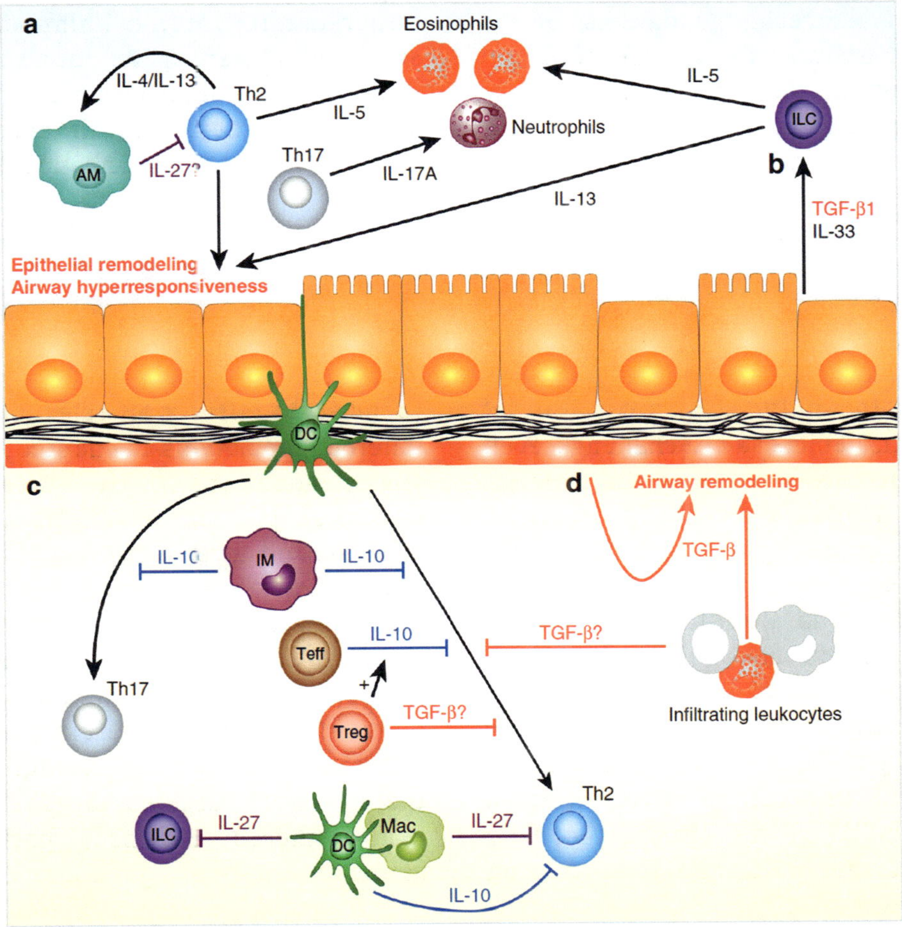

Figure 5.12. Cytokine regulation of allergic lung inflammation. a Type 2 cytokines (IL-4, IL-5, and IL-13) drive multiple pathogenic features of allergic airway disease (AAD), including eosinophilic inflammation, structural changes to epithelium, and activation of macrophages.

Source: https://www.researchgate.net/publication/331793985/figure/fig3/AS:736888369446912@1552699286091/Cytokine-regulation-of-allergic-lung-inflammation-a-Type-2-cytokines-IL-4-IL-5-and.png.

Current research has also illuminated the complex interactions between cytokines and the environment in triggering allergic responses. Single cytokine roles have formed the core of traditional models of allergy; however, the evidence suggests that their interactions may be equally crucial. For example, the presence of cytokine networks provides an environment in which allergic responses are either exacerbated or inhibited. The hypothesis of an inverse correlation between autoimmune disease and helminth infection illustrates this complexity, as highlighted by the immune modulation of these parasites through the secretion of immunomodulatory products (Pineda et al., 2014). Such findings encourage further research into how cytokine signaling may be utilized to make recommendations for the prevention and treatment of allergy, hopefully taking advantage of such immunomodulatory effects in the reversal of hyperresponsiveness in the allergic patient. Secondly, investigation into the genetic cause of allergic diseases encompasses examination of the relationship between genotype and cytokine expression. Current investigations suggest that there are some gene polymorphisms that predispose to elevated cytokine levels, thus predisposing to allergy. Though the multidisciplinary nature of atopic dermatitis depicts such a challenge, even though cytokines are the key to the process, the role of cornified envelope proteins in epidermal barrier disruption complicates the path to revealing the genetic underpinnings of this disease (Martyna, 2013). Future studies must delve further into the cooperation between the molecular processes of genetic variants and cytokine production to explain their synergistic impact on allergic diseases. This data will not just add to our understanding of allergies but may also influence the discovery of new biomarkers and therapy targets for increased patient gain (Figure 5.12).

5.4.3. Role of Gene Expression in Transplant Rejection

The function of gene expression in transplant rejection is underscored by its contribution to the alloimmune response, where the donor organ is perceived as foreign by the recipient's immune system. Alterations in gene expression patterns, particularly in immune activation, cytokine signaling, and cellular proliferation, can be the signals for the onset of acute rejection. These trends are significant in the determination of how grafts are recognized and attacked by the immune system. Genomic and proteomic profiling studies enable one to find biomarker candidate products that are capable of predicting rejection events before the onset of clinical manifestations. Subsequently, gene expression analysis not only contributes to the understanding of the immunological milieu surrounding transplants but also facilitates the development of improved monitoring tools that can lead to therapeutic interventions at the optimal time, thereby enhancing graft survival rates and patient outcomes as documented in recent research (Wang & Sarwal, 2015). Gene expression analysis also describes demographic differences in transplant outcomes. For instance, some gene expression patterns that are linked to racial and ethnic background have been reported to affect graft rejection rates among different populations. In one study tracking heart transplant outcomes, African American and non-Caucasian patients experienced higher acute rejection and adverse event rates compared with their Caucasian counterparts after being treated with similar doses of immunosuppressive treatments. These differences further highlight the need for personalized medicine in the field of transplantation, wherein gene expression analysis can render immunosuppressive therapy more targeted to genetic and ethnic factors, thereby enhancing patient care. The association between gene expression patterns and transplant outcomes highlights the need to integrate these analyses in clinical practice so as to enhance and characterize risks for transplant rejection (Khush et al., 2015). Within the world of the future transplant medicine, the integration of gene expression analysis into routine clinical practices holds enormous promise. Advances in computational biology and bioinformatics are enabling the development of predictive algorithms that can examine high-dimensional genomic information to determine key biomarkers of rejection. The use of these technologies can facilitate more precise evaluations of graft status, allowing clinicians to respond preemptively before rejection episodes occur. In addition, with further progress toward an understanding of the molecular processes that govern graft acceptance and rejection, the ability to engineer more biocompatible and acceptable grafts through lessons learned from the use of gene expression analysis becomes increasingly real. Thus, the role of gene expression is more than mere observation; it is increasingly being the basis upon which future plans are laid to overcome the challenge of transplant rejection and obtain superior long-term results for transplant patients (Wang & Sarwal, 2015).

5.5. Challenges in Gene Expression Analysis

Gene expression analysis presents a series of daunting challenges that can have a major setback on achieving progress in research on immunology. One of the biggest issues is the inherent biological heterogeneity among samples. Factors such as genetic background, tissue, and environmental conditions may produce striking differences in gene expression patterns. Such heterogeneity poses challenges to finding robust biomarkers or therapeutic targets across different populations or diseases. Furthermore, the effect of post-transcriptional regulation may obscure the actual level of gene expression measured by quantitative methods, and misleading interpretations. Without replication and controls, results can be equated with noise rather than actual biological signals and thus establishing reproducible and consistent results in research settings is challenging. Thus, addressing these sources of variance is critical to advancing our understanding of immune responses and developing new interventions in immunology. Another key problem of gene expression analysis is the choice of method employed for data collection. Various approaches, such as microarray analysis and RNA sequencing, have pros and cons. Microarrays are useful for profiling known sets of genes but often fail to capture new transcripts or deal with alternative splicing events. Conversely, RNA sequencing can provide in-depth information regarding the transcriptome, but can be challenging in terms of complex data processing and bioinformatics tools to interpret the vast volume of data generated. Moreover, high-throughput sequencing technology and financial inputs involved in it might be costly, especially for small laboratories. This disparity influences accessibility to high-level methods, which in turn may widen the immunology knowledge gap. Therefore, the selection of an appropriate method for specific research questions is paramount to produce reliable and relevant results. In addition to methodological and biological hurdles, the obstacle lies in interpreting and incorporating gene expression information into the immunological pathways. Correlation of gene expression changes with functionally immunologically meaningful outcomes in immune cells demands an intense understanding of complex signal networks and interactions. For example, studies using porcine intestinal epitheliocyte cell lines have demonstrated immune function modulation by probiotics through the use of transcriptomics to demonstrate complicated interactions between host and microbial cells (Kobayashi et al., 2016). These findings can be difficult to translate into other biological systems, including human immunity, due to species differences, immunity complexity, and differences in environmental context. Thus, researchers have to work around such complications with the utmost caution, such that conclusions from gene expression research are valid and applicable to the field of immunology. Overcoming complications is essential to leveraging gene expression analysis as a powerful instrument in uncovering new immunological discoveries.

5.5.1. Variability in Gene Expression Data

Gene expression variability research is important in unraveling the nuances of differences in immune responses among individuals. Gene expression can vary as a result of multiple factors, including genetic background, environmental elements, and physiological condition. For instance, research has shown that individuals have marked variation in their immune response to such immune challenges as infection or immunization. Such variation tends to come from baseline levels of expression of the central genes of the immunity pathways. Through the delineation of such differences, researchers can begin to discern patterns revealing disease susceptibility, which is necessary for the creation of targeted therapeutic regimens. For example, ascertaining the correlation between varying levels of the expression of specific genes and immune reactions can aid in making personalized medicine regimens for immunology, where treatment regimens can be adjusted on an individual-by-individual basis based on their personalized gene expression patterns (Wanelik et al., 2020). Furthermore, the coordination between single-cell environments and gene expression is significant in regulating immune responses. A recent, enlightening study on bone marrow mesenchymal stromal cells has elucidated some of this relationship by illustrating how alterations in gene transcription in the stroma can have a significant influence on hematopoietic stem cells. The heterogeneity observed in the expression of genes in such stroma cells has a direct impact on their interaction with hematopoietic stem cells and, in turn, the overall function and lineage production of the immune system. In particular, loss of a few genes in mesenchymal stromal cells can cause long-lasting changes in the cellular structure and gene expression profiles of these cells. These advances underscore the importance of the cellular microenvironment in organizing gene expression variability and demonstrate the intricate crosstalk necessary to maintain immune homeostasis, essential for long-term immunity (Derecka et al., 2020). Finally, an explanation of variability in gene expression data in immunology not only enhances our appreciation of human immune response but also illuminates more universal biological principles. It offers a framework for understanding how variant transcriptional activities shape immune cell behavior and the organism's general ability to respond to pathogens. Through an awareness of this heterogeneity, scientists are able to look for biomarkers that can potentially be used as indicators of an individual's immune status and prognostic outcomes. Thus, such knowledge lays the ground for novel therapeutic interventions that can modulate immune responses. With progress in the discipline, the application of sophisticated genomic approaches and high-throughput sequencing technologies will progressively clarify the complexity of gene expression variability, ultimately permitting more efficient immunotherapies tailored for heterogeneous patient populations (Wanelik et al., 2020).

5.5.2. Technical Limitations of Current Methods

The landscape of gene expression analysis in immunology is largely characterized by the method used, but the methods often encounter major technical limitations. One problem that is found on a consistent basis is overreliance on scRNA-seq data, which, while having high resolution, may not address well the nuances of bulk RNA-seq from sorted cell populations. Current methods demand excessive curation of results and application of extremely strict statistical thresholds, which can inadvertently suppress the true biological signals needed to uncover immune responses. Furthermore, the majority of available tools fail to effectively account for tissue background expression and, thereby, may misrepresent gene expression profiles. This methodological shortcoming not only prevents the identification of stable biomarkers but further complicates translation into clinical application, emphasizing the need to embrace sophisticated analytical methods that can overcome such a limitation (Chen et al., 2025). The development of approaches such as mastR is an important milestone in the transition toward addressing such challenges through offering an automated approach to marker identification in labeled bulk RNA-seq data. With this advance, however, there are still issues of ensuring that tools such as these provide consistent and reproducible outcomes under various experimental conditions. While mastR employs efficient statistical pipelines like edgeR and limma for explicit comparisons, inherent noise that is part of transcriptomic data may generate variation in marker selection performance. Additionally, the utility of such programs relies on the accurate assessment of signal-to-noise ratios, which play a significant role in minimizing background expressions. Hence, while mastR is encouraging when used in combination with traditional resources, the underlying complexity of the biological processes that are being studied calls for ongoing improvement and calibration of the approaches to ensure their efficacy under different immunological contexts (Chen et al., 2025). One more major limitation of gene expression research lies in the realm of post-transcriptional control, e.g., by alterations such as N6-methyladenosine (m6A). The techniques employed to investigate m6A and other modifications in RNA play a central role in deciphering how they operate in gene regulation, but are not without limitations. Much of today's mapping and measuring of m6A sites is still troubled by sensitivity and specificity. On top of that, as more is learned about such modifications, the demand for methods capable of examining more than one regulatory mechanism within a single framework becomes more pressing. Hence, as emphasized in recent reviews, ongoing evolution and integration of new technologies will be important to fill such existing gaps and promote research to effectively link gene regulation to immune function and disorder.

5.5.3. Ethical Considerations in Immunological Research

Just like in the case of expression analysis of genes in immunological research, ethical concerns become of great significance during the design and execution of experiments. Given that immunological data entails personal information, there must be adherence to very strict ethical principles in patient confidentiality and informed consent by researchers. The procurement of biological samples involves not only consent but also the explanation of potential risks and benefits in relation to research. Ethical protocols also necessitate the disclosure of findings to prevent the misleading of data that would lead to unjustified clinical application. The duty to uphold such standards of ethics becomes more imperative with the use of advanced technologies such as AI and machine learning in research processes. Such strategies generate large volumes of data, which increases the need for ethical consciousness in upholding secrecy and assuring proper utilization of information from gene expression studies. The complexity in gene expression data necessitates sophisticated computational techniques that may unintentionally create ethical challenges. For instance, while AI-based programs may improve the accuracy of immunological diagnosis, reducing computational complexity traditionally hinders interpretability and the validity of results. The application of methods like dimensionality reduction, while beneficial in data analysis simplification, might obscure critical biological variations necessary for the understanding of disease mechanisms. Furthermore, as researchers move for greater accuracy in diagnosing diseases such as cancer, ethical concerns of misdiagnosis or over-reliance on computer systems must be addressed. The imperative to harmonize the application of cutting-edge technologies with ethical balance renders the discussion on sound practices in immunological studies increasingly important as these technologies become increasingly prevalent in clinical practice. In addition, matters of equity and access with regard to immunological studies cannot be ignored. Genetic variation and reactions to immunotherapy can vary considerably in diverse populations, and this may have implications for health disparities if not adequately addressed. Researchers should take into consideration how the findings of gene expression analysis are communicated and utilized in different demographic populations. Immunological ethical standards need to prioritize inclusivity to guarantee research benefits are equitably distributed and vulnerable populations are not disproportionately harmed by research findings. As AI and machine learning technologies become increasingly utilized, as in recent studies, it is imperative that the focus of who partakes in such studies be expanded to allow for greater representation. Thus, ethical considerations in immunological research not only serve imminent needs for patient health but also encompass broader societal interests that impact future precision medicine and health equity (Figure 5.13).

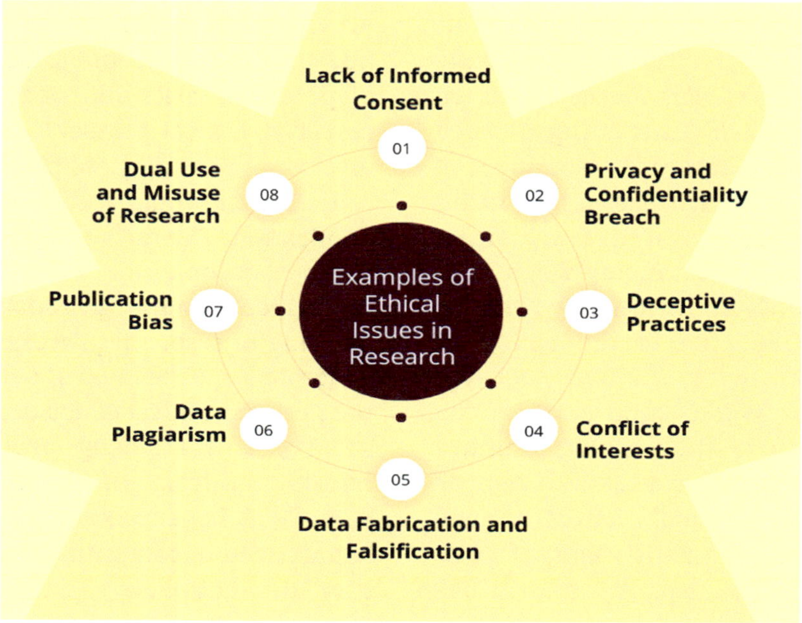

Figure 5.13. Examples of ethical issues.

Source: https://www.enago.com/academy/wp-content/uploads/2023/12/Examples-of-Ethical-Issues-1.png.

5.6. Future Directions in Gene Expression Research

Advances in the area of gene expression research hold tremendous potential for immunology advances. The identification of regulatory elements, such as enhancers and silencers, remains a prominent area of research, with a focus on their role in MHC determinant expression. As no surprise, research on CIITA, the MHC II transcriptional master switch, underscores the complexities of immune responses. Future research may explore post-translational modification of CIITA, which is not yet well characterized, as this could reveal new immune regulatory and dysfunction mechanisms. An improved understanding of such regulatory elements could identify novel therapeutic strategies in diseases like cancer and autoimmune disease, for which inappropriate immunity is the rule. With new gene expression profiling technologies, researchers are about to uncover the intricacies of immune system function and regulation. Another promising frontier in gene expression research is the combination of next-generation sequencing (NGS) and single-cell RNA sequencing (scRNA-seq) technologies. These technologies enable high-resolution analysis of gene expression patterns at unimagined scales, enabling investigators to study heterogeneous populations in innate and adaptive immunity. The application of scRNA-seq can shed light on cellular heterogeneity of responses to pathological stimulation and reveal how some immune cells engage within the general framework of the immune system. Data obtained by this investigation will undoubtedly guide the development of targeted immunotherapies. In addition, the understanding of expression patterns under various immune responses can allow the identification of novel biomarkers, enhancing diagnostic and prognostic capabilities in immunologic disease. The future of gene expression analysis in immunology will definitely be boosted by such superior technologies. As gene expression research expands, an integrated understanding of environmental factors that affect immune reactions will become paramount. The influence of external environments, such as pathogens and host organism interactions, needs to be included as well. Recent discoveries in the area of crustacean immunity reveal fundamental differences in innate immune responses between protostomes and deuterostomes, like vertebrates. This new area of science highlights the necessity for comparative immunology studies on a variety of disparate taxa. Beyond that, the breaking of issues like the lack of immortal cell lines as well as inadequate genomic resources will also be important in broadening our understanding of immune mechanisms. By addressing these issues, researchers have the ability to further develop our knowledge of host-pathogen interactions, which are critical to the design of efficient treatment strategies in aquaculture and other uses impacted by immunological constraints (Drozina et al., 2005; Hauton, 2012).

5.6.1. Advances in Technology and Methodology

Advances in technology and methodology over the past decade have completely transformed the field of gene expression analysis in immunology. High-throughput sequencing technologies, and RNA-seq in particular, have significantly enhanced the scope to profile gene expression with unprecedented depth and precision. Unlike other approaches, such as quantitative PCR, RNA-seq yields a snapshot of transcriptomes, which allows known and unknown transcripts, as well as splice variants, to be identified. This capability enables immunologists to study cellular responses to immune insult or infection at an unparalleled level, revealing insights that guide the development of immunotherapies and vaccines. Moreover, the application of bioinformatics tools in analyzing enormous data generated by RNA-seq makes it easier to identify biomarkers of possible clinical relevance, priming investigators to understand the complexities of immune responses at the molecular level. In conjunction with RNA sequencing, scRNA-seq is now a groundbreaking method in immunology. By facilitating the examination of gene expression at the single-cell level, scRNA-seq uncovers hidden heterogeneity among populations of immune cells that bulk analyses cannot resolve. This methodology breakthrough provides information on cell differentiation, activation status, and microenvironmental regulation of immune responses. This extent of specificity is especially significant in treatments like cancer, where the resolution of interactions between tumor and immune cells can uncover the optimal therapeutic targets. The design of sophisticated algorithms to process data also provides credence to deciphering intricate scRNA-seq profiles and thereby facilitating the integration of biological insights into the development of next-generation immunotherapies by means of accurate targeting of immune cell subsets. Besides, the integration of machine learning techniques into gene expression analysis protocols has stimulated the creation of novel understanding in immunological processes. Machine learning approaches make it possible to build patterns and predictive models from vast data sets, thereby utilizing maximum gene expression profile analysis. This is a boon in technology where immunologists can predict cellular responses to varied stimuli more rapidly and accurately. The potential of machine learning reagents to subclassify immune responses and predict treatment outcomes is particularly notable, for it brings together clinical knowledge and genomic insight, guiding individualized medicine approaches in immunotherapy. By continued refinement, these techniques stand to further dissect the complex functions of gene expression in disease and immunity, facilitating paradigmatic advances in immunological research and therapeutic development (Figure 5.14).

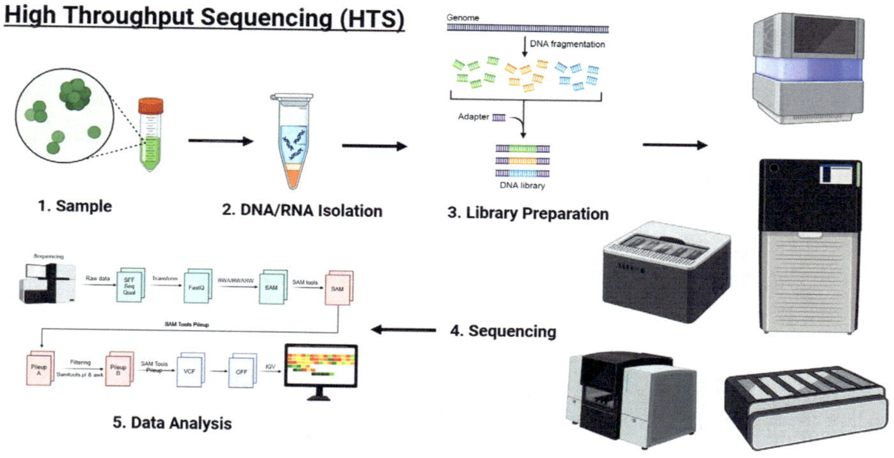

Figure 5.14. High-throughput sequencing (HTS).

Source: https://microbenotes.com/wp-content/uploads/2024/09/High-Throughput-Sequencing-HTS.jpeg.

5.6.2. Integration of Bioinformatics in Analysis

Bioinformatics integration in gene expression analysis is at the heart of the advancement of immunological science because it allows scientists to handle big data generated by high-throughput methods. By employing sophisticated computational tools, researchers have been able to decode complex biological information that would otherwise not be understandable using traditional methods. This integration makes it possible to identify differentially expressed genes, reveal molecular pathways involved in immune response, and determine possible targets for therapy. In addition, bioinformatics also helps in annotating non-coding RNAs (ncRNAs), which are principal players in gene control. Having access to complete databases and analysis tools enhances the validity of these analyses, which allows a better understanding of immune-related processes. With the growth of bioinformatics, its role in integrating diverse levels of biological data gains significance, imparting a broad overview of gene expression dynamics in immunology. An exemplary instance of bioinformatics impact upon the field can be found in the development of domain-specific ontologies, such as the Non-Coding RNA Ontology (NCRO). The NCRO exists to provide a shared terminology for annotating ncRNA data and thus satisfy a fundamental need for semantic consistency of biological data analysis.

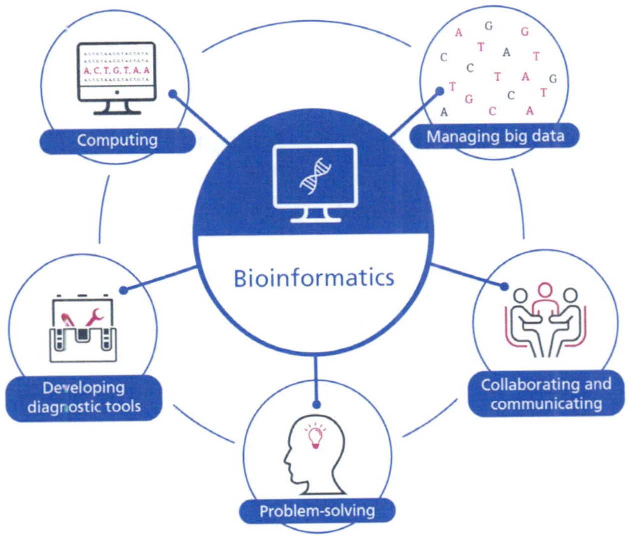

Figure 5.15. Bioinformatics graphic.

Source: https://www.genomicseducation.hee.nhs.uk/wp-content/uploads/2021/04/Bioinformatics-graphic-01-983x640.png.

By providing a solid foundation for exchanging and interpreting data, the NCRO allows researchers to compare findings and replicate studies on diverse platforms. This is particularly so in the field of immunology, where regulation of gene expression by ncRNA can have dramatic effects on immune processes. With bioinformatics, researchers are better placed to categorize and compare ncRNAs, and the outcome is the revelation of novel mechanisms that govern immune system function and disease, leading to unprecedented advances in the treatment and prevention of disease, hence demonstrating the critical interplay between computational and life sciences in immunological research. Moreover, the application of bioinformatics tools is spreading to the field of translational medicine, where it finds application in discovering biomarkers of immunological disorders. By application of computational algorithms on high-dimensional omics data, researchers can identify relevant biomarkers that facilitate diagnostics and drug development. The complexity of immunological responses implies that optimal sets of biomarkers must be selected, their selection being informed by mathematical theories and models in bioinformatics. Understanding such principles allows researchers to construct predictive models that hold promise to inform clinical decisions. In addition, multi-microarray data integration enhances the robustness of biomarker systems through the provision of complete information regarding expression patterns across different states of immunity. By bridging the gap between computational algorithms and clinical practice, bioinformatics is revolutionizing gene expression analysis in immunology, ultimately improving patient care and reducing the duration of biomedical innovation (Wang & Sarwal, 2015) (Figure 5.15).

5.6.3. Potential for Personalized Medicine in Immunology

Potential for personalized medicine in immunology is increasing, primarily as a result of improvements in gene expression analysis. By examining the unique expression patterns of genes involved in immune response, researchers are able to determine individual variation in resistance to disease, response to treatments, and overall health. Immunology increasingly uses genomic methods to divide patients into groups according to their expression profiles, allowing for personalized therapeutic regimens. As an illustration, individuals with a specific set of expression profiles for specific genes may respond to a specific type of immunotherapy more favorably, highlighting the need for personalized treatment approaches. This personalized approach not only optimizes effectiveness but also minimizes non-indicated side effects, a paradigmatic shift in the management of immunological disorders. In addition, as emphasized by the rise of pharmacogenetics, integration of gene expression profiling into individualized medicine has the potential to revolutionize therapeutic efficacy in immunology. Genetic variation can inform the selection of immunosuppressive therapy, leading to treatments that are aligned with the individual's genetic constitution. These advancements have already begun to impact clinical practice, but systematic application is still uneven. The remaining hurdles are inconsistent results of gene variant studies and the absence of consistent clinical guidelines. Progress towards these new developments thus necessitates the creation of standardized protocols for the effective use of these outcomes in the clinical domain, to realize the full potential of personalized medicine in immunology. Moreover, improvements in NGS technologies have been a vital factor in expediting the identification of personalized medicine in immunology. NGS allows high-throughput sequencing of large sets of genes, leading to in-depth information on immune-related gene expression. With its increasing capabilities, researchers are unraveling the complexities of immune responses at unprecedented speed and accuracy, enabling them to identify new biomarkers for disease progression and treatment response. The growing evidence base for these technologies highlights their importance in the generation of more effective immunotherapeutic strategies. However, it is important that quality control and the ethics of genetic testing receive attention to ensure patient safety and trust. In this fast-paced situation, open communication among the stakeholders is important to address challenges and enable the responsible implementation of NGS for personalized medicine in the field of immunology.

SUMMARY

Gene expression analysis has emerged as a major methodology in immunology for interpreting immune responses and their variation across different populations. The integration of gene expression profiling in immunologic studies reflects its significance in determining the mechanisms that regulate immune function. For instance, immune gene expression in threespine sticklebacks was studied, highlighting extensive differences in gene profiles between infected and uninfected populations due to condition and reproductive status. The findings indicate the interactional influence of environmental and biological factors on immune gene expression and, by proxy, the overall immune response of organisms. These discoveries not only reveal a better understanding of host-pathogen relationships but also open the way to the development of targeted immunotherapies, establishing the productive use of gene expression analysis in both basic and applied immunology. Moreover, the therapeutic potential of the understanding of gene expression is even illustrated dramatically in the regulation of regulatory T cells (Tregs), whose function in immune system balance and tolerance is fundamental. The newest developments have shown that Tregs may be grown *in vitro* without harming their functional integrity, so that more of these cells can be on hand for therapeutic use. The protocol that was proven used CD4+CD25 hi cells derived from human peripheral blood and confirmed that Tregs could be grown at length while retaining essential surface markers for the suppressive function. This highlights the profound importance of the analysis of gene expression for enhancing Treg-based treatments of autoimmune diseases. By recognizing and developing such valuable immune cells, researchers can anticipate new paradigms for treatment that promote tolerance and minimize the injurious features of autoimmunity, and this indicates the utilitarian consequences resulting from influential research on gene expression. Last but not least, gene expression research in immunology contributes both to theoretical insights and to a path for the translation of research to clinical application. The intricate relationship between gene expression profiles and immune reactions, as evidenced by experiments across a range of organisms, underlines the belief that a cure for immune disorders requires sensitive information about genetic elements. The immune gene expression profiles analyses, as seen in the findings of threespine sticklebacks and Treg expansions, pave the way for novel therapeutic intervention in line with personal response. With increasing science, there is a necessity for continued studies to build on these findings in powerful ways, propelling immunotherapy advancements founded on gene expression analysis that is its basis. Lastly, the future of immunology is inextricably linked to the further investigation of gene expression because it has the ability to unlock groundbreaking methods to treating and preventing diseases.

The regulation of gene expression is at the core of the science of immunology in terms of how transcriptional profiles within an organism influence immune responses. Cristina outlines key studies in relation to the importance of gene regulation for HSCs and their interaction with MSCs. It has been demonstrated through studies that the transcription factor Ebf1 plays a vital role in regulating the cellular composition of the bone marrow niche required to maintain good HSC function. Conditional deletion of Ebf1 illustrates deep alterations in gene expression profiles and composition of stromal cells, resulting in long-term modulation of HSC behavior, such as decreased quiescence and myeloid generation. It highlights the intricate relationship between regulation of gene expression and immune cell dynamics in health and disease, and suggests important pathways for future research into immunological therapies (Derecka et al., 2020). In addition to cellular communication, the gene expression analysis of pathogens provides critical insights into immune mechanisms. Bovine mastitis research demonstrates how systemic and local mechanisms might be followed through changes in gene expression. By employing next-generation sequencing to characterize mRNA and miRNA expression in CD14+ monocytes from infected bovine animals, researchers identified over 3,700 differentially expressed genes. Interestingly, genes with higher expression were related to inflammatory processes, with an emphasis on immune response induction in infection. Meanwhile, miRNAs seemed to be the important regulators of the activity of amplifying inflammatory signaling, fine-tuning the efficiency of immune responses. This overall investigation of gene expression is not merely helpful for broadening our knowledge about immune cell behavior during infection but also identifies some molecular networks that can be targeted as a matter of therapeutic interventions (Lawless et al., 2014). Lastly, the combination of results from these studies underscores the complexity of the immunological role of gene expression. The findings illustrate how alterations in gene expression can have widespread implications for immune cell function, stability, and disease susceptibility. For instance, the long-term consequences observed in HSCs following Ebf1 deletion show how genetic alteration in the bone marrow microenvironment can affect overall immunity. Meanwhile, the intricate regulatory roles miRNAs play in monocytes during infection reveal a depth in the immune system that must be investigated. Mapping gene expression studies to functional outcomes allows researchers to reveal the complexity of immunity, leading to new therapeutic avenues for the enhancement of immune response in various clinical situations (Lawless et al., 2014; Derecka et al., 2020).

A CLOSER LOOK

INNATE LYMPHOID CELLS (ILCS)

ILCs are a group of immune cells that play an essential role in both immunity and tissue homeostasis, acting as tissue sentinels and rapidly responding to infection or tissue damage signals. Unlike T cells, ILCs lack antigen-specific receptors but mirror T cell activities in cytokine release and regulation of immune responses. Five major subsets of ILCs are natural killer (NK) cells, ILC1, ILC2, ILC3, and lymphoid tissue inducer (LTi) cells (Figure 5.16).

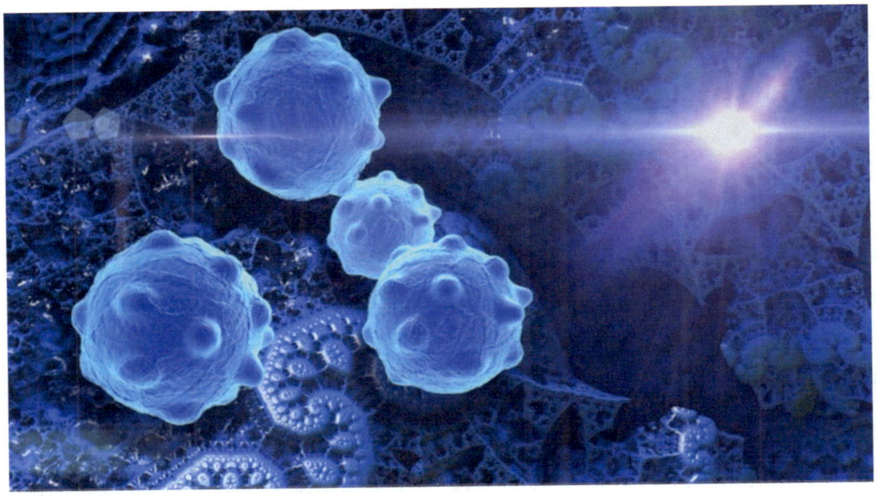

Figure 5.16. Innate lymphoid cells.

Source: https://blog.benchsci.com/hs-fs/hubfs/iStock-534404806-350963-edited.jpg?width=740&height=411&name=iStock-534404806-350963-edited.jpg.

1. Central Features of ILCs:

a. **Tissue Resident:** ILCs are predominantly tissue-resident, especially on mucosal tissues like the gut, lungs, and skin, where they act as sentinels.

b. **Rapid Response:** They react quickly to signals from infected or injured tissues, producing immune responses without sensitization.

c. **Cytokine Production:** ILCs produce a variety of cytokines, which are signal molecules that help to orchestrate immune responses, similar to T helper cells.

d. **No Antigen Receptors:** Unlike T cells, ILCs do not have T cell receptors (TCRs), meaning that they don't respond to specific antigens.

e. **Regulation of Homeostasis:** ILCs play critical roles in the maintenance of tissue health and homeostasis, as well as with the microbiota.

f. **Plasticity:** Some ILC subsets can change their characteristics depending on environmental cues to adapt to changing situations.

2. ILC Subtypes:

a. **NK Cells:** Similar to cytotoxic T cells, they target and kill infected or cancer cells.
b. **ILC1:** Released IFN-γ and TNF, and are involved in intracellular pathogen and tumor responses.
c. **ILC2:** Released cytokines IL-5, IL-13, and IL-4, and are involved in allergic response, tissue repair, and metabolic homeostasis.
d. **ILC3:** Released IL-22 and IL-17, important for mucosal immunity, gut health, and responses to extracellular pathogens.
e. **LTi Cells:** Only contribute to lymphoid tissue formation.

3. ILCs in Health and Disease:

a. **Infection Control:** ILCs help the body fight various pathogens, including bacteria, viruses, and parasites.
b. **Inflammation Regulation:** They are capable of triggering as well as inhibiting inflammatory responses and support tissue repair and homeostasis.
c. **Metabolic Homeostasis:** ILC2s support the regulation of fat storage and energy expenditure.
d. **Autoimmune and Inflammatory Disorders:** Dysregulation of ILCs can result in autoimmune conditions like inflammatory bowel disease (IBD) and atopic dermatitis.
e. **Cancer:** ILCs can support or suppress tumor development, depending on the context.

4. Future Directions:

a. Research has to continue to decipher the complex interactions between ILCs, other immune cells, and the environment.
b. Therapeutic targeting of ILCs can yield new opportunities for a host of diseases.

REFERENCES

1. Aburub, F., Al-Akayleh, F., Abdel-Rahem, R., Al-Remawi, M., & Agha, A. S. A. (2025). AI-driven transcriptomics: Advancing gene expression analysis and precision medicine. *2025 1st International Conference on Computational Intelligence Approaches and Applications (ICCIAA).* https://www.semanticscholar.org/paper/cf2ff47d6c01eeba89815fdd22810dd6801a60a3 (accessed on 27th June 2025).
2. Hauton C. The scope of the crustacean immune system for disease control. *J Invertebr Pathol.* 2012;110(2):251-260. doi:10.1016/j.jip.2012.03.005Ahmed, N., Heitlinger, E., Affinass, N., Kühl, A. A., Xenophontos, N., Jarquin, V. H., Jost, J., Steinfelder, S., & Hartmann, S. (2019). A Novel Non-invasive Method to Detect RELM Beta Transcript in Gut Barrier Related Changes During a Gastrointestinal Nematode Infection. *Frontiers in immunology, 10*, 445. https://doi.org/10.3389/fimmu.2019.00445(accessed on 27th June 2025).
3. Aghazadeh, A., Alho, C., Amitani, R., Anholt, R. R., et al. (2016). TSPO: Kaleidoscopic 18-kDa amid biochemical pharmacology, control and targeting of mitochondria. https://core.ac.uk/download/36779164.pdf (accessed on 27th June 2025).
4. Igata, M., Islam, M. A., Tada, A., Takagi, M., Kober, A. K. M. H., Albarracin, L., Aso, H., Ikeda-Ohtsubo, W., Miyazawa, K., Yoda, K., He, F., Takahashi, H., Villena, J., & Kitazawa, H. (2019). Transcriptome Modifications in Porcine Adipocytes via Toll-Like Receptors Activation. *Frontiers in immunology, 10*, 1180. https://doi.org/10.3389/fimmu.2019.01180(accessed on 27th June 2025).
5. Kobayashi, H., Albarracin, L., Sato, N., Kanmani, P., Kober, A. K., Ikeda-Ohtsubo, W., Suda, Y., Nochi, T., Aso, H., Makino, S., Kano, H., Ohkawara, S., Saito, T., Villena, J., & Kitazawa, H. (2016). Modulation of porcine intestinal epitheliocytes immunetranscriptome response by Lactobacillus jensenii TL2937. *Beneficial microbes, 7*(5), 769–782. https://doi.org/10.3920/BM2016.0095(accessed on 27th June 2025).
6. Pineda, M. A., Al-Riyami, L., Harnett, W., & Harnett, M. M. (2014). Lessons from helminth infections: ES-62 highlights new interventional approaches in rheumatoid arthritis. *Clinical and experimental immunology, 177*(1), 13–23. https://doi.org/10.1111/cei.12252(accessed on 27th June 2025).
7. Sanjurjo, L., Aran, G., Téllez, É., Amézaga, N., Armengol, C., López, D., Prats, C., & Sarrias, M. R. (2018). CD5L Promotes M2 Macrophage Polarization through Autophagy-Mediated Upregulation of ID3. *Frontiers in immunology, 9*, 480. https://doi.org/10.3389/fimmu.2018.00480 (accessed on 27th June 2025).
8. An, D. S., Baltimore, D., Bonifadno, A., Chen, I. S. Y., et al. (2007). Stable reduction of CCR5 by RNAi through hematopoietic stem cell transplant in non-human primates. https://core.ac.uk/download/4877409.pdf (accessed on 27th June 2025).
9. Khush, K. K., Pham, M. X., Teuteberg, J. J., Kfoury, A. G., Deng, M. C., Kao, A., Anderson, A. S., Cotts, W. G., Ewald, G. A., Baran, D. A., Hiller, D., Yee, J., & Valantine, H. A. (2015). Gene expression profiling to study racial differences after heart transplantation. *The Journal of heart and lung transplantation : the official publication of the International Society for Heart Transplantation, 34*(7), 970–977. https://doi.org/10.1016/j.healun.2015.01.987(accessed on 27th June 2025).

10. Anderson, J., Olafsdottir, T. A., Kratochvil, S., McKay, P. F., Östensson, M., Persson, J., Shattock, R. J., & Harandi, A. M. (2018). Molecular Signatures of a TLR4 Agonist-Adjuvanted HIV-1 Vaccine Candidate in Humans. *Frontiers in immunology*, *9*, 301. https://doi.org/10.3389/fimmu.2018.00301 (accessed on 27th June 2025).
11. Shaun Robertson, Janette E. Bradley and Andrew D.C. MacColl (2016). Parallelism and divergence in immune responses: A comparison of expression levels in two lakes. Evolutionary Ecology Research, 2016, 17: 1–16(accessed on 27th June 2025).
12. Tuccilli, C., Baldini, E., Sorrenti, S., Catania, A., Antonelli, A., Fallahi, P., Tartaglia, F., Barollo, S., Mian, C., Palmieri, A., Carbotta, G., Arcieri, S., Pironi, D., Vergine, M., Monti, M., & Ulisse, S. (2018). CTLA-4 and PD-1 Ligand Gene Expression in Epithelial Thyroid Cancers. *International journal of endocrinology*, *2018*, 1742951. https://doi.org/10.1155/2018/1742951(accessed on 27th June 2025).
13. Wanelik, K.M., Begon, M., Arriero, E. *et al.* Transcriptome-wide analysis reveals different categories of response to a standardised immune challenge in a wild rodent. *Sci Rep* **10**, 7444 (2020). https://doi.org/10.1038/s41598-020-64307-7(accessed on 27th June 2025).
14. Chirumamilla CS, Palagani A, Kamaraj B, et al. Selective Glucocorticoid Receptor Properties of GSK866 Analogs with Cysteine Reactive Warheads. *Front Immunol*. 2017;8:1324. Published 2017 Nov 1. doi:10.3389/fimmu.2017.01324(accessed on 27th June 2025).
15. Mathieu, M. G., Linley, A. J., Reeder, S. P., Badoual, C., Tartour, E., Rees, R. C., & McArdle, S. E. (2010). HAGE, a cancer/testis antigen expressed at the protein level in a variety of cancers. *Cancer immunity*, *10*, 2.(accessed on 27th June 2025).
16. Lawless, N., Reinhardt, T. A., Bryan, K., Baker, M., Pesch, B., Zimmerman, D., Zuelke, K., Sonstegard, T., O'Farrelly, C., Lippolis, J. D., & Lynn, D. J. (2014). MicroRNA regulation of bovine monocyte inflammatory and metabolic networks in an in vivo infection model. *G3 (Bethesda, Md.)*, *4*(6), 957–971. https://doi.org/10.1534/g3.113.009936(accessed on 27th June 2025).
17. Baldini, E., Carbotta, G., Catania, A., D'Armiento, M., et al. (2017). Vitiligo and autoimmune thyroid disorders. https://core.ac.uk/download/127588138.pdf (accessed on 27th June 2025).
18. Breda, J., Banerjee, A., Jayachandran, R., Pieters, J., & Zavolan, M. (2022). A novel approach to single-cell analysis reveals intrinsic differences in immune marker expression in unstimulated BALB/c and C57BL/6 macrophages. *FEBS letters*, *596*(20), 2630–2643. https://doi.org/10.1002/1873-3468.14478(accessed on 27th June 2025).
19. Bharanidharan, N., Chakravarthy, S., Venkatesan, V. K., Abbas, M., Ramakrishna, M. T., Ellappan, M., & Venkatesan, K. (2024). Local entropy-based remora optimization and sparse autoencoders for cancer diagnosis through microarray gene expression analysis. *IEEE Access*, *12*, 39285–39299. https://www.semanticscholar.org/paper/dbd8aa73a369458ff97660022e7b19603d585b8c (accessed on 27th June 2025).
20. Huang, J., Eilbeck, K., Smith, B., Blake, J. A., Dou, D., Huang, W., Natale, D. A., Ruttenberg, A., Huan, J., Zimmermann, M. T., Jiang, G., Lin, Y., Wu, B., Strachan, H. J., de Silva, N., Kasukurthi, M. V., Jha, V. K., He, Y., Zhang, S., Wang, X., ... Tan, M. (2016). The development of non-coding RNA ontology. *International journal of data mining and bioinformatics*, *15*(3), 214–232. https://doi.org/10.1504/IJDMB.2016.077072(accessed on 27th June 2025).
21. McLoughlin, K. E., Nalpas, N. C., Rue-Albrecht, K., Browne, J. A., Magee, D. A., Killick, K. E., Park, S. D., Hokamp, K., Meade, K. G., O'Farrelly, C., Gormley, E., Gordon, S. V., & MacHugh,

D. E. (2014). RNA-seq Transcriptional Profiling of Peripheral Blood Leukocytes from Cattle Infected with Mycobacterium bovis. *Frontiers in immunology*, *5*, 396. https://doi.org/10.3389/fimmu.2014.00396(accessed on 27th June 2025).

22. Richard H. Scheuermann et al. (2009). Ontology-based knowledge representation of experiment metadata in biological data mining. Prepublication version of chapter to appear in Jake Chen and Stefano Lonardi (eds.), Biological Data Mining, Boca Raton: Chapman Hall / Taylor and Francis, September 2009, 529-559.. https://core.ac.uk/download/131216239.pdf (accessed on 27th June 2025).

23. Derecka, M., Herman, J. S., Cauchy, P., Ramamoorthy, S., Lupar, E., Grün, D., & Grosschedl, R. (2020). EBF1-deficient bone marrow stroma elicits persistent changes in HSC potential. *Nature immunology*, *21*(3), 261–273. https://doi.org/10.1038/s41590-020-0595-7Chen, J., Mohamed, A., Bhuva, D. D., Davis, M. J., & Tan, C. W. (2025). mastR: An R package for automated identification of tissue-specific gene signatures in multi-group differential expression analysis. *Bioinformatics, 41*. https://www.semanticscholar.org/paper/7833006e90dfb0d30e25319cc3e0c085376606fd (accessed on 27th June 2025).

24. De Paepe, A., & Vanakker, O. (2013). Pharmacogenomics in children: Advantages and challenges of next generation sequencing applications. https://core.ac.uk/download/55848729.pdf (accessed on 27th June 2025).

25. Drozina, G., Kohoutek, J., Jabrane-Ferrat, N., & Peterlin, B. M. (2005). Expression of MHC II genes. *Current topics in microbiology and immunology*, *290*, 147–170. https://doi.org/10.1007/3-540-26363-2_7 (accessed on 27th June 2025).

26. Duan, J., Jiang, R., Shen, H., Xu, X., & Sun, D. (2024). Analysis of nitrogen metabolism-related gene expression in hepatocellular carcinoma to establish relevant indicators for prediction of prognosis and guidance of immunotherapy. *Computer Methods in Biomechanics and Biomedical Engineering.* https://www.semanticscholar.org/paper/3c614f922d7c14c91d88f2b7eb275adfe6a4a901 (accessed on 27th June 2025).

27. Sharma, S., & Eghbali, M. (2014). Influence of sex differences on microRNA gene regulation in disease. *Biology of sex differences*, *5*(1), 3. https://doi.org/10.1186/2042-6410-5-3(accessed on 27th June 2025).

28. Koido, S., Homma, S., Hara, E., Namiki, Y., Takahara, A., Komita, H., Nagasaki, E., Ito, M., Ohkusa, T., Gong, J., & Tajiri, H. (2010). Regulation of tumor immunity by tumor/dendritic cell fusions. *Clinical & developmental immunology*, *2010*, 516768. https://doi.org/10.1155/2010/516768(accessed on 27th June 2025).

29. Huang, S., & Tu, T. (2025). Integrating single cell analysis and machine learning methods reveals stem cell-related gene S100A10 as an important target for prediction of liver cancer diagnosis and immunotherapy. *Frontiers in Immunology, 15*. https://www.semanticscholar.org/paper/2c51e83afe3c6017f70dd4281e69a160f6cec35a (accessed on 27th June 2025).

30. Mikami, Y., Scarno, G., Zitti, B., Shih, H. Y., Kanno, Y., Santoni, A., O'Shea, J. J., & Sciumè, G. (2018). NCR$^+$ ILC3 maintain larger STAT4 reservoir via T-BET to regulate type 1 features upon IL-23 stimulation in mice. *European journal of immunology*, *48*(7), 1174–1180. https://doi.org/10.1002/eji.201847480(accessed on 27th June 2025).

31. Krol, E., & Martin, S. A. M. (2017). Nutrigenomics and immune function in fish: New insights from omics technologies. https://core.ac.uk/download/80685929.pdf (accessed on 27th

June 2025).

32. Martin, S. A. M., Pooley, N. J., Secombes, C. J., Tacchi, L., et al. (2013). Inflammatory responses in primary muscle cell cultures in Atlantic salmon (*Salmo salar*). https://core.ac.uk/download/20664098.pdf (accessed on 27th June 2025).
33. Sabins, N., & Storkus, W. (2013). Engaging the immune response to normalize the tumor microenvironment. https://core.ac.uk/download/16509411.pdf (accessed on 27th June 2025).
34. Wang, A., & Sarwal, M. M. (2015). Computational Models for Transplant Biomarker Discovery. *Frontiers in immunology*, *6*, 458. https://doi.org/10.3389/fimmu.2015.00458(accessed on 27th June 2025).
35. Seaman, W., & Whitehouse, J. H. (2001). *Florida Marine Biotechnology: Research, Development and Training Capabilities to Advance Science and Commerce.* https://core.ac.uk/download/11016354.pdf (accessed on 27th June 2025).
36. Tegowski, M., & Meyer, K. D. (2024). Studying m6A in the brain: A perspective on current methods, challenges, and future directions. *Frontiers in Molecular Neuroscience, 17*. https://www.semanticscholar.org/paper/4de6a4e2508a720d9eb1ab50b96feebaa49a3640 (accessed on 27th June 2025).
37. Tripet, F. (2009). Ecological immunology of mosquito-malaria interactions: Of non-natural versus natural model systems and their inferences. https://core.ac.uk/download/28874744.pdf (accessed on 27th June 2025).
38. Vaninov, N., & Samstein, R. (2023). Abstract B041: Defining the determinants of immune response in DNA homologous recombination deficient tumors. *Cancer Immunology Research.* https://www.semanticscholar.org/paper/81f29beaaebea82d04e5a00a2c3534a500f2415a (accessed on 27th June 2025).
39. Watkins, K., Diao, L., Crochiere, M., & Pinkas, J. (2024). Abstract 1373: Gene expression correlation of immune checkpoint molecules Siglec-15 and PD-L1 varies widely by cancer indication. *Cancer Research.* https://www.semanticscholar.org/paper/f1049a16d1fd7382f127deafaf6cee9c7d06b2e8 (accessed on 27th June 2025).
40. Wesserling, M. (2013). Role of genetic aspect in pathogenesis of atopic dermatitis. https://core.ac.uk/download/71976799.pdf (accessed on 27th June 2025).

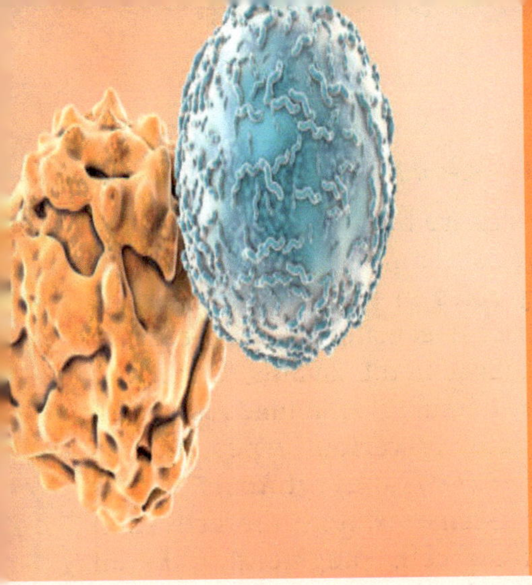

Chapter 6

T-CELL AND B-CELL BIOLOGY TECHNIQUES

Contents

Introduction

T-cell and B-cell biology are intricate biological processes that play a critical role in understanding adaptive immunity, and thus their study is critical for enhancing immunological understanding and therapeutic approaches. T-cells, which are thymus-derived cells, are responsible for guiding immune responses by various subpopulations, including helper and cytotoxic T-cells with distinct functions in immunity. Alternatively, B-cells, the antibody-producing cells, mature in the bone marrow and are at the forefront of humoral immunity. Their interaction not only aids in the recognition of pathogens but also in immune memory, making them the focus of vaccine and cancer immunotherapy development. Hence, learning the methods of T-cell and B-cell biology becomes essential to describe the mechanisms of immunity and to use that knowledge in practice, leading to breakthroughs in the treatment of infectious diseases and cancer. The research methods employed to study T-cells and B-cells have become increasingly advanced, integrating traditional and innovative approaches that allow researchers to dissect complex immune phenomena more effectively. Techniques such as flow cytometry and immunohistochemistry permit the characterization of cell populations and phenotypic markers with great specificity, providing insight into cellular functions and interactions. Moreover, mathematical models, particularly ODE-based models, are very useful for simulating biological systems and predicting reactions to interventions. Such experimental biology-mathematical modeling integration extends the analysis of immune dynamics towards an integrated understanding of T-cell and B-cell interactions within broader immunological contexts (MacLean et al., 2015). With further refinement of these approaches, new treatment options become available by tapping the full potential of the immune system.

As the dawn of an era broke where digital assets became even more prevalent than before, the use of e-learning environments and virtual microscopy in T-cell and B-cell biology techniques is transforming learning models fundamentally. Projects such as DMU e-Parasitology and DMU e-Biology are pioneering steps toward an improved mode of learning. The websites provide virtual exposure to tissue images and clinical slides through which students engage with sophisticated biological concepts actively (Peña-Fernández et al., 2019).

The ability to explore cellular morphology and pathology through digital platforms not only aids better comprehension but also boosts the learning of basic practical skills in present-day biomedical training. Furthermore, such technological advancement reflects the growing wave of integrative training in biomedical sciences that will equip future researchers and clinicians with a wide range of tools to combat the menace of immune-related diseases. Thus, the application of new education methods is crucial to foster future scientists in the area of immunology.

Overview of T-Cells and B-Cells

T-cells and B-cells are both components of the adaptive immune system, each with distinct but complementary roles in the protection of the body against disease-causing agents. T-cells, in turn most specialized in the thymus, function as the coordinators of multiple immune responses, discriminating among various types such as helper T-cells ($CD4^+$) and cytotoxic T-cells ($CD8^+$). Helper T-cells facilitate the activation of other immune cells, augmenting B-cell production of antibody and activating other immune responses. Cytotoxic T-cells, in contrast, kill infected or cancerous cells by direct cell-mediated cytotoxicity. Such ability to differentiate self from non-self is important in preventing autoimmune diseases, and hence the function of T-cells in immune self-tolerance and in the formation of protective immunological reactions. B-cells, which are derived from bone marrow and mature there, are the primary producers of antibodies that neutralize infections. Naive B-cells, upon encountering a specific antigen, possess the ability to become memory B-cells or plasma cells. Memory B-cells are crucial for long-term immunity because they allow for a prompt response to re-exposure to the same pathogen, while plasma cells are dedicated to antibody production. The antibodies secreted by plasma cells attach to antigens, allowing their neutralization and marking for destruction by other immune cells. B-cells' presentation of antigens is also important because they can present processed peptides to T-cells, again showing the coordination of these two cell types in immune response. Emerging techniques in T-cell and B-cell biology enhance our understanding of these building blocks of the immune system. Advances such as cryogenic electron microscopy and super-resolution microscopy play a pivotal role in deciphering the structural complexity of immune cell interactions. For example, individual nucleoporin copies were recently visualized successfully by DNA-PAINT microscopy, revealing the complex spatial structures of these immune cells (Schlichthaerle et al., 2019). Moreover, e-learning packages like DMU e-Biology, which make use of virtual microscopy, serve as valuable teaching material for students to explore cellular structures and dynamics in an interdisciplinary manner, adding to T-cell and B-cell biology (Peña-Fernández et al., 2019). With the help of these new technological methods, scientists can further understand the complexities of immune cell function and ultimately derive new therapeutic strategies for disease (Figure 6.1).

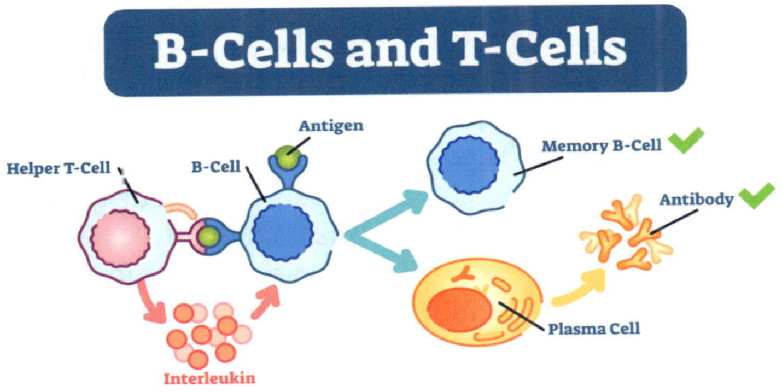

Figure 6.1. Illustration of B-Cell and T-Cell/

Source: https://kaleidoscopefightinglupus.org/wp-content/uploads/2021/04/B-Cell-and-T-Cell-Activation-diagram-scaled.jpg.

Importance of Studying T-Cell and B-Cell Biology

T-cell and B-cell biology is of extreme importance in comprehending the adaptive immune response, which plays a crucial role in the body's defense against disease. T-cells and B-cells have synergistic roles in the recognition and response to foreign invaders to acquire immunity. T-cells are primarily engaged in cell-mediated immunity, the recognition of infected cells, and the activation of other immune cells, while B-cells are critical for the production of antibodies that neutralize pathogens. Additionally, the research on these cells has revealed the wonders of immunological memory, explaining how vaccinations can establish a long-term immunity against some diseases. Continuing research in this area is important, as it not only makes us understand primary immunological principles better but also paves the way for the development of improved vaccines and therapeutic strategies against a large group of diseases, from allergies to autoimmune disorders. Moreover, technological and methodological innovations in the recent past have significantly enhanced our ability to conduct accurate studies on T-cell and B-cell dynamics. Techniques such as flow cytometry and single-cell RNA sequencing provide detailed information about cell populations and their functional status, and enable researchers to demystify the distinct functions of various T-cell and B-cell subsets. Such techniques also enable one to investigate how these cells engage with other immune components and respond to diverse stimuli and thereby get a clearer view of how the immune system works. For instance, there is recent research focused on non-classical major histocompatibility complex (MHC) class I molecules and their roles in innate and adaptive immunity that has the potential to radically change our perception of immunological interactions. The growing body of knowledge is not only essential for scientific research but also for guiding clinical strategies to modulate immune reactions in different therapies, particularly in oncology and chronic infections.

Lastly, understanding the biological mechanisms driving T-cell and B-cell function is key to the fight against public health concerns posed by infectious diseases and immune diseases. For example, amyloodiniosis imposes a broad impact on aquaculture, which causes severe economic loss as a result of severe mortality of fish. Research has begun to uncover the immune response of the affected species, such as the gilthead sea bream, by analyzing their plasma proteome and associated immunological markers, as identified in recent studies. These outcomes can be used to inform management practices and provide information on the production of effective vaccines or treatments to avert future outbreaks of disease within aquaculture systems. Ultimately, expanding our knowledge of B-cell and T-cell biology is not only required for the continuation of immunologic research but also to create solutions that can promote health globally, reinforcing the essential interface of basic science and practical application.

6.1. Fundamentals of T-Cell Biology

Biological functions of T-cells are central to understanding immunology and therapeutic applications. T-cells, which are the progeny of bone marrow-derived hematopoietic stem cells that mature predominantly in the thymus, are significant in adaptive immunity. Upon recognizing antigens, T-cells become clonally expanded and differentiated into effector and memory T-cells. Effector T-cells contribute significantly to orchestrating immune responses, whereas memory T-cells provide long-term immunity. The adaptive response allows for rapid and efficient responses against already encountered pathogens. An understanding of the sophistication of T-cell activation and the role of major histocompatibility complex (MHC) molecules in antigen presentation highlights the highly developed state of the immune system and the importance of T-cell biology (Guevara et al., 2016). Hence, the acquisition of T-cell biology not only provides insight into elementary immunological concepts but also determines therapeutic strategies against an array of diseases from cancer to autoimmunity. The most recent advancements in techniques to study T-cell biology have augmented our comprehension of their roles in function. Flow cytometry, for instance, is crucial to quantify and identify T-cell populations based on surface markers and intracellular cytokine production. The technique aids researchers in analyzing the activation and differentiation status of T-cells in high-throughput, enabling scientists to analyze intricate immune responses in disease and health. Furthermore, tools such as single-cell RNA sequencing allow the T-cell heterogeneity to be unraveled at a level of resolution that was previously unprecedented. Through such breakthroughs, scientists can analyze T-cell receptor (TCR) diversity and identify new T-cell subsets with distinct functional features. This new area of research will undoubtedly play its part in informing future therapeutic progress and our understanding of immune-mediated pathology, further emphasizing the significance of T-cell science to the broad discipline of immunology and clinical medicine (Cornell University, 1999). Moreover, the translation of the knowledge derived from T-cell biology to clinical use also involves an awareness of T-cell manipulation techniques. Techniques like CAR-T (Chimeric Antigen Receptor T-cell) therapy illustrate T-cell biology's impact on cutting-edge treatment. In this approach, T-cells are engineered to possess receptors that have the specificity for targeting specific cancer cells, a highlight of the capabilities of personalized medicine. Of equal importance is knowing the determinants of T-cell persistence and function after reinfusion for the optimization of treatment outcomes. Bringing together advances in bioinformatics with experimental approaches allows for enhanced predictions regarding patient response. As the biology of T-cells is increasingly advanced, multidisciplinary collaborations will be critical to the translation of these advances into effective therapies, filling the gap between laboratory research and bedside practice. Lastly, the fundamental principles of T-cell biology offer the platform upon which new approaches will have the potential to revolutionize therapeutic treatment of a wide array of health conditions.

6.1.1. Types of T-Cells: Helper, Cytotoxic, and Regulatory

The efficiency of the immune system relies largely on the multifunctional activities of T-cells, most importantly Helper T-cells, Cytotoxic T-cells, and Regulatory T-cells. The Helper T-cells, characterized by their CD4+ surface antigen, play the key role in coordinating the immune response. They activate B-cells to produce antibodies and enhance T-cell cytotoxicity and macrophage function. Coordination is crucial for creating a successful immune response against infection.

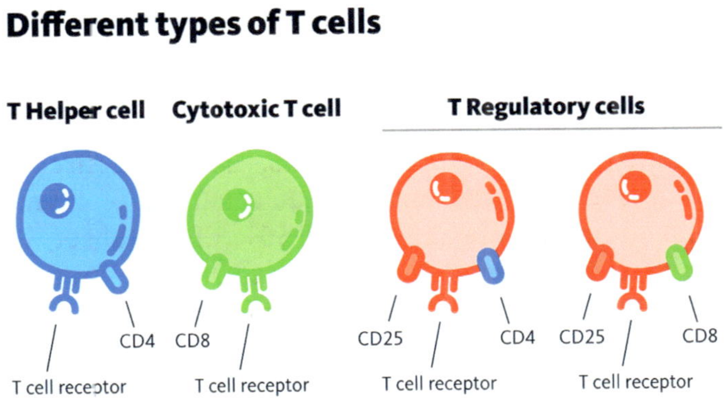

Figure 6.2. Different types of T cells.

Source: https://www.lipotype.com/wp-content/uploads/2022/07/different_types_of_t_cells-1024x623.png.webp.

The last decade or so has witnessed tremendous development in methods such as flow cytometry that have enabled researchers to quantify and analyze the different Helper T-cell populations with relative ease, thus better comprehending their complex roles in managing immunity and response processes. For instance, the identification of the various subsets of Helper T-cells, including Th1, Th2, and Th17 cells, has established their specific function in immunity and autoimmunity, and emphasized once again their importance in disease and health (Guevara et al., 2016). The CD8+ surface molecule defines cytotoxic T-cells, which are primarily involved in recognizing and destroying infected or cancer cells. Their activation is signal-restricted by Helper T-cells, which enhances the synergy behind the immune response. Once activated, Cytotoxic T-cells release perforins and granzymes that induce apoptosis in target cells and thus preserve tissue integrity in the presence of infections. Development of new biological techniques, such as single-cell RNA sequencing, has revealed the pathways of activation and the functional states of these T-cells, enabling scientists to characterize the variance in cytotoxic response between individuals. Interestingly, the efficacy of Cytotoxic T-cells is found to be determined by age, gender, and underlying disease presence, as much as it goes to highlight how complicated it is to tailor immunotherapies for illnesses such as cancer and viral infections (Zhang & Jin, 2023). Regulatory T-cells (Tregs), identified by their CD4+ and FOXP3+ antigens, are key immunological brakes whose function is to modulate immune responses and maintain tolerance to self-antigens. By suppressing other immune cells' proliferation and activation, Tregs prevent overactive immune responses leading to autoimmune disease. Recent advances in T-cell biology approaches have facilitated deeper exploration of Treg dynamics, including development and functional markers. Imaging and flow cytometric observations, for instance, have revealed perspectives on Treg migration patterns in tissue, influencing organ transplant and chronic inflammation discoveries. Furthermore, the balance between effector T-cells and Tregs is also critical in autoimmune diseases and cancer immunity, and therefore, such cells lie at the heart of the search for effective immunotherapies that are capable of releasing the immune system's regulatory capabilities (Guevara et al., 2016) (Figure 6.2).

6.1.2. T-Cell Development in the Thymus

The thymus is a specialized organ in the anterior chest and is critical for T-cell development. Being the central component of the adaptive immune system, the thymus is dedicated to the maturation of T cells from precursor cells that migrate from the bone marrow. The thymus develops a unique microenvironment where T cells undergo several critical phases, including positive and negative selection, to remain tolerant and functionally capable. In the thymus, there are distinct areas, such as the cortex and medulla, that handle distinct developmental processes. The cortex primarily facilitates positive selection of thymocytes since these cells express TCRs that are capable of recognizing self-MHC molecules. In this tightly controlled system, T cells that are capable of using self-MHC are stimulated to mature further, and others with non-functional receptors are induced to undergo apoptosis to arrive at a repertoire of T cells prepared to respond to pathogens. Negative selection is a physiological mechanism in the thymus that effectively deletes autoreactive T cells to maintain immune tolerance. This process occurs largely in the medulla and involves the presentation of self-antigens by thymic epithelial cells. Self-antigen high-affinity TCR-bearing thymocytes are triggered to undergo apoptosis, thus preventing potential autoimmune reactions. Balance in T-cell development is carefully regulated at a molecular level by necessary transcription factors and cytokines that orchestrate the process of maturation. Later studies have also revealed a fascinating facet of thymic biology: the existence of common progenitors that can differentiate into T cells and natural killer (NK) cells. Later research has identified directly that a subset of thymocytes, particularly the CD56+, CD5- subset, possesses characteristics akin to NK cells but with restricted capability to differentiate to T-cells, and this highlights the dynamic complexity of immune cell development and multifunctional function of the thymus (Sánchez et al., 1993). Moreover, thymic stroma-thymocyte interactions also play an important role in the successful maturation of T-cell and the development of functionally diverse T-cell subsets. Such interactions facilitate the development of different types of mature T cells, such as CD4+ helper T cells and CD8+ cytotoxic T cells, which have different functions in fighting infection. More knowledge of the thymic microenvironment can also enlighten the complexities of immune responses and potential targets of disease treatment, such as autoimmune diseases and lymphomas. Investigations of thymic function have uncovered the presence of several populations of thymocytes that possess unanticipated capabilities; that is, there are some cells with clonogenic potential and can contribute efficiently to T-cell reconstitution, suggesting that the thymus contains a reservoir of precursors fundamental to immune restoration (Saffrey et al., 2013). Thus, T-cell maturation in the thymus is not a simple linear affair but a complex interrelation of selection, lineage commitment, and maturation that plays an essential part in immunity competence in one's lifetime (Figure 6.3).

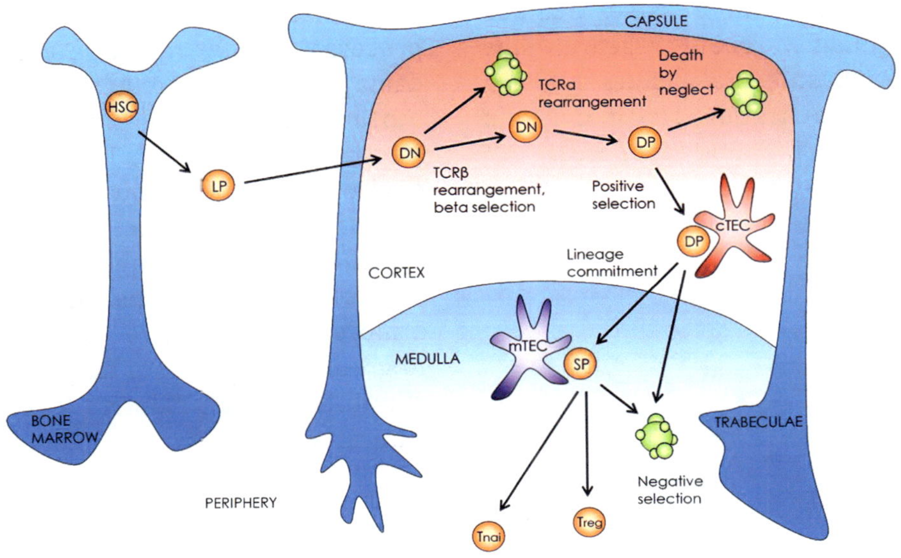

Figure 6.3. T-cell development in the thymus.

Source: https://www.researchgate.net/profile/Aleksey-Belikov/publication/303803545/figure/fig1/AS:369309240053760@1465061592136/T-cell-development-in-the-thymus.png.

6.1.3. Mechanisms of T-Cell Activation

The intricate mechanisms of T-cell activation are the signature of the adaptive immune response and involve a multi-step process guaranteeing specificity and efficiency in pathogen targeting. T-cell activation first occurs due to the recognition of antigen-presenting cells (APCs), primarily dendritic cells, presenting MHC molecules. The activation of the TCR by the peptide-MHC complex initiates cascades of signals that alter the T-cell functional status. This is supplemented by other signals derived from co-stimulatory molecules, such as CD28 activation of CD80/CD86 on the APCs, which is critical in initiating proliferation and differentiation of the T-cells. Explaining these pathways is important in developing strategies that control T-cell function, particularly in autoimmunity treatments or cancer immunotherapy, as the cellular signals determine the course of T-cell function in countless biological contexts. The role of the cytokine environment in determining T-cell activation cannot be overestimated. When activated, T cells release a variety of cytokines, like interleukins and tumor necrosis factors, that further modulate immune responses and influence the functioning of other immune cells. For instance, the production of interleukin-2 (IL-2) is essential for clonal growth of T cells and is of paramount significance in T-helper cell (Th cell) differentiation into specialized subtypes, e.g., Th1 and Th2 cells, each with distinct cytokine patterns and functional implications. Furthermore, dysregulated production of cytokines may lead to pathological immune responses that cause autoimmune pathology, as in the case of JDM, in which the immune microenvironment is dictated by the cross-talk among distinct immune cells, such as B cells that are regulated by T-cell interactions and cytokine signals (Wilkinson, 2018). Understanding thus becomes imperative the connection between T-cell activation and cytokine dynamics in deriving insights into immune homeostasis and disease. Besides classical mechanisms, recent research has identified that environmental factors are also significant in T-cell activation, broadening the classical definition of immune responses.

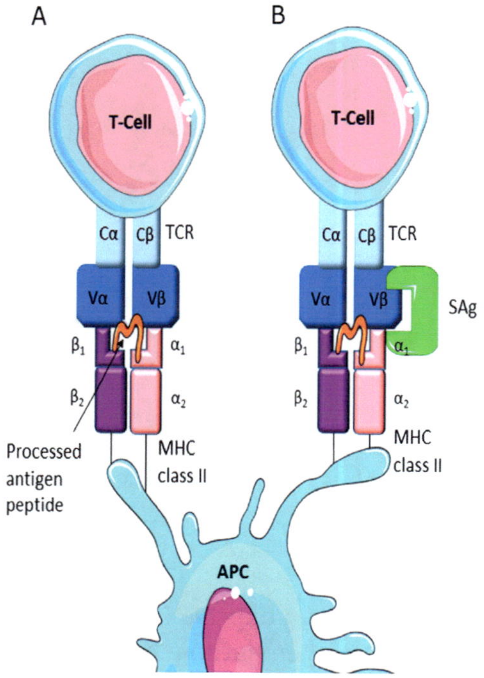

Figure 6.4. Mechanisms of T-cell activation: (A) Conventional T-cell activation by antigen-presenting cells (APC) and (B) the association of three proteins, *S. aureus* Sags, MHC class II, and the TCR β-chain, acts as an unconventional activation complex that triggers uncontrolled activation of T-cells.

Source: https://www.researchgate.net/publication/343787588/figure/fig1/AS:11431281420732108@1746255623190/Mechanisms-of-T-cell-activation-A-Conventional-T-cell-activation-by-antigen-presenting.tif.

For example, exposure to some antigens and related inflammatory signals can bias T-cell responses toward more Th17 cell differentiation, which has been linked with various autoimmune diseases and inflammatory disorders. Furthermore, ionizing radiation effect studies emphasize the complexity of T-cell activation processes in that radiation could induce DNA damage to influence cellular processes, including those related to T-cell activation and signaling (Jeggo & Lavin, 2009). These cellular process-environment signal interactions indicate that immune responses are not merely antigen-specific but also contingent upon more general physiological conditions. Such insights provide a more comprehensive paradigm upon which to ground the design of targeted therapies that may interact or modulate T-cell responses in clinical use (Figure 6.4).

6.2. Fundamentals of B-Cell Biology

B-cell biology is a critical part of the study of the adaptive immune response, where B cells are the focus of antibody formation. B cells begin life in the bone marrow and are characterized by their expression of unique surface proteins, including immunoglobulin (Ig) receptors. One B cell will only react to a specific antigen and, following activation, will clonally expand. This is a critical process to produce efficient immunological defense, allowing the creation of a tremendous array of antibodies that are tailored to the immense variety of pathogens. The ability of the B cells to class switch and somatically hypermutate enhances their efficacy at neutralizing menace, one of the specialties of the intricacies of adaptive immunity. In addition, the complex interactions between B cells and T cells play a central role in the development of long-term immunity and therefore, B-cell biology becomes an important subject of immunological research and drug discovery. B cells, aside from their potential for antibody production, possess the rare ability to present antigens to T cells and thereby to effect the shift between innate and adaptive immunity. Activation of B cells is normally a two-signal model: the first signal is antigen recognition through B cell receptors, and the second signal is normally supplied by T-helper cells. This interaction not only stimulates the proliferation of B cells but also leads to some B cells becoming memory cells.

Memory B cells play a crucial role in inducing long-term immunity and swift response to re-exposure to the same antigen, reflecting the immune system's complexity. Various techniques have been developed for studying the interactions of B cells, including flow cytometry and immunohistochemistry, which provide insight into their roles within the broader immune responses. These techniques advance our understanding of B-cell function and could impact the development of vaccine approaches in the future. The advances in microscopy and bioinformatics techniques have helped to advance the study of B-cell biology significantly, enabling researchers to closely study cellular interactions as well as behavior. Bioinformatics allows researchers to manage large quantities of data resulting from genomic and proteomic studies that provide information on signaling pathways in B cells as well as profiles of gene expression (Shamsir et al., 2012). Besides, high-technology microscopy techniques, such as immuno-gold transmission electron microscopy, have enlightened ultrastructural B-cell structural nuances (Fernando, 2007). With the aid of these high-technology tools, scientists can better understand mechanisms that regulate B-cell activation and differentiation and enable more targeted therapy. Their merging is a good example of the interdisciplinary nature of modern immunology, uniting biology and computational sciences to explain complex biological phenomena and improve our knowledge of B-cells' functions in the immune system.

6.2.1. Types of B-Cells: Plasma Cells and Memory B-Cells

B-cell-driven immune response is multifaceted, leading to the formation of essential subtypes: plasma cells and memory B-cells. Plasma cells, a by-product of activated B-cells, play a role in humoral immunity through the secretion of massive quantities of antigen-specific antibodies that neutralize the pathogen and tag it for killing by other immune cells. Notably, differentiation of plasma cells has a heavy dependence on a complex signaling cascade with a significant role for calcium signaling pathways. Intracellular calcium concentrations during the process regulate varied cell activities and determine plasma cell function and longevity. Interestingly, the same tools learned in the biology of T-cells, such as extracellular vesicles, are also utilized by plasma cells to communicate. The vesicles can transmit critical information, thus strengthening immune responses, as revealed in research where they played a role in the field of therapeutic uses, which implies the broader horizon of B-cell biology in medical technology (Kittel et al., 2013). Outside plasma cells, memory B-cells are also a significant component of adaptive immunity. They occur after the initial exposure to an antigen and persist for the long term, enabling faster and more effective response upon subsequent re-exposure to the same infection. Memory B-cells undergo somatic hypermutation, which enhances the affinity of antibodies to the respective antigen. This genetic adaptation illustrates the evolutionary importance of memory B-cells to allow stronger immunological recall. It is essential in the field of immunology to understand molecular mechanisms that govern the differentiation and survival of these cells. New data arising on calcium signaling research reveal that calcium-binding protein calmodulin is integral to the regulation of processes associated with B-cell maturation and function. The interaction between calcium level and memory generation of B-cells is thus central to improving vaccination strategies and treatment (Vaidyanathan, 2018). Plasma cells and memory B-cells show the flexibility of B-cell function in immune responses and mirror the significance of their biological mechanisms. These cell types not only characterize the adaptive arm of the immune system but also the intricate relationship between cell signaling and immunological function. Approaches that characterize the behaviors of these cells under various conditions can result in progress in the treatment of diseases that exploit or evade the immune system, such as cancer or persistent infections. The ability to leverage the profile of plasma cells and memory B-cells holds great promise for therapeutic progress. As researchers remain devoted to exploring the cellular and molecular pathways that govern B-cell behavior, targeted treatments are a rapidly developing front in immunology. A better understanding of these B-cell populations plays a role in our overall treatment of immunomodulation, thereby providing healthier outcomes (Kittel et al., 2013) (Figure 6.5).

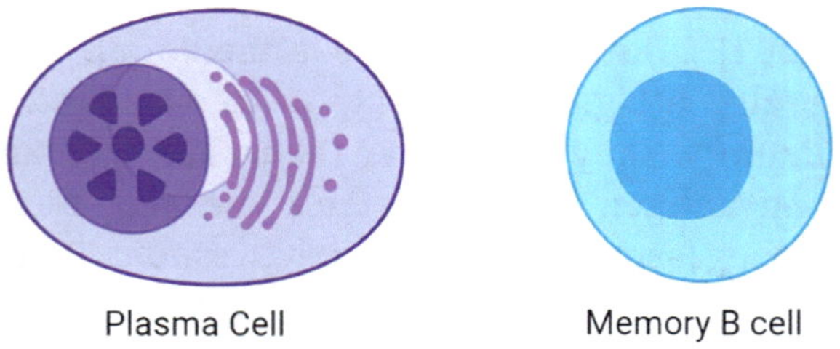

Figure 6.5. Illustration of plasma-cell and memory B-cell.

Source: https://microbenotes.com/wp-content/uploads/2021/04/Plasma-Cell-and-Memory-B-cell.jpeg.

6.2.2. B-Cell Development in the Bone Marrow

Bone marrow B-cell development is a multifaceted process involving various stages, of which the interactions with the bone marrow microenvironment are quite sophisticated. There are cytokine-rich stromal cells within the bone marrow microenvironment that help in the maturation of B-cells through cytokine signaling and cell contact. Early B-cell progenitors also undergo critical differentiation processes, transitioning from hematopoietic stem cells to common lymphoid progenitors and eventually to pre-B and mature B cells. Not only is the correct genetic rearrangement of immunoglobulin genes at fault for proper B-cell generation, but so are the supportive interactions with the bone marrow stroma, which are an essential part of propagating these nascent cells. It is essential to understand this complex paradigm to establish innovative approaches intended to control B-cell development in research and therapeutic processes. Advances in culture techniques for B-cells have revolutionized our understanding of the *in vivo* process governing their development. Traditional two-dimensional (2D) culture systems have failed for decades, being unable to reproduce the complex interactions that take place in the bone marrow. On the other hand, three-dimensional (3D) culture system development has allowed investigators to better mimic the complex bone marrow microenvironment, permitting growth and long-term survival of B-cell populations. The systems allow for maintenance of immunophenotypic features of fresh bone marrow, which may permit study of B-cell biology under conditions closely approximating physiological. With the ability to sustain mature B-cells for extended periods of time, the 3D culture platform holds new promise for the study of immunological response, immunogenicity of vaccines, and monoclonal antibody production, which are critical in therapeutic use (Wu & Bottaro, 2010). The possibility of successful *in vitro* development of B-cells has strong implications, particularly regarding their possible application in regenerative medicine and immunotherapy. As researchers move into such regions, understanding the intricacies of B-cell biology provides a foundation for tissue engineering approaches, enabling the use of patient-sourced cells to enhance immune responses or trigger tissue regeneration. Exploring endogenous tissue engineering approaches, which minimize *ex vivo* manipulation of cells, highlights the potential to harness patients' own B-cells towards therapeutic usage. This strategy not only addresses concerns related to the presence of autologous cells but also minimizes the risk associated with the transplantation of foreign cells. Through the support of advancements in B-cell culture technology, future research can pave the way for new treatments that integrate cellular therapies and regenerative strategies more harmoniously (Adam, 2012) (Figure 6.6).

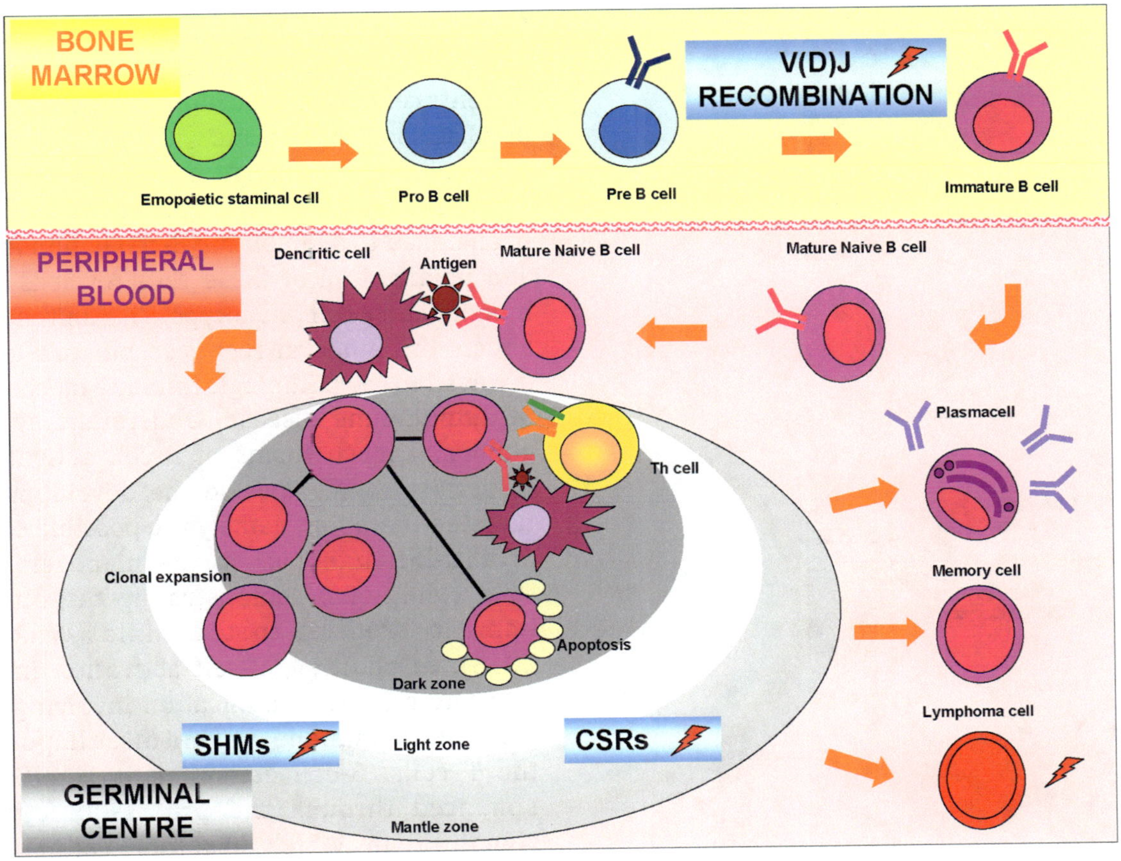

Figure 6.6. During B-cell development in the bone marrow, B-cell precursors are processed for V(D)J recombination.

Source: https://www.researchgate.net/profile/Paolo-Macor-2/publication/23159821/figure/fig1/AS:601764323667979@1520483203425/Fig-1-During-B-cell-development-in-the-bone-marrow-B-cell-precursors-are-processed.png.

6.2.3. Mechanisms of B-Cell Activation

B-cell mechanisms of activation play a crucial part in the adaptive immune response, primarily through interactions with T-helper cells and antigen recognition. B cells initially interact with particular antigens, which bind to the B-cell receptor (BCR) on their surface. This antigen-receptor interaction results in cascades of signals involving several protein kinases and adapter proteins to eventually activate central transcription factors such as nuclear factor kappa B (NF-κB) and activator protein 1 (AP-1). Co-stimulatory signals, generally provided by T-helper cells by CD40-CD40L interactions, are also essential for full activation of B-cells.

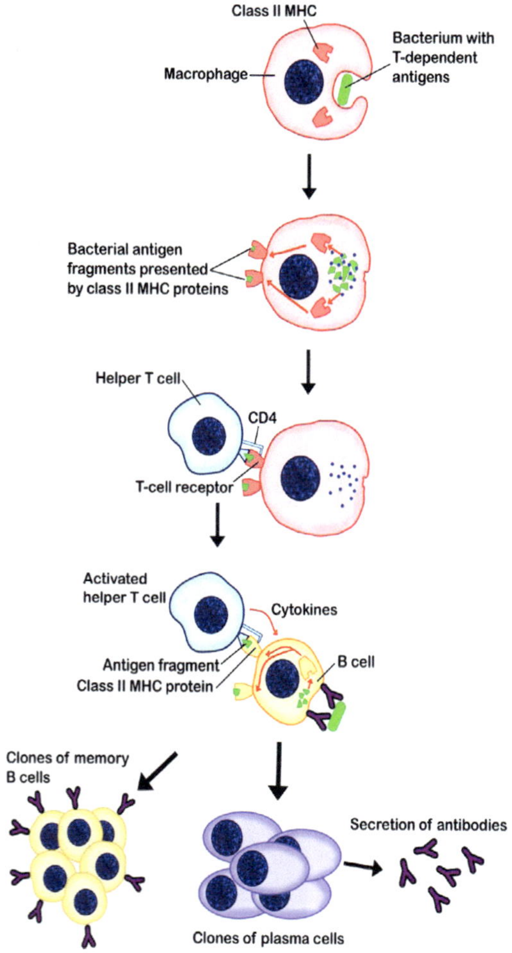

Figure 6.7. Mechanism of B cell activation and maturation by helper T-cell (Th) resulted in formation of specific antibody secreting plasma cells and memory B cells that have the ability to remember the infection.

Source: https://www.researchgate.net/profile/Mohd-Saad-3/publication/311795540/figure/fig1/AS:614518946275329@1523524142817/Mechanism-of-B-cell-activation-and-maturation-by-helper-T-cell-Th-resulted-in-formation.png.

This two-signal model highlights the requirement for antigen specificity as well as additional signals to generate proliferation and differentiation to antibody-secreting plasma cells, and the nuanced interaction required for effective humoral immunity. In autoimmune illnesses, such as juvenile dermatomyositis (JDM), abnormalities in the processes of B-cell activation may lead to pathogenic effects. Research of immune profiles in JDM patients reflects an elevation of immature B-cell populations that correlate with the augmentation of type I IFN signaling. As such, the activation of toll-like receptors (TLRs), particularly TLR7, has been linked to augmenting B-cell lymphocytosis and polarization of these cells towards a pro-inflammatory cell phenotype. This shift not only affects the humoral response but can also be involved in the pathologic immune mechanisms of autoimmune disease. Understanding these abnormal mechanisms of B-cell activation is of utmost significance to the development of targeted therapies, namely the possible efficacy of anti-IFN biologics in the management of such conditions, demonstrating the utility of immune profiling in the clinic (Wilkinson, 2018). In addition, B-cell activation involves intricate cross-communication involving other parts of the immune system, most importantly the T cells. B-cell activation is significantly enhanced through the process of cytokine signaling, in which T-helper cells release several cytokines that enable the proliferation and differentiation of B cells. Interleukin-4 (IL-4) and interleukin-21 (IL-21) are most critical among cytokines since they influence class-switch recombination through which B cells are able to produce different classes of antibodies. In addition to that, observations also indicate that environmental stimulation, such as ionizing radiation, interferes with regular B-cell activation pathways and has implications for tumorigenesis and genetic stability. Impairments of the DNA repair processes applicable to B-cell activation have the potential to lead not only to susceptibility to cancer but also to immune deficiencies, indicating the intricacies of B-cell biology and the need for advanced biology techniques to elaborate on these complicated mechanisms (Jeggo & Lavin, 2009) (Figure 6.7).

6.3. Techniques for T-Cell Isolation

T-cell isolation is a crucial component in immunology research and treatments. Various methods have been designed to ensure efficient separation of T-cells from peripheral blood mononuclear cells (PBMCs). One common method is density gradient centrifugation, in which the blood samples are layered over a specific medium, permitting the cellular components to be separated on the basis of density. It produces fairly large numbers of viable T-cells and is therefore widely favored for research as well as clinical purposes. The elegance of the approach is even supplemented by its effectiveness in maintaining cell integrity, which is so important for subsequent functional assays and further experimental manipulations. Overall, density gradient centrifugation is thus a model technique for T-cell isolation that enables researchers to delve into the complexity of T-cell biology and its applicability in immunotherapy. In addition to density gradient centrifugation, magnetic-activated cell sorting (MACS) has proved to be a new and highly successful method for isolating T-cells. MACS employs magnetic beads conjugated with antibodies against cell surface antigens for separating the T-cells from the other cells. Once labeled, the contents are placed in a magnetic field where the T-cells are trapped while other cells are washed away. The increased specificity of MACS not only enhances the purity of separated T-cells but also allows for simultaneous separation of different T-cell subsets, e.g., CD4+ and CD8+ T-cells. This is particularly beneficial for researchers investigating the roles of specific T-cell subsets in various contexts, i.e., autoimmunity or cancer immunology. Consequently, MACS gradually gains popularity as a result of its flexibility and stability in T-cell isolation procedures. Lastly, fluorescence-activated cell sorting (FACS) is a powerful technique that incorporates cell sorting with high specificity and flexibility. FACS uses lasers to read individual cells as they pass through a stream and fluorescence markers to tag specific T-cell populations. FACS provides not just quantitative data on cell populations but also functional data by allowing researchers to quantify the T-cell activation status and other functional markers in real time. FACS is particularly valuable for those applications that require very purified samples for subsequent assays or therapeutic uses. It is a highly valuable tool both in research and translational work, suggesting the interface of T-cell biology and disease processes. Employing these various methods in combination, researchers are able to determine a comprehensive understanding of the T-cell dynamics and their relevance in health and disease, enriching the scientific discipline of immunology to a great extent.

6.3.1. Density Gradient Centrifugation

Density gradient centrifugation is a central technique in cell biology, primarily employed for the isolation and study of lymphocyte types, e.g., T cells and B cells. The method involves the principle that different types of cells can be fractionated based on their density in a gradient medium when centrifuged. When a mixed cell population is spun at extremely high centrifugal force, cells are forced to move through a liquid medium of mixed densities. Cells will settle at points within the gradient that are a function of their individual densities, such that separation is extremely effective. This stratification has the advantage in immunological experiments that populations of lymphocytes can be collected with high purity and subsequent analysis and manipulation become appropriate for research and clinical applications. Other than its application for T and B cell isolation, density gradient centrifugation has the advantages of high integrity and viability of the sample. The method is comparatively gentle, involving little mechanical stress to cells, to help keep their functional attributes intact. This is particularly important within lymphocyte biology, where cell functionality plays a major role in downstream applications such as functional assays, cell culture, and therapeutic intervention.

For instance, CD4+ T lymphocyte isolation is crucial in monitoring immune responses in HIV patients, as exemplified in ongoing research studies. Such studies highlight the need for low-cost and simple technologies, thus proving the sustained relevance of density gradient centrifugation in multiple clinical applications (Kinahan et al., 2012). Furthermore, the variability of density gradient centrifugation is extended to encompass many other research applications aside from T and B cell separations. For example, the technique has been used *in vitro* to investigate the effect of protease digestion on particular receptors and whether or not cell membranes are structurally intact.

By this method, density gradient centrifugation can effectively separate receptor-rich membrane vesicles from the other components of the cytosol surrounding them so that scientists may investigate the biochemical processes associated with receptor efficiency. As shown in experiments that have utilized Torpedo californica electroplaques, experimental designs like these yield extremely useful information on receptor structure and function to contribute to a greater understanding of cellular processes (Klymkowsky et al., 1980). With the integration of density gradient centrifugation in their research methodologies, scientists continue to advance the frontiers of cellular and molecular immunology and make contributory advances toward therapeutic approaches and analytical equipment.

6.3.2. Magnetic-Activated Cell Sorting (MACS)

MACS is a technology-driven technique that enables the isolation and separation of target cells based on their surface antigens. This approach is particularly important in immunology, where T-cells and B-cells are components of the adaptive immune system. By employing magnetic beads pre-coated with antibodies against target cell surface antigens, researchers can employ a magnetic field to separate labeled cells from non-labeled cells. Such selectivity helps gain a greater understanding of T-cell and B-cell biology so that their unique functions and behavior under various physiological conditions can be studied. Furthermore, MACS is versatile and may be used to separate different kinds of immune cells, which have significant applications in the development of targeted immunotherapies and regenerative medicine solutions in clinics and research labs. The efficiency of MACS can be particularly useful while working on complicated immunological responses. It enables high-throughput analysis and can separate bulk amounts of cells needed for downstream experiments, such as functional assays and sequencing. As the immune system consists of heterogeneous cell populations that express distinctive gene features, MACS provides a means of selectively purifying individual populations for study. Insights gained from such separations can promote the characterization of complex interactions within the immune system, responding to fundamental queries into cell fate determination and immunological activation. Current research underlines the importance of selecting the right markers and procedures for the enrichment of the intended population, emphasizing how procedures like MACS are crucial in deciphering the intricacy of cellular heterogeneity in immunology (McClure & Southall, 2015). Moreover, MACS is especially essential for the construction of therapeutic applications of T-cells and B-cells towards the treatment of diseases like cancer immunotherapy.

By virtue of having the ability to isolate cells based on various markers, researchers are able to better strategize how they are going to target specific immune cells for maximal therapeutic outcome. For instance, isolated T-cells can be genetically modified *ex vivo* to enhance their anti-tumor activity before they are re-infused back into the patient's body. Studies on adhesive markers such as Stro-1, CD146, and CD105 demonstrate the potential to enhance methods of isolation so that populations are enriched for therapeutic targeting (Gothard et al., 2014). Enhanced cell sorting accuracy not only provides improved patient outcomes but also results in a better understanding of the cellular processes engaged in immune responses. Thus, MACS becomes a revolutionary tool at the interface of basic research and clinical application, serving to benefit both disciplines immensely (Figure 6.8).

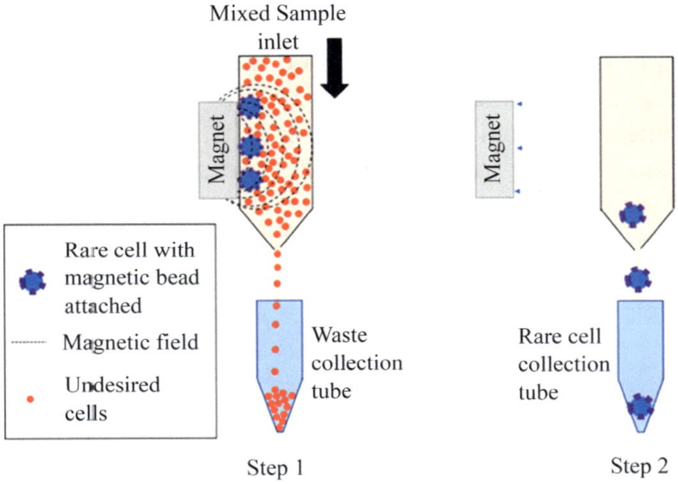

Figure 6.8. Magnetically activated cell sorting (MACS) is achieved by attaching antibody-coated magnetic nanometer-sized beads to the cells of interest.

Source: https://www.researchgate.net/profile/Shilpi-Pandey-3/publication/328137297/figure/fig3/AS:685175222566915@1540369911187/Magnetically-activated-cell-sorting-MACS-is-achieved-by-attaching-antibody-coated.png.

6.3.3. Flow Cytometry for T-Cell Analysis

Flow cytometry has emerged as an essential tool for the analysis of T-cells, giving correct quantitative and qualitative information regarding their nature. Using fluorescent antibodies, scientists can identify and quantify various surface antigens on T-cells, crucial for understanding their activation, differentiation, and overall immune response. This multi-parameter technique allows the simultaneous assessment of a number of different characteristics, including CD4 and CD8 densities, which are critical to the distinction between helper T-cells and cytotoxic T-cells. Flow cytometry can also report cytokine secretion and proliferation based on the physical attributes of single cells, thus enabling more precise characterization of T-cell function. The ability to analyze thousands of cells in a single second enhances the statistical power of the information and flow cytometry is consequently an anchor technology within immunological research and clinical use. Flow cytometry technology also significantly improved the capacity to recognize small T-cell populations, which are actually very often of interest in research and in the clinic. Using techniques like mass cytometry, researchers can analyze hundreds of markers simultaneously, thereby achieving a level of resolution that might be unattainable with conventional flow cytometry. This is particularly useful in the study of diseases characterized by cellular heterogeneity, such as autoimmune conditions or malignancies. For instance, the ability to detect a specific T-cell subset, such as regulatory T-cells or T-cell exhaustion markers, through flow cytometry has enabled an understanding of their disease-related functions. Enhanced analytical capability not only facilitates more sensitive detection of phenotypic heterogeneity but also identification of possible therapeutic targets and measurement of treatment response, which are important for optimizing patient benefit. The effectiveness of flow cytometry in T-cell analysis is further enhanced by its integration with molecular approaches. For instance, an integration of flow cytometry and gene expression profiling with single-cell RNA sequencing enables the comprehensive characterization of T-cell populations. Combined, this facilitates the quantitation not only of surface markers but intracellular signaling pathways and transcriptional profiles as well, thereby providing deeper insights into the functional status of T-cells. A prominent example of such an integrated approach is in the studies of T-cell responses in infectious and autoimmune diseases, wherein a demarcation between healthy and disease states can easily be made. Additionally, as discussed in recent research, the ability to phenotypically capture and sort T cells with the use of multicolor flow cytometry has the potential to directly translate into clinical strategies and treatment protocols, thereby highlighting the central role of the technology in contemporary immunology (Candia et al., 2013) (Figure 6.9).

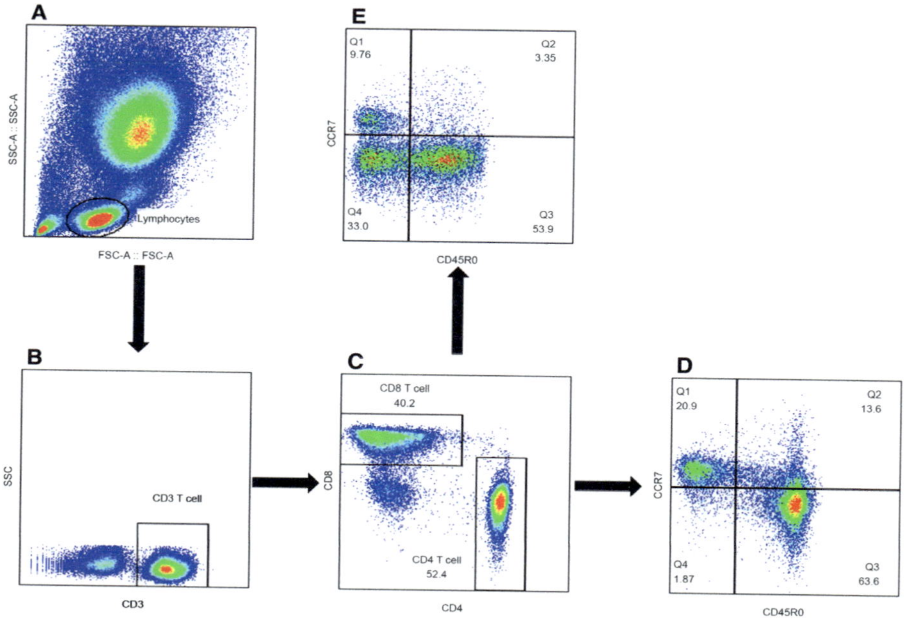

Figure 6.9. Flowchart of flow cytometry analysis to identify CD4 and CD8 T cells.

Source: https://www.researchgate.net/publication/334983113/figure/fig1/AS:788717031669760@1565056202991/Flowchart-of-flow-cytometry-analysis-to-identify-CD4-and-CD8-T-cells-a-The-flow.png.

6.4. Techniques for B-Cell Isolation

B-cell separation is a simple procedure in immunological research and treatment development. Various techniques have been created to purify and separate B-cells from mixed cell populations, each with advantages and limitations. One such method is density-gradient centrifugation, through which efficient B-cell separation can be achieved based on buoyancy, allowing enrichment from PBMCs. However, although this method is simple, it does not yield pure B-cells and therefore frequently requires follow-up purification protocols to exclude contaminating cell populations. An extremely powerful method that has been gaining popularity includes MACS, where antibodies directed against B-cell surface antigens are utilized, allowing rapid and selective recovery. This process not only raises the purity but also preserves cell viability, so it is ideally applicable for downstream usage, such as functional assays and studies on B-cell differentiation and activation under healthy and disease states. Of the evolving landscape of B-cell separation techniques, FACS stands out due to its efficiency and specificity. Using a similar antibody-based approach to MACS, FACS allows scientists to sort B-cells based on more than one surface marker at the same time. This is particularly beneficial when investigating heterogeneous populations, as in the immune system, with different subtypes of B-cells, each possibly playing unique roles in immune response. The ability to sort and analyze B-cells in an active state provides useful insight into their biology and interactions with other immune cells. Furthermore, sorting technology has been improved, which has allowed high-throughput systems to be developed, enormously increasing the amount and speed of B-cell isolation. Such technological advance broadens the potential for therapeutic use, including the manufacture of targeted B-cell therapies and vaccine manufacture. Emerging technology is also unveiling new methods in B-cell isolation, expanding the toolkit currently available to immunologists. For instance, the use of extracellular vesicles (EVs), such as exosomes, has been prominently advocated due to their capacity for cell communication and signaling. New findings emphasize the potential for the use of EVs as biomarkers for assessing B-cell function and status across various pathological conditions, including cancer and autoimmunity. Techniques for isolating such vesicles, while being developed, have the promise of use in combination with standard B-cell isolation methods. The integration of dynamic isolation techniques, such as microfluidics, allows live sorting and interrogation of B-cells based on functional responses in real time and offers a new way through which their biological function can be understood. In the end, such developments not only provide more insight into B-cell biology but can also enhance therapy by making the ability to target and manipulate B-cell populations more precisely possible, as the literature at present describes (Forte et al., 2016; Lawson et al., 2016).

6.4.1. Immunomagnetic Separation (IMS)

IMS is a major technique in the study and manipulation of immune cells, particularly T-cells and B-cells. This method utilizes magnetic beads with antibodies bound to them, targeted against cell surface markers, for the separation of desired cell populations from a heterogeneous population. By making use of the unique epitopes presented on the T-cell and B-cell surface, researchers can confidently delineate these populations for analysis, delineating their function and contribution to the immune system. In particular, IMS is now a requirement in clinical applications, such as in cancer immunotherapy, where the isolation of individual lymphocytes may enhance the therapeutic effect and monitor response to therapy. Therefore, IMS use has disclosed aspects of cellular biology that cannot be explored using traditional separation. Beyond simple separation, IMS use is imperative in the new field of circulating tumor cell (CTC) analysis. Prognostic and predictive analysis approaches in most cancers presently are concentrating on the significance of CTCs, which provide insight into tumoral dynamics as well as therapeutic responsiveness. In agreement with current studies, the CTC heterogeneity necessitates creative strategies over the traditional epithelial cell adhesion molecule (EpCAM) targeting, underlining the need for technologies like IMS that are capable of targeting a broader array of cellular phenotypes (Raimondi et al., 2015). This heterogeneity of IMS allows for the CTCs harvesting, which may have a different phenotype than the primary tumor, thereby maximizing the precision of molecular profiling that can inform real-time tumor biology-guided treatment choice, as has been demonstrated in breast cancer research (Forte et al., 2016). Further, the integration of immunomagnetic separation with advanced imaging and analytical tools enhances the understanding of T-cell and B-cell crosstalk within the tumor environment. Once these immunosubsets are isolated, researchers are better placed to understand how they migrate, infiltrate, and respond to tumor cells. This not only facilitates identification of potential immunotherapeutic targets but also assists in finding the immunological signature of various malignancies. With advancing technology, its combination with single-cell RNA sequencing and other high-throughput platforms will enable in-depth analysis of cellular states and provide us with the critical details of tumor-immune dynamics. Through such interdisciplinarity, IMS not only raises our investigative force but also raises the possibility of personal treatment and control of cancer under the evolving scenario (Figure 6.10).

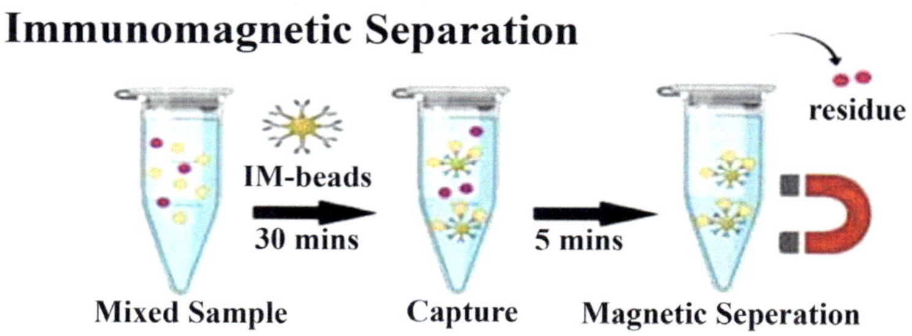

Figure 6.10. Illustration of immunomagnetic separation.

6.4.2. Fluorescence-Activated Cell Sorting (FACS)

FACS is a groundbreaking technique for the analysis and manipulation of cell populations that are heterogeneous, particularly in T-cell and B-cell biology. The technique exploits the properties of fluorescence to discriminate between various types of cells based on specific surface markers. By employing antibodies labeled with a fluorescent tag that bind to these markers, researchers can facilitate quantitation and purification of target subsets of cells. This capability is especially significant in immunology, where identification of individual T-cell and B-cell populations is the key to comprehension of immune response and the design of specific therapies. FACS makes a level of examination available that was not, enabling scientists to study cell functions and characteristics at a hitherto unimaginable level of resolution. The flexibility of FACS is once more exemplified by its application in the study of gene expression in specific cell types, particularly within intricate cellular interaction systems like Arabidopsis. FACS has been central to the understanding of the regulatory processes involved in cell type-specific expression of genes during various biological processes like root growth and stress (Grønlund et al., 2012). For instance, FACS experiments have shown us how the gene expression profiles are remarkably different in different cell types of a single organism and how these experiments enlighten us on cellular function and differentiation.

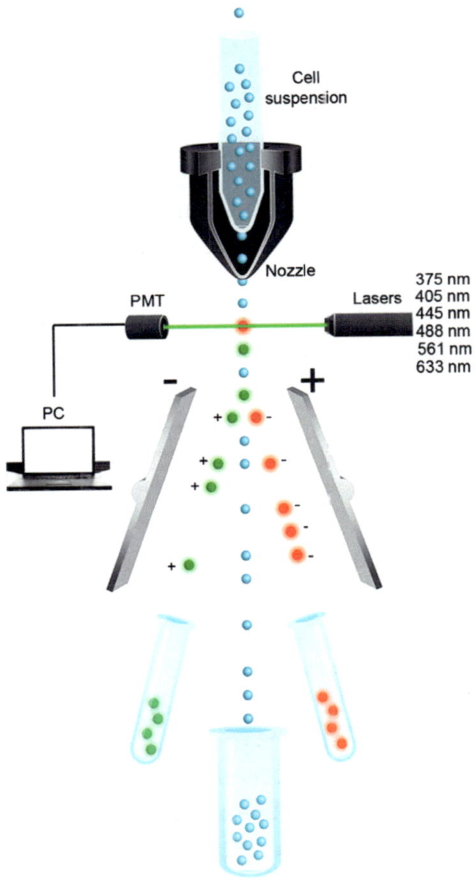

Figure 6.11. Fluorescence-activated cell sorting (FACS). The suspended cells are subjected to different fluorescent tags depending on the experimental set-up.

Source: https://www.researchgate.net/publication/283800102/figure/fig3/AS:667840646492164@1536237026218/Fluorescence-activated-cell-sorting-FACS-The-suspended-cells-are-subjected-to.jpg.

Such specificity of distinction not only brings us to attention regarding the multifaceted functions of different cell types in the immune system but also educates us on therapeutic intervention approaches, particularly in dysregulation-based diseases of the immune system. Beyond its applications in fundamental research, FACS also holds extensive implications for clinical applications, especially for cancer treatment and immunotherapy. FACS allows the isolation and identification of specific populations of cancer cells, facilitating the examination of tumor heterogeneity and therapeutic resistance behavior (Litzenburger et al., 2017). The technology enables scientists to separate cells based on their expression of surface markers that predict their responsiveness to treatment, thereby guiding the development of more effective therapeutic strategies. In addition, FACS also aids in monitoring immune cell populations following treatment, providing valuable information about patient response to therapy. By integrating FACS into the clinical process, personalization of disease treatment in leukemia and lymphoma is feasible, hence maximizing patient outcomes in the dynamic practice of oncology (Figure 6.11).

6.4.3. Enzyme-Linked Immunosorbent Assay (ELISA)

ELISA is a critical analytical technique widely applied in immunology, particularly in studying T-cell and B-cell biology. ELISA offers the capacity to measure specific proteins, including antibodies, cytokines, and antigens, through the utilization of enzymatic activity that creates measurable signals. By stabilizing antibodies or antigens on the surface of a microplate, researchers can selectively trap the target biomolecules from complex matrices such as plasma or serum. The secondary antibodies linked to an enzyme on binding enable colorimetric, fluorescent, or luminescent detection, thus enabling measurement of immune responses. The versatility and sensitivity of ELISA have made it an important tool in diagnostic disease, vaccine efficacy testing, and the assessment of therapeutic interventions in preclinical and clinical settings (Martinez et al., 1993). ELISA is one of the key applications in T-cell and B-cell biology to analyze cytokine release in immune response assessment. For instance, the quantification of interferon-gamma (IFN-γ) production has been at the core of understanding T-cell function, particularly in response to pathogen stimulation. Development of ELISA assays specific for some cytokines has played a key role in untangling immunity to various infections, with mycobacterial infections being most noteworthy. Clarke et al. (2017) illustrate the use of ELISA to measure IFN-γ and other cytokines to better understand immune interactions and pathogen responses within animal models. These methods assist in determining diagnostic cut-off values that aid in identifying healthy and infected populations (Clarke et al., 2017).

Furthermore, ELISA's specificity and reproducibility as a diagnostic tool highlight its application in both research and clinical diagnostics. Overall sensitivity of the tests into the upper 90s in certain applications highlights its value for detecting trace quantities of target analytes.

In the studies of serum samples in ruminants, for example, ELISA specificity was between 97% and 98.6%, which is a testament to its capacity to differentiate between actual positives and false positives across different species. Such precision is essential in the making of accurate diagnoses, further vindicating the possibility of ELISA to monitor disease progression and the therapeutic success in patients. To this end, ELISA is not only a standard tool in immunological research but also a tool that directly impinges upon clinical decision-making, significantly progressing T-cell and B-cell biology (Martinez et al., 1993).

6.5. Functional Assays for T-Cells

Functional assays for T-cells are significant assays utilized in immunology to determine the capabilities and reactions of these immune cells. Of the numerous approaches employed, antigen-specific stimulation methods such as ELISpot and proliferation assays are of high utility in comprehending T-cell reactivity. These classic approaches are typically handicapped by chronic infection when T-cell responses are being suppressed. For instance, the hepatitis C virus (HCV) utilizes mechanisms that suppress T-cell activation, rendering it challenging to comprehend the immunological landscape in infection. In this context, high-throughput sequencing (HTS) of TCRβ complementarity-determining region (CDR)3 sequences has been a significant breakthrough, which has the potential to enable researchers to track T-cell expansions without the stringent requirement for pre-existing knowledge of specific antigenic sequences (Robinson et al., 2016). This is a revolutionary shift in our approach to understanding T-cell dynamics during chronic infections. Besides, the functional integrity of separated T-cell populations can be tested by diverse *in vitro* tests, which elucidate their potential in immune responses further. Cell separation techniques such as free flow electrophoresis effectively separate antigen-positive from antigen-negative lymphocyte subpopulations with high yields of purified cell fractions. This kind of separation allows more targeted experimentation with individual T-cell subsets, making assays that assess T-cell functionality more efficient. For example, experiments on single-cell responses to stimuli such as monoclonal antibodies or polyclonal lectins allow investigation of drug or other variable effects on isolated T-cell subsets. Such approaches allow complex analyses of lymphocyte transformation and their subsequent roles in the regulation of antibody synthesis, allowing for a greater understanding of T-cell biology and therapeutic response (Hansen et al., 1989). Lastly, one important application of T-cell functional assays is in the determination of the effects of pharmacologic agents on immune function. By isolating the T-cell subsets and examining their response upon stimulation by varying factors, researchers can identify the effect of various drugs on specific immune functions. For instance, thiopental, an anesthetic, has been shown to depress lymphocyte functions in T-helper and T-suppressor cells, with non-cytotoxicity. This realization highlights the necessity of having accurate cell compositions in assays because changes in lymphocyte populations can be biased and lead to erroneous conclusions regarding immune competence. With the integration of new technology and the optimization of standard assays, more precise determinations of T-cell response in various clinical conditions can be achieved, and this can ultimately translate to better therapeutic approaches for the regulation of immune function (Hansen et al., 1989).

6.5.1. Proliferation Assays

Proliferation assays are critical to the investigation of T-cell and B-cell biology, allowing for an understanding of immune cell dynamics and the response of cells to stimuli. The assays measure cell growth and proliferation, revealing the functional competence of lymphocytes in various immune events such as activation, differentiation, and the formation of immune memory.

By employing cell growth-measuring assays, researchers can resolve the impact of various factors, such as cytokines or antigens, on lymphocyte proliferation. This is key to the development of vaccines and immunotherapies since it drives the requirement for successful immune responses. The suitability of proliferation assays relies on the conditions of optimizing cell cultures in most situations, and therefore, refinement in assay methods is important for sound interpretations of immune competence. Several proliferation assay techniques, such as [3H]-thymidine incorporation and flow cytometry with CFSE dye staining, have been developed to measure T-cell and B-cell proliferation. Each of the techniques has unique strengths to quantify cell division and to distinguish among different lymphocyte populations. For instance, [3H]-thymidine incorporation will measure DNA synthesis upon cell division, but will not be able to show individual cell division history. Conversely, CFSE allows one to trace cell divisions in real-time and provide data concerning cellular lineage and fate, which are extremely crucial in terms of explaining the clonal enlargement of a single T or B cell in an immune response.

Consequently, the diverse techniques allow the researchers to dissect the intricate biology of T-cells and B-cells and compile an integrated picture of their roles in immunity. Scientists are also embracing new techniques for optimizing proliferation assays. One example is the introduction of thin-layer angiogenesis assays, a compelling model for challenging not just lymphocyte function but their interactions with other cell types within the tissue environment. The benefits of reduced matrix volumes in proliferation assays not only conserve costs but also become more accessible to high-resolution imaging and molecular analysis. Furthermore, as advancements in stem cell biology progress, as reflected in the study of epidermal stem cells, researchers may unlock new therapeutic avenues that leverage lymphocyte proliferation dynamics. Understanding of the routes governing T-cell and B-cell proliferation will likely be employed in novel strategies that enhance immune responses or regulate over-proliferation in autoimmune diseases, thus elevating the role of new proliferation assays in modern immunological studies (Ghadially , 2012; Li et al., 2014) (Figure 6.12).

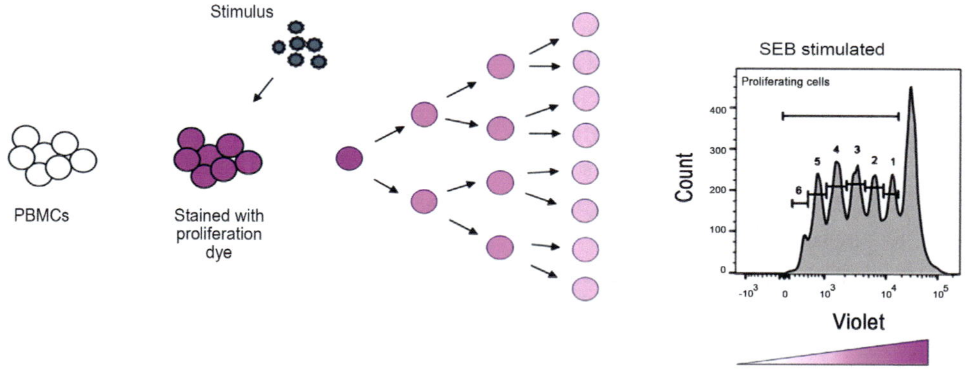

Figure 6.12. Proliferation assays.

Source: https://www.sanquin.org/binaries/content/gallery/content/en/products-services/diagnostic-services/immunomonitoring/proliferation-assay--flow-cytometry.png/proliferation-assay--flow-cytometry.png/sanquin%3Amedium.

6.5.2. Cytotoxicity Assays

Cytotoxicity assays are a basic group of immunological reagents that determine the ability of T-cells and B-cells to mediate cell killing against target cells, which is of crucial significance for the understanding of immune responses and the effectiveness of therapeutic drugs. The cytotoxicity assays measure the ability of immune cells to kill pathogen-infected cells or tumor cells, thereby providing information on immune surveillance mechanisms as well as cancer therapy efficiency. The most commonly utilized tests for cytotoxicity evaluation are the lactate dehydrogenase (LDH) release assay of cell membrane integrity and the Annexin V/PI staining test to differentiate between early and late apoptosis. The identification of cytotoxic mechanisms is not only significant for general research but also for the development of immunotherapies, according to the cytotoxic capacity of T-cells and B-cells against neoplastic cells and infected cells. In cancer studies, cytotoxicity assays are increasingly prominent because they provide valuable estimates of novel drugs. Essential oils, for instance, have been documented to possess potential cytotoxicity, as they induce apoptosis in cancer cells using multiple mechanisms (Lillestolen, 2020). Using cytotoxicity assays, scientists are able to measure the level of cancer cell death caused by these oils and thus assess their potential to serve as adjunct therapies in combination with conventional treatments. In addition, cytotoxicity assays can facilitate the identification of the pathways underlying the cytotoxic activity and thus lead to the development of maximized treatment strategies that maximize patient outcomes. The use of new compounds in cytotoxicity assays may provide more insight into immune cell interactions and their ability to drive antitumor responses. In addition, cytotoxicity studies in non-mammalian organisms, e.g., Botryllus schlosseri hemocytes, provide new insights into universal mechanisms of immune cell-mediated cytotoxicity (Franchi et al., 2015). The most prevalent circulating hemocyte in this organism, Morula cells, display intense cytotoxicity by releasing enzymes and generating reactive oxygen species that assist in eliminating incompatible cells from the animal. These findings highlight the conservation of cytotoxic mechanisms through evolution and also suggest the potential for cross-species application in the analysis of immune function. By establishing the cytotoxic activity of such cells, scientists are able to learn more about fundamental immunological processes, which in turn can direct the creation of new immune therapies and enhance our overall understanding of cellular interactions during disease and health (Figure 6.13).

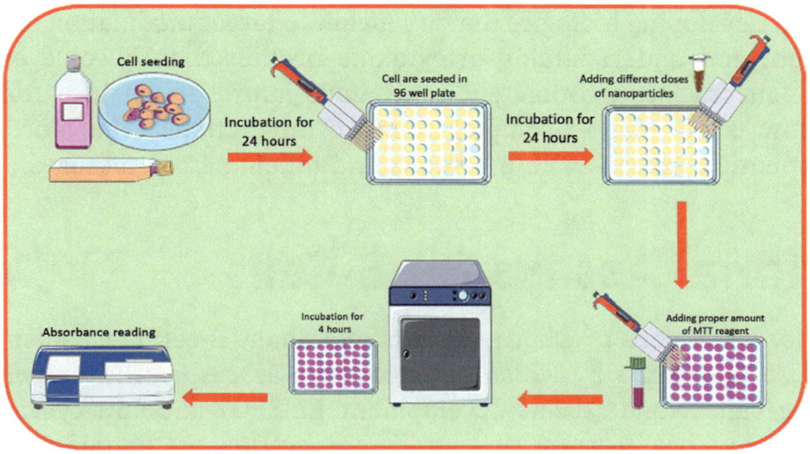

Figure 6.13. Schematic representation of the cytotoxicity assay.

Source: https://www.researchgate.net/publication/378711254/figure/fig2/AS:11431281238103815@1713837215494/Schematic-representation-ofthe-cytotoxicity-assay.png.

6.5.3. Cytokine Production Measurement

Cytokine production measurement is a core part of measuring T-cell and B-cell responses in immunology. Cytokines are important signal molecules that provide for interactions between immune cells, and the quantification of cytokine levels provides us with information about the activation and functions of lymphocytes. There are various ways to quantify cytokines, such as enzyme-linked immunosorbent assay (ELISA), flow cytometry, and multiplex bead assays. Each method has its own merits; for instance, ELISA is renowned for its specificity and sensitivity in the quantitative measurement of a single cytokine level. On the other hand, flow cytometry provides quick analysis in parallel of several cytokines at the single-cell level, which is especially useful when dealing with heterogeneous cell populations. Therefore, the preference between techniques depends on the research question being asked and the level of detail needed in the analysis to understand the immune response. In addition, disturbances in cytokine production can signal the occurrence of various pathologies, and their quantitation is therefore significant in the clinical context. In the context of T-cell and B-cell immunology, understanding of environmental impact, age, and state of disease on cytokine profiles enhances our comprehension of immune system dynamics. For instance, Namas et al. (2013) demonstrate how aging can have a significant impact on macrophage cytokine production, leading to altered inflammatory responses. Such insights are instrumental in the development of targeted interventions for age-related immune dysfunction and other dysregulated cytokine-producing diseases. Through the inclusion of data from these measurements, scientists are able to begin drawing more specific conclusions about the mechanisms involved in immune responses and the potential therapeutic avenues that may be derived from cytokine manipulation. In addition to their role in orchestrating the immune response, the use of cytokines also extends to therapeutic interventions for infectious diseases and immunotherapies. Quantifying cytokines is particularly vital in interpreting the immune response against pathogens such as *Mycobacterium tuberculosis*, where some cytokines may enhance protective immunity or cause pathology. As discussed in Marino et al. (2007), tumor necrosis factor (TNF) plays a vital role in sustaining tuberculosis and, therefore, is an essential factor in infection as well as treatment. During the process of developing biologics that are meant to target modulation of cytokine activities, precise measurement and understanding of cytokine profiles then become essential to ensure maximal treatment effectiveness. Ultimately, continuous improvement in cytokine measurement techniques will allow us to analyze complex immune interactions even more so and direct us towards new therapeutic approaches in infectious and inflammatory diseases.

6.6. Functional Assays for B-Cells

Functional assays form the core of what is understood about B-cell mechanisms in immunology. Functional assays are the means by which one is able to assess B-cell function in the setting of autoimmune disease, cancer, and vaccine development. ELISPOT and flow cytometry are two ways in which B-cell activation, proliferation, and antibody secretion can be quantified.

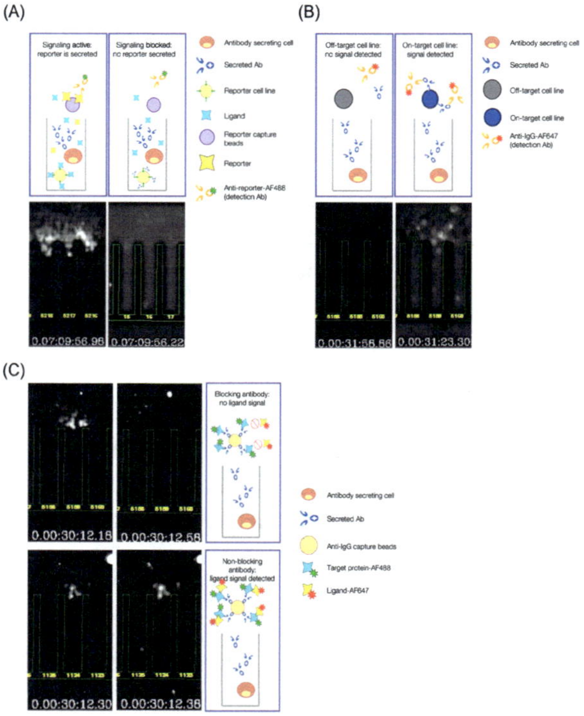

Figure 6.14. Functional assays for Beacon screening to determine biologically relevant properties of antibodies secreted from individual B cells. (A) Cell-based reporter assay. (B) Cell-binding assays. C) Ligand blocking assay.

Source: https://www.researchgate.net/publication/373630651/figure/fig1/AS:11431281187165108@1694141155570/Functional-assays-for-Beacon-screening-to-determine-biologically-relevant-properties-of.png.

For instance, identification of IL-10-secreting B regulatory phenotypes through functional assays has provided valuable information about their suppressive activities in the tumor microenvironment. These findings are essential, particularly regarding their involvement in post-operative recurrence of patients with non-small cell lung cancer (NSCLC), as evidenced by the correlation of increased circulating suppressive B cells with recurrence (Patel, 2023). Thus, the use of functional assays not only enhances our knowledge of B-cell biology but also has significant therapeutic implications and biomarker development. Moreover, combining functional assays with newer technologies has revolutionized our approach to the study of B-cell dynamics. New technologies in cancer immunology and high-throughput screening techniques have made it possible to explore the intricate interplay of B cells with other immune components, such as T cells. For instance, functional assays to measure B-cell reactions to checkpoint blockade therapies yield important insight into immune dysregulation and drug response. Functional impairments of B cells identified in NSCLC involved in immune-related adverse events point towards the importance of addressing the behavior of B cells in immunotherapy (Patel, 2023). This integrated approach will also help to detect auto-antibody signatures predictive of post-operative relapse and further consolidate the utility of functional assays as invaluable tools for clinical prognosis and targeted medicine. In addition, the utility of functional assays is further enhanced by the requirement for integration tools to capture the complexity of B-cell biology. As the field advances, the integration of multi-dimensional data, for instance, transcriptomic and proteomic profiles, with functional measures becomes increasingly important. The integration plays a central role in identifying key biological features and predicting clinical outcomes. Subsequently, approaches such as machine learning to analyze sophisticated datasets can reveal patterns and correlations beyond the reach of conventional techniques. By taking advantage of heterogeneous data, researchers can reveal new information on B-cell function, paving the way for new therapeutic interventions and expanding our understanding of immune mechanisms under health and disease. In that regard, functional assays are not simply stand-alone studies but also form part of a larger, more nuanced system for exploring B-cell biology (Figure 6.14).

6.6.1. Antibody Production Assays

Knowledge of the mechanisms involved in antibody production is necessary to advance immunological research and drug development. Antibody production assays are a central technique in B-cell functional investigation and a key tool for the detection of specific antibodies against pathogens or therapeutic agents. The assays typically consist of antigen stimulation of the B cells, resulting in proliferation and differentiation into antibody-secreting plasma cells. Various assay formats, such as ELISAs and flow cytometry, allow researchers to quantify the amount of antibodies and establish the specificity and affinity of antibodies produced. Such assays not only enhance the understanding of the immune system but also aid in vaccine efficacy assessment and the creation of monoclonal antibodies for therapeutic use, hence highlighting the importance of good and reproducible antibody production assays in immunology research. Moreover, advances in technology have significantly enhanced antibody production assays to improve high-throughput screening methodologies. As noted, limitations posed by traditional antibody screening processes, including low throughput and broken process sequences, have resulted in disparities. Modern-day practices have leveraged microscale bioprocess technologies and groundbreaking high-throughput platforms capable of automating and streamlining antibody discovery and engineering processes. These platforms enable the culture and manipulation of single cells in an organized setting, hence increasing efficiency in antibody production assays. The ongoing incorporation of lab-on-a-chip technologies is a paradigm shift that will reduce the time and cost of biologics development, a step that is crucial in the fast-paced world of current biomedical research, most notably in the building of therapies for complex diseases (Jorgolli et al., 2019). In addition, new biological applications to produce antibodies using production assays are in the pipeline to further enhance their application in basic and applied research. Recent research emphasizes the significance of molecular dynamics, such as recruitment and interaction of signal molecules, that govern B-cell response and antibody development. For instance, research on biomolecular pathways involved in enzyme activity, like soluble adenylyl cyclase (sAC), can uncover intricate mechanisms of regulation that influence immunoglobulin secretion and B-cell differentiation. As explained, the plasticity of sAC in different cellular contexts is evidence that the modulation of signaling pathways can enhance antibody responses, especially in a therapeutic context. Through the merging of thorough behavioral analysis of enzyme activity in antibody production assays, researchers can drive innovation in vaccine development, therapeutic antibody design, and disease intervention strategies, thereby enabling the critical role these assays play in advancing T-cell and B-cell biology methods (Tresguerres & Salmerón, 2018).

6.6.2. Class Switching Assays

Class switching of B cells is a critical process that enhances the diversity and specificity of the antibody response. Class switching assays are designed to quantify B cells switching from one class of immunoglobulin production, say IgM, to others, i.e., IgG, IgA, or IgE. It is essential for adaptive immunity since different classes of antibodies perform particular functions in combating various pathogens. Dynamics of class switching give scientists insight into the nature of B-cell versatility in responding to particular antigens. By employing techniques such as flow cytometry and ELISA, scientists are able to quantitatively detect the frequency and efficiency of class switching processes and compare the impact of various cytokines and co-stimulatory signals on B cell differentiation. Furthermore, analysis of mechanisms of class switching has demonstrated that the molecular signals and transcriptional regulation interact in a complex way. Single cytokines, like IL-4 and TGF-β, have been found to influence which class of immunoglobulin is most preferentially produced. Class switching assays may also be employed to study the roles of specific transcription factors, including Activation-Induced Cytidine Deaminase (AID), that must initiate the steps in recombination needed for class switching. In these instances, researchers employ genetic manipulation techniques to remove or overexpress these factors, and their functions in class switching become evident. The implications of such experiments are crucial to the development of targeted immunotherapies and vaccines to enhance immune responses against pathogens. Aside from their foundation in the determination of B-cell biology, class switching assays have substantial clinical significance. One of the main areas of investigation is the investigation of autoimmune diseases, where abnormal class switching can lead to the production of autoantibodies and cause pathology. Class switching assays will give a basis upon which to measure the mechanism causing aberrant B cell behavior, which will offer new therapeutic targets. In addition, advances in genomic technologies allow for high-throughput examination of class switching events to provide detailed insights into the antibody repertoire of individual patients. The approach holds promise to revolutionize personalized medicine, as clinicians could tailor interventions based on an individual's personal immune profile. Therefore, the assays not only enhance our understanding of immune responses but also establish avenues for new treatments in immunological conditions (Figure 6.15).

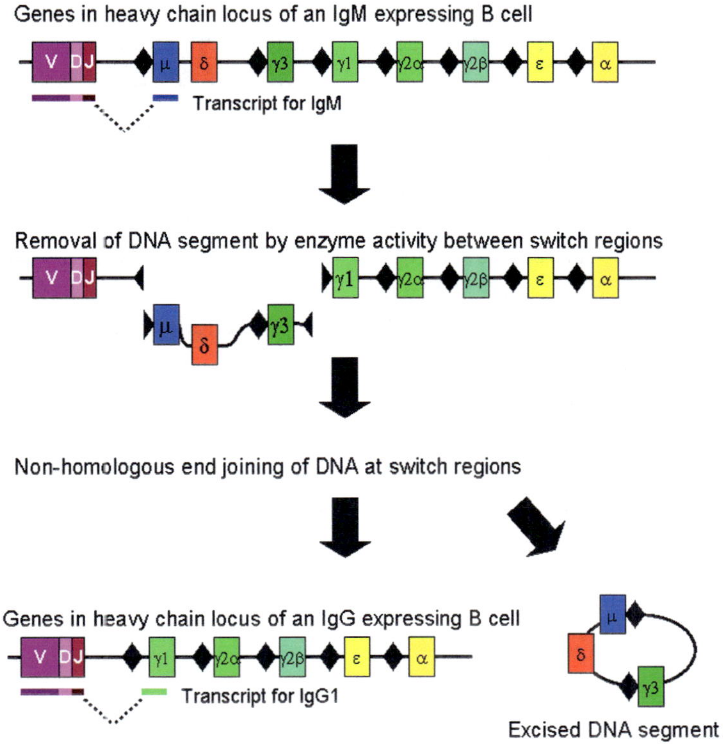

Figure 6.15. Mechanism of class-switch recombination that allows isotype switching in activated B cells.

Source: https://upload.wikimedia.org/wikipedia/commons/b/b3/Class_switch_recombination.png.

6.6.3. Memory B-Cell Response Evaluation

It is crucial to understand the measurement of memory B-cell responses in terms of driving the development of vaccines and therapy for infectious diseases. Memory B cells are the key component of the adaptive immune system since they can rapidly differentiate into antibody-secreting plasma cells on secondary exposure to previous antigens. Techniques used to analyze these memory responses typically include ELISAs and flow cytometry, which allow for the detection and quantification of the intended antibody response. By analyzing the affinity and class switch of the antibodies, the effectiveness of a memory B-cell response can be determined. In addition, new methods using high-throughput sequencing have given better insights into the specificity and diversity of antibody repertoires, thus facilitating more thorough assessments of how memory B cells play a role in long-term immunity and defense against pathogens. The relevance of memory B-cell response can be optimized by combining multiple biological approaches. This includes the integration of flow cytometry data with high-throughput omics techniques, where it is now feasible to quantify the functional state of memory B cells both at the proteomic and transcriptomic levels. Given the utility of high-performance computational algorithms, it is now viable to conduct integrative analysis that focuses on interactions and pathways employed by B-cell activation and differentiation. For instance, the understanding obtained using integrative analysis approaches indicates how single signaling pathways affect the functionality of memory B cells against specific antigens. Additionally, since vaccines are aimed at creating strong memory responses, determining how these memory B cells evolve in the long term, particularly against variant strains of pathogens, becomes more critical for long-term protective immunity (Choi et al., 2019). The most recent technological advances have contributed greatly to the general understanding of overall memory B-cell dynamics, thereby offering helpful insights into their immune response assessment. For instance, optogenetics was applied to spatially and temporally manipulate the behavior of memory B-cells in a way that real-time observations were achievable upon exposure to antigens. This technique addresses the earlier shortcomings of cell dynamics studies, where temporal specificity was typically sacrificed. Furthermore, the combination of optogenetic tools with standard immunological assays is a promising method for comprehensive investigation, as it makes simultaneous examination of cellular activity and functional outcome feasible. These sophisticated approaches enable comprehensive investigation of mechanisms of memory B-cell differentiation and maintenance of immunological memory, which can ultimately inform methods of enhancing vaccine efficacy and reorienting immunotherapy protocols to combat disease (Pinardo , 2018).

SUMMARY

In reviewing the developments and techniques covered in T-Cell and B-Cell biology, it is clear that contemporary immunological methods, including flow cytometry and immunohistochemistry, are central to advancing our knowledge of immune responses. Flow cytometry has been especially useful in the classification of different types of lymphomas through precise lineage determination by examining cell surface markers. As demonstrated, this technique can accurately diagnose cases of B-NHL, reinforcing its utility in clinical diagnosis and potential therapeutic intervention. Moreover, PCR detection of rearrangements in immunoglobulin heavy chain genes is a helpful adjunct in defining monoclonal populations, thus reinforcing the specificity of lymphoma classification as documented in recent research (Weber et al., 2019). This intricate dance between the various techniques indicates the degree of understanding to which one can arrive in the topic of T-Cell and B-Cell biology. In addition, the study of protein expression, and that of markers such as p53 and bcl-2, in particular, is of significant interest regarding the aggressiveness and behavior of the various grades of lymphomas. The immunohistochemical examination of these proteins is not only vital in prognosis but also in the tailoring of treatment strategies. Growing insight into how these markers correlate with tumor aggressiveness opens up the possibility of personalized medicine to allow clinicians to make decisions that are guided by the molecular profile of individual cases (Weber et al., 2019). As the swift development of these techniques continues to unravel, the inclusion of such techniques in routine clinical practice heralds a major turn towards a less obtrusive method of treating lymphoproliferative disorders.

Moreover, research using new experimental techniques, such as RNA interference in non-bilaterian animals, paves the way for an exciting area of research in the study of T-Cell and B-Cell biology. By applying techniques traditionally used in model organisms to sponge species investigations, researchers have been able to significantly describe the role of gene regulation in development and immunology. This demonstrates the potential for cross-disciplinary methods to the extension of our knowledge of immune mechanisms. As researchers go on to refine these approaches and hunt for their applications in other model systems, the dividend to immunology will automatically increase, with the potential for breakthroughs translatable into therapeutic advances on human diseases. The conjoining of diverse methodologies is therefore a central advance towards unravelling the complexities of T-Cell and B-Cell biology. T-cell and B-cell research is still at the core of immunology, and techniques are continuously being optimized to unravel their sophisticated roles in the immune system. Flow cytometry is one of the primary techniques employed for analyzing T-cell activities, where scientists analyze the surface antigens and intracellular cytokines of T-cells. With this technique, scientists can comprehensively characterize immune responses by measuring and sorting different populations of T-cells based on phenotypic and functional traits. Furthermore, advances in multiparameter flow cytometry allow for the exploration of multiple parameters at once to yield richer datasets for T-cell behavior understanding in various immunological contexts. This multidimensional data capture mirrors the rigor of benchmarking experiments, where the requirement for systematic comparisons is highlighted to draw sound conclusions from complex biological datasets (Weber et al., 2019). In the context of B-cells, techniques such as ELISA and hybridoma technology have proven to be very useful in producing and characterizing antibodies. ELISA allows one to measure specific antibodies present in a sample, and thus, it gives information on the humoral immune response that is useful. Hybridoma technology, on the other hand, allows for the combination of B lymphocytes with myeloma cells to produce monoclonal antibodies.

Such monoclonal antibodies are crucial diagnostic and therapeutic reagents that complement our understanding of antigen-specific immunity. In addition, model-informed design of biosensors, as reflected in corresponding principles of B-cell analysis, shows how new approaches can apply established paradigms to develop novel applications in synthetic biology (Gilbert et al., 2008). Lastly, the use of genomic and transcriptomic tools in T-cell and B-cell research has transformed our capability to examine these cells at the molecular level. Single-cell RNA sequencing, among others, provides unprecedented perspectives of the heterogeneity of T-cell and B-cell populations and of cell states buried in bulk analysis. This level of specificity provides us with a better understanding of how such immune cells are differentiated and what they do under various physiological and disease conditions. In addition, the application of computational methods to analyze such high-dimensional data is indicative of the dynamic nature of immunology research, looking back at the imperatives for firm benchmarking and methodological push in maximizing the inquiry into immune responses (Weber et al., 2019). As a result, follow-up studies on the biology of T cells and B cells continue to reveal intricate mechanisms necessary for designing targeted immunotherapies and vaccines.

A CLOSER LOOK

HEMATOPOIETIC STEM CELLS (HSCS)

HSCs are pluripotent bone marrow stem cells that are capable of giving rise to all types of blood cells, including red blood cells, white blood cells, and platelets. HSCs have significant roles in maintaining the output of blood cells throughout life and repairing damaged blood tissue. HSCs also form the basis of bone marrow transplantation, a lifesaving treatment for many blood diseases and cancers (Figure 6.16).

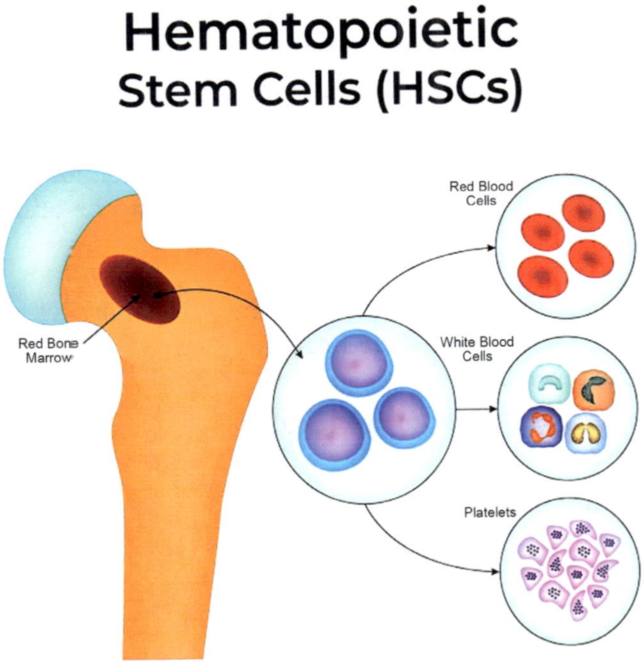

Figure 6.16. Illustration of hematopoietic stem cells (HSCs).

Source: https://img.freepik.com/premium-vector/hematopoietic-stem-cells-hscs-red-blood-cells-white-blood-cells-platelets-marrow_33402-972.jpg.

1. Key Features and Functions:

a. Self-renewal: HSCs can divide and sustain their own population, so there is a steady supply of stem cells.

b. Multilineage Differentiation: HSCs have the capacity to differentiate into numerous types of blood cells, both myeloid and lymphoid lineages, to restore all blood cell types.

c. Homeostasis: HSCs regulate the equilibrium of blood cell production, providing a constant supply of mature blood cells for numerous functions such as oxygen transport, immunity, and clotting.

d. **Regeneration:** HSCs have the capacity to regenerate damaged or disease-bearing blood-forming tissues and are, as a result, of great importance in the treatment of blood diseases.

2. Location and Isolation:

a. HSCs predominantly reside within the bone marrow but also reside in peripheral blood and umbilical cord blood.

b. They can be removed from these sites for therapeutic and research reasons.

3. Clinical Relevance:

a. **Bone Marrow Transplantation:** HSCs constitute the foundation of bone marrow transplantation, which is used in the management of various blood cancers (e.g., leukemia and lymphoma), aplastic anemia, and immunodeficiency.

b. **Gene Therapy:** HSCs are a potential candidate for gene therapy because their self-renewal capability allows for long-term and stable gene expression.

c. **Regenerative Medicine:** HSCs are also under investigation for their potential to regenerate injured tissue, like heart muscle, although this remains an area of research.

4. Niche Interactions:

a. HSCs have a distinct microenvironment in the bone marrow referred to as the "niche," which is made up of numerous varied cell types like stromal cells, endothelial cells, and other hematopoietic cells.

b. The niche plays a crucial role in the regulation of HSC behavior, such as self-renewal, differentiation, and survival.

5. Additional Considerations:

a. HSC heterogeneity is present, with different subsets possessing differing properties towards self-renewal and differentiation.

b. Clarification of the intrinsic and extrinsic factors regulating HSC behavior is crucial to optimize their use in regenerative medicine and gene therapy.

REFERENCES

1. Ghadially R. (2012). 25 years of epidermal stem cell research. *The Journal of investigative dermatology, 132*(3 Pt 2), 797–810. https://doi.org/10.1038/jid.2011.434 (accessed on 27th June 2025).
2. Tresguerres M, Salmerón C. Molecular, Enzymatic, and Cellular Characterization of Soluble Adenylyl Cyclase From Aquatic Animals. *Methods Enzymol.* 2018;605:525-549. doi:10.1016/bs.mie.2018.02.022(accessed on 27th June 2025).
3. A. Peña-Fernández, F. Izquierdo, L. Acosta, M.A. Peña, A. Magnet, M. Evans, G. Torrado, C. Young (2019) VIRTUAL LIBRARIES OF TISSUE AND CLINICAL SAMPLES: POTENTIAL ROLE OF A 3-D MICROSCOPE, INTED2019 Proceedings, pp. 9132-9138.(accessed on 27th June 2025).
4. Adam, C. (2012). Endogenous musculoskeletal tissue engineering–A focused perspective. https://core.ac.uk/download/10908942.pdf (accessed on 27th June 2025).
5. Jeggo, P., & Lavin, M. F. (2009). Cellular radiosensitivity: how much better do we understand it?. *International journal of radiation biology, 85*(12), 1061–1081. https://doi.org/10.3109/09553000903261263(accessed on 27th June 2025).
6. Allen, R. L. (2001). Non-classical immunology. Meeting report. https://core.ac.uk/download/9536591.pdf (accessed on 27th June 2025).
7. McClure, C. D., & Southall, T. D. (2015). Getting Down to Specifics: Profiling Gene Expression and Protein-DNA Interactions in a Cell Type-Specific Manner. *Advances in genetics, 91*, 103–151. https://doi.org/10.1016/bs.adgen.2015.06.003An, A., Babiskin, A., Andrianantoandro, E., Basu, A., Bayer, T. S., Beisel, C. L., et al. (2011). Engineering ligand-responsive RNA controllers in yeast through the assembly of RNase III tuning modules. https://core.ac.uk/download/4889928.pdf (accessed on 27th June 2025).
8. Miguel R. Guevara & Dominik Hartmann & Manuel Aristarán & Marcelo Mendoza & César A. Hidalgo, 2016. "**The research space: using career paths to predict the evolution of the research output of individuals, institutions, and nations**," Scientometrics, Springer;Akadémiai Kiadó, vol. 109(3), pages 1695-1709, December.(accessed on 27th June 2025).
9. Schlichthaerle, T., Strauss, M. T., Schueder, F., Auer, A., Nijmeijer, B., Kueblbeck, M., Jimenez Sabinina, V., Thevathasan, J. V., Ries, J., Ellenberg, J., & Jungmann, R. (2019). Direct Visualization of Single Nuclear Pore Complex Proteins Using Genetically-Encoded Probes for DNA-PAINT. *Angewandte Chemie (International ed. in English), 58*(37), 13004–13008. https://doi.org/10.1002/anie.201905685Franchi N., Ballarin L., Cima F., 2015. ***Insights on cytotoxic cells of the colonial ascidian Botryllus schlosseri***. Invertebr. Surv. J., 12: 109-117. https://core.ac.uk/download/53517180.pdf (accessed on 27th June 2025).
10. Candia, J., Maunu, R., Driscoll, M., Biancotto, A., Dagur, P., McCoy, J. P., Jr, Sen, H. N., Wei, L., Maritan, A., Cao, K., Nussenblatt, R. B., Banavar, J. R., & Losert, W. (2013). From cellular characteristics to disease diagnosis: uncovering phenotypes with supercells. *PLoS computational biology, 9*(9), e1003215. https://doi.org/10.1371/journal.pcbi.1003215(accessed on 27th June 2025).
11. Forte, V. A., Barrak, D. K., Elhodaky, M., Tung, L., Snow, A., & Lang, J. E. (2016). The potential for liquid biopsies in the precision medical treatment of breast cancer. *Cancer biology &*

medicine, 13(1), 19–40. https://doi.org/10.28092/j.issn.2095-3941.2016.0007(accessed on 27th June 2025).

12. Wu, J. H. D. , & Bottaro, A.(2010). Growing B lymphocytes in a three-dimensional culture system. NASA Tech Briefs, March 2010 https://core.ac.uk/download/pdf/10552636.pdf (accessed on 27th June 2025).
13. Weber, L. M., Saelens, W., Cannoodt, R., Soneson, C., Hapfelmeier, A., Gardner, P. P., Boulesteix, A. L., Saeys, Y., & Robinson, M. D. (2019). Essential guidelines for computational method benchmarking. *Genome biology, 20*(1), 125. https://doi.org/10.1186/s13059-019-1738-8(accessed on 27th June 2025).
14. Vale, R. D., Malik, F., & Brown, D. (1992). Directional instability of microtubule transport in the presence of kinesin and dynein, two opposite polarity motor proteins. *The Journal of cell biology, 119*(6), 1589–1596. https://doi.org/10.1083/jcb.119.6.1589(accessed on 27th June 2025).
15. Grønlund, J. T., Eyres, A., Kumar, S., Buchanan-Wollaston, V., & Gifford, M. L. (2012). Cell specific analysis of Arabidopsis leaves using fluorescence activated cell sorting. *Journal of visualized experiments : JoVE*, (68), 4214. https://doi.org/10.3791/4214(accessed on 27th June 2025).
16. Litzenburger, U. M., Buenrostro, J. D., Wu, B., Shen, Y., Sheffield, N. C., Kathiria, A., Greenleaf, W. J., & Chang, H. Y. (2017). Single-cell epigenomic variability reveals functional cancer heterogeneity. *Genome biology, 18*(1), 15. https://doi.org/10.1186/s13059-016-1133-7(accessed on 27th June 2025).
17. Kittel, A., Falus, A., & Buzás, E. (2013). Microencapsulation technology by nature: Cell derived extracellular vesicles with therapeutic potential. *European journal of microbiology & immunology, 3*(2), 91–96. https://doi.org/10.1556/EuJMI.3.2013.2.1(accessed on 27th June 2025).
18. Jorgolli M, Nevill T, Winters A, et al. Nanoscale integration of single cell biologics discovery processes using optofluidic manipulation and monitoring. *Biotechnol Bioeng.* 2019;116(9):2393-2411. doi:10.1002/bit.27024(accessed on 27th June 2025).
19. Choi, H., Chung, N. C., Mirza, B., Ping, Z., et al. (2019). Machine learning and integrative analysis of biomedical big data. https://core.ac.uk/download/323080394.pdf (accessed on 27th June 2025).
20. Cieniewicz, B., Danka, E. S., Haen, K. M., Hammel, J. U., et al. (2011). RNA interference in marine and freshwater sponges. https://core.ac.uk/download/12174125.pdf (accessed on 27th June 2025).
21. Martinez, D., Coisne, S., Sheikboudou, C., & Jongejan, F. (1993). Detection of antibodies to Cowdria ruminantium in the serum of domestic ruminants by indirect ELISA. *Revue d'elevage et de medecine veterinaire des pays tropicaux, 46*(1-2), 115–120.(accessed on 27th June 2025).
22. Saffrey, M.Jill & Premadasa, Prasanna & Davies, Heather & Colyer, Frances & Yeoman, Mark & Ranson, Rachel. (2013). Ultrastructural analysis of changes in neurons of the mouse internal anal sphincter during ageing. https://core.ac.uk/download/82978021.pdf (accessed on 27th June 2025).
23. Cornell University. (1999). *College of Veterinary Medicine.* https://ecommons.cornell.edu/bitstream/handle/1813/38459/COS_v90_1998_99_16.pdf?sequence=1&isAllowed=y (accessed on 27th June 2025).

24. Clarke, C., Patterson, S. J., Drewe, J. A., van Helden, P. D., Miller, M. A., & Parsons, S. D. (2017). Development and evaluation of a diagnostic cytokine-release assay for Mycobacterium suricattae infection in meerkats (Suricata suricatta). *BMC veterinary research*, *13*(1), 2. https://doi.org/10.1186/s12917-016-0927-x(accessed on 27th June 2025).

25. Kinahan, D. J., Glynn, M., Kearney, S. M., Ducrée, J., (2012). Concentration of white blood cells from whole blood by dual centrifuge-pneumatic siphoning with density gradient medium. https://core.ac.uk/download/11309830.pdf (accessed on 27th June 2025).

26. Fernando, D. (2007). Ultrastructural characterization (morphological and topochemical) of wood pulp fibers. https://core.ac.uk/download/11695137.pdf (accessed on 27th June 2025).

27. MacLean, A. L., Harrington, H. A., Stumpf, M. P., & Byrne, H. M. (2016). Mathematical and Statistical Techniques for Systems Medicine: The Wnt Signaling Pathway as a Case Study. *Methods in molecular biology (Clifton, N.J.)*, *1386*, 405–439. https://doi.org/10.1007/978-1-4939-3283-2_18(accessed on 27th June 2025).

28. Goldenberg, A., Hoffman, M. M., Leskovec, J., Nguyen, P., et al. (2018). Machine learning for integrating data in biology and medicine: Principles, practice, and opportunities. http://arxiv.org/abs/1807.00123 (accessed on 27th June 2025).

29. Gothard D, Greenhough J, Ralph E, Oreffo RO. Prospective isolation of human bone marrow stromal cell subsets: A comparative study between Stro-1-, CD146- and CD105-enriched populations. *J Tissue Eng*. 2014;5:2041731414551763. Published 2014 Sep 18. doi:10.1177/2041731414551763Raimondi C, Nicolazzo C, Gradilone A. Circulating tumor cells isolation: the "post-EpCAM era". *Chin J Cancer Res*. 2015;27(5):461-470. doi:10.3978/j.issn.1000-9604.2015.06.02(accessed on 27th June 2025).

30. Hansen, E., Wustrow, T. P., & Hannig, K. (1989). Antigen-specific electrophoretic cell separation for immunological investigations. *Electrophoresis*, *10*(8-9), 645–652. https://doi.org/10.1002/elps.1150100819 (accessed on 27th June 2025).

31. Klymkowsky, M. W., Heuser, J. E., & Stroud, R. M. (1980). Protease effects on the structure of acetylcholine receptor membranes from Torpedo californica. *The Journal of cell biology*, *85*(3), 823–838. https://doi.org/10.1083/jcb.85.3.823(accessed on 27th June 2025).

32. Houghton, C. J., et al. (2024). ET&C Best Paper of 2023. *Environmental Toxicology and Chemistry*, *43*. https://www.semanticscholar.org/paper/de84b02f4bb403319e71477fe2554c413fe02c71 (accessed on 27th June 2025).

33. Shamsir, M.S., Hussein, H., Hashim, S.Z., & Salim, N. (2006). Educating the educators: Incorporating bioinformatics into biological science education in Malaysia.https://core.ac.uk/download/11778588.pdf (accessed on 27th June 2025).

34. Marino, S., Sud, D., Plessner, H., Lin, P. L., Chan, J., Flynn, J. L., & Kirschner, D. E. (2007). Differences in reactivation of tuberculosis induced from anti-TNF treatments are based on bioavailability in granulomatous tissue. *PLoS computational biology*, *3*(10), 1909–1924. https://doi.org/10.1371/journal.pcbi.0030194(accessed on 27th June 2025).

35. Sánchez, M. J., Spits, H., Lanier, L. L., & Phillips, J. H. (1993). Human natural killer cell committed thymocytes and their relation to the T cell lineage. *The Journal of experimental medicine*, *178*(6), 1857–1866. https://doi.org/10.1084/jem.178.6.1857(accessed on 27th June 2025).

36. Lawson, C., Yellon, D. M., Gunduz, F., Headland, S. E., Joop, K., Jorgensen, C., et al. (2016). Macrovesicles and exosomes: New players in metabolic and cardiovascular disease. https://core.ac.uk/download/36779172.pdf (accessed on 27th June 2025).

37. Li, A., Pierce, A. D., Hibbert, A., Faulkner, A., Staton, C. A., et al. (2014). A thin layer angiogenesis assay: A modified basement matrix assay for assessment of endothelial cell differentiation. https://core.ac.uk/download/36778059.pdf (accessed on 27th June 2025).

38. Lillestolen, C. K. (2020). Possible roles for essential oils in chemoprevention and suppression of cancer. https://core.ac.uk/download/322850888.pdf (accessed on 27th June 2025).

39. Robinson, M. W., Hughes, J., Wilkie, G. S., Swann, R., Barclay, S. T., Mills, P. R., Patel, A. H., Thomson, E. C., & McLauchlan, J. (2016). Tracking TCRβ Sequence Clonotype Expansions during Antiviral Therapy Using High-Throughput Sequencing of the Hypervariable Region. *Frontiers in immunology*, *7*, 131. https://doi.org/10.3389/fimmu.2016.00131(accessed on 27th June 2025).

40. Patel, A. J. (2023). The immunobiology of B lymphocytes in non-small cell lung cancer. https://core.ac.uk/download/574733662.pdf (accessed on 27th June 2025).

41. Pinardo, H. (2018). Exploring adult hippocampal neurogenesis using optogenetics. https://core.ac.uk/download/215938323.pdf (accessed on 27th June 2025).

42. Porter, A. J., Barelle, C. J., Cornock, D., Donohoe, G., Steven, J., Saunders, K., et al. (2017). *In vitro* maturation of a humanized shark VNAR domain to improve its biophysical properties to facilitate clinical development. https://core.ac.uk/download/131025024.pdf (accessed on 27th June 2025).

43. Namas, R. A., Bartels, J., Hoffman, R., Barclay, D., Billiar, T. R., Zamora, R., & Vodovotz, Y. (2013). Combined in silico, in vivo, and in vitro studies shed insights into the acute inflammatory response in middle-aged mice. *PloS one*, *8*(7), e67419. https://doi.org/10.1371/journal.pone.0067419(accessed on 27th June 2025).

44. Vaidyanathan, U. (2018). Evolutionary covariant positions within calmodulin EF-hand sequences promote ligand binding. https://core.ac.uk/download/211334315.pdf (accessed on 27th June 2025).

45. Wilkinson, M. G. L. (2018). Investigating novel pathways in B cell mediated autoimmunity in the context of the disease juvenile dermatomyositis. https://core.ac.uk/download/158357476.pdf (accessed on 27th June 2025).

46. Gilbert, D., Heiner, M., Rosser, S., Fulton, R., Gu, X., Trybilo, M. (2008). A Case Study in Model-driven Synthetic Biology. In: Hinchey, M., Pagnoni, A., Rammig, F.J., Schmeck, H. (eds) Biologically-Inspired Collaborative Computing. BICC 2008. IFIP – The International Federation for Information Processing, vol 268. Springer, Boston, MA. https://doi.org/10.1007/978-0-387-09655-1_15(accessed on 27th June 2025).

47. Zhang, L., & Jin, D. (2023). Cytometry and analytical methods in COVID-19 diagnostics and potential treatment: A special issue on *Cytometry Part A*. *Cytometry Part A, 103*. https://www.semanticscholar.org/paper/3664cc09a636ea6b056c05d8a700277e055131eb (accessed on 27th June 2025).

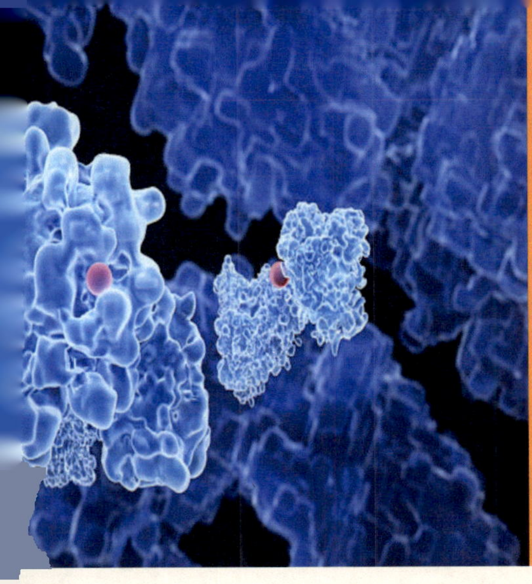

Chapter 7

PROTEIN-PROTEIN INTERACTION ANALYSIS IN IMMUNOLOGY

Contents

Introduction

Protein-protein interactions (PPIs) are most important to analyze for understanding immune mechanisms as well as disease processes in immunology. PPIs are essential for a number of immune functions, which immune cells perform, for perceiving danger as well as responding to it appropriately. PPIs facilitate the formation of complexes that define cellular signaling pathways relevant to immune response, e.g., the activation of transcription factors regulating gene expression when encountering pathogens. They are also an important determinant of immune cell function and behavior, including those of T cells and macrophages. Through the knowledge of the complexity of these interactions, researchers are able to discover how dysregulation leads to diseases like autoimmune diseases or cancer. To this end, systematic methods of PPI analysis have proved to be an essential part of immunology research, offering new opportunities for therapeutic target discovery and disease treatment. Advances in experimental techniques and bioinformatics have revolutionized the study of PPIs in immunology.

High-throughput techniques, such as yeast two-hybrid screening and co-immunoprecipitation, allow researchers to identify and characterize interacting protein networks in a systematic manner. Not only have high-throughput approaches demonstrated the dynamic nature of the interaction, but also supported evidence for how specific proteins help the immune system. For instance, the interactions between pattern recognition receptors (PRRs) and downstream signaling molecules are a critical area of research consideration, considering that the interactions play a crucial role in pathogen detection and initiating immune responses. Insight from such analyses goes towards the identification of potential targets for therapy, and hence the control of immune responses in diseases like viral infection and inflammatory disorders. With the application of these integrative approaches, the field continues to advance our knowledge of complex immunologic processes. The integrative research of PPIs also advances the boundaries of immunologic inquiry by providing insight into knowledge related to viral evasion mechanisms. The majority of pathogens have evolved sophisticated means of evading host immune responses, in certain instances by directly targeting core proteins within such interaction networks. For instance, African Swine Fever Virus (ASFV) employs proteins to capture immune signaling, which is a critical interface between immune regulation and viral pathogenesis. The intricate dynamic between immune evasion and PPI necessitates a comprehensive analysis that can tease apart mechanisms through which host-pathogen interactions are governed. This information not only reveals why pathogens are capable of thriving and producing disease, but it also provides new therapeutic avenues to enhance host defense mechanisms. Targeting certain studies, such as the K205R gene in ASFV, allows researchers the potential to unravel these mechanisms, thereby providing valuable feedback on the development of antiviral therapies.

Definition of Protein-Protein Interactions (PPIs)

PPIs constitute a phenomenon that forms the basis of most biological processes, particularly in immunology. Proteins, as biopolymers, need interaction for signal transduction, immune modulation, and coordination of metabolic pathways. These interactions are due to non-covalent affinities formed through specificity and dynamic equilibrium. The PPIs may be transient or stable and determine the formation of large multimeric complexes that are necessary in cellular function and survival. In the immune system, their comprehension is vital as they regulate the immune cell communication and antigen recognition. Therefore, the comprehension of PPIs' complexities makes it possible to comprehend further the immune mechanisms as well as determine the disease therapeutic targets, for example, autoimmune diseases and infectious diseases. Comprehension of PPIs entails sophisticated methods of their detection and analysis because of the complexity and variability of these interactions in biological systems. Biochemical methods, such as co-immunoprecipitation and yeast two-hybrid screening, have traditionally been employed to map these interactions. More recent advances, such as mass spectrometry and bioinformatics programs, have significantly encouraged the ability to delineate and quantify PPIs at an unprecedented scale. For instance, Folador et al. (2016) report a study to reconstruct presumptive interactomes for Corynebacterium pseudotuberculosis strains, identifying major proteins that could be drug targets. Such findings show that the mapping of PPIs is not only essential to understanding simple cellular functions, but to translating such information into useful practice in drug development and disease therapy. The utility of determining protein interactions transcends basic biology, influencing therapeutic strategies and diagnostic methods. Techniques that shed light on protein connections can identify potential therapeutic targets that are novel and specific. For example, approaches detailed in Ycart et al. (2013) introduce novel tools for the discovery of significant symbol relationships within genomic databases and reporting insights into PPI networks that are worth investigating. Such findings are of interest to immunology because they can lead to the development of targeted therapy for immune response regulation. Thus, concluding PPI analysis invites the possibility of more precise disease pathology intervention, ultimately resulting in improved patient care and novel models of treatment in immunology (Figure 7.1).

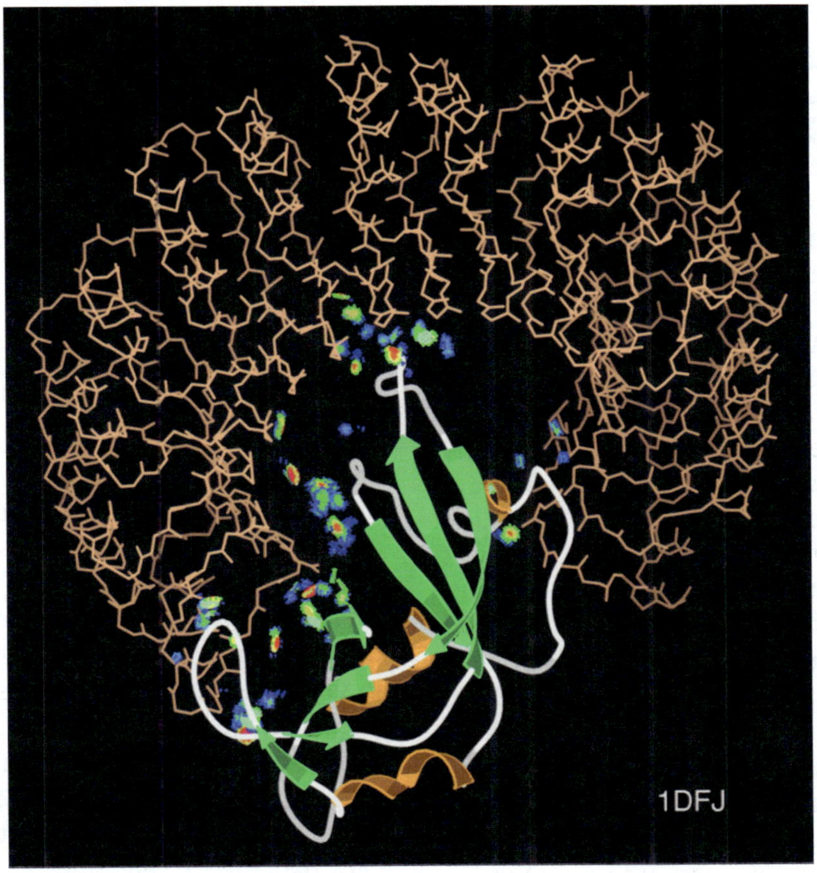

Figure 7.1. The horseshoe-shaped ribonuclease inhibitor (shown as wireframe) forms a protein–protein interaction with the ribonuclease protein. The contacts between the two proteins are shown as coloured patches.

Source: https://upload.wikimedia.org/wikipedia/commons/5/56/1dfj_RNAseInhibitor-RNAse_complex.jpg.

Importance of Protein-Protein Interactions (PPIs) in Immunology

The role of PPIs within the realm of immunology has increasingly become a focus of interest in research, particularly as researchers seek to understand the complex networks of cell-to-cell communication underlying immune responses. PPIs are the cause of the cascades of signaling that result in the activation and regulation of immune cells. Through the formation of discrete protein complexes, these interactions enable the transmission of signals that ultimately result in cellular activation, differentiation, and proliferation. This intricate web of interactions is vital to homeostasis and effective pathogen response. Just as with the advancements in selective glucocorticoid receptor agonists and modulators, further insight into individual PPIs can lead to the identification of more effective therapeutic molecules that stimulate immune response and minimize side effects (Chirumamilla et al., 2017). Thus, research on PPIs not only brings a better understanding of how the immune system works but also paves the way for new modes of therapy for immunology. Moreover, research on PPIs extends beyond the realm of traditional mammalian models to that of invertebrate immunology. By studying animals such as crustaceans, researchers have found unique immunological pathways unlike those found in vertebrates. Discovery of new recognition proteins and immune effectors reflects evolutionary diversity in immune systems. PPI analysis within these proteins can reveal how various immune pathways are functional and interact with one another, and ultimately determine responses to infectious organisms. Notably, the work can inform aquaculture disease resistance improvement strategies to address challenges of viral and bacterial infections in farmed stocks (Hauton, 2012). Research of PPIs in invertebrates thus not only increases our understanding of immune evolution but also informs practical applications for aquatic life control. The promise of PPIs has been identified in immunology to target therapies that would modulate the immune responses. As PPIs play a central role in cellular signaling, researchers are keen to tap this knowledge for the development of therapeutics that can selectively modulate immune processes. For example, therapeutic benefit from the knowledge of PPIs can potentially enhance vaccines or even come up with new therapies for autoimmune diseases. The novel field of PPI-based drug discovery is replete with promise; by cracking the specific interactions that form the basis of pathogen recognition or stimulation of immune cells, researchers can develop drugs that amplify or suppress these interactions. Not only is this a more targeted way to modulate the immune system, but it also meets the demand for increasingly targeted therapeutics with fewer side effects (Chirumamilla et al., 2017). Therefore, the general perception of PPIs is a groundbreaking avenue toward basic immunology development as well as clinical treatment.

7.1. Basics of Protein-Protein Interactions (PPIs)

PPI is a fundamental idea in immunology study because interactions between proteins are significant to mediating cellular processes and signal networks. Proteins do not prefer to function alone; rather, they rely on complex formation with other proteins to carry out biological processes efficiently. These interactions have been demonstrated to regulate a number of immune responses, including the activation and differentiation of immune cells such as T cells and B cells. The significance of PPIs is particularly significant in the context of cytotoxic CD8 T cells that play important roles in cytotoxicity towards infected cells. Recent advances in therapeutic strategies against such interactions indicate a need for increased focus on defining the molecular underpinnings of PPI networks, particularly in chronic infections and cancer, where T-cell responses are pivotal (Cosma & Eisenlohr, 2018). Thus, the understanding of the mechanisms of PPIs can give paradigm-shifting information to the development of vaccines and therapies in immunology. Protein stability, affinity, and specificity are all significant parameters in PPIs that have direct effects on the immune system's functioning. Techniques such as co-immunoprecipitation, yeast two-hybrid screening, and surface plasmon resonance have been employed to study these interactions in depth. These technologies allow researchers to catalog interaction networks and ascertain the level of association, thereby inferring dynamic changes in immune responses. For instance, changes in T-cell receptor (TCR) binding affinities for peptide-bound major histocompatibility complex (MHC) molecules can radically alter events downstream in signaling. Furthermore, the functional importance of disrupted or aberrant PPIs is used to highlight their importance in disease conditions, notably autoimmune conditions, where abnormal interactions lead to the inappropriate activation of immune cells or loss of tolerance. Therefore, thorough knowledge of PPIs is central to deciphering the complexities involved in immunological reactions. Moreover, the action of PPIs typically involves intricate biochemical and biophysical modifications, such as phosphorylation, ubiquitination, and glycosylation, that can affect immunological effects. In encounters with pathogens, such as trypanosomes, the interaction of these proteins with the immune components of the host has significant importance. These parasites employ PPIs for immune evasion by employing mechanisms such as antigenic variation and immune reaction modulation to acquire protection from host defenses (Magez et al., 2020). An investigation of such interactions not only improves our understanding of host-pathogen dynamics but also directs vaccine development through the identification of important immune intervention targets. Through the dissection of such complex interactions, scientists may engineer novel immunotherapies aimed at the amplification of immune response or the circumvention of immune evasion mechanisms by pathogens, thus driving the discipline of immunology towards the resolution of infectious disease and vaccine challenges.

7.1.1. Types of Protein-Protein (PPIs) Interactions

The paradigm of PPIs is at the heart of the discipline of immunology, as they control the functional dynamics of immune cells. There are various types of interactions, the basis of which is made up of electrostatic interactions, hydrogen bonds, and hydrophobic contacts. Electrostatic forces, which are produced by charged amino acid residues, play a key role in stabilizing the transient interactions, especially within signaling pathways where the responses should be rapid. In addition, protein structure significantly influences their potential to interact since any alteration in the structure can enable or hinder binding. This conformational plasticity allows proteins to adapt to various physiological states, and their dynamic partnership is optimized for immune function.

The complexity of these interactions attests to their importance in guaranteeing homeostasis and adaptability in the immune system. Another prominent category of protein-protein interaction is enabled by post-translational modifications (PTMs), which have drastic consequences for protein structure and stability. PTMs, including phosphorylation, glycosylation, and ubiquitination, can be used to introduce binding sites or change existing ones, thereby affecting protein-protein interactions. For instance, the phosphorylcholine-rich glycoprotein ES-62 secreted by the rodent filarial nematode Acanthocheilonema viteae interacts with immune cells like macrophages and lymphocytes through PTMs. Research indicates ES-62 interacts with other proteins on different immune cell types and the significance of these modifications within selective binding and immune modulation (Harnett et al., 2011). These small interactions may be stimulatory or suppressive of immune cell reactions, illustrating how PTMs are basic regulators of protein-protein interaction and thereby influence overall immune function. Additionally, the significance of protein complexes in enabling complex signaling networks cannot be overly stressed. These complexes are formed by numerous interactions and are generally transient so that cells can respond quickly to environmental signals. For instance, mitochondrial dynamics, including fusion and fission processes, are controlled by proteomic interactions that adjust according to the metabolic requirements of immune cells, displaying a relationship between structure and function in immunity (Rambold & Pearce, 2018). Apart from this, the formation of receptor-ligand complexes is also central to the initiation of signaling cascades and immune activation. Multi-protein complexes not only facilitate cross-talk between cellular pathways but also provide the ability to coordinate immune system responses based on spatial and temporal considerations, emphasizing the rich tapestry of protein-protein interactions as central to immunological processes (Figure 7.2).

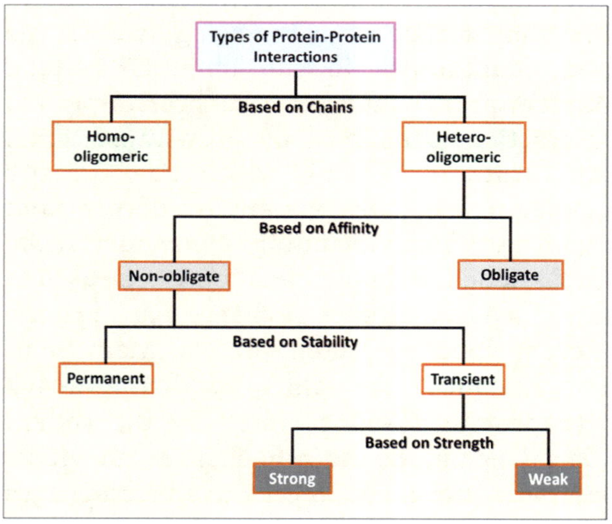

Figure 7.2. Diagrammatic representation of different types of protein–protein interactions.

Source: https://www.researchgate.net/publication/382827127/figure/fig2/AS:11431281282031776@1728095262200/Digrammatic-representation-of-different-types-of-protein-protein-interactions-The-types.png.

7.1.2. Mechanisms of Interaction

It is essential to know the mechanisms of protein-protein interaction to gain insight into the complex biological networks underlying immunological phenomena. Protein-protein interactions play a key role in signal transduction, particularly within the immune system, where they drive the critical processes of pathogen recognition and ensuing downstream signaling cascades. Pattern recognition receptors (PRRs) are central to this network of interactions as they perceive pathogen-associated molecular patterns (PAMPs) and initiate immune responses. This cascade will eventually translate into cytokine production and release, most notably interferons (IFNs), which serve as key mediators of host defense against viral infection. The intricate network of interactions demonstrates the importance of research into these mechanisms to design useful therapeutic interventions against many diseases, such as viral infections and other pathologies in which protein interactions fail to induce adequate immune responses (Costa, 2011).

Among the numerous proteins participating in immune signaling, optineurin (OPTN) has attracted considerable attention owing to its multifunctional character during inflammation and immunity. OPTN functions as a ubiquitin-binding protein to interact with various signaling pathways that play a central role in cellular functions such as autophagy. The ability of many partners to bind to optineurin allows immune response modulation, revealing one of the ways that cells can modulate inflammation and respond to pathogenic stressors. Notably, OPTN gene mutations result in disabling diseases, and thus protein interactions are important in health and disease. As additional research continues to unfold the complexity of OPTN in immune interactions, the unraveling of the mechanisms could unravel the possibility of novel therapeutic intervention strategies for the correction or modulation of these processes (Slowicka & van Loo, 2018). The host protein-virus protein interaction is yet another complexity of interaction mechanisms in immunology. For instance, the African Swine Fever Virus (ASFV) has learned to evade host immune mechanisms, revealing that viral proteins interact with host signaling pathways in order to evade detection and destruction.

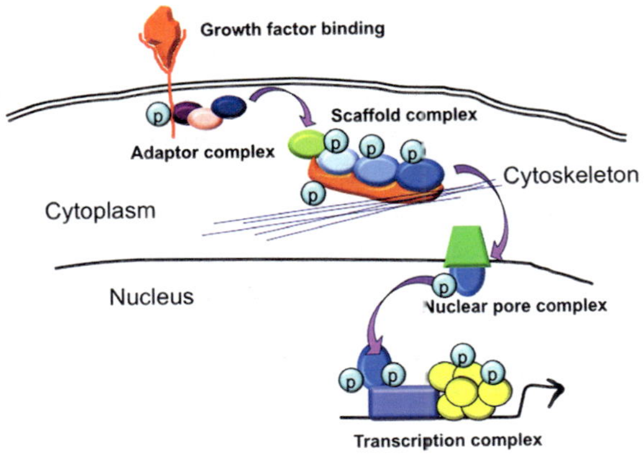

Figure 7.3. Protein interactions mediate cellular responses. A hypothetical signal transduction pathway where sequential and transient interactions between upstream and downstream components of this pathway are active. All depicted interactions, both between signaling proteins and with other cellular constituents, are critical for proper signaling. They are also potential targets for disease-causing alterations as well as for therapeutic targeting.

Source: https://www.researchgate.net/profile/Garry-Corthals/publication/236038026/figure/fig1/AS:393547128819734@1470840355678/Protein-interactions-mediate-cellular-responses-A-hypothetical-signal-transduction.png.

Research on early ASFV gene K205R reveals that it was able to inhibit interferon responses through precise interactions that dictate STAT1 phosphorylation, an integral part of IFN signaling pathways. These findings highlight the importance of unwinding the intricacy of the viral-host protein interactions, as they not only account for the virus's pathogenesis but also delineate potential targets against antiviral interventions. The understanding of these mechanisms provides insights into how the immune evasion occurs and may provide information regarding the development of treatments that can disrupt these deleterious interactions, thus bolstering the host's ability to combat infection (Costa, 2011) (Figure 7.3).

7.1.3. Techniques for Studying Protein-Protein Interactions (PPIs)

Understanding PPIs is key to dissecting molecular mechanisms of biological systems, especially in the realm of immunology. Different methodologies have been devised to analyze such interactions, each with its particular strengths and weaknesses. Co-immunoprecipitation (Co-IP) is a method by which scientists are able to purify certain proteins from a mixture and probe for their interaction. This technique relies on the use of antibodies to capture target proteins and any protein partners that they would most likely be bound to so that one can get insight into immunological pathway functional dynamics. However, Co-IP may fail to detect weak or transient interactions, so other methods must be used for an exhaustive analysis of PPIs. It is necessary to know these mixtures because intricate immune responses are likely to be composed of many interactions, which can be restrained by pathogen manipulation or genetics. Fluorescence resonance energy transfer (FRET) represents another novel technique employed to investigate PPIs, which is ideal to monitor interactions in the context of live cells. FRET relies on non-radiative energy transfer between two fluorescent dyes, allowing real-time observation of protein interactions under physiological conditions. This method has been especially useful in immunology, where the dynamics of signaling in immune cells are important for understanding effective responses (Figure 7.4).

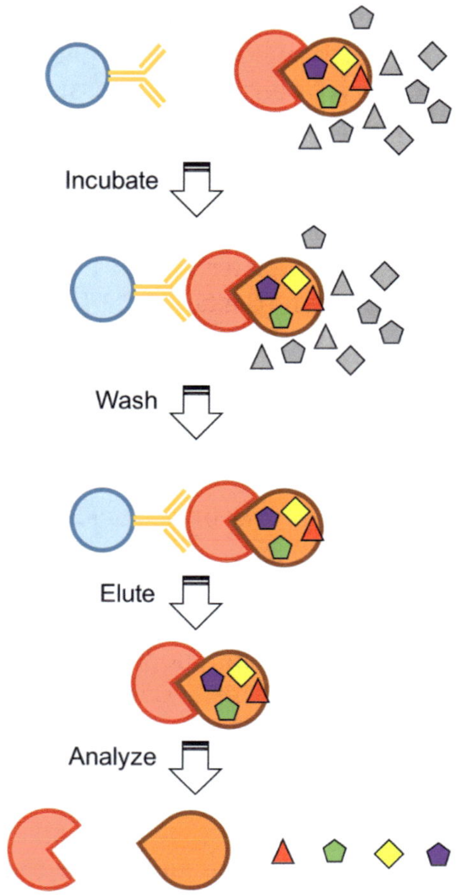

Figure 7.4. The workflow of a standard Co-immunoprecipitation (Co-IP) assay.

Source: https://www.lifeasible.com/wp-content/themes/v1/images/Co-immunoprecipitation-Assay-pic-1.png.

Although having powerful uses, FRET needs to be carefully calibrated and controlled experiments conducted in order to overcome issues of spectral overlap and background fluorescence. Ultimately, the application of FRET in immunology not only defines contacts but also plays a role in assessing the spatial and temporal aspects of cellular signaling events. Another recent approach to PPI research is in silico analysis, which employs computational models to predict and model interactions based on protein structure and sequence information. Statistical analysis and machine learning algorithms have revolutionized the prediction of PPIs, as a look at recent developments in B-cell epitope prediction approaches demonstrates. These computer-based methods have an initial screening function, determining potential candidates for interaction before laboratory verification. These methods are particularly valuable in large-scale studies, conserving time and money in the identification of significant PPIs. Of particular interest are new developments with new techniques employing molecular mechanics for epitope classification and prediction and thus furthering understanding of immune responses (Reitmaier, 2007). Importantly, findings in immunology experiments reflect PPI complexity as determined by research linking specific chromosomal regions with NKT cell function and thereby genotypes with immune function (Malagic, 2017) (Figure 7.5).

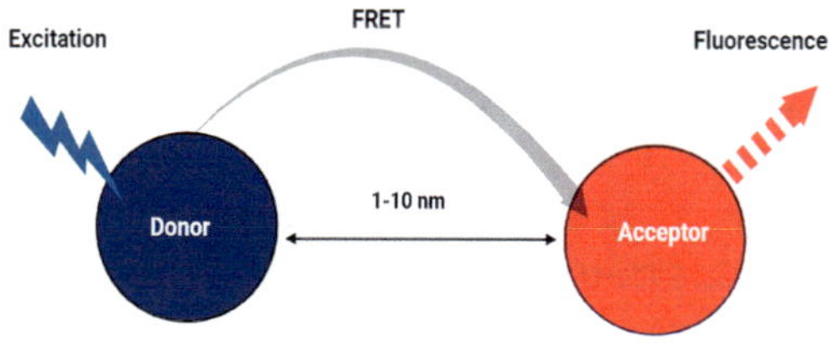

Figure 7.5. Fluorescence resonance energy transfer (FRET) basics.

Source: https://i.shgcdn.com/93555a25-e759-445a-a7bc-42ea91a8d9d7/-/format/auto/-/preview/3000x3000/-/quality/lighter/.

7.2. Role of Protein-Protein Interactions (PPIs) in Immune Response

PPIs in immunology are a key regulator of the immune response because they influence significant cellular pathways and signaling cascades. The interactions are accountable for pathogen sensing by receptors such as Toll-like receptors (TLRs), which are key components of the innate immune system. It has been established in research that TLRs recognize certain PAMPs, which trigger the immune reaction to infections. Activation of TLRs triggers a chain reaction of molecular interactions to activate transcription factors, including NF-kB and AP-1, that ultimately enhance the expression of pro-inflammatory cytokines. Such signaling pathways play important roles in amplifying the host's ability to mount an efficient immune response against invading microorganisms. Therefore, understanding PPI dynamics in this context is important to explaining immunity mechanisms and therapeutic intervention design for infectious diseases (Costa, 2011). Second, specificity of immune responses is also facilitated by the intricate networks formed by PPIs of numerous signaling proteins. For example, in adipocytes, TLR ligands Pam3csk4 and Poly(I:C) also control the transcriptome and immune-related gene function, consequently influencing lipid metabolism and inflammation. These interactions have been shown to lead to differential gene expression in immune response and metabolism-related genes, reflecting their proteomic impact on cellular behaviors. The discovery of key regulatory genes that emerge from PPI networks provides an understanding of the transcriptional landscape upon TLR activation. This can lead to the discovery of biomarkers required to analyze immunomodulatory effects in treatment approaches. The concept of including PPI analysis in the study of immunometabolism is promising to advance therapeutic intervention in veterinary and also human medicine (Igata et al., 2019). The far-reaching implications of PPIs in immunity are also in modulating antiviral defenses. For instance, host-virus protein interactions may strongly disrupt the immune signaling pathways. Research has suggested that viruses have methods to evade immunity through disrupting PPIs in the host, disabling the IFN response that is critical for antiviral immunity. Such studies have proven the function of certain viral proteins inhibiting STAT1 phosphorylation, an essential step in the IFN signaling cascade, showing the mechanism behind the survival and proliferation of viruses in the host. These findings show the importance of deciphering PPIs to clarify viral pathogenesis and mechanisms of immune evasion, thereby paving the way for targeted antiviral therapies. By understanding these interactions, researchers can develop innovative strategies to enhance host defense against virus infection, particularly relevant to current global health (Costa, 2011).

7.2.1. Antigen Recognition by Immune Cells

The mechanism by which immune cells recognize antigens is a complex mechanism that forms the core of the adaptive immune system. At the core of such recognition is the interaction between TCRs and peptide-MHC (major histocompatibility complex) complexes found on the surface of antigen-presenting cells. Not only does this interaction induce T cell activation, but it also determines the quality and magnitude of the immune response. Immune T cells must exert absolute discrimination, dividing self from non-self in a highly dynamic environment, a challenge met through sophisticated processes such as adaptive sorting. Immune cells can quantify several ligands in their environment and make a decision based on qualitative distinction rather than mere quantity. This subtle comprehension is required to mount an efficient defense against pathogens without encouraging the threat of autoimmunity, making the importance of protein-protein interactions in the immunological setting more prominent (François & Altan-Bonnet, 2015). In addition, the ability of the adaptive immune system to tailor its response by means of kinetic proofreading adds another level to antigen recognition mechanisms. Kinetic proofreading ensures that T cells become committed to activation only after the establishment of high-affinity interactions with foreign antigens. The immune system in this case exhibits phenotypic variation, and as a result, it enables a group of T cells to respond differently to the same antigenic challenge. Phenotypic variation is significant since it provides for a more focused immune response that can adapt to the changing nature of pathogens.

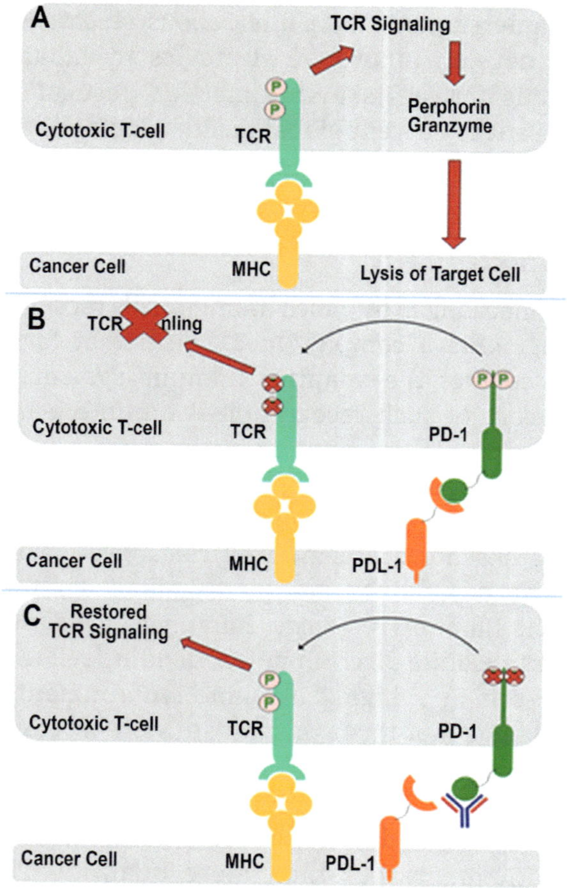

Figure 7.6. Antigen recognition through CTLs, TCR signalling and mechanism of action of immune checkpoint inhibitors.

Source: https://www.researchgate.net/profile/Fabian-Mairinger/publication/317716705/figure/fig1/AS:507568682434560@1498025213002/Antigen-recognition-through-CTLs-TCR-signalling-and-mechanism-of-action-of-immune.png.

These discussions highlight the nuanced interaction of protein-protein interactions that drive cellular decisions in immunology, demonstrating how TCR signaling may lead to high-impact consequences in immune capability and disease (François & Altan-Bonnet, 2015). In addition, research in antigen recognition branches into the study of oscillatory behavior in immune cell physiology, potentially reflecting underlying signaling consistency. Recent works on auditory steady-state responses (ASSRs) in immunology emphasize the importance of reliability throughout cellular responses when observing antigen interactions. The research demonstrated that consistent measurements of inter-trial phase coherence (ITPC) indicate a standard platform for describing antigen recognition fidelity. Such findings suggest that reliability in the oscillatory patterns of immune cells can be associated with effective immune responses, thus comparison between neuronal signaling mechanisms and T cell stimulation. Explaining these interactions in terms of protein-protein interactions may reveal new insights into therapeutic intervention involving amplified immune recognition and response (Figure 7.6).

7.2.2. Signaling pathways involving Protein-Protein Interactions (PPIs)

PPIs form the intricate network that is central to signaling pathways critical for immune response. These interactions enable various immune cells to interact, enabling them to adapt and respond to challenges brought by pathogens. A perfect example is the interaction of TLRs and their signal partners, which brings about downstream cascades required for pro-inflammatory cytokine expression. As evidenced by Rambold & Pearce (2018), TLR4 uniquely interacts with lipopolysaccharides, triggering signaling cascades that result in activating transcription factors like NF-κB. This activation is crucial for planning an effective immune response, and this underscores the role of PPIs in the immune signaling networks. Through the understanding of these interactions, researchers are able to potentially determine therapeutic targets to tailor immune responses in many diseases. Mitochondrial dynamics are becoming increasingly accepted as important regulators of immune cell function through the control of metabolic pathways and how they intersect with signaling cascades. Mitochondria, often referred to as the powerhouses of the cell, are responsible for the production of ATP and the supply of metabolites essential for cell function.

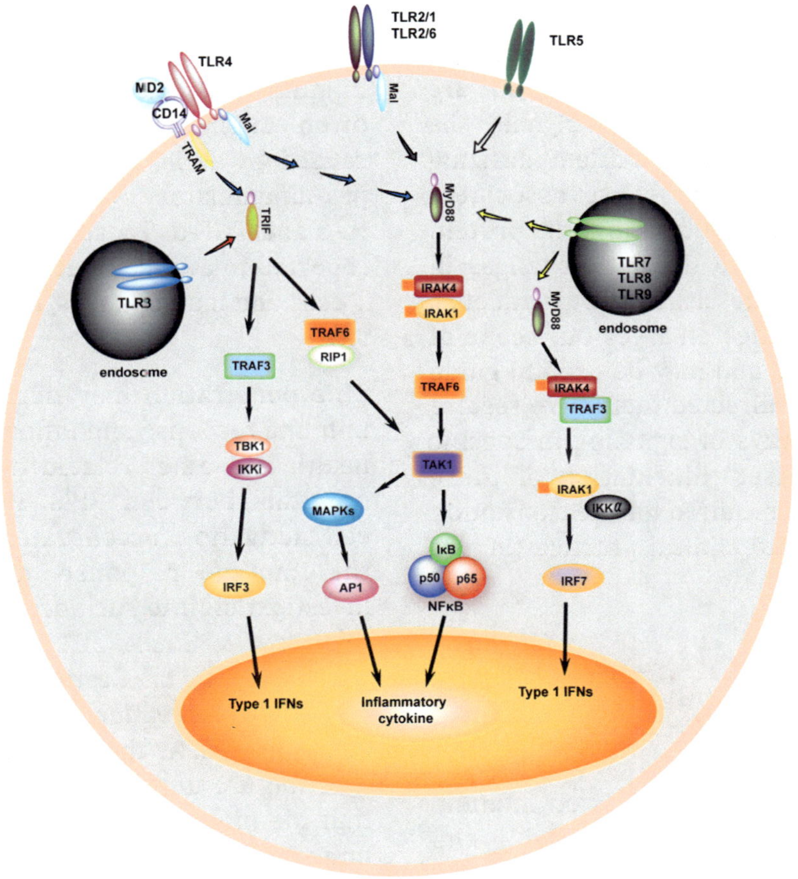

Figure 7.7. Toll-like receptor signaling pathways. Toll-like receptor (TLR) signaling is activated by stimulation of TLR ligands.

Source: https://www.researchgate.net/publication/273183697/figure/fig1/AS:294760309903381@1447287742977/Toll-like-receptor-signaling-pathways-Toll-like-receptor-TLR-signaling-is-activated-by.png.

The coordination between mitochondrial dynamics and PPIs plays a significant role in ensuring the efficiency of immunological function since metabolic adjustments have the potential to sculpt mitochondrial fission and fusion. According to Rambold & Pearce (2018), most current studies have suggested that mitochondrial morphology could regulate immune cell fate and function. This directs us to the necessity of exploring how PPIs that take part in mitochondrial proteins may affect the total signaling frameworks that decide immune cell action and extend our understanding of metabolic reprogramming in immunity. Moreover, interaction between PPIs and intracellular signaling mechanisms also signifies the complexity of immune regulation. The strength and specificity of signaling reactions, for instance, are decided by the interaction between adaptor proteins and receptor kinases. This is most applicable in restricting excessive inflammation, where tightly regulated PPIs are regulatory points in the cascade of signals. The data that is provided by research emphasizing genetic variation, such as those associated with TLR4, show how alterations in protein interactions can lead to dramatic changes in immune signaling, as described in Davoodi et al. (2012). This knowledge enlarges our scope of disease mechanisms and may be used to guide the development of directed therapy to restore dysregulated pathways of signaling in specific immunologic diseases. Elucidation of these mechanisms will be required for the translation of basic research into clinical practice (Figure 7.7).

7.2.3. Impact of Protein-Protein Interactions (PPIs) on Immune Cell Activation

Understanding the impact of PPIs on immune cell activation is crucial to identifying the mechanism by which drugs, such as proton pump inhibitors (PPIs), may unintentionally influence the immune system. In decreasing gastric acid production, PPIs effectively bring about alterations in gastrointestinal flora and nutrient digestion. This disruption will activate immune pathways because immune cells must become acclimatized to the changing microbiome and nutrient bioavailability that are essential to their activation and function. Mitochondrial dynamics regulated by PPIs are important to the metabolic programming of immune cells, influencing processes such as cell differentiation and inflammatory responses. According to existing research, some metabolic cues reach the mitochondrial machinery, thus influencing immune cell function, thus pointing towards an in-depth connection between PPIs and immune response modulation through metabolic pathways (Rambold & Pearce, 2018). Another point to consider is how PPIs cross-talk with the inflammatory functions of adipose tissues, such as perivascular adipose tissue (PVAT), which might further modulate immune cell activation. PVAT dysregulation, often augmented by systemic alterations caused by PPIs, leads to increased levels of pro-inflammatory cytokines and adipokines like IL-6 and TNF-α. These proteins have also been reported to attract other immune cells, such as T cells and macrophages, into the inflammatory site.

This penetration may determine the overall immune response and influence cardiovascular health and other related diseases. Therefore, crosstalk between PPIs, PVAT, and immune cell activation accentuates the intricacy in the immune response, demanding further investigation into such drug-induced pathways (Nosalski & Guzik, 2017). It is important to understand the implications of the use of PPIs on immune cell activation to offer better therapeutic interventions. As the intricacies of immune cell function are unraveled, it is increasingly clear that the interaction between PPIs and various immune pathways is worthy of intense scrutiny. In addition to their role in gastrointestinal disease, PPIs have the potential to facilitate, inadvertently, the modulation of inflammatory processes affecting well-being. Future research must tackle the task of deconstructing these interactions, shedding light on how PPIs alter not only immune cell activation but also the intricate systems of signaling mechanisms controlling immune function. Such research may reveal new avenues for inflammatory disease therapy, such as cardiovascular disease, where immune cell dynamics remain pivotal (Figure 7.8).

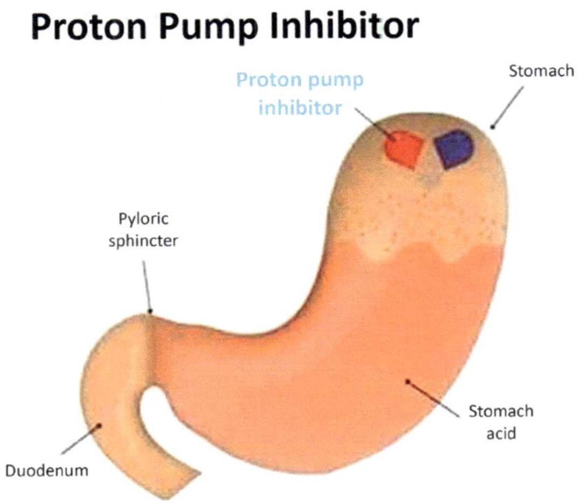

Figure 7.8. Proton pump inhibitor (PPI).

Source: https://speciality.medicaldialogues.in/wp-content/uploads/2017/04/proton-pump-inhibito-e1510139213555.jpg.

7.3. Methods for Analyzing Protein-Protein Interactions (PPIs)

PPIs must be elucidated in order to unravel immune responses and engineer bespoke immunotherapies. Co-IP represents one of the prevalent techniques for PPI analysis, allowing researchers to immunoprecipitate target proteins together with their interacting molecules from cell lysates. By exploiting antibodies against a target protein, Co-IP can be employed to enhance *in vivo*-assembled complexes and provide insight into functional interactions within a physiological context. After isolation, mass spectrometry can be used to determine co-precipitated proteins, allowing in-depth analysis of PPI networks. The technique has proved useful in immunology, specifically in research that seeks to understand receptor-ligand interactions and immune response signal pathways. Interestingly, the creation of imaging techniques such as FRET further optimizes understanding dynamic interactions in live cell settings and thus contributes to our understanding of PPI dynamics in immune systems (Chirumamilla et al., 2017). Yeast two-hybrid screening is another principal means of examining PPIs that utilizes a eukaryotic system in detecting protein-protein interactions by means of transcriptional activation. It is a high-throughput method that involves the creation of fusion proteins that combine a DNA-binding domain fused to one partner and an activation domain fused to another. Through interaction, the transcription of the reporter gene is activated, an indication of a PPI. The yeast two-hybrid system has played a crucial role in the identification of new interactions between immune-related proteins, especially in T cell activation and cytokine signal pathways. Although effective, this method has its shortfalls in the shape of false positives and a failure to probe the post-translational modification effect on interactions.

Nevertheless, when combined with other approaches, such as Co-IP or mass spectrometry, researchers can develop a more complete picture of the interactome (Costa et al., 2011). Surface plasmon resonance (SPR) is also a useful method to study PPIs in real time, allowing quantification of biomolecular interactions. This technique measures refractive index changes in close proximity to a sensor surface on which one of the two binding partners is immobilized and the interaction with the second partner is monitored as it traverses the surface. SPR allows kinetic data, and binding affinities, rates, and stability of complexes can be measured, all critical in studying immunological responses and therapy effectiveness. By integrating SPR with pharmacology, researchers can measure the interaction between immune receptors and their ligands and thus inform drug discovery. The ability to investigate PPIs under biophysical conditions further extends the relevance of findings to cellular environments and pushes the investigation of intricate immune regulatory processes and new therapies (Chirumamilla et al., 2017).

7.3.1. Yeast Two-Hybrid (Y2H) Screening

The Y2H system is a breakthrough method for the elucidation of protein-protein interaction, especially in the context of immunology. Through the use of a genetically modified yeast strain, target proteins are baited and putative interaction partners are determined. The technique exploits the fact that a two-protein interaction may drive transcription of a reporter gene so that interactions in a cell-based context can be detected. Due to the complexity of immune responses, understanding interactions can provide basic insights into how immune cells communicate and respond to pathogens. Further, Y2H screening not only detects direct interaction but also indirect interaction through complex formation, which sheds light on signaling pathways that are important for immune homeostasis and response variety. One of the significant applications of Y2H screening in the field of immunology is the ability to uncover novel interactions between viral proteins and host cell factors that influence infection processes. For instance, studies that explore the interactions between viral proteins and cellular targets identify the underlying mechanisms that govern the control of viral entry and replication. For this purpose, Yeast two-hybrid screening has been applied to investigate the interaction between the Severe Acute Respiratory Syndrome coronavirus (SARS-CoV) envelope glycoprotein Spike (S) and the ezrin protein, a host factor that restricts viral entry. Through the study of such pivotal interactions, Y2H screening has facilitated the elucidation of host-pathogen relationships through the identification of ezrin as a host protein that limits S-dependent membrane fusion, thus highlighting cellular factor contributions to viral pathogenesis (Chen et al., 2012). Besides, Y2H screening holds promise for the dissection of complex interactions within intracellular parasites with significant implications for immunological function.

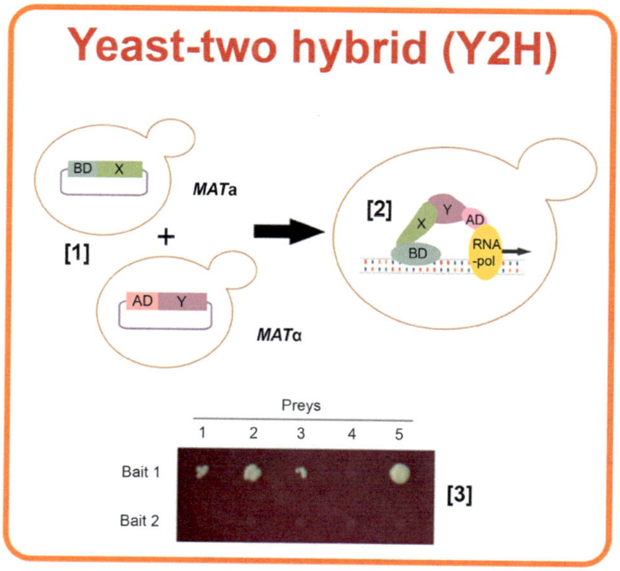

Figure 7.9. The yeast two-hybrid (Y2H) concept and a typical readout. [1] The BD domain fused to the bait protein (X) and the AD domain fused to the prey protein (Y) are expressed in yeast cells. [2] If proteins X and Y interact, BD binds DNA and AD activates RNA polymerase. An example readout [3] of a Y2H assay with two bait proteins (Bait 1 and Bait 2) and five prey proteins (1–5).

Source: https://www.ebi.ac.uk/training/online/courses/protein-interactions-and-their-importance/wp-content/uploads/sites/120/2020/07/fig3_new-2.png.

For example, dynamic properties of proteins implicated in mitochondrial morphology, such as Fis1, have been investigated using this platform to determine their correlations with other important proteins. Results from such a screen not only advance knowledge of the biological processes of mitochondrial function but also their broader implications for parasite fitness and the host's immune system. As such interactions occur, scientists can define how mitochondrial dynamics could affect immune signaling, thereby filling gaps in our understanding of host defense against different pathogens (Jacobs et al., 2020). Based on its applications both in viral and parasitic cases, Y2H screening proves to be a critical resource within the larger context of protein-protein interaction analysis in immunology (Figure 7.9).

7.3.2. Co-immunoprecipitation (Co-IP)

Co-IP stands as a pivotal technique in the exploration of protein-protein interactions, particularly in the field of immunology. This method allows researchers to isolate a specific protein along with its interacting partners from a complex mixture, such as cell lysates. By employing specific antibodies targeted against the protein of interest, co-immunoprecipitation easily precipitates not only the protein in question but also any molecule it is bound to, hence facilitating an improved understanding of the biological background under which such interactions are performed.

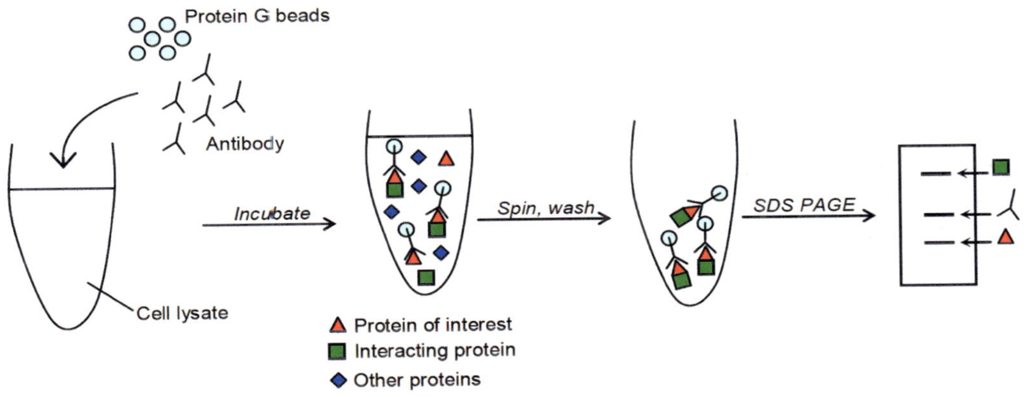

Figure 7.10. Principle of the co-immunoprecipitation technique.

Source: https://www.researchgate.net/profile/Anne-Sophie-Wavreille/publication/34179259/figure/fig3/AS:669572457852940@1536649922895/Principle-of-the-co-immunoprecipitation-technique.png.

The ability of these associations to be circumstantiated is vital, considering protein interactions' role in such processes as signal transduction, immune regulation, and pathogen recognition within the immunological framework. One of the major advantages of co-immunoprecipitation is its application to the study of the MHC molecules, which are central to T lymphocyte activation. Examination of how viral oncoproteins, such as the bovine papillomavirus (BPV-4) E5 protein, influence MHC class I molecules is used to highlight the importance of the interactions. The ability of the E5 protein to repress expression of traditional MHC class I molecules involves a specific interaction that inhibits transport of these molecules to the cell surface. The action is a viral immune evasion mechanism, a finding that was obtained through co-immunoprecipitation experiments demonstrating association of E5 with MHC heavy chains and inhibition of their normal pathway of trafficking (Araibi et al., 2006). In addition to classical MHC studies, co-immunoprecipitation has also played an important role in the study of interactions between tumor antigens like CLEC14A, which plays a role in tumor angiogenesis in the microenvironment. They can be validated by co-immunoprecipitation and mass spectrometry analysis, and the results could uncover new binding partners that are responsible for its biological activities. For instance, the capability of CLEC14A to interact with endothelial cells suggests a direct role in tumorigenesis-related vascular growth. By analyzing such interaction, scientists are able to advance their understanding of tumor biology and cellular processes, which may inform therapeutic strategy design for preventing tumor angiogenesis and improving cancer treatment outcomes (Lodhia, 2012) (Figure 7.10).

7.3.3. Mass Spectrometry (MS) Approaches

MS has proven to be a key instrument in the study of PPIs in the field of immunology, bringing a richness of detail and sensitivity to the analysis of intricate biological processes. The method enables the determination of protein complexes and their interactions by accurately measuring mass-to-charge ratios of ionized molecules. By application of various MS techniques, researchers can differentiate not only the presence of PPIs but also the specificity and affinity with which these interactions occur. Also, when combined with methods such as affinity purification, MS can enhance the understanding of dynamic interactions essential to immune responses, leading to concepts that may contribute to the development of targeted immunotherapeutics in a clinical setting. In particular, quantitative mass spectrometry techniques, stable isotope labeling, and label-free quantification have been made capable of carrying out comparative studies of protein interactions under varying experimental conditions. By quantifying protein complex abundance in the changed states, researchers are well equipped to decipher the regulatory impact of post-translational modifications and environmental factors on immune reactions. This is particularly pertinent in the context of diseases in which erroneous protein interactions are causally implicated, such as autoimmune disease and cancer. For instance, the interpretation of covalent modification of proteins by MS not only provides data on the functional implications of specific interactions but also raises the likelihood of designing biomarkers for disease progression and therapeutic response, enhancing our overall understanding of immune dynamics. Further, recent developments in mass spectrometry in sensitivity and resolution have extended the range of applications of this technology in immunology. High-resolution mass spectrometers can be employed to identify low-abundance proteins in PPIs that may play important regulatory roles in the immune system. Also, the integration of mass spectrometry with other approaches to biophysical investigations, such as nuclear magnetic resonance and X-ray crystallography, enables an in-depth exploration of protein interactions, uncovering structural insights that elucidate the mechanisms of action. For example, mass spectrometry in the identification of covalent interactions, such as glucocorticoid receptors research, illustrates the manner in which these methods can clarify molecular interaction topologies significant in the development of therapeutic protocols against diseases associated with inflammation (Mowers et al., 2013; Chirumamilla et al., 2017).

7.4. Computational Approaches in Protein-Protein Interaction (PPI) Analysis

The new field of computational methods for PPI analysis has revolutionized the manner in which scientists understand immunological response complexities. These approaches utilize advanced algorithms and bioinformatics tools to predict and predict interactions at the molecular level. As the pace of omics data, particularly genomic and proteomic data, has increased exponentially, computational strategies have become essential for defining the intricate networks of protein interaction necessary for immunity. Accurate prediction of these interactions not only enhances our understanding of the underlying biological processes but also facilitates the identification of candidate biomarkers and therapeutic targets. Computational platforms allow the integration of multi-dimensional data to conduct sophisticated analysis beyond simple interaction mapping to ultimately make discoveries that can transform clinical approaches in immunology and personalized medicine. The most critical aspect of applying computational methods to PPI analysis is that they can handle high-dimensional data and exploit sophisticated mathematical models. The application of machine learning techniques, for instance, has been effective in discovering patterns of interest from complex biological data. These techniques can predict PPIs by learning from existing interaction databases and integrating various sources of biological data, such as structural information and functional annotations. Furthermore, interpretation of such approaches requires an in-depth knowledge of the theoretical mathematics upon which they are embedded to identify the right algorithms for a specific research question. Familiarity with the strengths and limitations of various computational models, as highlighted in reviews, is crucial for maximum optimization of biomarker discovery and the translational merit of results in immunology research (Wang & Sarwal, 2015). Moreover, the application of computational analytics to PPI analysis assists not only in the discovery of new interactions but also aids in the refinement of current biological models. As the scientific world shifts to a systems biology focus, computational tools continue to become more important in bringing together varied data sets and making predictive models more plausible. This integration broadens the scale of immunological research through allowing for multi-faceted examination of protein interactions, such as pathways involved in immune processes. The creation of these computational methods illustrates their integral role in novel therapeutic target discovery and stratification of patient populations based on forecasted biomarker profiles. The advances in computational modeling are expected to drive extensive innovation in the field, providing a platform for future research activities seeking to solve complex immunological problems (Pappalardo et al., 2015).

7.4.1. Bioinformatics Tools for Protein-Protein Interaction (PPI) Prediction

The flexibility of bioinformatics tools has significantly improved the field of PPI prediction and has been at the forefront of shedding light on complex immunological processes. Some of these resources include databases like STRING and BioGRID, which enable the exploration of PPIs by integrating experimental data and computational prediction. STRING, in particular, leverages available biological knowledge by embracing a broad range of functional annotations and interactions from various organisms. This multi-parameter strategy enables scientists to identify biologically relevant interactions that contribute to immune responses and, therefore, guide the development of new therapeutic pathways. With the ongoing accumulation of big omics data, biologically relevant models may be built to predict the interactions that are not only central to basic understanding but also of clinical utility in immunology (Wang & Sarwal, 2015). Further, advances in machine learning have totally revolutionized PPI prediction approaches so that there are more efficient and precise analyses. By teaching algorithms with large datasets, such machine learning models can recognize hidden patterns and associations between proteins. Programmes like PyMOL and Cytoscape present graphical representations that make it easier for researchers to comprehend complex interaction networks, hence understanding the functional implications of such interactions in immunology. Furthermore, algorithmic implementation according to biological network properties enhances the predictive specificity, offering knowledge on the dynamic functions proteins exert during immune responses. In the interest of critical drug discovery and therapeutic design, where precise PPI prediction is of relevance, such advancements enable research to advance toward focused and effective immunotherapeutic interventions (Mengozzi et al., 2014). Finally, combining bioinformatics tools with experimental validation offers a robust platform for PPI discovery in immunology. On a starting note, computational predictions are then confirmed by experimental validation of the interactions by laboratory experiments, crucial to determining their biological relevance. This two-step strategy enhances the credibility of research findings and opens doors to more such breakthroughs in immunology. For instance, functional clustering applied in cytokine assessment demonstrates the role bioinformatics plays in guiding experimental design and hypothesis generation and finally leading to enhanced understanding of immune processes. Together, harmonization of bioinformatics and experimental methods ensures the solidity of immunological research basis, along with enhancing quick identification and characterization of crucial PPIs to the development of the field in both basic research and clinical application (Mengozzi et al., 2014) (Figure 7.11).

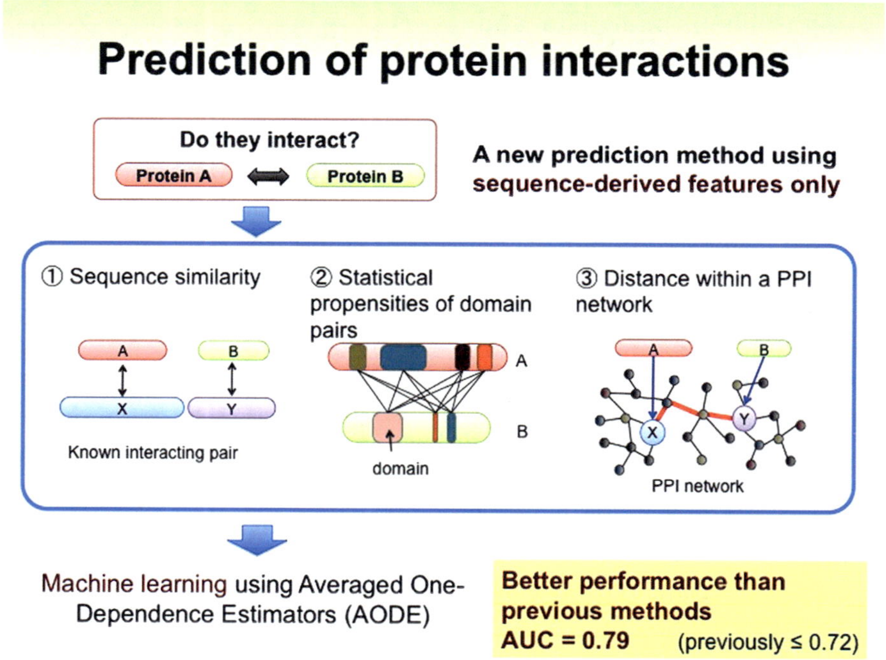

Figure 7.11. Prediction for protein interaction.

Source: https://archer.nibiohn.go.jp/sites/archer.nibiohn.go.jp/files/inline-images/PSOPIA-e.jpg.

7.4.2. Molecular Docking Simulations

Molecular docking simulations are key features of protein-protein interaction studies, particularly when applied to immunology. They are computational algorithms that enable scientists to predict the optimal orientation of the proteins as they interact with one another, a vital aspect of immune response studies. By mimicking the intricate molecular interactions between immunological proteins such as antigens and antibodies, docking simulations explain binding affinities and interaction dynamics. Of importance is that the accurate knowledge of these interactions can guide new therapeutic design as well as augment current treatment modalities. For example, improvement in the design of selective glucocorticoid receptor agonists, such as GSK866, has been achieved through docking studies that reveal conformational subtleties influencing their anti-inflammatory activity, which is depicted through their ability to bind receptors selectively and minimize side effects (Chirumamilla et al., 2017). In antibody engineering, molecular docking simulations provide essential insights into the selectivity and binding affinity of monoclonal antibodies to target antigens. High-throughput approaches enable researchers to highly define antibody-glycan complexes, which are notoriously recalcitrant to crystallization. By applying automated docking and molecular dynamics simulations, scientists can design thousands of viable 3D models for the complexes and determine their interactions. Not only does this method enable discovering key residues that are involved in binding, but it also allows scientists to further refine their designs in an attempt to boost efficacy. For instance, the specificity of mAb TKH2 was established employing such computer-based techniques, outlining its binding to the sialyl-Tn antigen (Amon et al., 2018). This is a comprehensive approach that allows for rational design of effective antibodies that are capable of targeting cancer markers based on carbohydrates. The incorporation of molecular docking simulations into protein-protein interaction analysis within immunology has the advantage of efficiency and accuracy. Through advanced algorithms and computing power, such simulations are able to calculate binding sites and affinities without recourse to exhaustive laboratory testing. This is extremely valuable in the context of rapid screening of lead drugs and the probing of complex immunological mechanisms. Through the use of molecular dynamics simulations, time-dependent protein interaction behavior is able to be investigated in more detail, information that static models may not be able to discover. With ongoing research in immunology, the applicability of such simulations in facilitating drug discovery and providing a clearer picture of protein interactions will be at the forefront, establishing their fundamental position in advancing biomedical sciences (Figure 7.12).

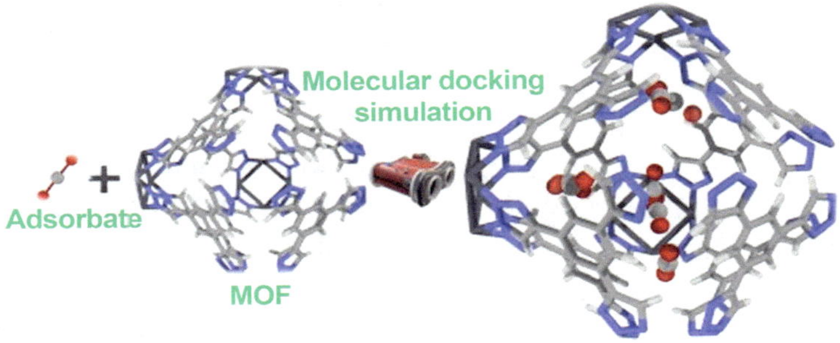

Figure 7.12. Illustration of a molecular docking simulation.

Source: https://ars.els-cdn.com/content/image/1-s2.0-S0927025623002513-ga1.jpg.

7.4.3. Network Analysis of Protein Interactions

It is crucial to know PPIs in the field of immunology because PPIs are the foundation for a wide range of physiological and pathological processes. The advent of advanced network analysis techniques has significantly enhanced our ability to analyze PPIs elaborately and systematically. With the help of tools such as STRING, scientists can map interaction networks that not only display direct interaction but also indirect association, as well, and are likely to be instrumental in immune regulation and response. The networks allow for the identification of hub proteins, which are the central actors in these biological interactions, regulating numerous signaling cascades and cellular functions. This approach enables a better overall view of the immune system to be obtained, enabling scientists to better understand complex processes such as cytokine signaling, receptor triggering, and pathways involved in autoimmune disease and infection. Recent studies have highlighted the role of specific proteins in mediating immune responses, particularly with regard to TLR signaling. For example, the listing of differentially expressed genes (DEGs) between porcine adipocytes after stimulation of TLR has identified potential genes of interest like EGR1, NOTCH1, and C3 involved in immune and metabolic functions (Igata et al., 2019). Network analysis reveals that these proteins do not work in isolation; rather, they are part of intricate networks of interactions that determine the end immune response. Also, the study of these networks clarifies potential therapeutic targets, since disruption of particular protein interactions may alter disease trajectory or enhance immunity. Thus, the use of network analysis not only informs our understanding of PPIs in immunology but also provides the basis upon which to construct new paradigms for treatment. The designation of cytokines as protective factors by network analysis also identifies the fine balance that the immune system maintains. Recent advances in functional clustering have made it possible for researchers to classify various cytokines based on their interactions and protective roles in tissue health (Mengozzi et al., 2014). This helps explain how certain cytokines, such as erythropoietin, can promote synaptic plasticity alongside immunomodulatory effects. Furthermore, research into how such proteins interact and cluster can lead to new forms of immunotherapy. Through the identification of specific cytokines that cluster with known protective factors, researchers may be able to unlock new avenues for treating diseases characterized by immune deregulation. Overall, network analysis is a powerful tool in the continued battle to unravel the complexity of protein interactions in the immune system, culminating in the development of targeted interventions.

7.5. Case Studies in Immunology

The identification of PPIs has become a mainstay of immunological investigation, offering profound insights into mechanisms of immune response. A useful case study is the design of selective glucocorticoid receptor agonists (SEGRAs) to optimize therapeutic potential and reduce adverse effects. Current investigations of GSK866 analogs have shed light on how covalent-binding strategies can modulate GR potency and selectivity. Through biochemical and cellular assays, researchers have demonstrated that certain analogs of the GSK866 exhibit favorable anti-inflammatory activity, pointing to the potential of PPIs in the design of personalized immunomodulation therapies. The sophisticated methods employed, including the GR immuno-localization and mass spectrometry, divulged the unique conformations that result from such interactions, and it has been suggested that selective PPI modulation can yield new therapies with improved safety profiles (Chirumamilla et al., 2017). Alternatively, case studies on autoimmune-poly-endocrinopathy-candidiasis-ectodermal-dystrophy syndrome (APECED) describe the role of PPIs in autoimmune disease mechanisms. The description of novel mutations in the autoimmune regulator (AIRE) gene, the c.396G > C (p. Arg132Ser; p. R132S) mutation, illustrates how alterations at the protein level are able to disrupt normal cell function. Effects of such mutations propagate to affect nuclear import pathways, thereby blocking the protein's transcriptional regulatory function. This particular case illustrates the delicate interaction between genetic mutations, protein conformation, and abnormal immune responses. The insights gained from the study of AIRE mutations not only enhance our understanding of autoimmunity but also underscore the critical role of PPIs in the maintenance of immunological homeostasis (Pellegrino et al., 2018). Overall, these case histories illustrate the core importance of protein-protein interactions in advancing immunological research. By investigating the dynamic, complex web of PPIs, scientists are uncovering novel therapeutic strategies for inflammatory diseases and autoimmune conditions. The employment of advanced techniques such as molecular dynamics simulations and coregulator interaction profiling has provided important insights into how these interactions give rise to immune responses at a molecular level. Such inter-disciplinary approaches not only enhance our comprehension of the mechanisms involved, but they also facilitate the development of targeted therapies that can potentially alter the therapy landscape for most immunological conditions. Ongoing research involving PPIs in immunology places scientists in a good position to make significant progress in theoretical insights and practical use of immunotherapies.

7.5.1. Protein-Protein Interactions (PPIs) in T-cell Receptor Signaling (TCR)

PPIs in TCR signaling play crucial roles in comprehending molecular processes of T-cell activation as well as immune responses. The TCR plays an essential role in T lymphocytes, enabling them to recognize and react against respective antigens presented on the MHC molecules of antigen-presenting cells. After recognition of the antigen, the TCR conveys a complex signal transduction process involving several intracellular proteins. Critical PTKs such as Lck and ZAP-70 also interact with the phosphorylated immunoreceptor tyrosine-based activation motifs (ITAMs) in the CD3 complex to facilitate downstream processes. The interactions are critical for the recruitment and activation of adaptor molecules such as LAT and SLP-76, which coordinate signaling complexes that ultimately lead to T-cell proliferation and effector function. Effectively, the precise orchestration of PPIs during TCR signaling determines the quality and quantity of the T-cell response. Moreover, the dynamics of PPIs in TCR signaling are not passive but controlled by post-translational modifications such as phosphorylation and ubiquitination. For instance, binding of the ligand to the TCR is capable of inducing conformational changes to reveal new interaction sites with signaling molecules to amplify the signaling cascade. Furthermore, OPTN proteins have also been shown to have significant roles in modulating these interactions and downstream signaling. Through binding to ubiquitinated proteins, OPTN may control the localization and stability of signaling complexes, enabling control of inflammation and immune activation. Subsequent studies highlight the role of OPTN in autophagy, further involving PPIs in not only the regulation of TCR signaling but also more general immune processes, showing a multi-modal approach to understanding immunological response (Slowicka & van Loo, 2018). In the realm of immunology, the comprehensive characterization of PPIs in pathways of TCR signaling holds paramount therapeutic value. Aberrations in the signaling process can lead to immune deficiencies or dysregulated immune responses, such as autoimmunity or cancer. By means of an understanding of the intricate network of PPIs involved in TCR signaling, researchers can identify potential candidates for pharmacological intervention. For instance, low-molecular-weight molecules that interfere with specific PPIs can potentially be used as immunomodulators and regulate the activation of T-cells as and when needed. In addition, understanding these interactions can potentially unlock new pathways for novel immunotherapies based on the potential of T-cells to combat malignancies. Overall, research on PPIs in TCR signaling not only illuminates further T-cell biology but also identifies promising avenues for the development of immunotherapy and improving patient management of many immune-mediated diseases (Figure 7.13).

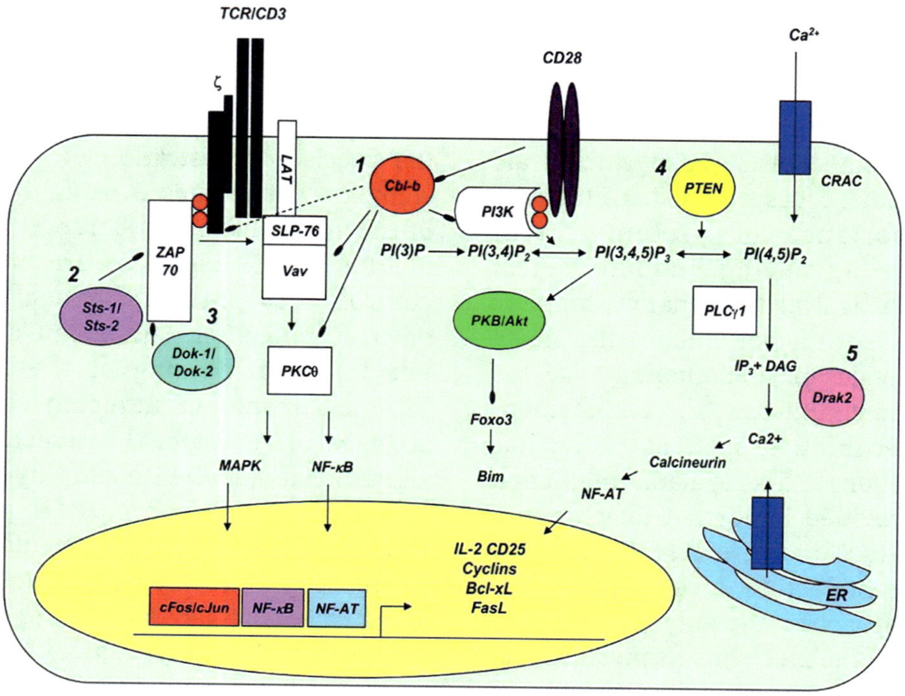

Figure 7.13. T cell receptor (TCR) signaling pathways and key effectors of negative regulators of TCR signaling are implicated in immunological tolerance.

Source: https://www.researchgate.net/profile/Martina-Gatzka/publication/233619111/figure/fig1/AS:651500908990465@1532341329462/Fig-1-T-cell-receptor-TCR-signaling-pathways-and-key-effectors-of-negative.png.

7.5.2. Interactions in Antibody Production

Antibody production is fundamentally dependent on intricate protein-protein interactions among various immune cells, the most significant being T and B lymphocytes. Antigens, after entering the body, are recognized by antigen-presenting cells (APCs), which process and present antigens to naïve T cells. This is a critical interaction because it results in T cell activation and proliferation. Activated CD4+ helper T cells play a critical function in providing necessary signals, such as cytokines, that enhance the differentiation of B cells into antibody-secreting plasma cells. T cell-B cell interactions are critical because they render the immune response specific and effective, leading to the generation of high-affinity antibodies that can effectively neutralize pathogens. To this, the role of co-stimulatory molecules, including OX40 ligand, during the activation of T cells, cannot be presumed. OX40L binding to its receptor on T cells enhances their activation and survival, subsequently affecting the activation of B cells in an indirect manner. Activation of OX40L enhances the immunogenicity of some antigens, leading to an enhanced antibody response. In model systems, OX40L fusion protein injection was shown to augment the proliferation of cytotoxic T lymphocytes (CTLs) that can attack tumor-associated antigens, and thus the therapeutic value of the manipulation of such interactions is also evident. The downstream effects of such interactions can not only enhance innate and adaptive immunity but also influence the strategies for cancer immunotherapy, exemplifying the high level of complexity of protein-protein interactions in antibody production.

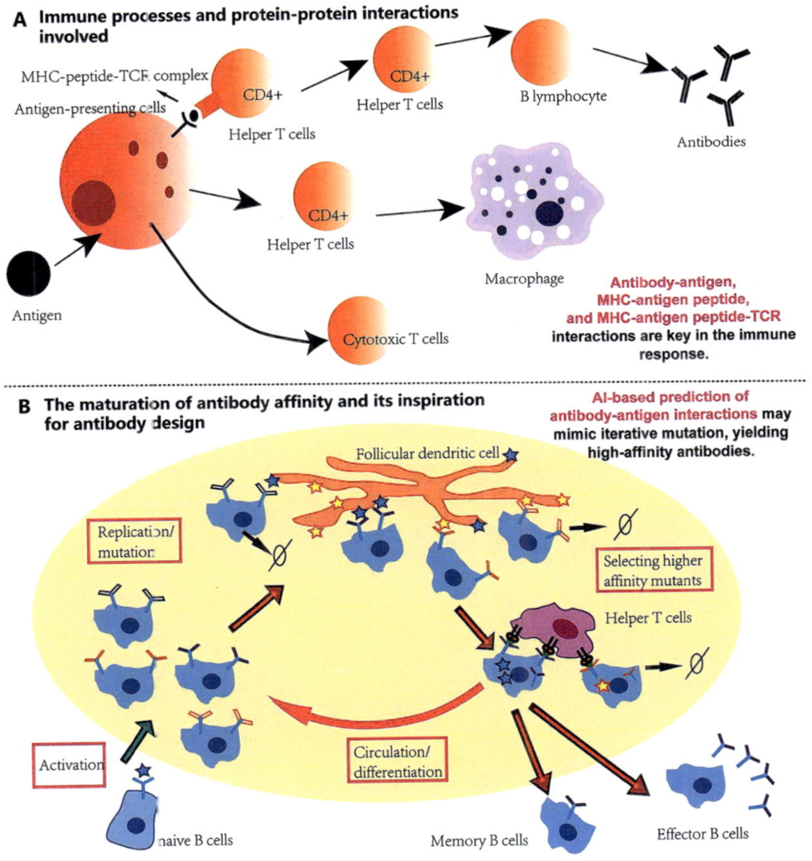

Figure 7.14. Protein interactions during immune processes and maturation of antibody affinity. (A) Immune processes involve numerous protein-protein interactions, especially specific interactions. (B) The maturation process of antibodies and its inspiration for developing antibody design methods.

Source: https://www.researchgate.net/publication/384589828/figure/fig1/AS:11431281282301859@1728276214506/Protein-interactions-during-immune-processes-and-maturation-of-antibody-affinity-A.jpg.

In antibody production, understanding the mechanisms of such protein-protein interactions is important for the creation of novel immunotherapeutic approaches. There has been emphasis in recent studies on the need for the stability and reliability of the ASSR in quantifying immune function. By the study of such oscillatory signatures, one can elicit an understanding of the dynamics of T and B cell interactions that are crucial in orchestrating the antibody response. High intraclass correlation coefficients shown for ASSR measurements across various studies indicate excellent reproducibility of methods, which provides a solid ground for using them in both basic and clinical research. This reinforces the central role of precise protein interactions in effective immune system function and the exploitation of these interactions in the development of therapeutic strategies against many diseases (Figure 7.14).

7.5.3. Role of Protein-Protein Interactions (PPIs) in Autoimmune Diseases

The study of PPIs has been a core area in identifying autoimmune diseases, whereby interactions have been shown to dictate immune system behavior. Autoimmune conditions typically present as a consequence of immune dysregulation, leading to failure of the body's discrimination between self and non-self antigens. Crucial proteins that are involved in immune signaling have a tendency to interact with one another in close proximity, with ramifications for pathways that regulate T cell activation and differentiation. For example, mutations within the AIRE gene have been identified in conditions such as APECED, and these show how disrupted PPIs can lead to the onset of autoimmune conditions. By investigating such interactions, researchers can uncover molecular mechanisms of disease pathology and identify possible therapeutic targets for the restoration of normal immune function (Pellegrino et al., 2018).

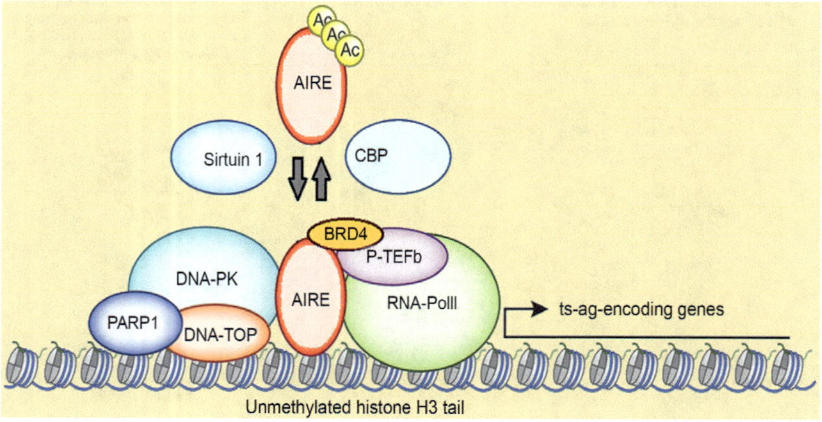

Figure 7.15. Schematic representation of autoimmune regulator (AIRE)-containing multimolecular complexes involved in initiation and post-initiation events of gene transcription.

Source: https://www.researchgate.net/publication/323137342/figure/fig3/AS:11431281250271425@1717826344365/Schematic-representation-of-autoimmune-regulator-AIRE-containing-multimolecular.tif.

In addition to genetic factors, environmental determinants play a strong role in cellular signaling processes as well as the interaction between immune proteins. The rapid rise of autoimmune disorders in the Western world reflects an interaction between environmental determinants and genetic susceptibilities (Harnett et al., 2010). Parasitic infections, for instance, have shown a protective role against the hyperactive immune processes involved in some autoimmune disorders.

Understanding how helminth products modulate immune responses and influence PPIs yields insight into potential therapeutic strategies for treating autoimmune disease. These observations can lead to novel treatments that leverage the immunomodulatory effects of these interactions, highlighting the significance of PPI analysis both in understanding disease processes and in guiding clinical interventions. Furthermore, comprehension of PPI activity in autoimmune disease is important for the design of inhibitors that can block pathogenic interactions without disturbing protective immune mechanisms. Such research has employed high-throughput screening methods to identify small-molecule inhibitors of specific PPIs involved in autoimmune signaling cascades. By blocking or attenuating such interactions, scientists are optimistic about developing more targeted therapies with fewer side effects characteristic of broad-spectrum immunosuppressive therapy. Such specificity highlights the significance of PPIs not only in revealing the mechanistic facts of autoimmune diseases but also in opening up a new drug discovery platform. The integration of PPI analysis in immunology, therefore, presents an overall solution to address the problem of autoimmune diseases effectively and innovatively (Harnett et al., 2010) (Figure 7.15).

7.6. Challenges in Protein-Protein Interaction (PPI) Analysis

PPI analysis is fraught with numerous challenges that have a profound influence on the understanding of immunological responses. The most significant challenge is the native complexity of biological systems, whereby proteins participate in dynamic interactions that are determined by many variables like post-translational modifications and cell conditions. Given the diversity of immune pathways and the corresponding proteins, isolating these interactions requires highly specific approaches to produce qualitative results. Furthermore, conventional laboratory procedures, although reliable, are prone to capturing the transient nature of PPIs, leading to incomplete or misleading datasets. These limitations undermine the ability of researchers to fully delineate the network of the immune system, which in turn affects the design of therapeutic interventions for diseases, including infections and autoimmune diseases. Another important challenge in PPI analysis concerns the constraints brought by available genomic and proteomic resources. The lack of high-quality and comprehensive databases can restrict the exposure of researchers to important information regarding known interactions and thus render the validation process necessary for novel findings an obstacle. For instance, as highlighted in previous descriptions in recent reviews, past success in knowledge of the crustacean decapod immune system indicates important but currently unexplored areas in invertebrate immunology. The current lack of available genomic resources in the public domain for most organisms increases these challenges to an extent that leads to a dependence on possibly outdated or incomplete data. Improved characterization methods and the development of integrated databases are critical to overcoming these problems since they would enable more thorough investigation of PPIs in the context of immunology, contributing to research progress. Moreover, as immunology moves toward big data, the reproducibility of PPI research becomes a problem. Open-access repositories like the ImmPort data repository represent a significant step toward addressing this problem by allowing researchers to reproduce existing methods and assess the robustness of their outcomes. But whereas such platforms offer a lot of advantages, smooth integration and re-purposing of the diverse datasets for meta-analyses remain tricky issues that are marred by many challenges. Such immense heterogeneity in data collected in different studies may complicate comparison and the making of meaningful conclusions. Hence, stimulating further collaboration and standardization within the research community is essential to enhance the reliability and usefulness of PPI analyses in order to make more well-founded discoveries in the field of immunology, particularly in immune responses and disease regulation (Hauton, 2012; Bhattacharya et al., 2018).

7.6.1. Complexity of Protein Networks

Protein network complexity has a complicated pattern of interactions that regulate cellular functions, particularly in the immune system. Proteins don't function independently; rather, they engage in intricate interactions that are categorized into numerous types, such as direct binding, cooperative behavior, and feedback loops. Interconnectedness of this nature is necessary for establishing homeostasis and responding to external stimuli such as pathogens. The ability of proteins to fulfill numerous roles highlights an aspect referred to as networked buffering, where redundancy within the system facilitates resilience to perturbations. Such resilience is vital to immune responses, which must respond to a range of challenges without tumbling into dangerous consequences, such as autoimmunity. The control of these intricate protein networks thus informs us about how the immune system balances between activity and successfully utilizes defense mechanisms against a range of threats (Whitacre et al., 2010). Besides, using the principles of systems biology can improve our comprehension of the complexity of protein networks in the field of immunology. By integrating high-throughput data that are derived from omics technologies, researchers can create models explaining how various proteins interact within the immune system. Such an integrated approach is rather the opposite of reductionist methods, examining components in isolation. Instead, systems biology reiterates dynamic protein interactions and reveals emergent behavior that cannot be predicted from the components themselves. Applying these methods, scientists are able to reveal pathways that are responsible for immune responses and might have novel therapeutic implications. These findings also might illuminate the molecular underpinnings of disease, a state brought about by dysregulation of these networks. By adopting this complete perspective, the immunology discipline is capable of accessing a degree of complexity in protein interactions to propel novel clinical applications (Woelders et al., 2011). Protein network research is not purely an intellectual pursuit but is instead a vehicle for advancing seminal change in immunotherapy and vaccine design. Unraveling the protein-protein complexity layers, scientists may find the best-regulated nodes in the immune network that may serve as a target for therapy. Therapeutic interventions might optimize the vaccine's efficacy or control individualized medicine approaches to immune diseases. Protein interactions' malleability points to the need for an integration effort, multi-disciplinary in nature. Therefore, as the field progresses, integrating computationally utilized devices and experimental information into one framework will be essential to deconstruct the intricate web of protein networks. Doing so will not merely illuminate the immune mechanism on the molecular level but also create a platform for developing innovative healthcare solutions in harmony with the dynamics of biological processes (Whitacre et al., 2010).

7.6.2. Limitations of Current Methodologies

PPIs in immunology are severely impeded in research by the methods currently available, which are not very sensitive and specific. Traditional approaches, such as yeast two-hybrid systems and Co-IP, fall short in identifying dynamic protein interactions in living cells. These methods are usually founded on isolated states that may not truly represent the *in vivo* state and thus provide partial information on how these interactions influence immune responses. In addition, they fail to differentiate between specific and non-specific interactions, which conceals valuable information concerning regulatory mechanisms in immune pathways. Therefore, the efficacy of these methodologies in uncovering the intricacies of immune responses remains limited, and it is necessary to have more advanced and context-aware methods to cover the whole spectrum of PPIs that are relevant to immunity. In addition to the limitations of sensitivity, application of *in vitro* systems also presents a tremendous challenge with regard to understanding the multi-dimensional interactions between the immune system. For example, the application of *in vitro* assays, while beneficial for initial screenings, is prone to neglecting the dynamic interaction of cellular milieus and external signals that govern protein interactions. AOP-based methods aim to provide a coherent framework for allergenic responses but are susceptible to neglecting the cellular context in allergic sensitization events (Lozano-Ojalvo et al., 2019). Currently available assays more precisely target mechanisms involved in innate immune responses than in adaptive immunity, reflecting a tragic limitation of methods that fail to account for the biological realities of immune interactions. Addressing these problems is central to advancing our understanding of immunological dynamics. Moreover, the isolation of individual proteins for analysis remains a daunting challenge, particularly with regard to post-translational modifications that have the potential to affect protein-protein interactions. The need for the right quantities of glycoproteins is also a challenge since standard extraction methods yield suboptimal samples for extensive PPI studies. New developments in chemical and enzymatic synthesis, however, provide new ways to improve access to complex carbohydrates and their conjugates (Park et al., 2018). These innovations can aid in the development of highly advanced methods for the measurement of protein interactions, possibly with the incorporation of new biological contexts and therapeutic significance. Ultimately, to enhance our understanding of PPIs in immunology, there must be a paradigm shift towards even more convergent and flexible methodologies filling the gaps left unattended by existing methods (Figure 7.16).

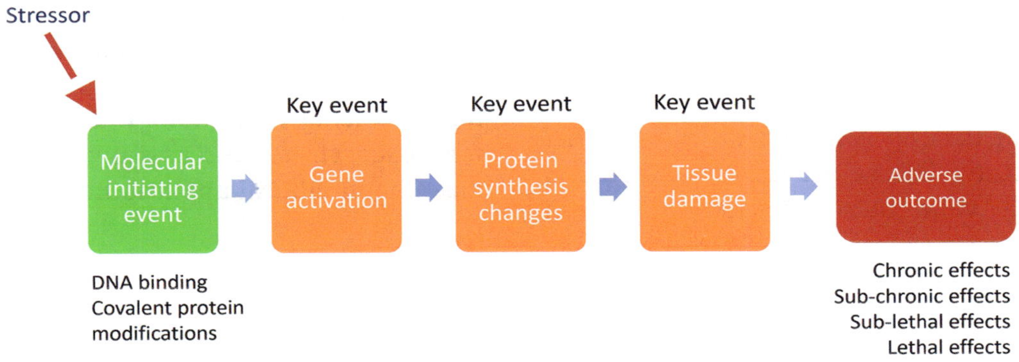

Figure 7.16. Adverse outcome pathway (AOP) framework.

Source: https://www.researchgate.net/profile/Sebastian-Hoffmann-10/publication/350795254/figure/fig1/AS:1027230901739538@1621922340995/Adverse-outcome-pathway-AOP-framework.png.

7.6.3. Need for Standardized Protocols

PPIs analysis is a key aspect of research in the development of immunology, such as the examination of immune responses and therapeutic strategies. Despite becoming increasingly essential over time, it remains threatened by a shortage of standardized protocols. Variations in experimental conditions, reagents, and protocol can lead to irreproducible results, which interfere with reproducibility that promotes scientific progress. The need for standard protocols is attained through introspection of combining heterogeneous immunological assays, where variability can mislead data interpretation and hamper comparability of outcomes between studies. This variance lowers drug discovery at early stages and progress in therapeutic intervention, necessitating a concerted effort to come up with guidelines that enhance the reliability of PPI studies in immunology. Reliance on universal methodologies will be necessary to build a paradigm upon which groups of researchers can collaborate. This paradigm would foster the sharing of best practices and common effort among immunologists. For example, standard protocols permit the identification and validation of biomarkers for immunological disorders, such as those of protein interactions during T-cell activation or antibody responses. Such consistency is essential in making certain that experiments aimed to study disease processes yield results not merely valid but also interpretable in clinical scenarios (Roedder et al., 2011). With increasing concern with personalized medicine, as seen with the recent translational work on biomarkers in transplantation, the application of standardized methodology can go a long way towards making immunological therapies accurate and effective. This facilitates a broader view of PPIs in immunology and their application in clinical settings in real life. Furthermore, standardization is not limited to experimental procedures and also extends to data analysis, interpretation, and reporting. Different computational tools applied in analyzing PPI are based on a common vocabulary regarding methodologies and parameters for assessing the data. By establishing uniform parameters for the analysis of PPI networks, researchers are able to have a more systematic assessment of immunological interactions that could pave the way for revolutionary therapeutic strategies. Integration of frontier technologies, such as the use of bioluminescence imaging that is being referred to in the context of fibrosis research, underlines the potential advantage of standardization in terms of the magnitude and quality of immunological research. With a focus on exact correlation of findings, such methodology aligns with the broader picture of optimizing patient outcomes based on excellent scientific evidence (Stellari et al., 2017). Standard protocol making is thus not a procedural improvement; it is required for advancing immunology as a science and for research to successfully translate into meaningful clinical applicability.

SUMMARY

As PPI analysis in immunology continues to advance, it is evident that interactions form an integral part of the comprehension of numerous immune responses and pathologies. Identification and characterization of PPIs can provide insight into mechanisms of action for immune-regulatory proteins, and this is highly relevant to therapeutic approaches. SEGRAs have also emerged as a recent interest for the possible treatment of inflammatory disease, and GSK866 analogs are one example of how covalent binding can change protein interactions. This might result in new methods of treating inflammatory diseases that have fewer side effects (Chirumamilla et al., 2017). Thus, understanding of PPIs not only contributes to basic immunological research but also unveils prospects for discovering novel therapeutic strategies. The role of Tregs in immune homeostasis highlights another extremely critical aspect of PPIs in immunology. Tregs are crucial for coordinating immune responses with tolerance-autoimmunity. The successful expansion of Tregs has been demonstrated with aimed protocols and has established the capability of PPI manipulation to enhance therapeutic qualities against autoimmune conditions. This is critical because the limited number of peripheral Tregs decreases their treatment potential in clinical applications. Reports of Treg expansion *ex vivo*, with the preservation of suppressive function, highlight the position of PPIs in therapeutic treatments aimed at maximizing patient responsiveness to conditions such as graft-versus-host disease (Earle et al., 2005). Thus, research on PPI dynamics yields information that has direct application in clinical practice with cellular immunotherapy. In conclusion, the confluence of immunology and protein-protein interaction analysis comes of age as an essential area of research illuminating the complexity of immune regulation. From insights into how SEGRAs propel their therapeutic efficacy to enhancing the viability of Tregs for therapy, the implications are profound. Through continued advances in the research area, the introduction of advanced techniques for analyzing PPIs will yield a greater understanding of disease and immune processes, with the promise of delivering revolutionary therapies. Continued research into PPIs will also be certain to reveal novel biological pathways and regulatory systems governing the immune landscape, ultimately driving both preclinical immunological research and clinical immunotherapy. This multifaceted approach has a promising horizon in the manipulation and understanding of immune responses for therapeutics.

PPI analysis forms a core in interpreting immunological responses, particularly autoimmune disease. Evolving evidence points to the function of heat shock proteins (HSPs), which are also damage-associated molecular patterns (DAMPs) and form a key component in regulating the immune response. Not only are they involved in tissue repair after cellular damage, but they also modulate inflammatory mediators. It has been observed that the role of HSPs in tendinopathy and their potential contribution to tissue recovery processes within tendon pathology have been acknowledged. By illustrating the molecular processes behind such events, the present study offers promising avenues for therapeutic intervention in PPI dynamics, thus increasing our understanding of immune responses in disease situations, particularly against the backdrop of autoimmune diseases in soft tissues (Millar & Murrell, 2012). Apart from HSPs, more recent findings have unraveled the fairly polyvalent function of mitochondrial antiviral signaling (MAVS) in the context of systemic lupus erythematosus (SLE). The MAVS oligomerization under oxidative stress conditions has been a central mechanism to drive the innate immune response, inducing tremendous amounts of type I interferon production. The MAVS-mediated activity in SLE patients is amplified and is a major cause of the disease's characteristic type I IFN signature. Studies into the dynamics of MAVS have offered insights into its relationship with mitochondrial integrity and reactive oxygen species (ROS) production. Through the analysis of how oxidative stress and MAVS interact, we are given informative data about pathophysiological mechanisms behind SLE and its manifestations, once again highlighting PPI involvement in immune deregulation (Buskiewicz et al., 2016). Furthermore, research on MAVS variants, like the MAVS-C79F mutation prevalent in the sub-Saharan population, is enlightening regarding genetic determinants of immune responses in SLE. This allele appears to lower MAVS oligomerization and is linked with less severe disease expression in affected subjects. Not only do these findings emphasize the utility of genetic diversity to immunological processes, but they also show promise for candidate therapeutic options that can minimize overactive immunity in SLE. By integrating both knowledge of HSP dynamics and MAVS interactions, protein-protein interaction research may significantly enhance our ability to design specific immunotherapies. Collectively, these findings provide a complex view of the biological processes responsible for immune regulation and disease onset in autoimmune disorders, indicating the hallmark control exerted by PPIs over immunological outcomes (Millar & Murrell, 2012; Buskiewicz et al., 2016).

A CLOSER LOOK

CO-IMMUNOPRECIPITATION (CO-IP)

Co-IP is a method of determining and investigating the interactions of proteins. It takes place where an antibody is used to purify a target protein (the "bait") and any other proteins attached to it (the "prey") from a lysate of cells. This helps one study protein complexes and learn about how proteins interact with one another in a cell (Figure 7.17).

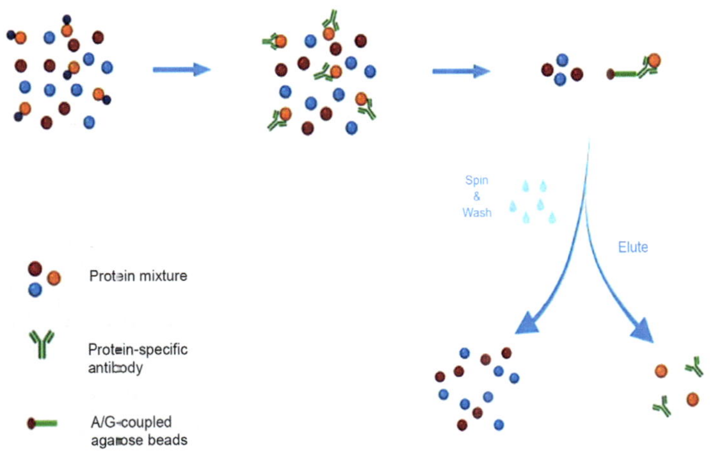

Figure 7.17. Co-immunoprecipation (Co-IP) principle.

Source: https://i.shgcdn.com/ca65ffc4-4dc6-4095-9ac1-90b31ab1956d/-/format/auto/-/preview/3000x3000/-/quality/lighter/.

1. How Co-IP Works:

a. **Lysis of the Cell:** The process begins with cell breaking (lysis) so that the proteins can be extracted.

b. **Incubation with Antibodies:** A specific antibody against the protein in question (the "bait" protein) is added to the cell lysate.

c. **Bead Binding:** The antibody-protein complex is then mixed with beads that carry a tag for the antibody (e.g., protein A or G beads).

d. **Washing:** The beads are washed to remove any free proteins, retaining the target protein and its partners behind.

e. **Elution and Analysis:** The proteins bound to the beads are eluted and can be analyzed by techniques like Western blotting, mass spectrometry, or other appropriate techniques to identify the interacting proteins.

2. Key Applications:

a. **Discovery of Protein-Protein Interactions:** Co-IP is a useful method to determine which proteins interact with each other within the context of a cell.

b. **Analysis of Protein Complexes:** It helps determine protein complex composition and dynamics that are significant for many cellular processes.

c. **Analysis of Signaling Pathways:** Co-IP can be used to study the interactions of proteins in signaling pathways, indicating how signals are passed through a cell.

d. **Disease Research:** Disease research also makes use of Co-IP to study how protein interactions are modified during disease conditions, such as in cancer.

3. Key Considerations:

a. **Antibody Specificity:** The choice of an antibody is crucial for the success of Co-IP. It should be extremely specific for the target protein and non-cross-reactive with other proteins.

b. **Native vs. Denaturing Conditions:** Co-IP may be performed in native conditions (preserving protein-protein interactions) or denaturing conditions (preventing interactions), depending on the question to be answered.

c. **Low Affinity Interactions:** Co-IP may not be the best method for the identification of very weak or transient protein interactions.

d. **Indirect Interactions:** It should be noted that the identified interactions can be direct or indirect with other proteins.

REFERENCES

1. Whitacre JM, Bender A. Networked buffering: a basic mechanism for distributed robustness in complex adaptive systems. *Theor Biol Med Model.* 2010;7:20. Published 2010 Jun 15. doi:10.1186/1742-4682-7-20(accessed on 27th June 2025).
2. Chen, A., Roumier, A., Wise, A. G., Fievet, B., Nal, B., Treanor, B., Treanor, B., et al. (2012). Ezrin interacts with the SARS coronavirus spike protein and restrains infection at the entry stage. https://core.ac.uk/download/18488580.pdf (accessed on 27th June 2025).
3. Hauton C. The scope of the crustacean immune system for disease control. *J Invertebr Pathol.* 2012;110(2):251-260. doi:10.1016/j.jip.2012.03.005Akiba, A., Ali, S., Bretscher, A., Carreno, M., Entwisle, C., McLean, C. S., et al. (2004). Anti-tumor therapeutic efficacy of OX40L in murine tumor model. https://core.ac.uk/download/30647676.pdf (accessed on 27th June 2025).
4. Igata, M., Islam, M. A., Tada, A., Takagi, M., Kober, A. K. M. H., Albarracin, L., Aso, H., Ikeda-Ohtsubo, W., Miyazawa, K., Yoda, K., He, F., Takahashi, H., Villena, J., & Kitazawa, H. (2019). Transcriptome Modifications in Porcine Adipocytes via Toll-Like Receptors Activation. *Frontiers in immunology, 10,* 1180. https://doi.org/10.3389/fimmu.2019.01180(accessed on 27th June 2025).
5. Harnett, W., Goodridge, H. S., Allen, J. M., & Harnett, M. (2012). Receptor usage by the Acanthocheilonema viteae-derived immunomodulator, ES-62. *Experimental parasitology, 132*(1), 97–102. https://doi.org/10.1016/j.exppara.2011.09.001(accessed on 27th June 2025).
6. Harnett, M. M., Melendez, A. J., & Harnett, W. (2010). The therapeutic potential of the filarial nematode-derived immunodulator, ES-62 in inflammatory disease. *Clinical and experimental immunology, 159*(3), 256–267. https://doi.org/10.1111/j.1365-2249.2009.04064.x(accessed on 27th June 2025).
7. François, P., Altan-Bonnet, G. The Case for Absolute Ligand Discrimination: Modeling Information Processing and Decision by Immune T Cells. *J Stat Phys* **162**, 1130–1152 (2016). https://doi.org/10.1007/s10955-015-1444-1(accessed on 27th June 2025).
8. Amon, R., Chen, X., Fleishman, S. J., Glushka, J., et al. (2018). A combined computational-experimental approach to define the structural origin of antibody recognition of sialyl-Tn, a tumor-associated carbohydrate antigen. https://core.ac.uk/download/323068873.pdf (accessed on 27th June 2025).
9. Araibi, E. H., Marchetti, B., Dornan, E. S., Ashrafi, G. H., Dobromylskyj, M., Ellis, S. A., & Campo, M. S. (2006). The E5 oncoprotein of BPV-4 does not interfere with the biosynthetic pathway of non-classical MHC class I. *Virology, 353*(1), 174–183. https://doi.org/10.1016/j.virol.2006.05.031(accessed on 27th June 2025).
10. Mengozzi M, Ermilov P, Annenkov A, Ghezzi P, Pearl F. Definition of a Family of Tissue-Protective Cytokines Using Functional Cluster Analysis: A Proof-of-Concept Study. *Front Immunol.* 2014;5:115. Published 2014 Mar 17. doi:10.3389/fimmu.2014.00115(accessed on 27th June 2025).
11. Jacobs, K., Charvat, R., & Arrizabalaga, G. (2020). Identification of Fis1 Interactors in Toxoplasma gondii Reveals a Novel Protein Required for Peripheral Distribution of the Mitochondrion. *mBio, 11*(1), e02732-19. https://doi.org/10.1128/mBio.02732-19(accessed on 27th June 2025).

12. Chirumamilla CS, Palagani A, Kamaraj B, et al. Selective Glucocorticoid Receptor Properties of GSK866 Analogs with Cysteine Reactive Warheads. *Front Immunol.* 2017;8:1324. Published 2017 Nov 1. doi:10.3389/fimmu.2017.01324(accessed on 27th June 2025).
13. Folador EL, de Carvalho PV, Silva WM, et al. In silico identification of essential proteins in Corynebacterium pseudotuberculosis based on protein-protein interaction networks. *BMC Syst Biol.* 2016;10(1):103. Published 2016 Nov 4. doi:10.1186/s12918-016-0346-4(accessed on 27th June 2025).
14. Woelders, H., Te Pas, M. F., Bannink, A., Veerkamp, R. F., & Smits, M. A. (2011). Systems biology in animal sciences. *Animal : an international journal of animal bioscience*, *5*(7), 1036–1047. https://doi.org/10.1017/S1751731111000036(accessed on 27th June 2025).
15. Pellegrino, M., Bellacchio, E., Dhamo, R., Frasca, F., Betterle, C., & Fierabracci, A. (2018). A Novel Homozygous Mutation of the *AIRE* Gene in an APECED Patient From Pakistan: Case Report and Review of the Literature. *Frontiers in immunology*, *9*, 1835. https://doi.org/10.3389/fimmu.2018.01835 (accessed on 27th June 2025).
16. Daniel Lozano-Ojalvo, Sara Benede, Celia M. Antunes, Simona L. Bavaro, Grégory Bouchaud, et al.. Applying the adverse outcome pathway (AOP) for food sensitization to support in vitro testing strategies. Trends in Food Science and Technology, 2019, 85, pp.307-319. ⟨10.1016/j.tifs.2019.01.014⟩. ⟨hal-02623081⟩(accessed on 27th June 2025).
17. Bhattacharya, S., Butte, A., Chen, J., Dunn, M., et al. (2018). ImmPort, toward repurposing of open access immunological assay data for translational and clinical research. https://core.ac.uk/download/153326602.pdf (accessed on 27th June 2025).
18. Earle, K. E., Tang, Q., Zhou, X., Liu, W., Zhu, S., Bonyhadi, M. L., & Bluestone, J. A. (2005). In vitro expanded human CD4+CD25+ regulatory T cells suppress effector T cell proliferation. *Clinical immunology (Orlando, Fla.)*, *115*(1), 3–9. https://doi.org/10.1016/j.clim.2005.02.017(accessed on 27th June 2025).
19. Pappalardo, F., Brusic, V., Pennisi, M., & Zhang, G. (2015). Advances in Computational Immunology. *Journal of immunology research*, *2015*, 170920. https://doi.org/10.1155/2015/170920(accessed on 27th June 2025).
20. Buskiewicz, I. A., Montgomery, T., Yasewicz, E. C., Huber, S. A., Murphy, M. P., Hartley, R. C., Kelly, R., Crow, M. K., Perl, A., Budd, R. C., & Koenig, A. (2016). Reactive oxygen species induce virus-independent MAVS oligomerization in systemic lupus erythematosus. *Science signaling*, *9*(456), ra115. https://doi.org/10.1126/scisignal.aaf1933(accessed on 27th June 2025).
21. Mowers, J., Uhm, M., Reilly, S. M., Simon, J., Leto, D., Chiang, S. H., Chang, L., & Saltiel, A. R. (2013). Inflammation produces catecholamine resistance in obesity via activation of PDE3B by the protein kinases IKKε and TBK1. *eLife*, *2*, e01119. https://doi.org/10.7554/eLife.01119(accessed on 27th June 2025).
22. Cosma, G. L., & Eisenlohr, L. (2018). CD8+ T-cell responses in vaccination: Reconsidering targets and function in the context of chronic antigen stimulation. https://core.ac.uk/download/213438552.pdf (accessed on 27th June 2025).
23. ENOQ Costa (2011). Viral modulation of interferon (IFN) responses to African swine fever virus (ASFV). https://core.ac.uk/download/12424877.pdf (accessed on 27th June 2025).

24. Davoodi, H., Hashemi, S. R., & Seow, H. F. (2012). Increased NFκ-B activity in HCT116 colorectal cancer cell line harboring TLR4 Asp299Gly variant. https://core.ac.uk/download/52204755.pdf (accessed on 27th June 2025).

25. Stellari, F. F., Ruscitti, F., Pompilio, D., Ravanetti, F., Tebaldi, G., Macchi, F., Verna, A. E., Villetti, G., & Donofrio, G. (2017). Heterologous Matrix Metalloproteinase Gene Promoter Activity Allows *In Vivo* Real-time Imaging of Bleomycin-Induced Lung Fibrosis in Transiently Transgenized Mice. *Frontiers in immunology*, *8*, 199. https://doi.org/10.3389/fimmu.2017.00199(accessed on 27th June 2025).

26. Bernard Ycart, Frederic Pont, Jean-Jacques Fournie. (2014). Statistical Data Mining for Symbol Associations in Genomic Databases. International Journal of Genetics and Genomics, 2(6), 97-104. https://doi.org/10.11648/j.ijgg.20140206.11(accessed on 27th June 2025).

27. Park, S. S., Hsieh, H.-W., & Gervay-Hague, J. (2018). Anomeric *O*-Functionalization of Carbohydrates for Chemical Conjugation to Vaccine Constructs. *Molecules*, *23*(7), 1742. https://doi.org/10.3390/molecules23071742(accessed on 27th June 2025).

28. Nosalski, R., & Guzik, T. J. (2017). Perivascular adipose tissue inflammation in vascular disease. *British journal of pharmacology*, *174*(20), 3496–3513. https://doi.org/10.1111/bph.13705(accessed on 27th June 2025).

29. Roedder, S., Vitalone, M., Khatri, P., & Sarwal, M. M. (2011). Biomarkers in solid organ transplantation: establishing personalized transplantation medicine. *Genome medicine*, *3*(6), 37. https://doi.org/10.1186/gm253(accessed on 27th June 2025).

30. Lodhia, P. (2012). Investigating the interaction between the tetracaine CD82 and gangliosides, and, the binding partners of CLEC14A and the function of the CLEC14A extracellular domain. https://core.ac.uk/download/16292601.pdf (accessed on 27th June 2025).

31. Magez, S., Obishakin, E. T., Pinto Torres, J. E., Radwanska, M., et al. (2020). Infections with extracellular trypanosomes require control by efficient innate immune mechanisms and can result in the destruction of the mammalian humoral immune system. https://core.ac.uk/download/288817508.pdf (accessed on 27th June 2025).

32. Malagic, M. (2017). Genetic regulation of NKT cell function. https://core.ac.uk/download/215152759.pdf (accessed on 27th June 2025).

33. Millar, N. L., & Murrell, G. A. C. (2012). Heat shock proteins in tendinopathy: Novel molecular regulators. https://core.ac.uk/download/9651505.pdf (accessed on 27th June 2025).

34. Rambold, A. S., & Pearce, E. L. (2018). Mitochondrial Dynamics at the Interface of Immune Cell Metabolism and Function. *Trends in immunology*, *39*(1), 6–18. https://doi.org/10.1016/j.it.2017.08.006Reitmaier, R. (2007). Review of immunoinformatic approaches to *in-silico* B-cell epitope prediction. https://core.ac.uk/download/pdf/287415.pdf (accessed on 27th June 2025).

35. Wang, A., & Sarwal, M. M. (2015). Computational Models for Transplant Biomarker Discovery. *Frontiers in immunology*, *6*, 458. https://doi.org/10.3389/fimmu.2015.00458(accessed on 27th June 2025).

36. Slowicka, K., & van Loo, G. (2018). *Opt*ineurin Functions for *Opt*imal Immunity. *Frontiers in immunology*, *9*, 769. https://doi.org/10.3389/fimmu.2018.00769(accessed on 27th June 2025).

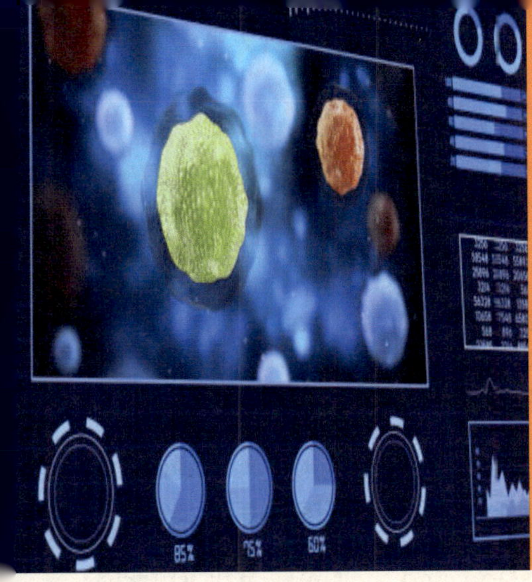

Chapter 8

SINGLE-CELL ANALYSIS TECHNIQUES

Contents

Introduction

The past few years have witnessed incredible advancement in the science of molecular immunology, some of the most significant of which have been the emergence of single-cell analysis techniques. Such techniques allow for cell heterogeneity in the immune system to be studied and even complex immune reactions to be deconstructed at levels never seen before. By observing single cells rather than populations in large quantities, scientists can disentangle the heterogeneity of the functional states and transcriptional profiles of various immune cells. This is particularly relevant when it comes to illnesses like asthma, where the action of immune cells can be very disparate based on variables like obesity. With new studies beginning to recognize unique transcriptional signatures between different phenotypes, single-cell tools are becoming increasingly critical in treatment choice and refinement of treatment models for diseases with immune dysregulation (Tejwani et al., 2025). Single-cell analysis is one of the best examples of the potential of single-cell analysis in its application in analyzing immune profiles of populations in a state of variable health. In asthma-obesity, an overweight child was recently found to have unique CD4+ T-cell transcriptional profiles that are different from non-overweight children. Single-cell RNA sequencing not only identified numerous gene expression differences but also identified divergent enriched pathways that were linked to more severe asthma phenotypes. The research illustrates the potential of single-cell technology to decipher pathological processes and disclose new therapeutic targets. Furthermore, in-depth information obtained by such analysis can also be a base for designing more individualized treatment protocols to address diversified patient populations through greater sophistication in their immune topography (Tejwani et al., 2025). Single-cell analysis is also incorporated in tumor immunology research, where immune reactions at the single-cell level are known to have extremely important implications in cancer therapy. For example, in colon cancer, the investigation of ICD has been transformed by bioinformatics and single-cell RNA sequencing technology. They have revealed typical ICD-associated gene expression profiles, which have enabled new subtyping classifications of cancer based on their respective immune signatures. It not only enhances the comprehension of tumor microenvironments but also offers possibilities for novel delivery of therapy, e.g., new combinatorial therapy with ferroptosis agents. Lastly, investigation of single-cell methods drives development in precision medicine, offering important insight into how immune mechanisms may be utilized successfully to increase the success of treatment for most conditions, particularly concerning the boundary between immune dysregulation and cancer.

Definition of Single-Cell Analysis

Single-cell analysis is a collection of techniques enabling one to analyze individual cells at a proximal level and expose their unique biological characteristics and actions, usually masked in bulk tissue investigations. Single-cell analysis is a significant molecular immunology method, enabling one to separate multicomponent tissues' heterogeneous cell populations. Through this technique, scientists are capable of anatomically resolving heterogeneity at the cell-to-cell level in gene expression, protein content, and metabolism. By isolating cells one by one and analyzing each individually, researchers can pick up on slight differences that are imperative for identifying immune responses, disease progression, and therapies, particularly in cancer and autoimmunity. Furthermore, advances in technology in tools such as single-cell RNA sequencing and mass cytometry have increased the resolution and information depth available at the cellular level by many orders of magnitude, enabling vigorous interrogation of the immune landscape and the impact on disease and health. Single-cell analysis becomes even more valuable by virtue of the ability of its high-resolution three-dimensional (3D) imaging of the biological tissue. Techniques such as 3D histology and single-cell spatial omics uncover new information, giving the researchers in-depth analysis of cell-cell interactions within their *in vivo* microenvironment. Not only do these techniques unveil how each cell is engaged in tissue structure and function, but they also indicate their regulatory mechanisms and spatial organization within the immune system. For instance, single-cell technologies coupled with high-tech imaging may be able to show in real-time how immune cells are responding to tumors or pathogens, uncovering cellular dynamics beyond the reach of bulk analysis. This information is significant since it may be able to reveal new targets for therapy and the improvement of clinical responses to immunotherapy (Xu et al., 2025). In addition, uniting single-cell analysis with artificial intelligence and computational biology can potentially change the course of treatment and disease diagnosis, specifically cancer. Cell gene expression data predictive modeling can predict the patients' survival rates and tailor treatments based on cell-by-cell profiles (Li et al., 2025). This model of precision medicine demonstrates the way in which single-cell analysis not only divulges fundamental biological secrets but also connects this information to clinically meaningful conclusions. As the science develops further, overcoming challenges such as standardization of protocols and result interpretation will be key to the fulfillment of advancement. Therefore, the uses and meaning of single-cell analysis extend far beyond observation itself, driving innovation that may one day push our understanding of immunological mechanisms and disease mechanisms (Figure 8.1).

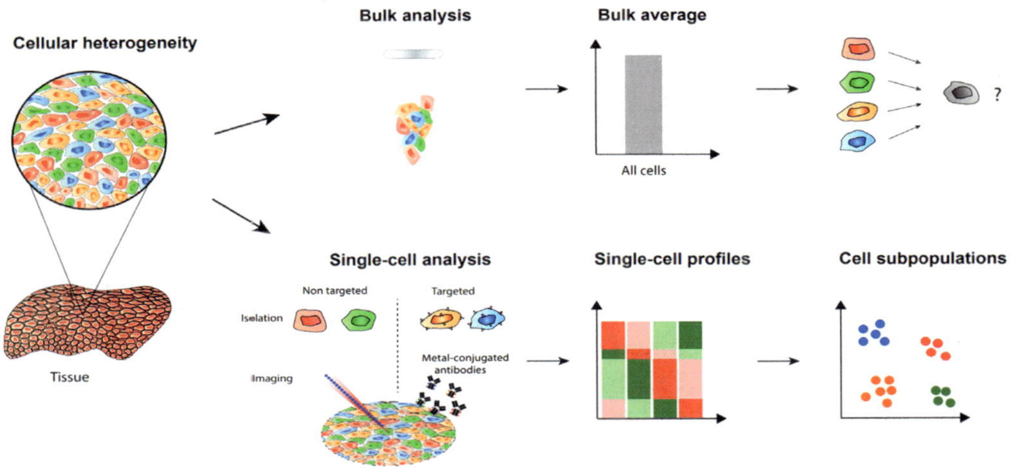

Figure 8.1. Single-cell analysis and imaging reveal cellular heterogeneity not seen by bulk analysis methods.

Source: https://www.mdpi.com/biology/biology-12-00395/article_deploy/html/images/biology-12-00395-g001.png.

Importance of Molecular Immunology

Molecular immunology is crucial in an effort to understand immune responses at the cellular level. By studying interactions between various immune cells and molecular mechanisms of their action, scientists are able to assess how the immune system responds to infections and diseases. This is especially important in chronic infections when traditional analytical methods prove insufficient. For example, in HCV disease, traditional methods usually fail to profile T cell responses due to the fact that effector functions are inhibited. Emerging technologies, such as high-throughput sequencing, enable thorough exploration of T cell populations. Quantification of such transient changes in T cell responses, presented in the chapter, opens a way for enhanced antiviral treatment and immunotherapy and therefore renders the contribution of molecular immunology to ongoing research and medical therapy valid (Robinson et al., 2016). The ability of single-cell methodology increases the value of molecular immunology further, revealing data central to advancing personalized medicine. An approach, such as adaptive immune receptor repertoire sequencing (AIRR-seq), represents one of the ways in which single-cell techniques can clarify the mystery of immunity through the investigation of T-cell receptor and antibody diversity and specificity. This analytic platform enables characterization of immune repertoires, enabling researchers to uncover the evolution and dynamics of adaptive immunity in conditions such as cancer and autoimmunity. The combination of high-level computational approaches with AIRR-seq data not only removes the aura of immune receptor landscapes' intricacy but also accelerates our understanding of immune interactions, promising novel therapeutic interventions as well as immunodiagnostics (Miho et al., 2018). Finally, the utilization of single-cell analytical approaches in molecular immunology exemplifies the utility function of the field in contemporary biomedical science. The understanding of the immune system at the cellular level makes it possible to identify new immunotherapeutic targets and biomarkers. This innovation is particularly valuable where the immune response is regulated, for instance, in cancer or chronic infections, where traditional therapeutic interventions might be limited. With the ability of single-cell technologies, researchers can now follow the fine differences between immune cells over time and therefore create improved and specific therapeutic strategies. The integration of molecular immunology and single-cell analysis not only enhances our understanding of the immune mechanisms but also represents a key step towards novel solutions for everyday diseases.

8.1. Historical Background of Single-Cell Analysis

The history of single-cell analysis goes back to the onset of cellular biology and microscopy, which laid the ground for the discovery of the complexity of cellular heterogeneity. The past is in the sense that it was limited by the equipment scientists had when analyzing cells individually. Fluorescence microscopy, which became widely used in the middle of the 20th century, was the breakthrough period when researchers became capable of observing and studying individual cells on the basis of some markers. The technological leap altered the view of cellular interactions and moved towards understanding how different cell types contribute to immunological reactions. As immunology advanced, it also became evident that the operation of single cells needed to be tackled, and doors opened for new ways of understanding the mechanisms of the immune system. In the next decades, single-cell analysis expanded with the development of flow cytometry, a technique of analyzing large populations of cells by their physical and chemical characteristics. This technique transformed the discipline of immunology because it made it possible for investigators to separate various immune cells and their activities within seconds. Flow cytometry identified infrequent cell populations, such as stem cells and some immune cell populations, and such discoveries explained the role of such cells in disease and health. Also, as the function of the glycocalyx in immunity came to be recognized by scientists, studies then shifted to knowing how certain profiles of sialic acid, like the absence of Neu5Gc, would affect cell-to-cell interaction during immune responses. This integration of single-cell analytical technologies provided more insight into evolutionary adjustments to regulate immune responses between groups (Altman & Gagneux, 2019). The emergence of single-cell RNA sequencing (scRNA-seq) in the late 20th and early 21st centuries was a transformative era for single-cell analysis that enabled extensive profiling of gene expression on a per-cell basis. scRNA-seq elevated the understanding of cellular heterogeneity within the immune system, uncovering new cell types and states not previously detectable using bulk analysis tools. Researchers were able to define immune cells' transcriptional landscapes, enhancing understanding of their developmental pathways and functional potential. Integrating single-cell methods with other approaches, such as mass cytometry and spatial transcriptomics, also enhanced molecular immunology analysis tools. The multi-dimensional perspective has produced more robust models of immune behavior, ultimately paving the way to therapy based on the individual cellular complexities of disease (Carbone et al., 2020).

8.1.1. Early Techniques in Cell Analysis

The methods of cell analysis have revolutionized immunology, at least in the documentation of single-cell complexities. Flow cytometry and microscopy are two of the ancient techniques that have paved the way for sophisticated methods. Microscopy, being capable of unveiling cellular morphology, allowed scientists to identify and study different immune cells and their respective morphologies and localizations. These methods, nevertheless, could not supply quantitative data on cell activities or their interaction with other cells in mixed cell populations. Flow cytometry was a developing method that allowed the rapid analysis of hundreds of thousands of cells based on some surface antigens. By applying fluorescently tagged antibodies, flow cytometry permitted multi-parameter quantitation of many cell characteristics and thus made it more sophisticated to analyze immune cell populations and their role in disease as well as health. The merging of genomics with the original cell analysis methods further propelled the technology, revealing genetic regulation of immunity. Once scientists began applying methods like quantitative polymerase chain reaction (qPCR) and microarray analysis, the focus then shifted towards gene expression patterns within immune cells. These technologies shed light on molecular mechanisms that regulate cellular functions, such as cytokine production, proliferation, and apoptosis. While these bulk assays had a tendency to mask heterogeneity within populations and gave an averaged response that did not mirror cell behavior. This constraint created the birth of scRNA-seq, the revolutionary technology that allowed scientists to analyze gene expression at the cellular level. This capability has subsequently provided the discipline with limitless understanding into immune cell population diversity and functional status, revolutionizing how scientists research the immune system. Integration of early cell analysis techniques into the single-cell analysis platform has brought unprecedented advancements in the understanding of disease pathology and response to treatment. For instance, application of scRNA-seq to query high-grade serous ovarian cancer (HGSOC) has revealed insights into tumor heterogeneity and the interaction with the immune system and hence prognosis and therapeutic approaches (Zhao et al., 2025). Similarly, initial biomarker identification via gene expression profiling of prostate cancer has described the advantage of integrating molecular and cellular information in optimizing treatment strategy (Karoii et al., 2025). The study shows the importance of early methods because they are the background against which modern single-cell approaches, not only dissecting cell populations but also characterizing the associated molecular pathways critical in the optimization of immunotherapy, are developed. The balance between emerging techniques and ongoing innovations spells the way for cell analysis as a prime driver towards molecular immunology, releasing robust platforms for upcoming breakthroughs.

8.1.2. Evolution of Technology in Immunology

Technology development in immunology has basically transformed our capability to investigate immune reactions on a level of resolution unparalleled to date. Historically, immunology research was characterised by bulk population analyses concealing cell actions at the single-cell level. Whereas, with the advent of single-cell analytical technologies, this paradigm has changed, with scientists now being able to interrogate immune cell heterogeneity and function with unparalleled resolution. Procedures like single-cell RNA sequencing and mass cytometry have risen as indispensable platforms, which have the ability to interrogate thousands of cells in parallel. This resolution not only defines the multilayered cellular organization within immune cohorts but also sheds light on cellular communication and differentiation. The future potential of personalized medicine is tremendous, as these technologies enable the identification of novel drug targets and biomarkers not previously accessible. Apart from single-cell sequencing, other imaging technologies have similarly expanded the immunological window. Highly advanced microscopy techniques, such as super-resolution microscopy and multiphoton microscopy, provide the ability to visualize immune responses in real time within their native tissue environments. These techniques allow researchers to observe dynamic interactions of immune cells and pathogens and have revealed information that is not available with traditional imaging modalities. With the conjunction of these imaging techniques and single-cell transcriptomics, it becomes possible to understand how cellular functionality is influenced by spatial context, and this is what accounts for the intricacy of immune responses in infection and disease states. As the technologies become increasingly sophisticated, they give new windows into understanding the complexities of immune pathogenesis and regulation that underlie new approaches to the generation of new immunotherapies. Expanded technology input to immunology also involves computing and analysis platforms, which are central to addressing the enormous amounts of data provided by single-cell analyses. The flood of high-throughput methods brings an imperative for advanced bioinformatics tools to deconvolute complex biological information and translate the enormous diversities of immune cell profiles. Machine learning and artificial intelligence are rapidly entering the limelight here to assist in corroborating experimental findings and enhancing the predictive power of immunology. These computational advances not only facilitate easier processing of data but also make interdisciplinarity possible, culminating in improved hypotheses and experiments. Collectively, the path of technology in immunology—various levels from single-cell analysis to high-level imaging and high-end data analysis—powers greater understanding of the immune system that will propel new therapeutic modalities to disease prevention and cure (Figure 8.2).

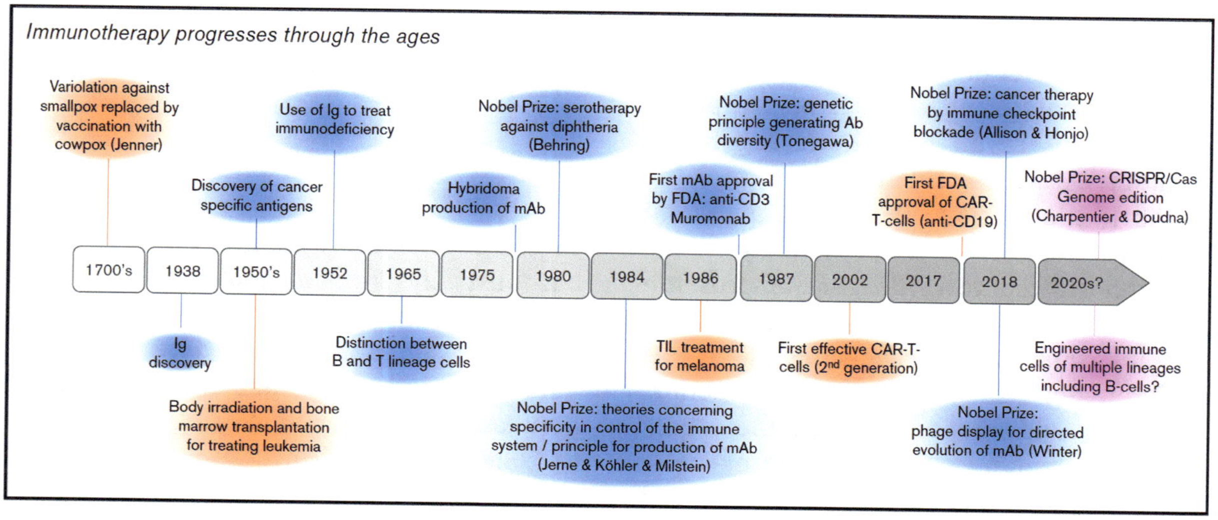

Figure 8.2. A timeline of the history of immunotherapy.

Source: https://www.researchgate.net/profile/Jerome-Moreaux/publication/350329540/figure/fig1/AS:1006550839750657@1616991829280/A-timeline-of-the-history-of-immunotherapy-Although-based-on-old-medical-practices-such.png.

8.1.3. Key Milestones in Single-Cell Research

Single-cell research has been characterized by a series of important milestones that have contributed significantly to the topic of molecular immunology. Perhaps the most significant among them was the creation of scRNA-seq during the early 2010s. This technique revolutionized the level of analysis of gene expression to an unprecedented resolution, enabling researchers to determine the heterogeneity between different individual cells in complicated tissues. Therefore, scRNA-seq has opened up the possibility to discover novel immune subpopulations of cells and acquire valuable insights on the immune response during tumorigenesis and infection. In addition, the continuous improvement in scRNA-seq technologies has made it feasible to establish multiple computational frameworks and statistics tools, which are crucial for effectively interpreting the massive data being produced by these technologies.

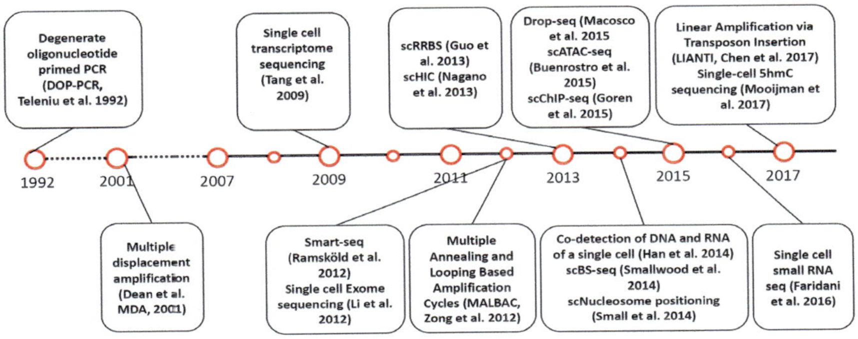

Figure 8.3. Timeline of single-cell sequencing methods milestones.

Source: https://www.researchgate.net/publication/323747793/figure/fig1/AS:11431281246787707@1716470604616/Timeline-of-single-cell-sequencing-methods-milestones.tif.

This accomplishment has permitted molecular immunologists to investigate immune signaling cascades and cell dynamics during disease and health. Spatial transcriptomics integration is another milestone in single-cell science that reduces the gap between cellular inspection and tissue architecture. Tools like multiplexed error-robust fluorescence *in situ* hybridization (MERFISH) and Slide-seq allow researchers to map the cellular landscape in tissues, while parallel gene expression profiling is possible. This spatial context is important in molecular immunology, with interactions of immune cells within their microenvironment influencing functional outcomes. Through the integration of transcriptomic data and histological information, investigators can dissect intricate interactions that enable immune responses, such as those observed in cancer. High-resolution three-dimensional (3D) tissue imaging is a case in point, with high resolution enabling specific characterization of spatial arrangement and molecular composition at single-cell resolution. Further improvement and innovation in these technologies are needed in the understanding of our knowledge regarding immune cell behavior in increasingly more complex biological systems (Xu et al., 2025). In cancer science, single-cell technologies have come a long way with a great emphasis in colorectal cancer, where precision medicine increasingly sets the agenda for treatment. For instance, ongoing studies employ single-cell sequencing to unveil gene expression patterns related to patient survival and treatment outcomes. By unraveling the immune landscape of immune cells within colorectal cancer, researchers have built predictive models that incorporate immune status and personalized lifestyle factors to enhance the prognosticability. Such breakthroughs underpin the viability of using artificial intelligence in conjunction with single-cell analysis for precision-directed refinement of therapy in accordance with individual patient profiles. Progress in gene expression analysis, as seen in the study using NCAM1 and CADM1 genes, exemplifies the potential of single-cell research to yield landmark information regarding immune regulation and disease formation (Li et al., 2025). Such progress mirrors significant milestones that have far-reaching implications in molecular immunology, shaping future outlooks in cancer therapy and beyond (Figure 8.3).

8.2. Techniques for Single-Cell Isolation

Single-cell isolation techniques are a defining point in the evolution of molecular immunology that further our understanding of cellular heterogeneity and competency. Protocols such as fluorescence-activated cell sorting (FACS) and magnetic-activated cell sorting (MACS) are now preferred due to the fact that they allow for efficient separation and enrichment of target cell populations from endogenous markers. FACS sorts and identifies cells using a laser system, allowing scientists to choose high-purity populations and in real time. MACS utilizes magnetic antibody-coated beads to capture target cells, which is a simpler and cheaper approach for scientists. Both approaches provide a solid platform for cellular interrogation, enabling downstream applications such as RNA sequencing and proteomics, and thus enabling additional research of the immune landscape, along with furthering our understanding of disease mechanisms behind immune responses (Xu et al., 2025). In parallel, advances in microfluidic devices have revolutionized single-cell isolation by enabling scalable high-throughput devices that can deal efficiently with large quantities of samples. These systems support the manipulation of single cells in micrometer-scale chambers with a controlled environment that minimizes contamination and preserves cellular integrity. Techniques such as acoustic focusing and droplet-based microfluidics enable the sorting and compartmentalization of individual cells with high precision, which is particularly useful for analyzing rare cell populations in heterogeneous samples. Further, by integrating such isolation strategies with spatial omics, researchers can gain unprecedented insights into the cellular tissue-in-housing architecture. Such technological breakthroughs have ushered in a new frontier for single-cell dissection with significantly enhanced capabilities to mechanistically deconstruct tissue-resident immune responses and tumor microenvironments (Chen et al., 2024). Furthermore, new methods such as laser capture microdissection (LCM) and optoelectronic tweezers are cutting-edge tools for capturing individual cells. LCM uses a focused laser beam to isolate single cells or regions of interest from tissue sections, thereby allowing intense study of individual cellular functions or molecular profiles. This is particularly valuable in molecular immunology, where a comprehensive understanding of immune cell interaction with their microenvironments is critical. On the other hand, optoelectronic tweezers employ light and electric fields to grasp and move cells with high precision, enabling single cell types to be isolated based on their physical properties. Such novel techniques are continually expanding the range of possibilities available to researchers, advancing our understanding of immune responses and cellular behavior in sickness and in health (Chen et al., 2024; Xu et al., 2025).

8.2.1. Microfluidics and Its Applications

Microfluidics is a new technology that has been a revolutionary power in the analysis of single cells, particularly in molecular immunology. Microfluidics allows researchers to manipulate infinitesimal amounts of fluid on a microscale, providing a significant advance in the ability to monitor cell behaviors and interactions. One of the most renowned applications of microfluidics is the Lab on a Chip technology, which allows one to accelerate and economically conduct experiments. These microfluidic devices are able to simulate the intricate dynamics of biological systems, crucial for the analysis of phenomena such as leukocyte extravasation. By utilizing a microfluidic chip, researchers can create a controlled system mimicking physiological conditions, rendering their results more accurate and ultimately enabling better comprehension of immune responses (Navarrete, 2018). One of the key strengths of microfluidics is its ability to manipulate and analyze single cells, which uncovers heterogeneity within populations of cells.

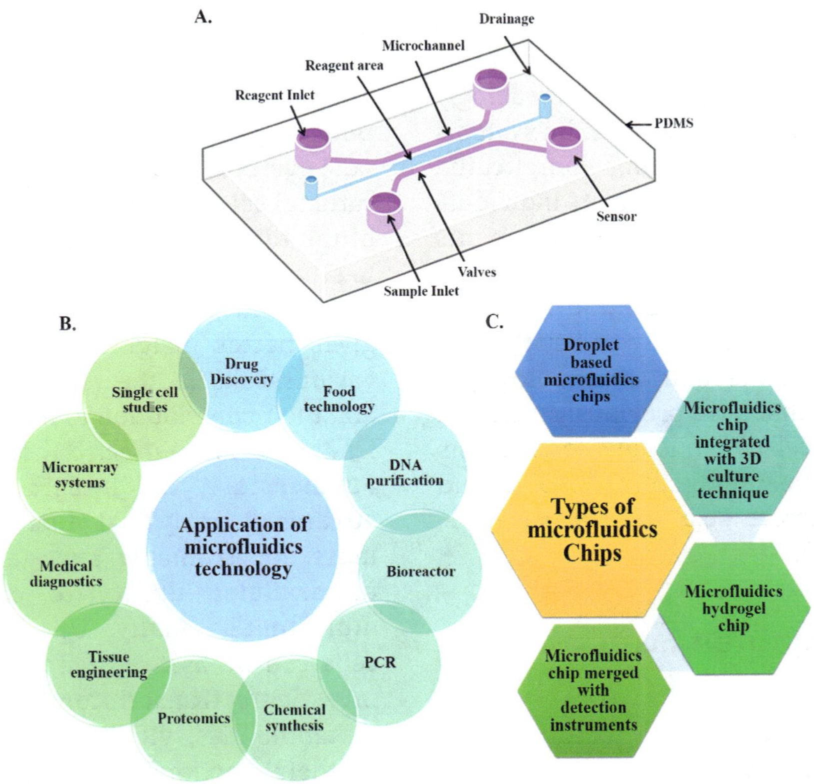

Figure 8.4. A Diagrammatic representation of the microfluidic chip; B type of microfluidic chips and C application of microfluidic chips.

Source: https://www.researchgate.net/publication/355657151/figure/fig1/AS:1143128136088798 3@1744106343288/A-Diagrammatic-representation-of-the-microfluidic-chip-B-type-of-microfluidic-chips-and.png.

Such resolution is crucial in pushing the understanding of immune function and dysfunction across diseases. For instance, combining droplet microfluidic technology and fluorescence lifetime imaging microscopy enables scientists to measure metabolic states of single cells without the need for invasion. These approaches are essential for distinguishing among different cell types, such as proliferative and quiescent cells, with specific roles in immune responses and the initiation of cancer.

Connecting these metabolic signatures with genomic data, microfluidics not only enhances our understanding of cellular behaviors but also provides a strong platform for targeted therapy and personalized medicine approaches (Ma et al., 2019). Additionally, the adaptability of microfluidic devices also carries forward to their possible use in high-throughput screening and diagnostic testing. The small size of such devices allows for the simultaneous measurement of multiple samples, opening up many avenues for enhanced efficiency and throughput in laboratories. With continuous advances in this field by researchers, there is an increasingly focused effort on creating microfluidic systems that are capable of performing complicated biological assays. The ability to isolate individual cells and control finely the microenvironments into which they are placed has the potential to reveal the mechanisms of immune response and disease processes. Lastly, microfluidics will revolutionize molecular immunology by providing insights that have previously not been possible on single-cell dynamics and interactions that will enable novel therapeutic strategies and diagnostics (Navarrete et al., 2018; Ma et al., 2019) (Figure 8.4).

8.2.2. Laser Capture Microdissection (LCM)

LCM has been found to be a major tool in molecular immunology for the isolation of specific cell types from complicated tissue samples. This technique utilizes focused laser beams to dissect and trap cells of interest, allowing for the analysis of gene expression, protein content, and other molecular characteristics on a single-cell level. LCM is particularly useful when analyzing tissues that contain cellular diversity that is robust, since it allows for the enrichment of particular cells that may be critical in elucidating disease pathologies. For instance, in Alzheimer's disease, the ability to isolate amyloid plaques from brain tissue using LCM makes it possible for scientists to investigate their proteomic content, improving our knowledge about the root pathophysiology (Jiao, 2024). Thus, LCM is a foundation technique in the armory of single-cell analysis techniques. The use of LCM is not only for neuroscience but also for other complex diseases such as pancreatic cancer, with the technique helping in unraveling tumor heterogeneity. Pancreatic cancer's aggressive nature typically complicates treatment and its course further since it typically has no symptoms at early stages and is diagnosed late. Bulk tissue analysis is not adequate in delivering vital information about the tumor microenvironment and the unique molecular phenotypes between tumor subpopulations. LCM overcomes this shortcoming by enabling the rational selection and characterization of some of the tumor cells, thereby better preparing us to study cancer development pathways at a very high resolution (Rao et al., 2022). This precision gives better insights into the interaction of various cells in the tumor microenvironment and their contribution to malignancy, eventually leading to more precise therapeutic strategies. Furthermore, the integration of LCM with advanced analytical technologies such as mass spectrometry and genomics offers an unparalleled ability to characterize cells multidimensionally. Once captured, single cells can be assayed using multiple assays to investigate transcriptomics, proteomics, and metabolomics, yielding detailed information on their functional state and interactions. This combined view not only illuminates the roles of each cell type in disease and immunity but also informs potential biomarkers for therapy and diagnosis. By increasing the resolution at which immunological events may be accessed, LCM completely changes our understanding of single-cell dynamics in health and disease. As science develops, LCM can potentially make a much greater contribution to the field of molecular immunology, illuminating the pathways hidden hitherto in complex tissues (Figure 8.5).

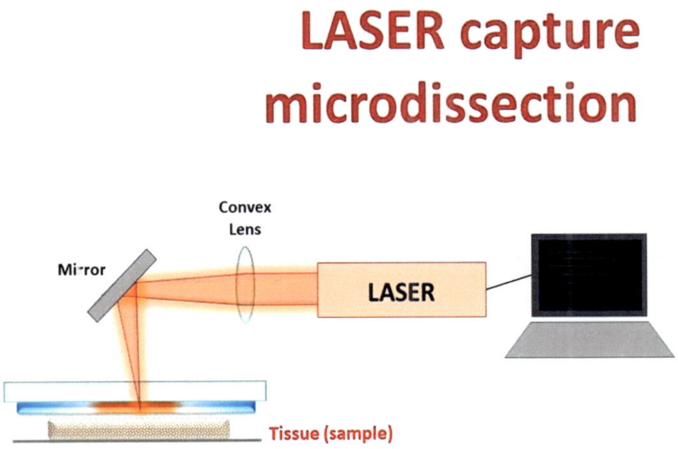

Figure 8.5. Laser capture microdissection.

Source: https://i.ytimg.com/vi/I5G7x52D1PE/maxresdefault.jpg.

8.2.3. FACS (Fluorescence-Activated Cell Sorting)

FACS is one of the most important techniques of single-cell analysis, particularly within the field of molecular immunology. This strong methodology is capable of distinguishing between populations of distinct cells by using markers that are tagged with fluorescence, thereby enabling many downstream applications. The precision of FACS enables discrimination between cellular heterogeneity, which is paramount in the understanding of complex immune response dynamics. Through combining laser technology and sophisticated fluidics, FACS enables a high-throughput method of sorting live cells while preserving their functional integrity. The implication of such potential for T cell activation research, B cell lineage tracing research, and memory cell identification highlights the significance of FACS as a necessary facility in current immunology research. Moreover, the combination of FACS with other single-cell analytic technologies increases its utility in molecular immunology. For instance, FACS can be applied to enrich the populations of scarce cells, such as activated T cells, before scRNA-seq. The combination makes it possible to perform multiple transcriptome analyses describing the gene expression profiles characterizing various states of immune cells. It provides scientists with the ability to study complicated signaling cascades and discriminate cellular responses to vaccinations or infections. Furthermore, advances in FACS technology and techniques, such as the utilization of additional fluorescent labels and enhanced sorting efficiency, also have a pivotal impact on the comprehension of complex immune interactions. All this contributes to the value of FACS in target identification of therapeutic interventions and mechanisms of disease in immunological conditions. Advancements in methodology have recently been demonstrated by studies illustrating increasing sophistication in FACS to further facilitate single-cell analysis. For instance, the application of FACS in the induced reprogramming of astrocytes to neurons highlights its utility in non-conventional immunological applications. By subjecting successfully transfected cells to enriching and subsequent scRNA-seq, researchers were able to map the transcriptional landscape of reprogramming of the cell and thereby reveal important pathways and gene interactions involved in the process. The ability to achieve high sorting efficiency without affecting cell viability is a testament to the role

FACS plays in making single-cell experiments possible. As researchers continue to fine-tune FACS applications across various fields of biological science, the method will remain at the forefront of unveiling new knowledge in molecular immunology and beyond, ultimately translating to the development of precision medicine and therapeutic strategies (Qin et al., 2024; Wang et al., 2025) (Figure 8.6).

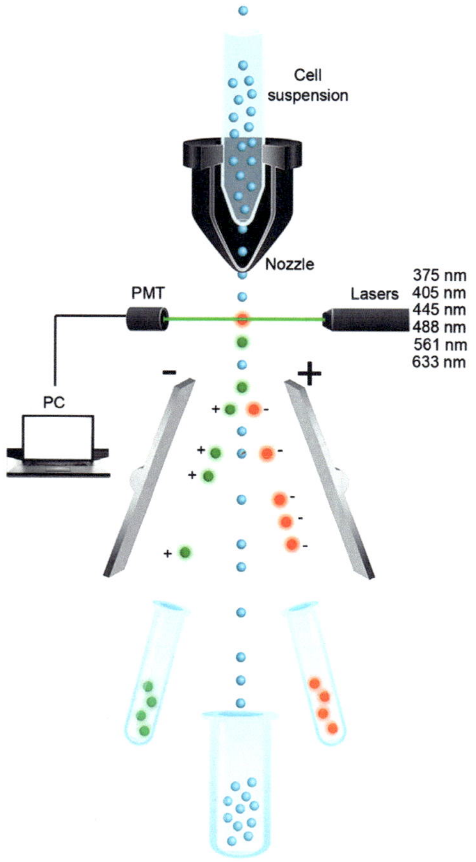

Figure 8.6. Fluorescence-activated cell sorting (FACS). The suspended cells are subjected to different fluorescent tags depending on the experimental set-up.

Source: https://www.researchgate.net/publication/283800102/figure/fig3/AS:667840646492164@1536237026218/Fluorescence-activated-cell-sorting-FACS-The-suspended-cells-are-subjected-to.jpg.

8.3. Genomic Analysis at the Single-Cell Level

The advent of single-cell genomic analysis has revolutionized the field of molecular immunology, making it possible for researchers to dissect the intricate complexity of cellular heterogeneity. Traditional genomic methods are used to average the signal across populations of cells, concealing the unique characteristics of individual cells. Using methods such as scRNA-seq, scientists can now capture transcriptomic profiles at unprecedented resolution. This allows rare cell types to be isolated, cellular states to be described, and dynamic mechanisms that control immune responses to be revealed. Moreover, the ability to derive vast amounts of data from individual cells to analyze cellular interactions presents a powerful possibility for uncovering disease mechanisms at their origin, for example, in cancer or autoimmune disorders. Therefore, single-cell analysis is not only a technical breakthrough but a revolutionary approach that transforms our understanding of immunological processes. In disease modeling, single-cell genomic dissection has a key role to play in untangling the microenvironmental impact on immune cells. For instance, crosstalk between HSCs and MSCs has an important function in hematopoietic homeostasis, as evidenced by studies that demonstrate transcriptional changes in MSCs to dramatically affect the behavior of HSCs. The role of transcription factors like Ebf1 in influencing bone marrow niche structure and function has been highlighted in the latest findings. Ebf1 disruptions in MSCs resulted in impaired adhesion and differential gene expression, impacting HSC quiescence and myeloid output. These results illustrate how single-cell genomic technologies not only find heterogeneity in immune cell populations but also illuminate the central role of cellular interactions in shaping immune responses and how these might have therapeutic implications (Derecka et al., 2020). The specificity and sensitivity of single-cell genome analysis also enhance detection and identification of pathogens that pose important immunological challenges. For instance, efforts to find *Mycobacterium avium* subsp. paratuberculosis have underscored the necessity for refining diagnostic approaches using advanced DNA amplification techniques. Progress in molecular biology techniques that improve the detection of this pathogen, especially in subclinically infected animals, demonstrates the promise of single-cell analysis techniques for transforming diagnosis. Through discrimination between mycobacterial species that are very closely related, such as those present in paratuberculosis, these techniques improve our insights into pathogen evolution, immune evasion, and disease pathology. Hence, single-cell-level genomics is not only advancing basic research but also has tremendous translational significance in disease diagnosis and infectious disease control (Englund, 2002).

8.3.1. Single-cell RNA Sequencing (scRNA-seq)

scRNA-seq revolutionized the field of molecular immunology by allowing the study of gene expression at the level of a single cell.

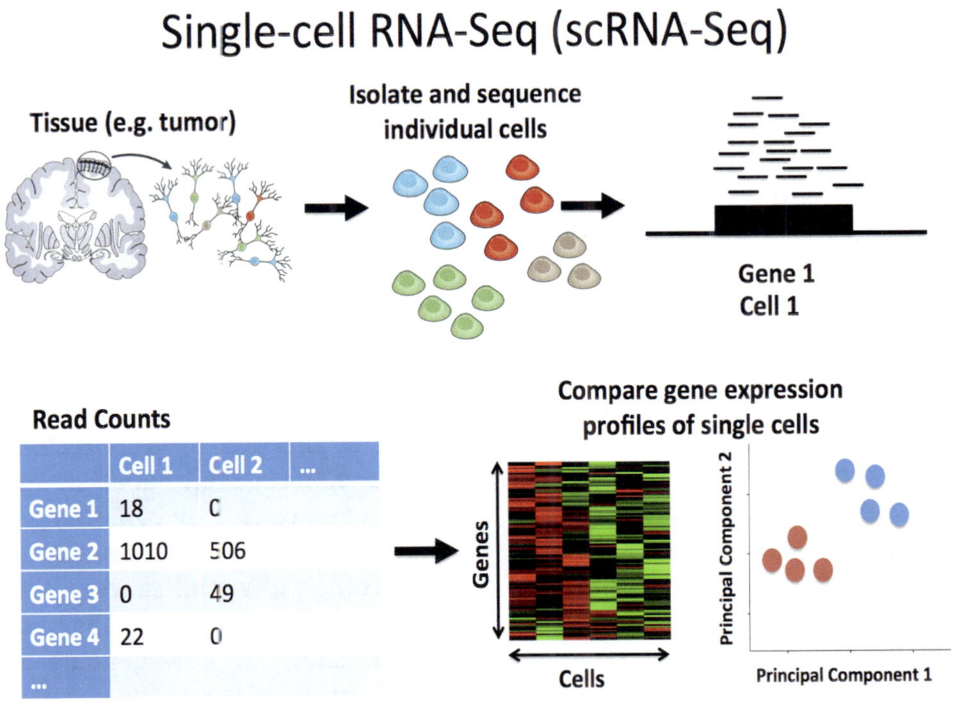

Figure 8.7. The advent of single-cell RNA sequencing (scRNA-seq) has revolutionized the landscape of molecular immunology by enabling the analysis of gene expression at the individual cell level.

Source: https://learn.gencore.bio.nyu.edu/wp-content/uploads/2018/01/scRNA-overview.jpg.

This technology bypasses the limitations of bulk RNA sequencing, which averages and pools gene expression profiles of heterogeneous populations of cells and may suppress critical biological information. By providing its fine-grained view of transcriptomic variations, scRNA-seq allows researchers to detect unique cellular states as well as identify rare subtypes of immune cells that might be important in immune responses. With its potential for the breakdown of complex immune milieus, scRNA-seq enables the deciphering of immune system processes in health and disease, paving the way for personalized immunotherapies and targeted therapies in oncology and autoimmune diseases. As applications of scRNA-seq evolve, the meaning of data integration and interpretation has become increasingly important. Its high dimensionality makes it one of the most difficult data sets to analyze, necessitating advanced computational techniques for analysis. Methods such as dimension reduction, clustering, and trajectory analysis are employed to find important biological patterns in very large data sets. Detection sensitivity and inference accuracy can also be influenced by the platform used for sequencing, as indicated in recent comparisons of several different methods for TCR sequencing. Noticeably, Looney et al. (2019) suggest that differences in sequencing technology can influence the assessment of TCR convergence, foregrounding the necessity for methodological rigour in scRNA-seq experiment design and analysis. Such considerations serve to underscore the necessity for continuous methodological advancement throughout the field. Furthermore, scRNA-seq has far-reaching effects on the comprehension not only of infectious disease but also of chronic disease, such as bovine tuberculosis, as exemplified by associated work. The infected and non-infected gene expression profiles comparisons illustrate the vast potential of scRNA-seq in disassembling complicated immune responses and host-pathogen relationships. For instance, McLoughlin et al. (2014) illustrate that RNA-seq platforms have greatly enhanced the identification of differentially expressed genes to better elucidate immune function against pathogens. This skill is priceless in immunology, where the need to examine complex cell-to-cell contacts and the molecular cause of disease takes precedence. With continued advances in scRNA-seq, its capacity to highlight new therapeutic targets and biomarkers for application in immune-related disorders is at the forefront of scientific inquiry, holding the key to future progress in both experimental and clinical immunology (Figure 8.7).

8.3.2. Whole-Genome Amplification (WGA) Techniques

WGA approaches have emerged as game-changing tools in the realm of molecular immunology for researching single cells. Since the human immune system is so intricate and certain cell populations rarely occur, WGA allows comprehensive genomic profiling by the amplification of minimal quantities of DNA from single cells. Amplification is needed to allow downstream analyses, such as sequencing and qPCR, to detect variations, mutations, and other genomic features using sufficient DNA material. With the application of WGA, researchers can determine the immunity complexities in people at a resolution that was impossible to date, and light up the activity of rare cellular subsets responsible for immunity and disease, particularly in situations such as cancer and autoimmune disease. An example of the application of WGA technique includes cellular heterogeneity analysis in tumors, that is, in breast cancer. By combining WGA with the analysis of the targeted proteome, researchers can profile individual cancer cells for genomic as well as proteomic properties in parallel. For instance, the new genome and proteome (G&P) protocol introduced recently enables the quantification of gene copy numbers and protein expression levels in individual cancer cells. This bidirectional analysis allows for a better understanding of how genetic alterations, such as those in the ERBB2 locus, correlate with protein expression levels, i.e., HER2. The response to drugs like lapatinib can also be examined by this dual approach, which allows scientists to observe responses of cells to drugs.

Such methods are a prime example of how WGA plays a crucial role in correlating genomic information with functional cellular responses in cancer immunology (Alyasin et al., 2024). Furthermore, WGA methods are also being found useful beyond the field of oncology, specifically for the investigation of pediatric low-grade gliomas (LGGs). The application of highly sensitive screening assays that are WGA-based enables the identification and molecular characterization of tumors in liquid biopsy samples such as cerebrospinal fluid and plasma. The approaches can be utilized to identify circulating tumor DNA, which is vital for early detection and decision-making on treatment. As an example, the existence of multiplexed droplet digital PCR assays has made it possible to evaluate certain genomic alterations, e.g., BRAF duplication and KIAA1549::BRAF fusion junctions, in pilocytic astrocytoma patient CSF samples. As an adjuvant tool, WGA methods enhance our ability to profile low levels of cell-free DNA (cfDNA), releasing precious insights into the molecular phenotype of LGGs, potentially leading to greater improvements in non-invasive diagnosis and patient management in pediatric neuro-oncology (Krynina et al., 2024) (Figure 8.8).

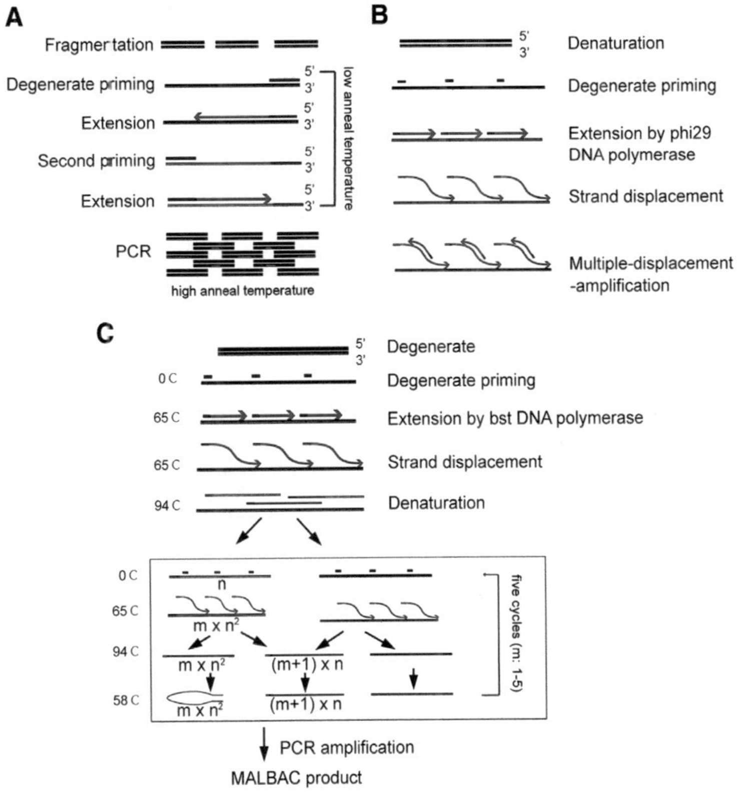

Figure 8.8. Whole-genome amplification methods for single-cell sequencing. a Degenerate oligonucleotide-primed PCR (DOP-PCR). b Multiple displacement amplification (MDA). c Multiple annealing and looping-based amplification cycles (MALBAC).

Source: https://www.researchgate.net/publication/327632896/figure/fig4/AS:963411378700300@1606706580581/Whole-genome-amplification-methods-for-single-cell-sequencing-a-Degenerate.png.

8.3.3. Applications in Understanding Immune Responses

The application of single-cell analysis techniques has significantly accelerated the understanding of the immune response, particularly through immune repertoire studies. These repertoires include a vast repertoire of antigen-binding antibodies and T-cell receptors, essential to recognize a variety of pathogens. Through Adaptive Immune Receptor Repertoire Sequencing (AIRR-seq), researchers are able to molecularly and quantitatively define these immune repertoires, revealing their complex dynamics in meeting diseases such as autoimmunity and cancer. The analytical approaches set for processing data of AIRR-seq, including diversity analysis, clustering, and phylogenetic analysis, have deciphered profound understandings of adaptive immunity's evolutionary history and resilience to different challenges. Such specificity in the data eases the likelihood of strategizing targeted immunotherapies and vaccines, which play pivotal roles in bolstering patient outcomes in various immunological disorders (Miho et al., 2018). Furthermore, continued probing of immune responses through single-cell analysis also entails the vigorous probing of innate immunity, such as in invertebrate models, for example, crustaceans. Such organisms' new immune systems, which are unique and distinct from vertebrate systems, present new pathways and recognition proteins of utmost significance to understanding pathogen interaction. New discoveries have facilitated the identification of novel classes of immune effectors and regulatory processes, improving our understanding of innate immunity responses. Investigation of such novel immunological processes not only aids in uncovering the processes of diseases in aquaculture but also contributes to understanding broader ecological and evolutionary issues. Through the analysis of immune responses in such organisms using single-cell approaches, scientists can discover about that can be used to inform strategies for managing disease in commercially relevant species both in the sea and in fresh waters (Hauton, 2012). The integration of single-cell analytical methodologies has the potential to revolutionize immunological research by enabling scientists to dissect the intricate details of immune responses at resolutions previously unattainable. Computational immunology is developing, underpinned by the enormous amounts of data that methods like AIRR-seq are generating, in an effort to de-mystify immune systems in different species and contexts. This facilitation of cross-disciplinary interaction between computational and wet-lab scientists will not just elucidate immune dynamics but also power the discovery of new immunotherapeutics. Future studies within this field would involve applying machine learning and other data-mining techniques to predict immune and treatment responses and ensure that what single-cell work uncovers is translated into effective real-world applications that benefit public health and disease control (Miho et al., 2018).

8.4. Proteomic Analysis Techniques

Advances in proteomic analysis techniques have significantly enhanced the volume of information on molecular mechanisms of immune responses. Proteomics is focused on high-scale protein research, particularly in structures and function. In single-cell evaluation, data-independent acquisition (DIA) proteomics, for instance, supports whole-proteome protein expression profiling at the level of a single cell. This type of approach is critical for the determination of heterogeneity in immune cell populations, providing information regarding how individual cells contribute to immune responses. Of particular interest, the coupling of these proteomic technologies with single-cell

RNA sequencing has generated more informative data, demonstrating relationships between gene expression profiles and protein levels that may provide insights into therapeutic potential and vaccine development in immunology research. Furthermore, proteomic methods are critical in the identification of biomarkers that relate to different states of disease, e.g., cardiovascular diseases. For instance, extensive proteomic profiling of carotid atherosclerotic plaques has identified different proteins that are predictive of plaque stability and inflammatory reactions. Such data are crucial; some of these proteins, such as CD44 and IL-6R, have been linked with atherogenesis and risk of ischemic stroke (Wang et al., 2025). Detection of such biomarkers by proteomic techniques not only enhances our understanding of disease pathophysiology but also reveals potential targets for therapeutic intervention. Future advances in proteomics with single-cell analysis will drive the discovery of new biomarkers and permit more personalized treatment schemes. Proteomic analysis is not restricted to the analysis of biological processes but is applied to a multitude of other biological contexts, further emphasizing its application in molecular immunology. Tissue compartmentalization and structural specificity approaches have been increasingly advanced to allow molecular exploration of regions that dictate disease pathogenesis. For instance, advanced label-free quantitative proteomic pipelines can identify the distinctive molecular signatures in kidney compartments where kidney diseases occur (Barati et al., 2025). By applying such cautious methods, researchers are able to reveal the intricate pathways of immune-related disorders, further bridging the discrepancy between gene expression and proteomics of functions at the individual cell level. While these technological developments become widespread, they can change the landscape of immunology and enhance therapeutic interventions.

8.4.1. Mass Spectrometry (MS) in Single-Cell Proteomics

Single-cell proteomics has increasingly become a key strategy in unraveling the intricacies of cell behavior and heterogeneity in various biological systems, particularly in molecular immunology. MS is a prime technology that is a trendsetter in this group by virtue of enabling the identification and quantification of proteins in single cells.

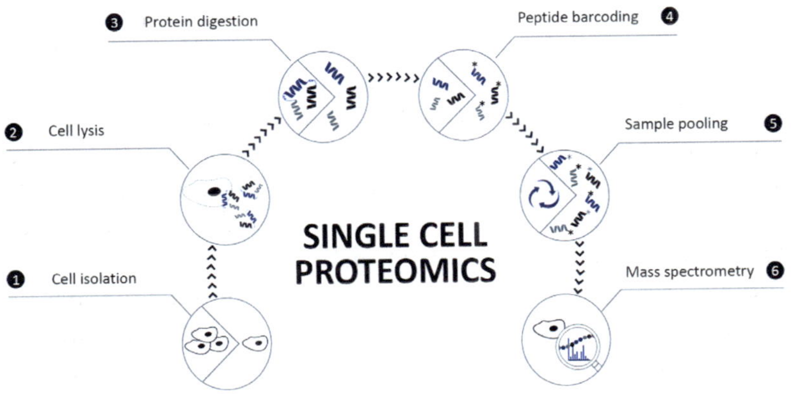

Figure 8.9. Single-cell proteomics.

Source: https://www.cellenion.com/wp-content/uploads/2021/06/Workflow-SCP.png.

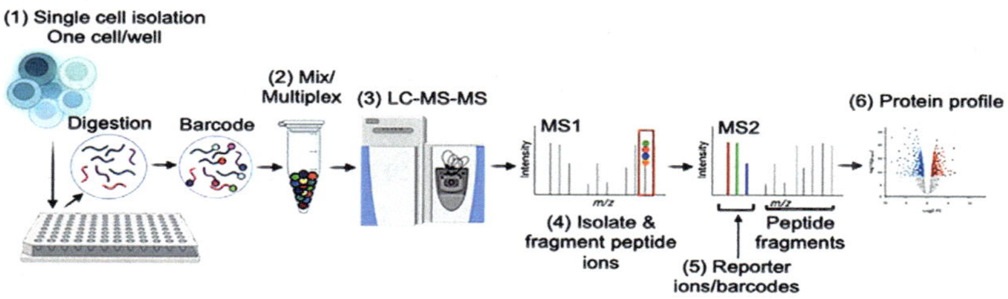

Figure 8.10. Basic overview of single-cell mass spectrometry workflow. Single-cell proteomics tends to use a "bottoms-up" approach.

Source: https://www.researchgate.net/publication/365429725/figure/fig1/AS:11431281254477662@1719198273783/Basic-overview-of-single-cell-mass-spectrometry-workflow-Single-cell-proteomics-tends-to.tif.

Traditional proteomic techniques disregard cellular heterogeneity and thus a knowledge of immune responses derived from them is incomplete. With a focus on single-cell analysis, mass spectrometry provides a more nuanced characterization of protein expression, post-translational modifications, and interactions and therefore reveals information essential for designing targeted therapies and disease mechanism insights. As method development for sample preparation and analysis has evolved, the accuracy and sensitivity of mass spectrometry have increased exponentially, and it has become an extremely useful tool in questioning the proteomic landscape of single cells. Current advancements in mass spectrometry have accelerated the field of single-cell proteomics to new levels, particularly by integrating advanced sample processing techniques and data analysis procedures (Figure 8.9). Techniques such as microdissection using laser capture and microfluidics have emerged as key features in the separation of individual cells, enabling more detailed proteomic content analysis. In addition, the development of ultra-high-resolution mass spectrometers enabled enhanced detection of low-abundance proteins and post-translational modifications, which is vital for understanding immune cell differentiation and function. For instance, the application of label-free quantitation tools has permitted scientists to compare protein expression levels in a single cell, independent of biases introduced by labeling agents and therefore collect more reliable data. Such a methodological breakthrough demonstrates the strength of mass spectrometry in mapping the complex protein networks that govern immune responses at the cellular level. Mass spectrometry in single-cell proteomics has its weaknesses, too (Staunton et al., 2013). Achievement of high sensitivity and specificity amidst the natural variability of single cells requires innovative approaches in experimental design and execution. Protein extraction and preparation from individual cells require optimal optimization for close replication of the proteome of the cell without significant loss or alteration. To boot, computational analysis of the enormous amounts of data generated by mass spectrometry needs to decipher and handle the complex information obtained from single-cell proteomic profiles with the aid of robust bioinformatics resources. As in the case of *Streptococcus sanguinis,* when the proteome extraction pipeline enabled the analysis of cellular response to stress, the same may be applied to immune cells to determine their functional state and regulatory states under health and disease (El-Rami et al., 2017). As such, the ongoing development of mass spectrometry and its use in single-cell analysis has huge potential to improve our knowledge of molecular immunology (Figure 8.10).

8.4.2. Antibody-Based Assays for Protein Detection

Antibody-based assays are part and parcel of the scene of protein detection in the context of single-cell analysis methods in molecular immunology. These assays utilize the specificity and affinity of antibodies to detect and quantify proteins in the single-cell level, providing valuable information about cellular function and heterogeneity. Quantitative protein expression analyses are offered by enzyme-linked immunosorbent assay (ELISA) and Western blotting, while more advanced methodologies such as flow cytometry and multiplex assays enable the simultaneous detection of multiple proteins in individual cells. The ability to quantify proteins in a particular manner allows researchers to disentangle complex signaling cascades and immune responses, thereby broadening our understanding of cellular behavior during health and disease. In particular, the versatility of antibody-derived technologies allows us to study cellular signaling within a dynamic and space-resolved context. Antibody-based assays are also versatile to use with various forms of samples, e.g., cultured cells and tissue sections, which would enable researchers to elucidate the functional roles of the protein in various milieus. Single-cell analysis using these assays for proteins can uncover protein expression heterogeneity in seemingly homogeneous cell populations, which will provide insight into the pathogenesis mechanisms of diseases such as cancer and autoimmune diseases. The combination of high-throughput screening technologies with antibody-based assays also allows for the discovery of novel biomarkers, hence advancing precision medicine initiatives and therapeutic strategies. Improved techniques in the past decade in antibody engineering, along with the streamlining of assay protocols, have allowed for the specificity and sensitivity of protein detection to improve, hence raising the overall usefulness of these types of approaches. For example, the identification of nanobodies and other small antibodies holds promise for providing unprecedented resolution into cellular interactions. In addition, the incorporation of antibody-based methods into high-content imaging systems has enabled visualization of complex cellular microenvironments and interactions. In addition to enhancing the detection of proteins in individual cells, these developments also promote an enhanced understanding of immune dynamics. Ultimately, the role of antibody-based assays in single-cell analysis will redefine molecular immunology's future and transform therapeutic planning for many diseases, ranging from infectious diseases to cancer.

8.4.3. Challenges in Single-Cell Proteomics

Single-cell proteomics is faced with a number of challenges that negatively impact global protein analysis within single cells. One of the major issues arises from the intrinsic heterogeneity and complexity of biological samples, which normally contain a rich blend of cell types with differentiated protein profiles. The heterogeneity of cell types makes it difficult to draw firm conclusions because classic bulk proteomics techniques cannot recognize the subtlety that exists at the single-cell level. Furthermore, the sensitivity and specificity of current proteomic techniques also make the challenge all the more daunting, as most proteins may potentially be present in astoundingly low amounts and hence go undetected. Therefore, researchers must employ advanced techniques and equipment capable of untangling proteomic data accurately without compromising cellular information fidelity, since the success of stratifying information is crucial to identifying essential biomarkers for molecular immunology. Another significant challenge of single-cell proteomics is data integration and interpretation of high-throughput data generated by advanced methods such as mass spectrometry and imaging-based proteomics. As highlighted in recent studies, the integration of proteomic data with other omics data, such as genomics and transcriptomics, is a significant computational challenge due to the nonuniformity of structure and formats of data. This complexity necessitates the development of standardized computational pipelines that are capable of not just analyzing but also seamlessly integrating such datasets. Integration of machine learning and artificial intelligence techniques has emerged as a desirable solution, considering the fact that such algorithms are better able to visualize the intricate interdependencies between various biological variables.

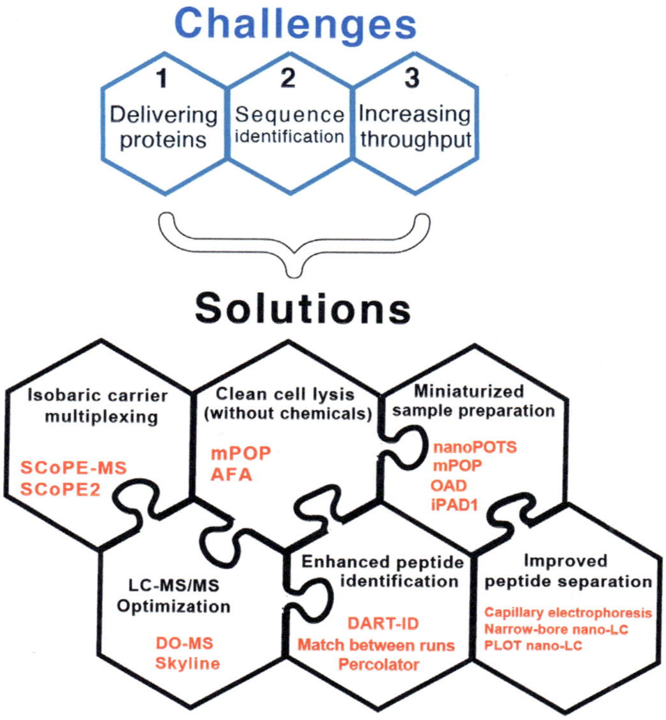

Figure 8.11. Major challenges to single-cell protein analysis by mass-spectrometry and their solutions Single-cell proteomics.

Source: https://www.researchgate.net/profile/Nikolai-Slavov/publication/340475438/figure/fig1/AS:877527161634821@1586230187246/Major-challenges-to-single-cell-protein-analysis-by-mass-spectrometry-and-their.png.

However, the successful implementation of these strategies relies heavily on efficient algorithms and sufficient computational capabilities, an entry barrier for the majority of research laboratories (Dezem et al., 2024). Also, technical limitations surrounding current single-cell proteomic techniques remain to hinder their cross-laboratory reproducibility and common usage. Methods such as mass spectrometry imaging and multiplexed immunofluorescence are full of high-resolution protein analysis potential but also create significant analytical and methodological hurdles. For instance, mass spectrometry imaging, by allowing accurate information on protein localization, typically struggles in terms of spatial resolution and sensitivity in complex tissue environments. Similarly, multiplexed immunofluorescence is also subject to cross-reactive antibody problems, which preclude accurate protein quantitation within single cells. To address these issues, novel solutions in the form of improved reagents and novel imaging technology must be conceptualized and engineered. Convergence of single-cell analysis and spatial proteomics can possibly lead to improved research in the area of molecular immunology, allowing for personalized treatment strategies and diagnostic tools (Liyanage & Guo, 2024) (Figure 8.11).

8.5. Applications in Disease Research

The development of single-cell analysis techniques has revolutionized the landscape of disease exploration with unparalleled accuracy of cellular heterogeneity in complex biological systems. Such fineness is particularly important in probing the immune system, as various cells can do very dissimilar things that together constitute the disease pathology. By investigating cellular behavior at the single-cell level, researchers can identify and characterize new cell populations contributing to diseases ranging from autoimmune disease to cancer. Such advanced analyses allow researchers to design targeted therapies, elucidating the mechanisms of disease development and response to treatment, ultimately leading to the development of personalized medicine approaches. Besides, the technologies of single cells allow not only the identification of heterogeneous cell types but also the investigation of their interactions with the immunological microenvironment. As an illustration, understanding how various immune cells interact in the presence of tumor cells or infections can uncover integral pathways that can be targeted for therapy. For infectious diseases, understanding generated through single-cell analysis can be pivotal in uncovering immune evasion strategies employed by pathogens. In the case of diseases like African trypanosomiasis, immunity manipulation is a hallmark aspect of disease survival and virulence, as outlined in Stijlemans et al. (2017). Using these approaches, our approach to de-mystifying complex disease mechanisms, therefore, can be significantly enhanced. Finally, integrating single-cell analysis with advanced immunological studies has revealed new avenues towards diagnostic and therapeutic strategies. With the use of high-throughput sequencing and imaging technologies, scientists are now able to create accurate maps of cellular activity in disease to reveal new biomarkers at an accelerated rate. This is demonstrated in nanobody design for disease diagnosis and treatment, which are highly advantageous over conventional antibodies from their unique characteristics, as detailed in Stijlemans et al. (2017). The implications are vast, not just for the outcomes of research but also for clinical practice, in that these single-cell insights hold open the promise of innovation in early diagnosis and targeted therapeutic treatment of various diseases and, thus, revolutionizing how we tackle and combat various diseases.

8.5.1. Role in Cancer Immunology

Investigating the potential of applying single-cell analysis techniques in cancer immunology holds profound implications for insight into tumor-immune dynamics. Classic bulk analysis is prone to smearing valuable cellular heterogeneity and providing oversimplified data on the immune status of cancer. Through the employment of single-cell omics, researchers can delineate discrete immune cell populations within the tumor and enumerate disparate phenotypes and functional states. This level of resolution permits identification of rare yet informative cell types that could play a significant role in tumor growth or response to therapy. Higher resolution enables a deeper insight into the mechanisms through which tumors are hidden from the immune system, thus providing new avenues for therapeutic intervention to re-activate the immune system against cancer. What insights can be gained through such analysis can be applied in the construction of more effective immunotherapies specifically tailored to the specific makeup of a patient's tumor microenvironment, leading to personalized medicine in oncology. The application of single-cell multi-omics approaches further illuminates the field of cancer immunology by integrating various molecular levels of cellular understanding.

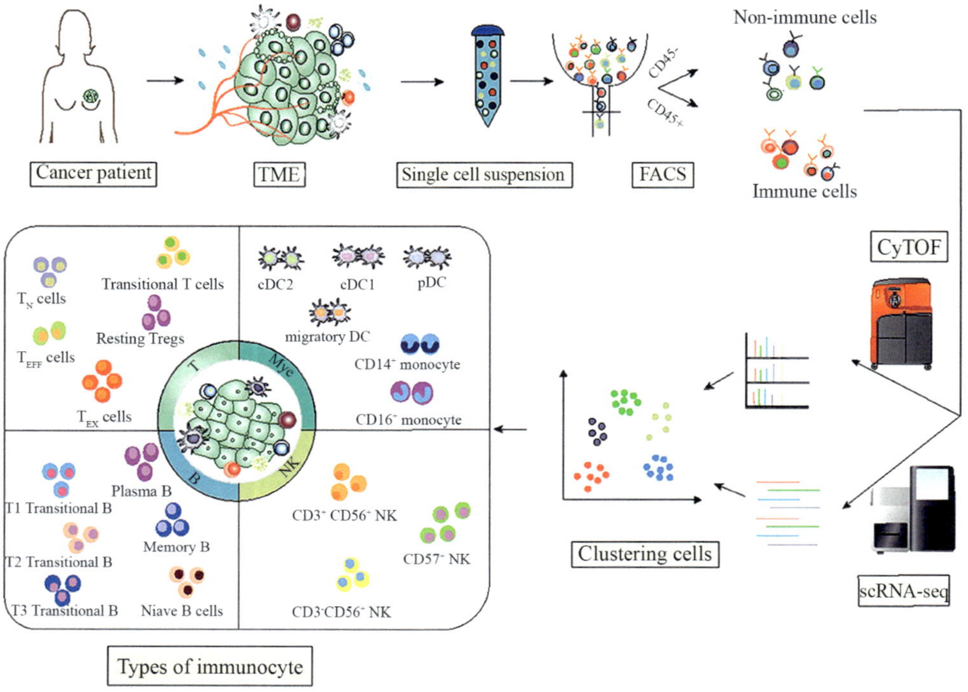

Figure 8.12. State of the art of single-cell technology and its application in breast cancer studies.

Source: https://www.researchgate.net/publication/349635005/figure/fig1/AS:1143128125102107 8@1718119804146/State-of-the-art-of-single-cell-technology-and-its-application-in-breast-cancer-studies.tif.

It not only reveals gene expression and protein production but also accounts for the interactions and regulatory networks that influence immune responses against cancers. By deconvolving the intricate pathways of interaction within the tumor microenvironment, researchers can identify major checkpoints that govern immune activation or suppression. Such integrated analyses broaden the understanding of tumor immune evasion mechanisms and offer invaluable information about how tumors develop as they adapt to therapeutic stresses. Single-cell analysis, for instance, became pivotal to understanding how immune checkpoint inhibitors reconstitute the cellular structure of tumors and thereby modulate the efficacy of the treatment. Such discoveries are likely to guide subsequent therapeutic regimens and tailor those to specifically target subpopulations of immune cells, thereby optimizing treatments for overall cancer immunotherapy. In addition, single-cell analysis incorporation within cancer immunology is a valuable platform for the discovery of new biomarkers and therapeutic targets. Researchers utilize the high-resolution information obtained from single-cell approaches in order to uncover novel expression patterns linked to tumor immunogenicity, ultimately resulting in the identification of immunogenic neoantigens that can be targeted in vaccine development. For example, the technology of single cells has made it possible to analyze T-cell receptor repertoires, linking specific T-cell functions with clinical outcomes in cancer therapy. These discoveries are groundbreaking because they have enabled the development of individualized cancer vaccines dependent on an individual's immune profile. Furthermore, as demonstrated through some of the new developments in live cell imaging technologies allied with single-cell technologies, it is possible to visualize dynamic interactions between tumors and immune cells in real time, providing further insight into live tumor microenvironments. These are complemented by the technologies emphasizing the single-cell analysis technologies' revolutionary impact in driving cancer immunology as a discipline and enhancing therapeutic strategy in cancer therapy (Figure 8.12).

8.5.2. Insights Into Autoimmune Diseases

The complexity of autoimmune diseases provides in-depth insights that result in innovations in molecular immunology. Autoimmune diseases result from an abnormal immune response system that attacks the body's tissue by mistake, leading to inflammation and tissue damage. The genetic underpinning of such conditions, such as the association of particular alleles of human leukocyte antigen (HLA) with disorders like Ankylosing Spondylitis (AS), is an indicator of the large role played by genetic predispositions in the aetiology of autoimmune disorders. For instance, the prevalence of HLA-B27 in patients with AS is very high, which reflects a strong genetic underpinning for the disorder. This connection highlights the value of pioneering single-cell analysis techniques, which can reveal how genetic markers interact with immune responses to provide information on disease mechanisms and potential therapeutic targets (Paladini et al., 2019). Moreover, the analysis of somatic hypermutation (SHM) of immunoglobulin variable-region genes sheds light on the adaptive immune response in autoimmune diseases. By applying lineage tree analysis of autoimmune disease patients' B cell clones, such as Myasthenia Gravis and Rheumatoid Arthritis, researchers gain informative data regarding the mechanism of antibody diversification and selection in autoimmune responses. By quantifying the characteristics of the lineage trees, researchers are able to compare SHM dynamics in different lymphoid tissues, thus offering insight into how tissue-specific mechanisms may influence the onset of autoimmune diseases. Forming these connections has tremendous implications for developing targeted therapies, since understanding the chronic nature of the disease can direct treatment paradigms toward modulating such processes (Steiman-Shimony et al., 2006). Single-cell analysis techniques not only enhance our understanding of autoimmune diseases, but they also enable us to detect new biomarkers and therapeutic targets. By interrogating single cells from tissue microenvironments, researchers can reveal autoimmunity's intricate signaling pathways and cell-to-cell interactions that orchestrate disease. At this level of detail, one can reveal unique cellular profiles that underlie disease states, providing new opportunities for precision medicine. Also, as immune cell populations evolve in time through SHM and other mechanisms, it may become feasible to track these changes at a single-cell level and thus offer vital information for disease progression and routes to relapse. In this context, the inclusion of single-cell analysis in autoimmune disease research has the potential to change our approaches towards diagnosis, monitoring, and treatment (Steiman-Shimony et al., 2006; Paladini et al., 2019) (Figure 8.13).

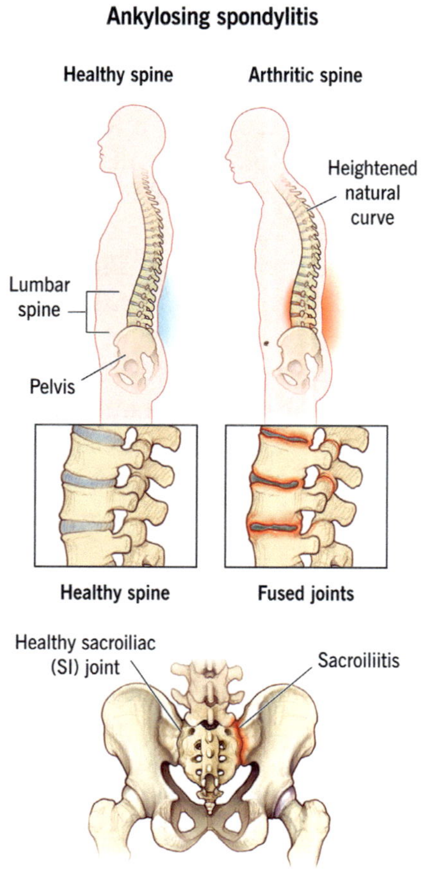

Figure 8.13. Illustration of ankylosing spondylitis (AS).

Source: https://my.clevelandclinic.org/-/scassets/images/org/health/articles/ankylosing-spondylitis.jpg.

8.5.3. Potential in Infectious Disease Studies

The identification of infectious diseases has been greatly enhanced by advances in single-cell analysis techniques within molecular immunology. Such advanced techniques allow scientists to interrogate the heterogeneity of immune responses at a previously unattainable level, which might improve the understanding of pathogen-host cell interactions. Through techniques such as scRNA-seq, scientists are able to untangle the complex cellular responses elicited by infection, revealing the specifics of how different immune cells respond uniquely to pathogens. This specificity permits us to more fully understand disease mechanisms, particularly in heterogeneous infections where responses can vary immensely between hosts. By identifying specific cellular pathways and recognition modes, such investigations pave the way for specific therapeutic intervention to boost immune responses against diverse infectious pathogens, thereby leading to improved patient management in infections that have been recalcitrant to treatment. Recent breakthroughs in the identification of pattern recognition receptors (PRRs) have also placed emphasis on their core role in host defense during infection. PRRs contribute to the initiation of immune responses by recognizing certain molecular patterns associated with pathogens and thus bridging innate and adaptive immunity. Single-cell response mapping upon PRR activation has the promise to uncover how infections hijack such pathways to evade host immunity. Recent research indicates the effectiveness of interrogating PRR pathways in clarifying how different immune cells respond to infections and implies insights into their potential therapeutic role in disease (Li et al., 2021). This may inform the design of vaccines and therapeutic agents that can better employ the immune system, offering new approaches to combat infectious diseases that exhibit variable immune responses across populations. Finally, the potential of postbiotics in infection research represents an intriguing horizon of molecular immunology. Since preparations of dead microorganisms or their components with health impacts, postbiotics can modulate immune reactions and serve as a second-choice therapeutic strategy in disease treatment involving infections. As mechanisms of how postbiotics work become clearer with more studies, there is a growing potential to leverage these compounds with single-cell analysis methods to track immune system changes following postbiotic treatment (Salminen et al., 2021). By characterizing cellular and molecular changes resulting from postbiotics, scientists can identify new immune protection mechanisms for enhancing immune protection as well as designing new therapeutic models for infectious diseases, expanding the horizon of molecular immunology against health challenges posed by pathogens.

8.6. Future Directions in Single-Cell Analysis

Exploring future directions in single-cell analysis suggests enormous potential for molecular immunology research. New approaches not only aim to enhance the resolution of and selectivity between molecular analysis but also to improve cellular heterogeneity. Single-cell endoscopy is one such novel method that offers a least-invasive method for interrogating single cells without perturbing their physiological state. Facilitating flexible single-cell manipulation and ultrasensitive detection, this technique might revolutionize how intracellular processes are investigated by scientists. As described in contemporary studies, single-cell endoscopy holds promise for applications ranging from targeted drug delivery to precise molecular sensing and thus becomes an important tool in deconstructing complex immunological responses and aiding therapeutic innovation (Xue et al., 2025). Moreover, single-cell sequencing (SCS) continues to soar as a backbone method in the field because of its ability to recover genomic and transcriptomic data to levels of unprecedented depth. Studies using bibliometrics have indicated a rising trend of SCS-related publications every year, which is indicative of a mounting trend towards incorporating this technology in numerous fields of research, including immunology (Chen et al., 2024). Through the analysis of immune responses on the single-cell level with the help of SCS, researchers acquire important insights into the dynamics of cellular interactions and cellular populations in the immune system. Guidance for future research can be directed towards streamlining sequencing protocols to achieve maximum throughput and precision and towards the extension of applications to studies of epigenomics. This is required for the understanding of disease and the development of new immunotherapeutic strategies. Finally, the future of single-cell analysis in molecular immunology depends on the continuing development of hybrid approaches that combine prevailing methodologies with new techniques. Technologies that integrate single-cell sequencing with imaging and proteomics will likely yield more insightful datasets, enabling researchers to relate different cellular biomarkers and responses. By adopting the building of artificial intelligence and machine learning, researchers will likely more accurately interpret dense datasets, identifying new cell types and states that enable immune responses. These integration strategies not only have the potential to extend our understanding of disease and health, but also position single-cell analysis at the forefront of precision medicine and immunology-targeted treatment (Chen et al., 2024; Xue et al., 2025).

8.6.1. Integration of Multi-Omics Approaches

The coming together of multi-omics approaches is now a revolutionary tool in molecular immunology, which generates insight into complex cellular processes that are potentially lost when analyzing through single-omics alone. Through the concurrent analysis of genomic, transcriptomic, proteomic, and metabolomic data within an individual cell, researchers are able to make comprehensive biological profiles that identify the interactive functions of biomolecules in immunity. This holistic perspective emphasizes the dynamic functions played by cellular systems, where crosstalk between different omic layers has a critical impact on cellular outcomes, including differentiation and activation states. Utilization of advanced computational algorithms and systems biology models for interrogation of such heterogeneous data sets enables new biomarkers and therapeutic targets and ultimately leads to a better understanding of immunological mechanisms underlying disease and health. The value of multi-omics is not merely in its potential to provide a more intricate view of biological systems but also in the potential role it can play in personalized medicine and targeted therapy. A primary challenge to the integration of multi-omics is the requirement for a robust computational infrastructure that is able to handle large, high-dimensional data. Traditional analytical methods are poor at capturing complexity and interactions within multi-omics data. Therefore, new mathematical models and bioinformatics tools are critical to bring together information from separated omic layers.

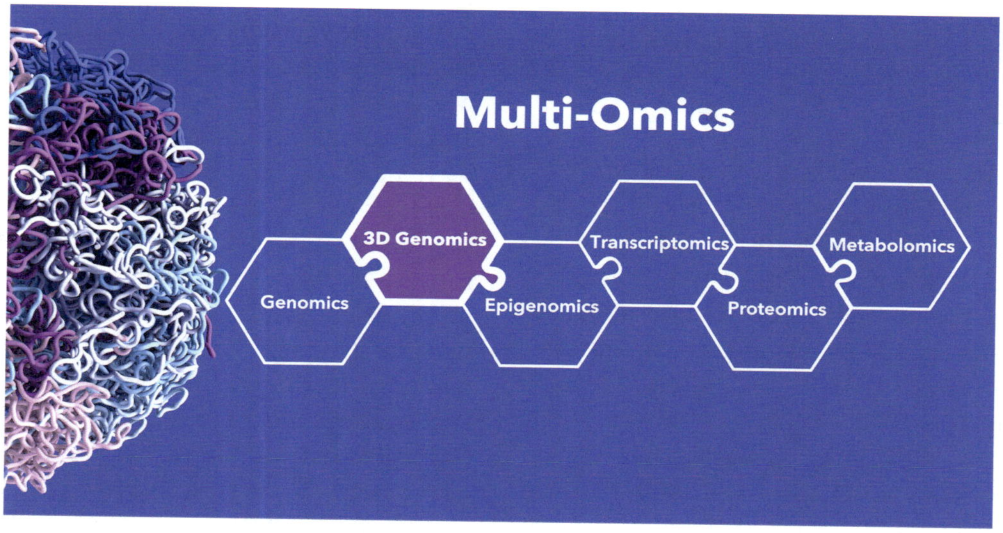

Figure 8.14. Multi-omics approaches: An overview.

Source: https://dromicslabs.com/multi-omics-an-overview/.

These models facilitate the prediction of biological behavior through the interaction of varying molecular components instead of singling out individual contributions. For instance, as discussed in recent advancements, maximal integration of proteomic and genomic data can identify immune regulation mechanisms that, otherwise, remain unaccounted for by individual analysis. One needs to grasp the mathematical concepts behind these computational approaches because they are solely responsible for whether the finding of clinically relevant biomarkers and therapeutic targets becomes possible or not, based on the integration perspective in multi-omics approaches (Wang & Sarwal, 2015). Within the field of single-cell technologies, the use of multi-omics approaches not only enriches our understanding of immune cell function but also provides access to new lines of inquiry into cellular heterogeneity and plasticity. Systems biology concepts distill an inherently holistic framework in which individual cell information is positioned within larger biological contexts. Through methodologies that integrate empirical data and theoretical modeling, scientists can see how immune cells dynamically communicate under various immunological stresses, such as infection or inflammation. The integrative approach also allows the examination of how environmental conditions can influence cellular states at various levels of omics. Therefore, with the continued advancement of multi-omics and its incorporation into next-generation single-cell analytical technologies, capabilities for the discovery of immune system function and disease processes complexity will undoubtedly increase, eventually culminating in immunological research and therapy advancement (Woelders et al., 2011) (Figure 8.14).

8.6.2. Advances in Computational Analysis

Computational analysis advances have had a remarkable influence on single-cell analytical techniques in molecular immunology by introducing imaging flow cytometry (IFC) into the fold. By the union of flow cytometry's capacity to enumerate cell populations nimbly with high-resolution fluorescent microscopy, researchers can now perform enriched multiparametric analysis on single cells. The latest advent of light-field microscopy (LFM) has further supplemented this approach, enabling 3D cellular structures to be imaged with hitherto unprecedented spatial resolution. By contrast, conventional approaches generally did not cut it, for the requirement for high resolution and high throughput often consigned data quality to the starting gate. The development of a light-field flow cytometer (LFC) is the breakthrough here, harnessing cutting-edge optofluidics and stroboscopic illumination to deliver near-diffraction-limited imaging at unprecedented speeds. These advances have broad implications for the understanding of cellular mechanisms in health and disease and mark a significant advancement in biomedical science and clinical diagnostics (Hua et al., 2025). Moreover, advances in computational methodology have revolutionized the manner in which scientists interpret and examine richly detailed datasets generated from single-cell technologies. The application of machine learning algorithms, for instance, has enabled automatic identification of high-dimensional data and derivation of meaningful biological insights from large datasets from single-cell experiments. Traditional analysis techniques cannot cope with the brute force of data and its complexity, but computational frameworks provide solutions to these issues through the identification of patterns and relationships that are otherwise hard to see. With these algorithms, researchers are able to gain a better understanding of cellular heterogeneity and dynamics to more precisely investigate immune responses at the single-cell level. These analyses hold importance in numerous domains, from finding new targets for therapeutics to building new treatments in immunology and cancer biology (Xu et al., 2025). Lastly, the application of computational analysis to single-cell analysis cannot be overstated, as it enables researchers to achieve high-resolution three-dimensional (3D) measurements of tissue structure and cell-to-cell interactions. Such 3D visualization techniques enable more intuitive comprehension of tissue organization and function, eventually giving way to critical insight into the microenvironments governing immune responses. Modern computing capabilities can integrate data from multiple imaging modalities and couple it with spatial omics approaches to give an integrated view of cellular functions within their physiological context. Progress of the field into the future will necessitate that current challenges—standardization of methodologies and improving data robustness—be overcome. By overcoming these challenges, the full potential of advanced computational analysis in single-cell research is put into prominence, and additional innovation in molecular immunology and precision medicine is facilitated (Xu et al., 2025).

8.6.3. Ethical Considerations in Single-Cell Research

Ethical concerns in single-cell studies are central to preventing innovation in molecular immunology coming at the expense of moral integrity. While single-cell investigations reveal intricate mechanisms at the cellular level, researchers must navigate a landscape of issues with ethical considerations, particularly when human tissues are utilized. This is especially so in the case of allogeneic hematopoietic stem cell transplantation (allo-HSCT) where donors, including children, may be under grave risk. Ethical practice focuses on the safety of donors taking precedence in the donation procedure, demanding that informed consent be obtained, and that the potential benefits to recipients surpass the risks. This approach emphasizes the need for ethical control, where researchers not only adhere to institutional practice but are also required to meet broader societal issues related to their research and specifically in consent processes and safeguarding of the donor (La Russa et al., 2017). Apart from donor-specific issues, single-cell research also presents ethical concerns on a general level in terms of data privacy and use implications of using cellular data. As single-cell technologies generate enormous data on single cells, including epigenetic and genetic data, scientists need to be vigilant about maintaining participant anonymity and confidentiality. Single-cell data analysis typically presents challenges regarding handling sensitive data, particularly in human subject research. The potential misuse of genetic data or its impact on family privacy can have a lasting ethical impact. Therefore, researchers must institute robust data governance mechanisms to counter the problem, achieving equilibrium between path-breaking research and adherence to human rights as well as scientific ethics (Salvatore et al., 2015). In addition, the intersection of technological progress and ethical issues in single-cell analyses invites an argument for the general social implications of such discoveries produced by these analyses. Single-cell analysis techniques have the potential to revolutionize disease diagnosis, but researchers are also called to ensure that applications of their findings do not contribute to existing inequalities or reinforce biased health interventions. The ethical principle of justice mandates that scientific advances in single-cell research benefit a diverse populace and not aggravate health inequalities. Scientists thus have to critically analyze their research with respect to social justice issues, actively involving oppressed groups in the research process and facilitating fair distribution of the benefits accrued from scientific advancements (Salvatore et al., 2015).

SUMMARY

In pointing out the advances and conclusions of single-cell analysis techniques in molecular immunology, it is observed that such techniques have greatly changed our understanding of immune cell function and heterogeneity. Through the capability of measuring cell behaviors and properties on an individual basis, single-cell methods allow a high-resolution picture that bulk analysis techniques are unable to achieve. This is particularly crucial in the examination of paucicellular immune populations, such as Tregs, whose activities are critical to the maintenance of immunological homeostasis and tolerance. As an example, such experiments have demonstrated that the expansion of Tregs can be successfully generated with preservation of suppressive function, illustrating the utility of single-cell analysis to engineer enhanced therapeutic strategies to autoimmune disease and graft-versus-host disease (Earle et al., 2005). Lastly, the conclusions of these studies provide avenues for more advanced immunotherapeutic treatments and enhanced immunological understanding of immune response dynamics. Single-cell analysis implications also extend beyond therapy in medicine and have an impact on fundamental immunological investigations. An understanding of the molecular and cellular networks governing immune responses can shed light on the etiology of numerous diseases, including allergies and autoimmune diseases. The inclusion of ideas such as the adverse outcome pathway (AOP) framework in analytical procedures is critical to developing a comprehensive understanding of immune processes (Lozano-Ojalvo et al., 2019). Apart from making the identification of the sensitizing capacity of food proteins and other compounds systematic, it also helps direct research agendas aimed at reducing immune-related disease. By basing current testing methodologies on the more established features of the AOP, investigators are more effective in surmounting the immune system's complexities in finer detail, ultimately to develop a more refined approach to risk evaluation and therapeutic treatment. Single-cell analysis methodologies overall constitute a paradigm shift in molecular immunology, closing the gap between basic and clinical applications. The capacity to interrogate the immune landscape at the single-cell level enhances the capacity to identify and characterize heterogeneous immune cell populations, leading to precise and personalized therapeutic interventions. Ongoing progress in this direction will undoubtedly identify additional biomarkers and therapeutic targets as the sophistication of such techniques continues to enhance, with a greater understanding of immune reactions to different stimuli. The ongoing integration of advanced methodologies, such as those created in response to the AOP framework, will not only enhance research effectiveness but also ensure new treatments are safe when applied to modify immune responses. In the future, the joint contributions in single-cell analysis will undoubtedly shape the future of immunology and push innovation development in research and therapeutic applications faster.

The field of molecular immunology has witnessed revolutionary advancements with the emergence of single-cell analysis tools, making them pivotal to cell heterogeneity and functional diversity within immune populations. The tools allow researchers to break down the individualized profiles of single cells that belong to the immune system, where their function in health and disease can be dissected. With the growing understanding of the human microbiome's contribution to immune function, the inclusion of single-cell analysis is now imperative in the examination of these complex interactions. By allowing scientists to gain deep insight into immune cell interactions at the single-cell level, researchers are better able to create more accurate therapies and interventions and, ultimately, improve patient outcomes and propel personalized medicine projects in oncology and elsewhere in immunology (Pizzo, 2019). Single-cell data analysis is particularly daunting, considering the immense amount of biological information generated through high-throughput methods. Traditional analytical tools have been seen to fail in accommodating the complexity and heterogeneity inherent in such data sets. New cluster algorithms and bioinformatics software have played key roles in the successful interpretation of single-cell RNA sequencing data. For instance, new algorithms like GExposer have been designed in order to enhance the detection of differentially expressed genes and mitigate bias induced by sequencing artefacts. Ongoing development of these analytical tools is imperative in order to advance our knowledge of immune functions and enhance the precision of therapeutic applications in molecular immunology (Wu et al., 2015). Furthermore, the application of single-cell analysis extends beyond characterization alone to the real-time adjustment of treatment for hematologic malignancies and other complex diseases. What is obtained from single-cell research has an important bearing in characterizing disease mechanisms, identifying novel biomarkers, and facilitating the development of targeted therapies. For instance, differential coexpression analysis is now an essential tool in the unraveling of the regulatory networks for diseases like Type 2 diabetes and cancers. By revealing how different cellular pathways interact and function independently or synergistically, such approaches greatly enhance the practice of precision medicine, whereby treatment is individually tailored to an individual's own cellular landscape, ensuring greater efficacy of treatment and fewer side effects (Pizzo, 2019).

A CLOSER LOOK

SOMATIC HYPERMUTATION (SHM)

SHM is a significant mechanism of the adaptive immune response in which B cells introduce mutations into their immunoglobulin (antibody) genes, especially in the variable regions. The mechanism, occurring in germinal centers (GCs) of lymph nodes, is a prerequisite for affinity maturation, enabling B cells to produce antibodies with greater affinity to a specific antigen. SHM utilizes the activation-induced cytidine deaminase (AID) enzyme to create DNA lesions that are then processed by DNA repair processes (Figure 8.15).

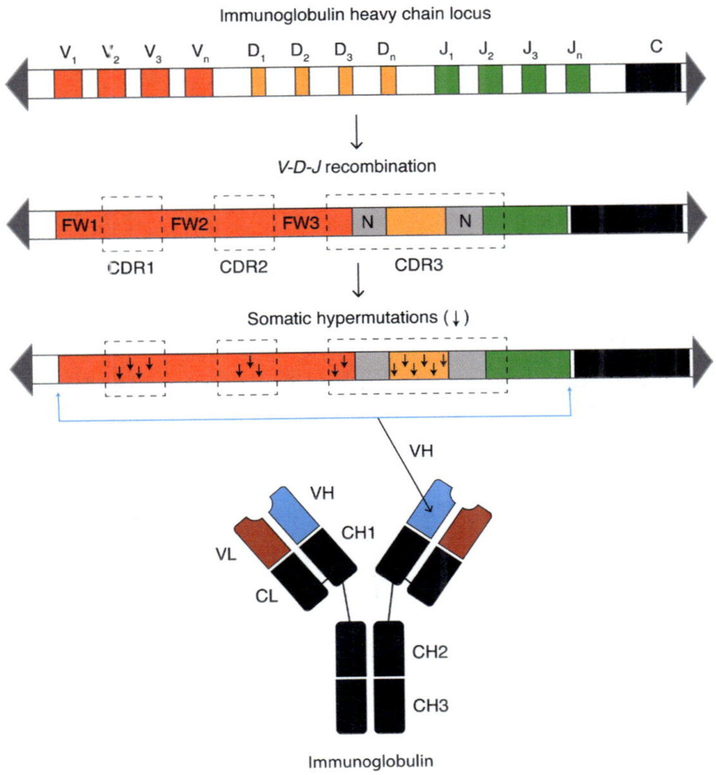

Figure 8.15. Simplistic overview of V(D)J recombination and somatic hypermutations at the immunoglobulin heavy chain variable region.

Source: https://upload.wikimedia.org/wikipedia/commons/thumb/b/bc/Somatic_hypermutation_v5.png/800px-Somatic_hypermutation_v5.png.

- **AID's Function:**
  - AID is a cytidine deaminase and the major SHM enzyme.
  - Deaminates cytosines in DNA to uracil.

- This creates a U:G mismatch in the DNA.

- **Uracil Lesion Processing:**
  - The uracil can be detected by a range of DNA repair processes.
  - One of the mechanisms involves uracil-DNA glycosylase (UNG), which removes the uracil, resulting in an abasic site.
  - This site may be processed by different DNA polymerases, leading to mutations.
  - The second mechanism involves mismatch repair (MMR) proteins, causing mutations upon their repair of the U:G mismatch.
- **Variable Region Targeting:**
  - SHM primarily targets the variable (V) regions of immunoglobulin heavy and light chains.
  - These regions are responsible for antigen binding.
  - Mutations in such areas are capable of altering the shape and binding ability of the antibody.
- **Affinity Maturation:**
  - B cells acquire mutations in their antibody genes via SHM.
  - B cells possessing antibodies with higher affinity are selected and amplified in the germinal center.
  - Such a process, also known as affinity maturation, results in antibodies binding more strongly to the antigen.
- **Importance in Immunity:**
  - SHM is critical for the generation of a diverse repertoire of high-affinity antibodies.
  - High-affinity antibodies have a pivotal role in effective immune responses against pathogens.
  - Through enhancing antibody affinity, SHM participates in long-term protection provided by the immune system.

REFERENCES

1. Steiman-Shimony, A., Edelman, H., Barak, M., Shahaf, G., Dunn-Walters, D., Stott, D. I., Abraham, R. S., & Mehr, R. (2006). Immunoglobulin variable-region gene mutational lineage tree analysis: application to autoimmune diseases. *Autoimmunity reviews*, *5*(4), 242–251. https://doi.org/10.1016/j.autrev.2005.07.008(accessed on 27th June 2025).

2. Hauton C. The scope of the crustacean immune system for disease control. *J Invertebr Pathol.* 2012;110(2):251-260. doi:10.1016/j.jip.2012.03.005Miho E, Yermanos A, Weber CR, Berger CT, Reddy ST, Greiff V. Computational Strategies for Dissecting the High-Dimensional Complexity of Adaptive Immune Repertoires. *Front Immunol.* 2018;9:224. Published 2018 Feb 21. doi:10.3389/fimmu.2018.00224(accessed on 27th June 2025).

3. Ma, N., Kamalakshakurup, G., Aghaamoo, M., Lee, A. P., & Digman, M. A. (2019). Label-Free Metabolic Classification of Single Cells in Droplets Using the Phasor Approach to Fluorescence Lifetime Imaging Microscopy. *Cytometry. Part A : the journal of the International Society for Analytical Cytology*, *95*(1), 93–100. https://doi.org/10.1002/cyto.a.23673(accessed on 27th June 2025).

4. Altman, M. O., & Gagneux, P. (2019). Absence of Neu5Gc and Presence of Anti-Neu5Gc Antibodies in Humans-An Evolutionary Perspective. *Frontiers in immunology*, *10*, 789. https://doi.org/10.3389/fimmu.2019.00789 (accessed on 27th June 2025).

5. Alyasin, A., Weidele, K., Botteron, C., Klein, C. A., & Czyż, Z. (2024). Abstract 3704: Whole genome and targeted proteome analysis of single cancer cells. *Cancer Research*. https://www.semanticscholar.org/paper/85b068a1fd2372360460a2b42717e69b2db6a81f (accessed on 27th June 2025).

6. Woelders, H., Te Pas, M. F., Bannink, A., Veerkamp, R. F., & Smits, M. A. (2011). Systems biology in animal sciences. *Animal : an international journal of animal bioscience*, *5*(7), 1036–1047. https://doi.org/10.1017/S1751731111000036(accessed on 27th June 2025).

7. Barati, M., Wilkey, D., Klein, J. B., & Cummins, T. (2025). Comparative proteomic analysis of whole kidney, medulla, and cortical tubules in diabetic pathogenesis of kidney injury in mice. *Journal of Visualized Experiments: JoVE, 219*. https://www.semanticscholar.org/paper/762778a2f0bfe386c429667329519312434687d3 (accessed on 27th June 2025).

8. Daniel Lozano-Ojalvo, Sara Benede, Celia M. Antunes, Simona L. Bavaro, Grégory Bouchaud, et al.. Applying the adverse outcome pathway (AOP) for food sensitization to support in vitro testing strategies. Trends in Food Science and Technology, 2019, 85, pp.307-319. ⟨10.1016/j.tifs.2019.01.014⟩. ⟨hal-02623081⟩(accessed on 27th June 2025).

9. Earle, K. E., Tang, Q., Zhou, X., Liu, W., Zhu, S., Bonyhadi, M. L., & Bluestone, J. A. (2005). In vitro expanded human CD4+CD25+ regulatory T cells suppress effector T cell proliferation. *Clinical immunology (Orlando, Fla.)*, *115*(1), 3–9. https://doi.org/10.1016/j.clim.2005.02.017(accessed on 27th June 2025).

10. McLoughlin, K. E., Nalpas, N. C., Rue-Albrecht, K., Browne, J. A., Magee, D. A., Killick, K. E., Park, S. D., Hokamp, K., Meade, K. G., O'Farrelly, C., Gormley, E., Gordon, S. V., & MacHugh, D. E. (2014). RNA-seq Transcriptional Profiling of Peripheral Blood Leukocytes from Cattle Infected with Mycobacterium bovis. *Frontiers in immunology*, *5*, 396. https://doi.org/10.3389/fimmu.2014.00396(accessed on 27th June 2025).

11. Stijlemans B, De Baetselier P, Caljon G, Van Den Abbeele J, Van Ginderachter JA, Magez S. Nanobodies As Tools to Understand, Diagnose, and Treat African Trypanosomiasis. *Front Immunol.* 2017;8:724. Published 2017 Jun 30. doi:10.3389/fimmu.2017.00724(accessed on 27th June 2025).

12. Carbone, E., D'Oro, U., De Felice, M., Di Rosa, F., et al. (2020). Serafino Zappacosta: An enlightened mentor and educator. https://core.ac.uk/download/323077038.pdf (accessed on 27th June 2025).

13. Salvatore F, Cariati F, Tomaiuolo R (2015) Facts, Challenges, Difficulties and Hopes in Single-Cell Biology: Physiopathological Studies. Single Cell Biol 4: 121. doi:10.4172/2168-9431.1000121Derecka, M., Herman, J. S., Cauchy, P., Ramamoorthy, S., Lupar, E., Grün, D., & Grosschedl, R. (2020). EBF1-deficient bone marrow stroma elicits persistent changes in HSC potential. *Nature immunology, 21*(3), 261–273. https://doi.org/10.1038/s41590-020-0595-7Paladini, F., Fiorillo, M. T., Tedeschi, V., Cauli, A., Mathieu, A., & Sorrentino, R. (2019). Ankylosing Spondylitis: A Trade Off of HLA-B27, ERAP, and Pathogen Interconnections? Focus on Sardinia. *Frontiers in immunology, 10,* 35. https://doi.org/10.3389/fimmu.2019.00035(accessed on 27th June 2025).

14. Chen, H. C., Ma, Y., Cheng, J., & Chen, Y. C. (2024). Advances in single-cell techniques for linking phenotypes to genotypes. *Cancer Heterogeneity and Plasticity, 11.* https://www.semanticscholar.org/paper/b1bb0534cf6f72176c966878e2924974c47306ed (accessed on 27th June 2025).

15. Chen, L., Wan, Y., Yang, T., Zhang, Q., Zeng, Y., Zheng, S., Ling, Z., et al. (2024). Bibliometric and visual analysis of single-cell sequencing from 2010 to 2022. *Frontiers in Genetics, 14.* https://www.semanticscholar.org/paper/d0c40805ff8a219816bbb9396911b30ecf7ad464 (accessed on 27th June 2025).

16. Looney, T. J., Topacio-Hall, D., Lowman, G., Conroy, J., Morrison, C., Oh, D., Fong, L., & Zhang, L. (2020). TCR Convergence in Individuals Treated With Immune Checkpoint Inhibition for Cancer. *Frontiers in immunology, 10,* 2985. https://doi.org/10.3389/fimmu.2019.02985(accessed on 27th June 2025).

17. Dezem, F., Morosini, N. S., Arjumand, W., DuBose, H., & Plummer, J. T. (2024). Spatially resolved single-cell omics: Methods, challenges, and future perspectives. *Annual Review of Biomedical Data Science.* https://www.semanticscholar.org/paper/fd2180e6d1ea32e2b561a660e1623766ccf3ec7c (accessed on 27th June 2025).

18. El-Rami, F., Nelson, K., & Xu, P. (2017). Proteomic Approach for Extracting Cytoplasmic Proteins from *Streptococcus sanguinis* using Mass Spectrometry. *Journal of molecular biology research, 7*(1), 50–57. https://doi.org/10.5539/jmbr.v7n1p50(accessed on 27th June 2025).

19. Englund, S. (2002). Molecular biology techniques as a tool for detection and characterization of *Mycobacterium avium* subsp. *paratuberculosis.* https://core.ac.uk/download/11694594.pdf (accessed on 27th June 2025).

20. S., O., Staunton, L., FitzGerald, O., & R., S. (2013). Biomarkers of Inflammatory Arthritis and Proteomics. InTech. doi: 10.5772/54218(accessed on 27th June 2025).

21. Hua, X., Han, K., & Jia, S. (2025). High-throughput, high-resolution volumetric imaging with light-field flow cytometry for multiparametric 3D single-cell analysis. *13330,* 1333002–1333002-8. https://www.semanticscholar.org/paper/62863822e0e07ee50214244a8cb1d2

52572e9060 (accessed on 27th June 2025).

22. Jiao, Y. (2024). Spatial proteomic analysis of single amyloid plaques in brain tissue using laser capture microdissection and mass spectrometry. *Alzheimer's & Dementia, 20.* https://www.semanticscholar.org/paper/a47383752e2fc78d4ef0416ec1b66d4da1975e63 (accessed on 27th June 2025).

23. Karoii, D. H., Abroudi, A. S., Forghani, N., Bavandi, S., Djamali, M., Baghaei, H., Shafaeitilaki, S., et al. (2025). Analysis of microarray and single-cell RNA-seq identifies gene co-expression, cell–cell communication, and tumor environment associated with metabolite interconversion enzyme in prostate cancer. *Discover Oncology, 16.* https://www.semanticscholar.org/paper/cfa0f09862c96ff9cec51a61499fdcc67366281e (accessed on 27th June 2025).

24. Krynina, O., de Ståhl, T., Jylhä, C., Arthur, C., Giraud, G., Nyman, P., Fritzberg, A., et al. (2024). The potential of liquid biopsy for detection of the *KIAA1549-BRAF* fusion in circulating tumor DNA from children with pilocytic astrocytoma. *Neuro-Oncology Advances, 6.* https://www.semanticscholar.org/paper/28c283a78373183003eeca6ee2a900b9625cb9d8 (accessed on 27th June 2025).

25. La Russa, R., Liso, A., Pascale, N., Riezzo, I., et al. (2017). Donor selection for allogenic hemopoietic stem cell transplantation: Clinical and ethical considerations. https://core.ac.uk/download/141694739.pdf (accessed on 27th June 2025).

26. Lei, M., Xiao, M., Long, Z., Lin, T., Ding, R., & Quan, Q. (2024). Prognosis of colorectal cancer, prognostic index of immunogenic cell death associated genes in response to immunotherapy, and potential therapeutic effects of ferroptosis inducers. *Frontiers in Immunology, 15.* https://www.semanticscholar.org/paper/9db03dd2d9c7081d5e57b96873900ea952f94958 (accessed on 27th June 2025).

27. Li, D., & Wu, M. (2021). Pattern recognition receptors in health and diseases. *Signal Transduction and Targeted Therapy, 6.* https://doi.org/10.1038/s41392-021-00687-0 (accessed on 27th June 2025).

28. Li, L., Jiang, J., Guo, L., Santos, J., González, A. M., Li, S., & Qin, Y. (2025). Clinical diagnosis and treatment system for neurological psychological gastrointestinal diseases based on multimodal artificial intelligence and immunology. *Current Pharmaceutical Biotechnology.* https://www.semanticscholar.org/paper/1396156732c4698216b6abcf0a7b339f7e0c5f79 (accessed on 27th June 2025).

29. Liang, A., Kong, Y., Chen, Z. H., Qiu, Y., Wu, Y., Zhu, X., & Li, Z. (2023). Advancements and applications of single-cell multi-omics techniques in cancer research: Unveiling heterogeneity and paving the way for precision therapeutics. *Biochemistry and Biophysics Reports, 37,* 101589–101589. https://doi.org/10.1016/j.bbrep.2023.101589 (accessed on 27th June 2025).

30. Lim, J., Park, C., Kim, M., Kim, H., Kim, J., & Lee, D. S. (2024). Advances in single-cell omics and multimers for high-resolution molecular profiling. *Experimental & Molecular Medicine, 56,* 515–526. https://doi.org/10.1038/s12276-024-01186-2 (accessed on 27th June 2025).

31. Liyanage, S., & Guo, J. (2024). Single-cell spatial proteomics. *Histology and Histopathology.* https://www.semanticscholar.org/paper/3e246658cce5e2fd94a91119dea5d454cd0c14aa (accessed on 27th June 2025).

32. Navarrete, P. M. (2018). Development of flow focusing device for the visualization of leukocyte rolling adhesion. https://core.ac.uk/download/214845386.pdf (accessed on 27th June 2025).

33. Robinson, M. W., Hughes, J., Wilkie, G. S., Swann, R., Barclay, S. T., Mills, P. R., Patel, A. H., Thomson, E. C., & McLauchlan, J. (2016). Tracking TCRβ Sequence Clonotype Expansions during Antiviral Therapy Using High-Throughput Sequencing of the Hypervariable Region. *Frontiers in immunology*, *7*, 131. https://doi.org/10.3389/fimmu.2016.00131/42370434.pdf (accessed on 27th June 2025).

34. Pizzo, P. (2019). Management of patients with fever and neutropenia through the arc of time. *Annals of Internal Medicine, 170*, 389–397. https://www.semanticscholar.org/paper/230391e07a5738835a59c2f1a9997846bf05c34b (accessed on 27th June 2025).

35. Qin, R., Zhang, Y., Yang, Y., Chen, J., Huang, L., Xu, W., Qin, Q., et al. (2024). Decoding single-cell molecular mechanisms in astrocyte-to-iN reprogramming via Ngn2- and Pax6-mediated direct lineage switching. *European Journal of Medical Research, 29*. https://www.semanticscholar.org/paper/11f217995bbe1b34f9aeac0d831228d08545af9e (accessed on 27th June 2025).

36. Rao, B. H., Souček, P., & Hlaváč, V. (2022). Laser capture microdissection: A gear for pancreatic cancer research. *International Journal of Molecular Sciences, 23*. https://www.semanticscholar.org/paper/c0fc82fcfb8d5a5631e8639a4e9b30d22a53ad92 (accessed on 27th June 2025).

37. Salminen, S., Collado, M. C., Endo, A., Hill, C., Lebeer, S., Quigley, E. M. M., Sanders, M. E., et al. (2021). The International Scientific Association of Probiotics and Prebiotics (ISAPP) consensus statement on the definition and scope of postbiotics. *Nature Reviews Gastroenterology & Hepatology, 18*, 649–667. https://doi.org/10.1038/s41575-021-00440-6 (accessed on 27th June 2025).

38. Wang, A., & Sarwal, M. M. (2015). Computational Models for Transplant Biomarker Discovery. *Frontiers in immunology*, *6*, 458. https://doi.org/10.3389/fimmu.2015.00458(accessed on 27th June 2025).

39. Seaman, W., & Whitehouse, J. H. (2001). Florida marine biotechnology: Research, development and training capabilities to advance science and commerce. https://core.ac.uk/download/11016354.pdf (accessed on 27th June 2025).

40. Tejwani, V., Wang, R., Villabona-Rueda, A., Suresh, K., Wu, T., Adcock, I., Kermani, N., et al. (2025). Distinct single cell transcriptional profile in CD4+ T-lymphocytes among obese children with asthma. *American Journal of Physiology. Lung Cellular and Molecular Physiology*. https://www.semanticscholar.org/paper/7d09d49de69b60a4250435d69e9d843f52330412 (accessed on 27th June 2025).

41. Wang, C., Feng, Y., Liu, X., Sun, H., Guo, Z., Shao, J., Li, K., et al. (2025). Molecular landscape of atherosclerotic plaque progression: Insights from proteomics, single-cell transcriptomics and genomics. *BMC Medicine, 23*. https://www.semanticscholar.org/paper/c39e290db360c6ce446141f00bdb8d5f253ea1cf (accessed on 27th June 2025).

42. Wang, Y., Xue, Y., Wang, H., Qu, Y., Zhang, K., Shang, L., Liang, P., et al. (2025). Automated laser-assisted single-cell sorting for cell functional and RNA sequencing. *ACS Sensors*. https://www.semanticscholar.org/paper/82f70550450f836a0cf650d660d76c32636993ff (accessed on 27th June 2025).

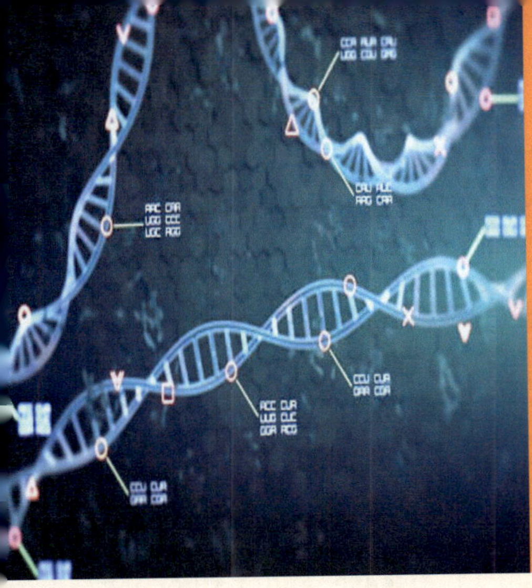

Chapter 9

GENE EDITING IN IMMUNOLOGY

Contents

Introduction

Gene editing reagent evolution has revolutionized immunology, opening up possibilities for disease treatment and management never previously encountered. Gene editing, particularly with reagents like CRISPR-Cas9, permits exquisite genome manipulation, thus facilitating novel ideas in immunological research and therapeutic regimes. This potent technology allows scientists to study the complex interplay between genes and immune response and propose solutions to a range of diseases, from autoimmune diseases and infectious diseases to cancer. With these technologies being employed by scientists, it has never been more vital to be mindful of their power and limitations when employed in the framework of immune system modulation, outlining some of the potential clinical usefulness and ethical ramifications of gene editing in immunology. The application of gene editing is not only of theoretical importance but also holds real problems with therapeutic safety and effectiveness. Engineered Extracellular Vesicles (EVs) as a new vector to deliver therapeutic payloads, like gene editing machinery, is one such example. Due to their favorable safety profile and low immunogenic nature, EVs have the promise of targeting specificity and effective delivery *in vivo* for gene-editing cargos. Existing research indicates that human Expi293F cell-derived EVs can function without producing robust immune responses *in vitro* and do not exhibit significant adverse effects when delivered *in vivo*. These features indicate the application of state-of-the-art methods for enhancing the efficacy and safety of gene editing therapeutics, providing a platform for extending similar research with EVs towards biomedical applications in immunology (Askeland et al., 2019). In addition to that, gene editing technologies are now very important in deciphering and interpreting the gene etiology of immune disorders, which is of great importance in developing targeted treatment mechanisms. Genomic and proteomic profiling is not only helpful in disease gene identification but also in investigating gene interactions and their roles in immune responsivity. Specifically, the use of bioinformatics programs provides for the identification of such complicated systems at a higher level to facilitate the identification of potential targets for therapy and biomarkers. While the debate still rages regarding the implications of gene editing, particularly in chronic disease and in cancer, the convergence of genomics and immunology has much in store for future study. The joint research across all these fields ensures that scientific advances get translated into practice as new therapeutic regimens capable of directly addressing the patient outcomes (Falus, 2006).

Definition of Gene Editing

Gene editing is a revolution in the field of molecular biology, which allows precise alteration of an organism's genome. The method utilizes a number of tools such as CRISPR-Cas9, TALENs, and ZFNs to introduce targeted alterations that could enhance, disable, or erase selected genes. The effect of gene editing is linked to the ability to assist with research and treatment. Scientists can create new drugs for previously non-functional disease as they discover the genetic cause of diseases. Thus, gene editing is no longer a process of thinking; it is now at the frontline of science, particularly in fields like immunology, where it holds enormous potential for the development of novel therapeutic interventions against immune diseases. Gene editing has opened up new avenues for enhancing the body's defense mechanism against disease and pathogens, like cancer, in immunology. As an example, researchers are now exploring the use of gene editing as a method of engineering immune cells, such as T cells, to more specifically and effectively kill cancer. This is achieved through editing the genes that regulate the manner in which T cells function, thereby making them more effective. Gene editing also creates customized immunotherapies, crafted from an individual patients genetic makeup. By facilitating the development of a more responsive immune system, gene editing can potentially bridge the gap between existing treatments and the demand for more potent, patient-specific drugs. The swift development of gene editing technology is thus offering essential tools to address daunting problems in immunology. Gene editing also raises delicate ethical and regulatory challenges, irrespective of its potential for therapy. As this technology continues to develop, risks of unpredictable genetic consequences, such as off-target or ecosystem-disruptive effects, become increasingly relevant. Problems surrounding germline editing, which involves the irreversible modification of DNA in embryos or reproductive cells, also present long-term implications for future generations. The scientific and regulatory communities should issue guidelines ensuring the safety and effectiveness of gene editing technologies for immunology and for all other applications. The achievement of a consensus about definitions, i.e., therapeutic assertions and safety protocols, is an utmost priority to facilitate trust and facilitate the responsible development of gene editing methods in both clinical and scientific applications (Falzone et al., 2018; Salminen et al., 2021) (Figure 9.1).

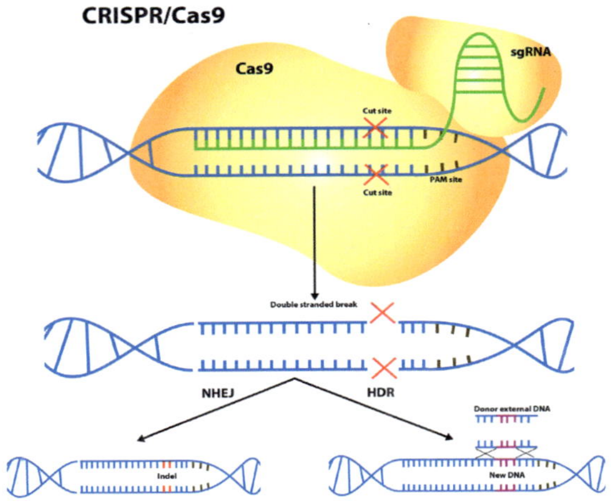

Figure 9.1. CRISPR-Cas9 mediated gene-editing mechanisms.

Source:https://www.researchgate.net/profile/Adam-Cribbs/publication/322251194/figure/fig1/AS:579073518256128@1515073293608/CRISPR-Cas9-mediated-gene-editing-mechanisms-A-single-guide-RNA-sgRNA-recognizes-a.png

Overview of Immunology

Immunology, the biomedical science to investigate the immune system, is the secret to learning how organisms defend themselves from infection. The immune system is an intricate set of cells, tissues, and organs working in concert to identify and reject external invaders such as viruses and bacteria. Advanced knowledge about natural and adaptive immunity is critical in the context of evolving new therapeutic interventions, e.g., gene editing. Natural immunity is the first line of defense and comprises physical barriers and immune cells that react nonspecifically to pathogens. Adaptive immunity, however, occurs over time and relies on lymphocytes, i.e., T and B cells, that are specialized for responses to a single antigen, creating long-term immunity. This fundamental knowledge is the foundation for immunomodulatory strategies through mechanisms of gene editing, with the trend headed toward personalized medicine and vaccines. An example of the fundamental intersection of gene editing and immunology is the creation of neoantigens, new antigens produced by mutation that are tumor-specific. These neoantigens are recognized by the immune system as foreign and hence can induce powerful immune responses that can be harnessed for cancer immunotherapy. These neoantigens have been identified and characterized extensively with the advances in next-generation sequencing and bioinformatics resources. This has brought about the generation of patient-specific cancer therapies that are targeted towards cancer neoantigens, exemplifying the potential of gene editing to control immunity to allow greater anti-tumor immunity. There is a need to know how to use neoantigens effectively to generate immunotherapies, including cancer vaccines and adoptive cell therapy, as it offers new targets that can be utilized in combination with gene editing technologies. The face of cancer treatment is evolving at a speed never previously witnessed as immunologists and geneticists come together to further develop these modes of therapy towards improved patient outcomes. In addition, the creation of Chimeric Antigen Receptor (CAR) T cell therapy represents an intriguing application of immunologic concepts and a demonstration of the utility of gene editing to maximize immune capacity. CAR-T cell therapy has transformed the treatment of a few types of blood cancer, especially B-cell cancer, by genetically modifying patients' T cells to express receptors capable of targeting specific cancer cells. The modification allows the immune system to more effectively recognize and eliminate the cancer cells, typically leading to very excellent clinical outcomes, for instance, a cure in some cases when other treatments have not worked. Despite these successes, significant challenges remain in applying CAR-T cell therapy to solid tumors and other malignancies, since the tumor immunosuppressive microenvironment complicates treatment. Continued investigation into gene editing reagents like CAR construct optimization and target strategy optimization holds much promise to surmount such hurdles as well as extend the use of CAR-T therapy to more cancers, pointing to synergy between immunology and gene editing in modern medicine (Charrot et al., 2019; Xie et al., 2023).

Importance of Gene Editing in Immunological Research

Gene editing technology, e.g., CRISPR/Cas9, has transformed immunology by providing previously unmatched specificity in gene engineering of immunity-related genes. This enables scientists to explore the function of individual genes in immune cells like T cells and B cells in disease and health. By making targeted manipulation possible, CRISPR/Cas9 illuminates mechanisms of autoimmune disease, allergic diseases, and other immunopathies. Its ability to create knockout models—organisms where a specific gene is knocked out—is also utilized in explaining the mechanisms through which gene alterations result in immune deficiency. These studies form knowledge utilized in formulating new therapy strategies aimed at restoring proper immune function or enhancing immunity against cancer and pathogens. Beyond enhancing immune function and cell biology, gene editing is at the center of advancing immunotherapeutic strategies. Researchers are increasingly using CRISPR/Cas9 to edit immune cells to function better in cancer treatment. For instance, the method is used to engineer T cells to improve their efficiency in recognizing and killing tumor cells. By removing genes that inhibit T cell activity or adding genes that construct tumor-targeting receptors, researchers aim to improve the accuracy and effectiveness of immunotherapies. This approach is not only poised to reduce off-target effects typical of traditional therapies but also presents the potential of personalized medicine efforts targeted to an individual patient's genetic uniqueness in the war on cancer and other immunological disorders. Another area where the gene editing technology is of importance is in vaccine development, an important area of immunological investigation. The prospect of developing vaccines with unprecedented efficacy is surely tantalizing. CRISPR/Cas9 technology offers the potential to have a better understanding of genetic contributions towards immune reaction to vaccines and how individuals react differently against the same vaccine. By targeting individual genes that allow for immune diversity, researchers are able to identify biomarkers that predict vaccine efficacy, especially against the rapidly mutating pathogens, such as pandemic-causing viruses. In addition, the technology will be utilized to speed up vaccine development with the incorporation of genetic material encoding antigens known to induce effective immune responses. The novel approach can streamline vaccine design processes, which in return will lead to safer and more effective vaccines for addressing new global health challenges.

9.1. Historical Background of Gene Editing

The historical context for gene editing is also firmly rooted in molecular biology milestones that have shaped modern science. Gene editing has its beginnings way back in 1953, when the discovery of the DNA structure provided a platform for learning about genetic information. Breakthroughs such as the discovery of restriction enzymes in the 1970s made it possible to cut and reassemble DNA sequences with accuracy. These enzymes would soon be the tools of choice for molecular cloning, allowing scientists to edit and assemble pieces of DNA with great precision. The shift from crude gene manipulation to sophisticated editing opened the door for its use in immunology today. After scientists grasped the potential of precise targeting, the requirement for quicker and more precise mechanisms created improvements in gene editing tools. The next few decades saw gene editing revolutionized by the identification of programmable nucleases. The discovery of zinc-finger nucleases (ZFNs) and transcription activator-like effector nucleases (TALENs) was a paradigm shift in genetic engineering. These technologies enabled the induction of mutations in specified loci or the repair of genetic malformations with unprecedented precision. However, the most significant breakthrough ever achieved in the area arrived with the discovery and utilization of the CRISPR-Cas9 system in 2012. This new tool, which is founded on bacterial adaptive immunity, has transformed gene editing and rendered it infinitely more reachable to scientists all over the world. The ease with which CRISPR can target and modify genes has caused enthusiasm and hope in many fields, from immunology, where it has the potential to enhance vaccine science as well as therapy. The timeline for gene editing has changed numerous times over the decades to result in ethical and regulatory considerations that continue to affect its application. Though the promise of gene editing technologies is unrivaled for disease cure and scientific advance, safety, efficacy, and ethical concerns have been raised. Human germline editing capacity is especially troubling due to the ethical implications the prospect poses for unforeseen effects, as well as the social implications of designer genes. These are added to by the rate of technological advancement, which in the majority of instances has outpaced the development of adequate regulatory frameworks. As the gene editing science revolution unfolds, there is a need that scientific investigation to be responded to with ethical responsibility, making the breakthroughs useful to society and preventing harm from new therapies.

9.1.1. Early Techniques in Gene Manipulation

The creation of gene manipulation techniques was a revolutionary period in the domain of molecular biology that still depends largely on the achievements that were made. Recombinant DNA technology formed one of the first methods that were developed in the 1970s when researchers could cut and splice DNA from different organisms to design novel gene combinations. This revolutionary approach was employed to precondition bacteria to produce insulin, a genetic engineering revolution that would revolutionize the face of medicine. Aside from that, the discovery of plasmid vectors enabled one to transfer a particular gene into host organisms, which in turn gave birth to advancements in the areas of gene therapy and gene editing. It was only with researchers exploring more into genetic manipulation that the fundamental methods came about that would go on to lead to even more accurate approaches in immunology, and in turn open up the applicability of the original gene manipulation techniques in teaching future disease prevention and treatment methods (Dunbar et al., 2018).

The effects of early gene manipulation techniques extend beyond mere production of recombinant organisms and encompass their application in the understanding of gene function and interaction. For instance, techniques such as polymerase chain reaction (PCR), developed during the 1980s, were a testament to the need for effective and efficient DNA amplification technologies. This made it possible for researchers to study individual genes in detail, illuminating their role in immunity and disease pathogenesis. As these initial techniques became available, researchers could examine genetic aspects of disease and thereby pursue intentional immunologic investigation. By molecular characterization of genetic variation and mutation in immunologic diseases, the stage was laid for individualized medicine approaches in immunology. Therefore, the legacy of previous gene modification technology is inherited by the present uses of gene editing technologies aimed at further therapeutic progress in immunodisorders (Sies et al., 2017). In conclusion, gene manipulation technology development illustrates a line of successor innovations culminating in further greater developments in immunology and therapy. Early techniques paved the way for increasingly advanced methods, including the development of CRISPR-Cas9, now used in direct genome editing with unprecedented precision. Looking back at the first success in gene manipulation, it is clear that these early methods were not only adding to increased genetic research; they were also establishing a greater understanding of cellular immune process mechanisms. Currently, ancient traditions lie behind many of the applications across the board, from cancer therapies applied to boost immune function to inherited immunodeficiency management. These advancements mark the position of early gene manipulation techniques in the increasingly expanding horizon of gene editing in immunology, paving the way for expectations of future treatments (Dunbar et al., 2018) (Figure 9.2).

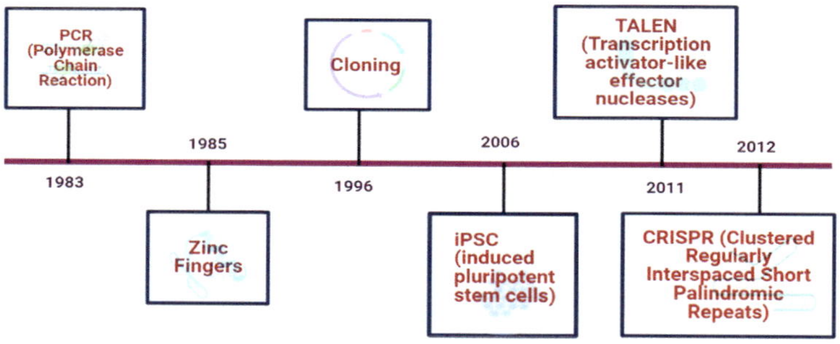

Figure 9.2. Timeline of gene alteration techniques: genetic manipulation started in the 19th century when PCR was first invented by Kary B. Mullis for gene amplification.

Source: https://www.researchgate.net/profile/Dr-Ahmad-18/publication/351888280/figure/fig1/AS:1143128117214482@1675395482593/Timeline-of-gene-alteration-techniques-genetic-manipulation-started-in-the-nineteenth.png.

9.1.2. Development of CRISPR Technology

The evolution of CRISPR technology has revolutionized the editing of genes, particularly in immunology. Initially derived from the natural defense mechanisms of bacteria, CRISPR was employed by researchers to create a universal tool for genetic modification at a specific locus. This tool has enabled researchers to explore complex genetic interactions in immune responses, which have provided insight into pathways that are crucial for the understanding of cancer and autoimmune diseases. Following the development of CRISPR technology, it has found application in advancing unprecedented breakthroughs in immune cell manipulation to more effectively target malignancies and infections. Simplified use of the technology to experiment on readily initiates a thriving research culture that propels advances and applications in immunotherapy. Thus, CRISPR not only represents a significant milestone in genetics but also becomes a building block for novel therapeutic methods of modulating immune responses. Moreover, the combination of CRISPR technology with current computational methods magnifies its possible uses in immunology. In combining CRISPR with high-throughput screening technologies, researchers are able to assess gene function in various disparate biological contexts and finally generate wide datasets. Such datasets are a valuable resource for artificial intelligence applications and computational modeling of immunological research.

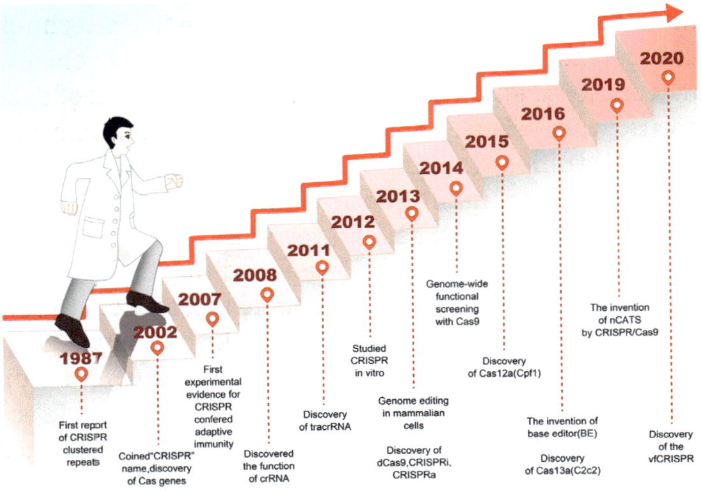

Figure 9.3. Development history of the CRISPR/Cas9-based gene editing tools.

Source: https://www.researchgate.net/publication/355004264/figure/fig3/AS:1074336836354053@1633153270496/Development-history-of-the-CRISPR-Cas9-based-gene-editing-tools-The-CRISPR-repeat.png.

Single-cell CRISPR tools further advanced immune cell population profiling so that researchers could demarcate fine-grained differences in cells and their responses to therapies. As testified by Menon et al. (2025), this powerful synergy offers unprecedented insights into human biology, revealing basic mechanisms of disease and potential therapeutic avenues. Such further advancement of CRISPR, combined with computational science, then reiterates its central role in shaping the future trajectory of immunological research and treatment. In the future, ongoing advances in CRISPR technology promise to make further breakthroughs in focused immunotherapy and the field of personalized medicine. Recent innovations such as CRISPR gene drives and precision editing techniques have the potential to provide highly targeted interventions in immune cells, paving the way for genome-customized treatments based on individual genetic fingerprints. As Dhar (2025) highlights, the intersection of immunology, computational biology, and machine learning is consolidating the therapeutic landscape, enhancing diagnostic accuracy and treatment approaches. Upcoming wearable technology for real-time immune monitoring and federated learning to safeguard patient information is just the beginning of the future of immunological investigation instigated by CRISPR technology. Combined, these developments are revolutionizing standards of care and entering a new era where personalized healthcare solutions become real, emphasizing the major impact of CRISPR technology on the field of immunology (Figure 9.3).

9.1.3. Milestones in Gene Editing Applications

The CRISPR/Cas9 gene editing technology discovery has revolutionized the field of genetic research, particularly immunology. First found to be a bacterial immune defense mechanism, CRISPR has emerged as a workhorse for targeted genome editing. Easy to use, inexpensive, and effective, high-throughput studies looking for gene functions of relevance to immune responses have been quickly conducted. This has yielded precious information on how specific genes influence immune system behavior and disease susceptibility. The ability to undertake large-scale genomic experiments allows researchers to uncover complex interactions among immune pathways, ushering in the potential for revolutionary treatments and diagnostic technologies. As increased studies continue to expand, CRISPR incorporation into high-throughput sequencing techniques continues to advance our understanding of immune cell dynamics, marking a milestone juncture point in the use of gene editing that continues to shape modern immunological research (Menon et al., 2025). In addition to CRISPR, other advances in gene editing have also had large roles in shaping therapeutic strategies in immunology. One such development is that of CAR T-cell therapy, which involves genetically engineering a patient's T cells to enhance how well they are able to identify and destroy cancer cells. This groundbreaking approach has been shown to be truly successful in the eradication of some types of leukemia and lymphoma, and marks a big step towards personalized immunotherapy. Furthermore, the use of gene editing to engineer bispecific antibodies has opened up the possibility of targeting two distinct antigens, thus enhancing therapeutic specificity and minimizing off-target activity. All these advances not only enhance anti-tumor activity but also show how gene editing can be used to generate personalized therapies based on the unique requirements of specific patients. These landmarks highlight the evolving imprint of gene editing in clinical immunology to demonstrate its potential to overcome age-old issues in disease management (Dhar, 2025). The synergy between artificial intelligence (AI) and gene editing technologies is also poised to revolutionize the field of immunology further. By analyzing vast sets of data generated by genomic studies and immune profiling, AI can identify novel biomarkers and predictive markers significant for the understanding of immune responses. When coupled with CRISPR and other gene-editing tools, machine learning algorithms enable researchers to reveal intricately complex networks of immune regulation, allowing them to dissect never-before-seen interactions. Further, advances in computational biology will enable optimizing gene-editing experiments and forecasting likely outcomes by modeling immune interactions with high fidelity. Such collaborations promise to accelerate drug discovery, improve the accuracy of diagnostics, and ultimately result in personalized therapeutic regimens that better target patient populations. Emphasizing the intersection of immunology and technology, such milestones mark a new era of personalized medicine in which the care of each individual patient can be tailored uniquely to achieve maximum efficacy with minimum side effects (Dhar, 2025; Menon et al., 2025).

9.2. Mechanisms of Gene Editing

The intricate mechanisms of gene editing have profoundly revolutionized the discipline of immunology, enabling researchers to edit and modify specific genes with unprecedented precision. Techniques such as CRISPR-Cas9 allow for precise control of the genome, including knocking out genes that play roles in immune functions or augmenting pathways that are key to the detection of pathogens. By directing the Cas9 enzyme to specific locations within DNA with guide RNA, researchers can induce DNA cuts that are repaired using various cellular mechanisms. This particular editing allows for research into immune processes and the development of therapeutic strategies against diseases like cancer and autoimmune disease. Perhaps most importantly, understanding how the immune system adapts to these gene-modification technologies can lead to improved outcomes and reduced off-target effects and thus the overall safety of gene editing in immunological applications. In addition, the use of gene editing extends beyond treating and understanding genetic diseases and includes enhancing adoptive cell therapies, particularly T cells, against diseases such as cancer. Through designing T cells to have certain receptors or eliminate suppressive checkpoints, researchers expect that immunotherapies can be made more effective. For instance, CRISPR has been employed to eliminate genes that repress the activity of T cells, effectively making them more effective killers of tumor cells. Gene editing can also be employed for the production of engineered T cells that are immune to tumors' avoidance mechanisms. As these techniques continue to advance, a greater appreciation of the interplay between mechanisms of gene editing and the immune system will be necessary when creating therapy that not only amplifies the immune response but also restricts off-target side effects, thereby maximizing the benefits of the patient. Further, the new technologies in gene editing have sparked immense interest in treating chronic immune dysfunctions, wherein the conventional regimens fail. Researchers are also increasingly interested in the role of immune cells, such as neutrophils, in chronic illnesses such as atopic dermatitis, characterized by persistent itch and inflammation. Recent research has identified that neutrophils play a central role in generating and sustaining chronic itch since they regulate the expression of key signaling molecules and inflammatory cytokines. Investigating the gene-editing potential to control neutrophil activity can unveil new doors of therapy for chronic itching syndromes. Through gene editing techniques, it is possible to selectively target specific neutrophil activities and inhibit the mechanisms that cause itching, with potential for more effective treatment in immunology (Roberts et al., 2019). Lastly, the extensive applications of gene editing have revolutionary potential for improving immunological health and pushing therapy boundaries.

9.2.1. Overview of CRISPR-Cas9

The revolutionary technology of CRISPR-Cas9 has revolutionized the art of gene editing, particularly in immunology. Initially discovered as a bacterial defense mechanism against viruses, CRISPR-Cas9 has unparalleled precision and efficiency in editing genomic sequences. This system comprises two major components: a guide RNA that is targeted to a specific DNA sequence and the Cas9 nuclease that induces a double-strand break at the target site. The following DNA repair mechanisms can be employed to either knock out gene function or introduce new genetic material. This disruptive capability of CRISPR-Cas9 has offered new opportunities for understanding immune responses and the regulation of immune cells, thereby significantly influencing therapeutic interventions in cancer and autoimmune diseases. With more studies on CRISPR-Cas9, its application in immunology has become increasingly sophisticated. Recent studies demonstrate its capability to generate genetically engineered immune cells, such as CAR T-cells, which are designed to identify and kill cancer cells. For instance, with the use of CRISPR-Cas9, the affinity of T-cell receptors can be enhanced, thus improving the efficacy of immunotherapies. CRISPR-Cas9 is also key in exploring gene functions that are involved in immune modulation and may reveal novel therapeutic avenues. The efficiency of multiplexed gene editing systems also provides significant advantages through the capability to perturb genes that are associated with the immune response simultaneously. Therefore, it is crucial for researchers to keep pursuing the significance of CRISPR-Cas9 in the immunological context to advance knowledge and treatment techniques. However, the application of CRISPR-Cas9 technology in immunology is fraught with challenges and ethical concerns. Despite its groundbreaking importance, issues such as off-target effects, where areas outside the target parts of the genome are affected, are still a significant threat. Also, the long-term effects of gene changes, particularly in germline editing, need to be adequately analyzed ethically and regulated. Researchers are engaged to address such issues by generating high-fidelity Cas9 variants and employing advanced delivery methods, e.g., lipid nanoparticles, to enhance precision and reduce off-target activity. Research with CRISPR-Cas9 in animal models, for example, generating genome-targeted knock-in mice, illuminates the complex relationships of genes within the immune system and hence provides new direction for innovative uses in immunotherapy and beyond (Tang et al., 2024; Elkord, 2025).

9.2.2. Other Gene Editing Technologies (Transcription Activator-Like Effector Nucleases (TALENs) and Zinc Finger Nucleases (ZFNs))

Of the array of gene editing technologies, TALENs and ZFNs also occupy significant positions alongside the more familiar CRISPR/Cas9 system. TALENs and ZFNs both utilize engineered nucleases to direct double-strand breaks in specific DNA sequences, so that subsequent modifications can be made via cellular repair mechanisms. TALENs are unique in their capacity to have their DNA-binding domains customized, which means that precise genes can be targeted with excellent specificity. This specificity might be particularly valuable in immunological uses, such as gene therapy targeted to immune deficiency or editing immune cell receptors for enhanced recognition of cancer cells. Precision editing is crucial in immunology, where specific alterations can have profound effects on the treatment of numerous conditions. While effective, the application of TALENs and ZFNs has been tempered by certain limitations compared to the CRISPR/Cas9 system. For instance, the expense and complexity of ZFN and TALEN design might pose barriers to their widespread application (Figure 9.4).

TALENs, although more convenient, need two distinct constructs per target site. But both ZFNs and TALENs have been promising in therapeutic use, particularly in treating monogenic disorders like Sickle Cell Disease and Beta-Thalassemia, as reported in studies on their potential to edit genes in gene modification for model organisms and cell lines (Khare, 2021). Their potential to edit a single gene is highly promising in immunological paradigms, especially in making patient-specific therapies. In general, while CRISPR/Cas9 is now widely used for its ease and efficacy, TALENs and ZFNs remain indispensable tools in the gene editing arsenal. Both of these systems have varying advantages which can be employed for different applications in immunology, particularly in the continued efforts to understand and master immune responses. As ongoing research continues to explore the potential of these tools, important insights are being gained into not only gene editing technologies themselves but also their implications for treating complex immune-related disorders. The application of TALENs and ZFNs in existing frameworks can lead to novel therapeutic strategies that increase our understanding of immunity and improve patient outcomes, reflective of greater promise in the field of gene editing (Keul et al., 2022) (Figure 9.5).

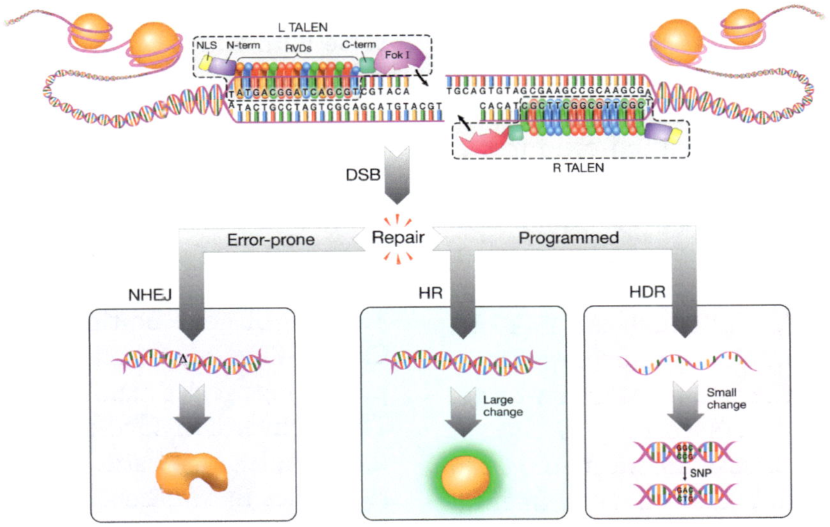

Figure 9.4. Overview of transcription activator-like effector nuclease (TALEN) genome engineering.

Source: https://www.researchgate.net/profile/Xiaolei-Xu-4/publication/255957098/figure/fig1/AS:297944289955845@1448046862347/Overview-of-transcription-activator-like-effector-nuclease-TALEN-genome-engineering.png.

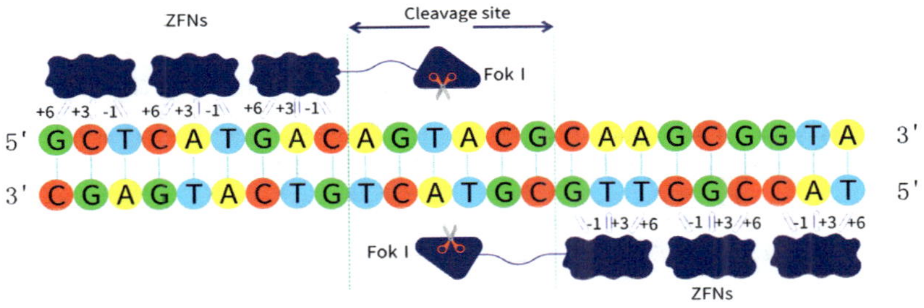

Figure 9.5. The schematic diagram of zinc finger nucleases (ZFNs).

Source: https://upload.wikimedia.org/wikipedia/commons/thumb/5/56/The_schematic_diagram_of_ZFNs.png/1920px-The_schematic_diagram_of_ZFNs.png.

9.2.3. Comparison of Gene Editing Methods

The landscape of gene editing technologies has shifted significantly in recent years, especially in the field of immunology. Tools such as CRISPR-Cas9 have revolutionized the precision of genomic changes so that targeted modifications are achievable with unprecedented facility. In particular, ease of use and flexibility of CRISPR have made it the preferred method for researchers interested in probing mechanisms of immune response or creating novel therapeutic approaches. However, other methods like TALENs (Transcription Activator-Like Effector Nucleases) and ZFNs (Zinc Finger Nucleases) have different advantages, particularly in off-target effects and delivery problems. Immunologists should understand these relative advantages and disadvantages when choosing the optimal tools to use in investigation, as the dependability of each method can directly impact experimental outcomes and resulting therapeutic uses (Yao et al., 2025). Comparison of these methods is another critical factor when determining gene editing efficiency. Various methods, such as T7 Endonuclease I (T7EI) and Tracking of Indels by Decomposition (TIDE), allow researchers to measure on-target efficiency of gene edits. According to current analyses, the choice of assessment method can have profound implications on experimental design. For instance, while ddPCR (droplet digital PCR) is very sensitive, it may be costly and difficult to operate, so less available to some laboratories. By contrast, methods such as ICE (Inference of CRISPR Edits) are quicker at reporting on editing outcomes but perhaps less informative in measuring all off-target alterations. Every evaluation method thus carries inherent trade-offs that need to be prudently avoided by immunologists to make precise genomic alterations (Permyakova & Deineko, 2024). Apart from conventional gene editing methods, advances in human gene editing technologies redefine the boundaries of immunological research. The development of base editing, where one can introduce single-base changes in a targeted manner without inducing double-strand breaks, is proof of the ability to be more precise and less toxic. The novel approach holds enormous promise for therapeutic intervention in immunology, including autoimmune diseases and cancer treatment. Furthermore, the application of these newer techniques in conjunction with conventional methods can result in enhanced precision therapy, enabling scientists to study complex networks of genes that determine immune mechanisms. With the advancement of science, continued refinement of these gene editing technologies will offer new avenues for optimizing immunotherapeutic approaches and allowing scientists to use the most effective tools with which to tackle major diseases (Yao et al., 2025).

9.3. Applications in Immunology

The use of gene editing technologies, namely CRISPR-Cas9, has revolutionized immunology by permitting precise manipulation of immune cells. This conversion facilitates investigation into the complex roles and interactions of immune responses in disease. For instance, researchers have cultured conditionally immortalized macrophages that retain characteristics of primary cells but simplify genetic modification. This is a new approach permitting studies on host genetics during bacterial infection, as demonstrated in the study of pathogens like Listeria monocytogenes and *Mycobacterium tuberculosis*. The ease of applying gene editing on these models not only accelerates research but also enhances the potential for developing new therapeutic approaches based on immune modulation, hence treating infectious and autoimmune diseases effectively (Roberts et al., 2019). Gene editing is also at the center of enhancing therapeutic strategies, especially those of antibody production. Mechanisms of somatically rearranged antibody variable gene hypermutation exhibit a valuable evolutionary adaptation. Through the use of AID deaminase for DNA modification and mRNA editing by ADAR1 deaminase, researchers are able to study immune response evolution under environmental stress. Reverse transcription, which targets DNA polymerase eta, allows for additional insight into antibody variability and selection. Hence, knowledge gained by applications of gene editing is crucial in designing accurate therapies that modulate the immune recognition and activation against pathogens, ultimately opening up for the improvement in vaccine development and immunotherapy (Steele, 2009). Gene editing implications extend beyond their therapeutic application; they offer a valuable insight into the evolution of the immune system. The study of feedback loops between somatic mutations and germline sequences is contrary to the traditional concepts of genetic inheritance, i.e., Weismann's Barrier. Lamarckian feedback represents a new perspective on how future generations of immune responses can be molded by adaptive responses. This information is important for the understanding of how developed mechanisms within the immune system can be harnessed with the help of gene editing in order to build resistance to emerging infectious diseases and normalize responses under immunotherapy protocols. These advancements ultimately position gene editing as the focal point of modern immunology research and its therapeutic applications, with the possibility of having revolutionary impacts on the health outcomes of the world.

9.3.1. Gene Editing for Vaccine Development

The evolution of gene-editing technologies, particularly CRISPR/Cas9, has revolutionized vaccine development, with unparalleled speed and precision obtained in the process. Vaccine development has been conventionally a laborious and multi-step process, involving detailed characterization of the pathogen and safety evaluation. Gene editing, however, facilitates scientists in realizing the rapid design of vaccine candidates by permitting direct targeting and modification of the key genes responsible for pathogenicity.

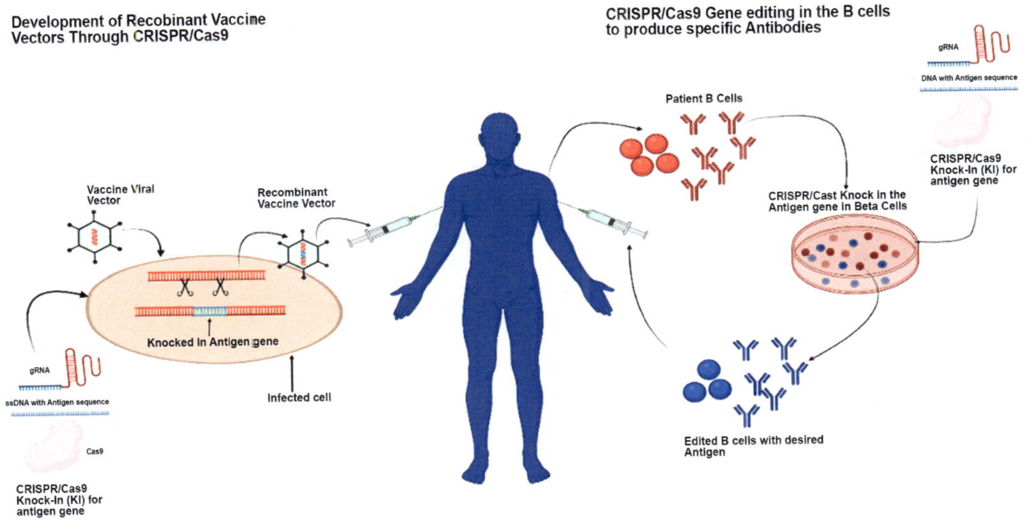

Figure 9.6. Abstract overview of the use of CRISPR/Cas9 to generate recombinant vaccine vectors and engineer B-cells to produce specific antibodies.

Source: https://www.researchgate.net/profile/Amjad-Khalil-2/publication/363803157/figure/fig1/AS:11431281086463403@1664217044741/Abstract-overview-of-the-use-of-CRISPR-Cas9-to-generate-the-recombinant-vaccines-vectors.png.

This enhancement of efficiency, beyond accelerating the timeline for vaccine availability, can also lead to the development of more effective and safer vaccines, focusing on significant public health issues, such as reemerging and emerging infectious diseases. The precision of gene editing minimizes off-target mutations, thus paving the way for vaccine design against specific pathogens and improving the overall efficacy of immunization programs (Fang, 2025). Furthermore, gene editing contributes significantly to improving the safety profiles of vaccines. Through the ability to allow for precise targeting of disease-causing genes, scientists can incapacitate pathogens without compromising their ability to stimulate an immune response. This approach is particularly critical for the development of live-attenuated vaccines, which must be preserved with sufficient virulence to stimulate a sufficient immunological response but prevent harmful effects. Further, applications of gene editing are not merely confined to the development of various vaccine modalities, including nucleic acid vaccines, viral vector vaccines, and subunit vaccines.

All these new strategies benefit from gene editing techniques, leading to customized immunity with fewer side effects. This flexibility secures gene editing as an essential technology in vaccine research and production, capable of enhancing the effectiveness of immunization and safety protocols in numerous clinical uses (Fang, 2025). The future of gene editing for vaccine development remains in search of discovery and innovation.

While the current success exists, concerns such as off-target effects and the cost of gene editing tools persist, encouraging ongoing research to better maximize accuracy and predictive capability. In addition, there is growing interest in employing multivalent vaccine constructs that can target multiple pathogens simultaneously, further enhancing the efficiency of vaccination efforts. Further future studies can investigate high-throughput screening strategies facilitated by gene editing, which have the potential to accelerate vaccine candidate identification and validation processes. Gene editing's horizon of new strategies and applications holds a revolutionary promise beyond current methods and has the potential to eliminate future infectious disease pandemics (Figure 9.6).

9.3.2. Modifying Immune Cells for Cancer Therapy

In recent years, advances in gene editing technology, particularly CRISPR-Cas9, have hastened the progression of immunotherapy. The modification of immune cells is the focus of investigators to enhance the efficacy of cancer therapy by avoiding the evasion strategies of tumors and the tumor immunosuppressive microenvironment (TME). Traditional treatments are lacking in their ability to target the cancer cells effectively due to their immuno-evasion and plasticity. Immunomodulation of cells, for instance, T cells, allows them to target cancer cells more effectively. This approach not only aims to mirror the immune response but also targets tumor-specific antigens, providing a form of precision in cancer treatment previously impossible (Gupte et al., 2024). The application of CRISPR-Cas9 has been particularly revolutionary for directing immune cells towards specific objectives in the tumor environment. By editing genes encoding immune checkpoint proteins and immunoregulatory pathways, researchers are able to enhance T cell activity and block inhibitory signals used by cancer cells. This allows for a heightened and longer duration of immune activation that is needed for effective anti-tumor activity. As an example, immune checkpoint manipulation by CRISPR has the ability to induce T cell expansion and cytotoxicity, thus leading to a more potent attack on tumor cells. However, while the promise of CRISPR technology is enormous, there are also tremendous challenges in store, including safety and specificity of gene editing to prevent unintended consequences resulting from these alterations (Gupte et al., 2024). The therapeutic efficacy of infused edited immune cells is also highly dependent on surmounting the technical hurdles of gene editing technologies. Some of the areas for improvement include optimizing delivery procedures for CRISPR components and precise targeting to minimize off-target effects. Clinical trials have also highlighted the requirement for designing safe and effective regimes for delivering such edited immune cells into patients. Moreover, combinatorial implementation of CRISPR-Cas9 approaches with existing immunotherapies can potentially provide synergistic advantages, collectively enhancing therapeutic efficacy. As additional proof from preclinical models comes to light, researchers are becoming increasingly optimistic about designing personalized cancer therapies that take advantage of gene editing to reprogram immune cells, eventually changing the therapeutic model for cancer patients (Feng et al., 2024) (Figure 9.7).

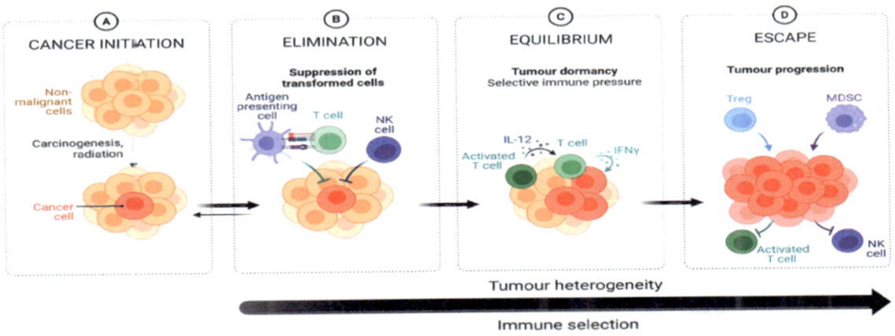

Figure 9.7. Cancer immuno-editing. By killing tumor cells with high immunogenicity, the immune system puts pressure on cancers for tumor cell variants with low immuno-stimulating profiles to emerge and proliferate preferentially.

Source: https://www.researchgate.net/publication/363752205/figure/fig4/AS:11431281208198448@1701378755130/Cancer-immuno-editing-By-killing-tumor-cells-with-high-immunogenicity-the-immune-system.jpg.

9.3.3. Gene Therapy for Autoimmune Diseases

The use of gene therapy for the treatment of autoimmune diseases is a major milestone in immunological science and clinical practice. It seeks to repair intrinsic genetic faults, enhance immune regulation, and reestablish tolerance to self-antigens. For example, therapeutic interventions utilizing regulatory T cells (Tregs) have become increasingly popular as a result of their pivotal role in immune homeostasis under conditions of autoimmune reactions. Enlarged Tregs from peripheral blood can be used to suppress auto-reactive immune cells effectively. As demonstrated in Earle et al. (2005), the expansion protocol for CD4+CD25 hi Tregs proves one's ability for *in vitro* manipulation to enhance curative activity. This specific protocol displays a remarkable increase in the numbers of Treg cells, which may represent a promising route for eradicating autoimmune pathology by way of targeted cell-based approaches. Gene editing technologies, particularly CRISPR/Cas9, have revolutionized the ability to edit with precision the genetic material of immune cells. For autoimmune disorders, such techniques can be applied to selectively eliminate or repair genes for the inappropriate immune response characteristic of such conditions. For instance, correction of mutations in genes responsible for T cell activation or cytokine production could lead to a more improved immune response and alleviate symptoms. The capabilities of CRISPR technology are also evidenced through research focused on discovering how molecular processes contribute to autoimmune diseases, as seen with immune phenotype and immune response studies involving gene editing and systemic modulation therapies. Enhanced knowledge garnered from such findings will ideally allow for the development of novel therapeutic regimens for sufferers of long-term autoimmune disease. Furthermore, the complexity of autoimmune diseases, which often involves numerous immune mechanisms, necessitates an approach that integrates various gene therapy methods. A disease such as uveitis shows this complexity, where regulatory mechanisms can fail and lead to inflammation and tissue damage as described in Amadi-Obi et al. (2014). An understanding of how maladaptive immune responses arise is essential to the development of effective gene therapies. Advances in immunology are beginning to unpack these intricate mechanisms and define a path towards the use of directed gene editing technologies that can reverse the normal immune and induce tolerance. Through addressing the root causes of autoimmunity through gene therapy, doctors can not only alleviate the symptoms but also achieve long-term stability and improved quality of life for those suffering from it, ushering in a new era of treatment for autoimmune disorders (Figure 9.8).

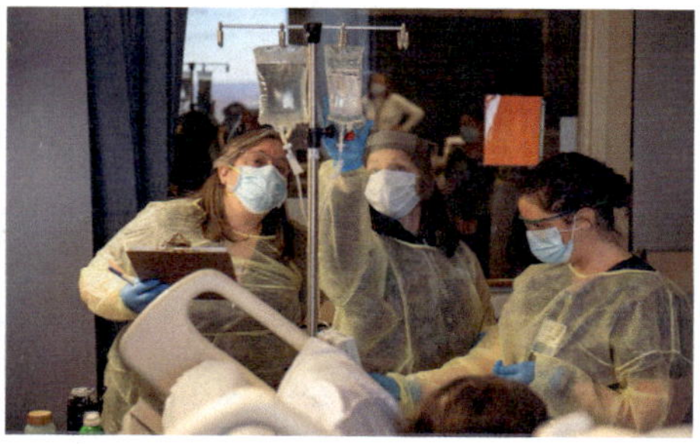

Figure 9.8. Gene therapy as a treatment for autoimmune diseases.

Source: https://today.uconn.edu/wp-content/uploads/2022/01/gsd-trial_UCH_2022-01-18_8566-1200x800-1-998x665.jpg.

9.4. Ethical Considerations

The entry of gene editing tools in the form of CRISPR/Cas9 is accompanied by a host of ethical problems that cannot be overlooked in immunology. While scientists strive to find out the extent of these tools in modifying the human genome to cure diseases, there is concern regarding unwarranted effects, especially off-target effects. The implications of inadvertently editing genes that participate in other biological processes are severe problems of long-term safety and genetic integrity. Moreover, the possibility of heritable changes requires an ethical consideration of whether it is permissible to modify the human germline, potentially affecting future generations in unforeseeable ways. As gene editing becomes increasingly close to clinical applicability, these issues raise the call for robust ethical guidelines to oversee research and application within the discipline of immunology (Nicholson & Pepper, 2016). Moreover, accessibility and equity issues in how gene editing technologies are being used must be addressed. The potential to develop revolutionary treatments has ethical ramifications on who has access to these innovations and on the way social disparities might be exacerbated. If gene editing is left in the control of rich individuals or groups, it could lead to a world in which people are genetically modified based on groups, possibly causing further discrimination or division of society. Ethically, issues also arise as to how research activity must be regulated, including informed consent and the potential manipulation of vulnerable groups. Creating fair access to advanced immunological therapy demands careful discussion and policymaking that guarantees that advantages are shared fairly and justly across all affected communities (Meiliana et al., 2017). Finally, the influence of public opinion cannot be overemphasized in the ethics of gene editing. Engaging the public in a discussion of CRISPR and its implications for immunology will allow for a full appreciation of the technology and its potential implications. This is important for developing a socially responsible gene editing system because it provides space for dissenting views to be heard and incorporated into policy-making. Additionally, transparency of research processes and open discussion of risk and benefit will increase the credibility of scientific activities. Ethically sound gene editing in immunology thus does not only rely on scientific rigor, but also on a commitment to involve society in the formulation of such breakthrough technologies (Nicholson & Pepper, 2016).

9.4.1. Ethical Implications of Gene Editing in Humans

The development of gene editing technologies has revolutionized the discipline of possible medical interventions. The ethical implications of the use of such methods on human beings cannot be overstated. The ability to manipulate the genes of human embryos raises profound ethical issues about how far we should extend the manipulation of human development. Unlike prior manipulations such as *in vitro* fertilization or preimplantation genetic diagnosis, addressing already established embryos, CRISPR/Cas9 implies direct gene alteration, essentially introducing new genetic information.

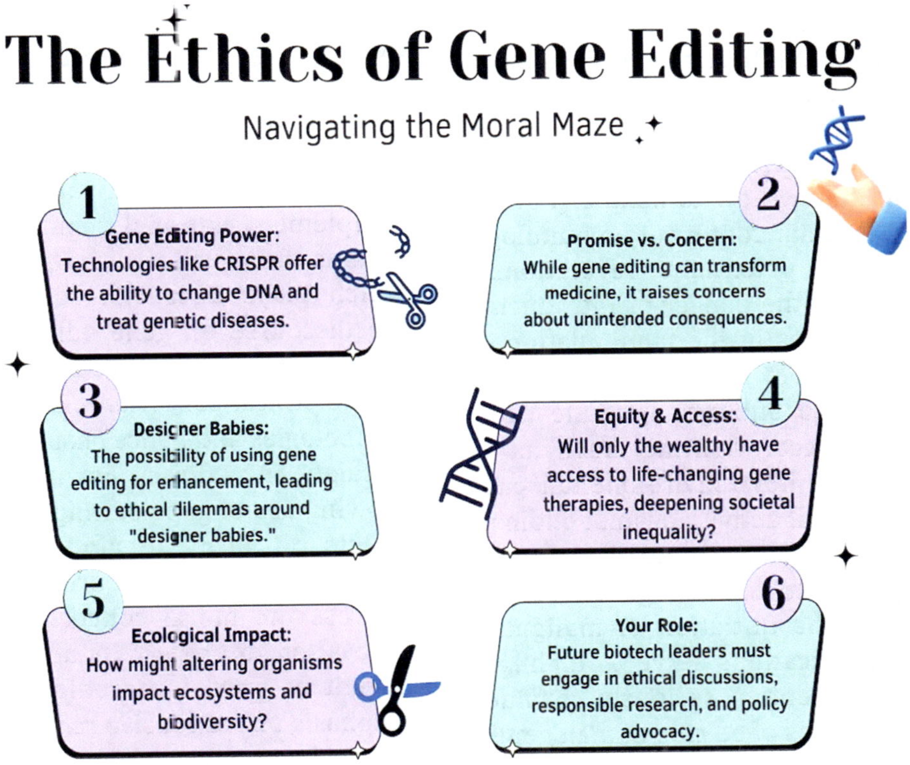

Figure 9.9. The ethics of gene editing.

Source: https://digianalix.com/blog/wp-content/uploads/2024/09/The-Ethics-of-Gene-Editing.webp.

This power to shape human genetics poses ethical issues, such as the slippery slope of eugenics and the social effects of designer babies, raising issues of inequality and access to these technologies.

Therefore, the debate over gene editing cannot just be about its scientific worth but must take into account the moral responsibilities of wielding such huge power over human biology (Powell, 2017). In addition, the jurisprudence of gene editing complicates the ethical argument. Current medical malpractice laws within most jurisdictions do not treat embryos as separate patients, leaving a gray area for liability in the event of outcomes from gene editing practices. As argued in recent discussions of CRISPR/Cas9 therapies, the lack of legal obligation to embryos suggests a dangerous precedent, one in which genetic modifications are possible with minimal regulation or consequence. This raises serious ethical concerns about potential misuse of the technology, especially if government leaders prioritize scientific advances over the welfare of future generations. Without proper regulatory checks on these techniques, the potential of gene editing to fulfill the promise of disease cure can open up unexpected ethical pitfalls that society does not know how to handle (Powell, 2017). In the particular context of immunology, gene editing has the potential to revolutionize treatment but holds the danger of introducing new ethical challenges in the manipulation of the immune system. For instance, gene editing can be employed to enhance immune cells' capabilities for cancer fighting, such as in research illustrating how environmental cues can guide myeloid cell activity against gliomas. Immune cells are indeed modified at some risk, including the possibility of off-target effects like autoimmunity or the initiation of malignant tumors. These implications serve to highlight the moral requirement to seriously consider long-term implications of editing human genes, particularly within immune pathways whose roles are absolutely essential in maintaining homeostasis. While medical science ventures into these new and uncharted waters of genetic manipulation, it is important to have firm ethical discourse to balance innovation with safeguarding human dignity and well-being (Figure 9.9).

9.4.2. Regulatory Frameworks Governing Gene Editing

Regulatory frameworks behind gene editing are intricate and evolving. They are crucial to enabling the safe application of gene editing technologies, such as CRISPR, which promise a significant level of hope in the treatment of immunological disorders. Regulators globally vary in their approach; the U.S., for instance, the Food and Drug Administration (FDA) has implemented stringent regulations to oversee gene therapy trials, while the European Medicines Agency (EMA) emphasizes an in-depth risk assessment process. The disparity among agencies complicates the task of researchers and clinicians conducting international work. By overlapping regulatory principles, the industry can better navigate complex ethics and ensure that gene editing therapies are given safely and efficiently to patients, hence motivating trust in gene editing technologies by healthcare systems. International agencies complement national regulation, and among them is the World Health Organization (WHO), which plays a crucial role in determining the discourse on gene editing. WHO's expert advisory committees give important suggestions on the ethical concerns related to gene editing technologies and hence ensure world standards of safety and efficacy. For instance, due to the growing use of gene editing technologies, their effects on germline modification in human beings are a concern. Current legislation must address the moral concerns related to such innovation to prevent its abuse. Moreover, the advent of precision medicine places greater emphasis on responsive regulatory approaches that are capable of keeping pace with rapid technology advancements as well as pinpointing the advantages and risks to patients in a delicate balance. This is particularly applicable in immunology since gene editing holds the potential to overhaul therapy approaches in autoimmune diseases and immunodeficiency. The increase in regulatory stages also reflects the degree of intricacy in grappling with the convergence of gene editing and transdisciplinary life sciences. As shown through advancements in xenotransplantation, the creation of multi-gene altered organisms such as Gal-knockout pigs shows how gene editing has progressed towards addressing significant medical challenges. With emerging methods increasing the viability of creating multi-gene altered animals, regulatory mechanisms must evolve to assess not just safety but also the ethics of these studies. The impact of gene editing on immune tolerance in xenotransplantation has raised issues regarding the limits allowed on genetic modification in animals and the impact on human well-being. This must be dealt with to provide guidelines for safe research protocols and ensure that biotechnological advances beneficially affect health outcomes without compromising moral principles, which is all the more necessary in immunological advancements (Ekser et al., 2017) (Figure 9.10).

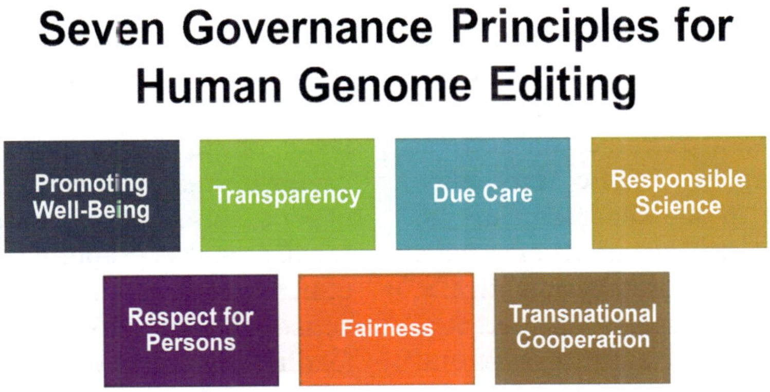

Figure 9.10. Seven governance principles for human genome editing.

Source: https://assets.weforum.org/editor/4u9HF1_QEcu2kIXVtKgQAgjkveFc4-xZcLWJI05F65Q.jpg.

9.4.3. Public Perception and Societal Impact

Public perception of gene editing technologies, and particularly those in the field of immunology, directly influences the acceptability and moral values of such advancements. With advancements such as CRISPR-Cas being a subject of continuous media waves, public discourse gains greater significance. The complexity of gene editing, and especially human germline gene editing (HGGE), stirs up diverse opinions and emotions in the public's discussion. It is required that underrepresented populations be included to confirm that divergent perspectives are heard within the discussion. Public engagement research indicates that inclusive conversation that not only addresses safety and effectiveness but also ethics and societal implications is a necessity that is needed immediately. Mass public discussion can make a significant difference to the social effect of gene editing by generating a sense of responsibility in societies who care about the decision-making concerning their well-being and health (Geuverink et al., 2024). In addition, the social effect of gene editing can be directly connected to whether or not the public perceives it as safe and ethically acceptable. Recent research indicates that knowledge of gene editing technologies is connected with positive opinions related to their safety, particularly when applied in medicine. Surveys have confirmed that individuals with some type of knowledge of gene editing are bound to have positive opinions regarding its use, which is correlated with improved comprehension of the technology's advantages and downsides. This familiarity puts at the forefront of prominence the necessity for initiative communication actions towards the education of the masses. Through the dissipation of confusion and fostering knowledge, stakeholders can cultivate an enlightened society that can meaningfully participate in discourse on the moral and utilitarian implications of gene editing (McFadden et al., 2024). Finally, public opinion about gene editing in immunology needs to be incorporated on a multi-dimensional basis that unites scientific objectivity and social values. Gene editing has immense repercussions beyond the research laboratory, reaching into human daily life and influencing health outcomes and societal welfare. With widespread public acceptance levels being critical to the successful use of gene editing technologies, the impact of various opinions needs to be evaluated systematically. In-depth communication possesses the potential to bridge the gap between scientific groups and the general public, establishing trust as well as understanding. Such an approach will not only make gene editing technologies more acceptable in general but will also allow individuals to participate in broader social discourse regarding their possibilities and ethics and thereby shape future immunology policies and practices (Geuverink et al., 2024).

9.5. Challenges and Limitations

With gene editing in immunology, there are some significant challenges and limitations that occur and must be given due attention. One of the principal ones is the very nature of biological systems that regulate immune responses. Their coordination among genetic differences and environmental stimuli complicates the identification of specific genomic loci for immune diseases. Despite the advancement toward genome-wide association studies (GWAS), which have been successful in identifying numerous loci involved in a variety of diseases, most of these associations are not characterized functionally. It is this lack of mechanistic data that tends to cloud the translation of genetic findings into therapeutic intervention, and this is a disconnect that exists between genetic association and clinical use. Also, as increased research relies on complex genetic models, such as the Collaborative Cross and Diversity Outbred populations of mice, the challenge of accurately representing human disease through these models is always a question (Saul et al., 2019). Another major drawback in gene editing studies is the ethical issue of its application to human subjects, primarily immunological interventions. The use of gene editing techniques, such as CRISPR-Cas9, is a high-stakes proposal that creates significant ethical questions around potential unintended consequences. Off-target effects, potentially leading to detrimental mutations, represent an especially concerning risk in the case of the human genome. Long-term consequences of such alterations, including potential impacts on generations to come, ignite intense controversy within science and society. Thus, science not only needs to labor to improve the precision and efficacy of gene editors but also to develop strong ethics that can serve to direct their use. It is important that discussion concerning the ethics of gene editing remain in tandem with technical advancements to facilitate responsible scientific innovation (Bhattacharya et al., 2018). The data management and reproducibility issues then limit the utility of gene editing research in immunology further. As the field advances, the sheer scale of data generated through genomic research necessitates robust data-sharing and analysis infrastructure to facilitate collaboration among scientists. Such initiatives as ImmPort have been launched subsequently to enhance data access as well as promote reuse of immunology data, but data integration continues to be impaired.

Variation in study design, standardization of data collection processes, and interoperability of multiple data systems may render the utilization of acquired wisdom for secondary analysis or meta-study challenging. This fragmentation not only hampers scientific progress but also denies research the benefits of shared understanding that can progress the therapeutic application of gene editing technologies in disease therapy for immunological disorders. These data challenges will be overcome by being key to realizing maximal benefit for gene editing in immunology (Saul et al., 2019).

9.5.1. Technical Challenges in Gene Editing

Gene editing techniques, such as the CRISPR-Cas9 system, have revolutionized the field of immunology by providing the ability to make precise changes to the genome. Broad application of this technology, however, is severely restricted by a number of technical limitations.

One significant issue is off-target effects, where the scope of genome changes becomes unintended and thus has the potential to hurt normal cells or cause undesirable outcomes on gene function. Such imprecisions complicate therapeutic activity, particularly in immunotherapy, where the accuracy of immune cell alteration is at stake. While scientists attempt to optimize therapeutic usage, avoidance of these off-target effects is still a primary goal for enhancing reliability and safety in gene editing's clinical use (Zou, 2025). Other than off-target effects, the technical specificity of the gene editing reagents continues to be a challenge.

Use of CRISPR-Cas9 requires precise delivery systems that can transfer the intended change to the correct genomic target. These include factors like the delivery system option, i.e., viral vector or lipid nanoparticles, which can dramatically affect gene editing efficiency and accuracy. The relative deficiencies of these delivery platforms can restrict their application in certain cellular contexts, making the design of effective treatment strategies problematic. Enhanced precision of editing—necessary to successful immunological interventions—is underpinned by continuous innovation and experimentation with new nucleases and vehicles for delivery to offset these intrinsic challenges (Huang, 2024).

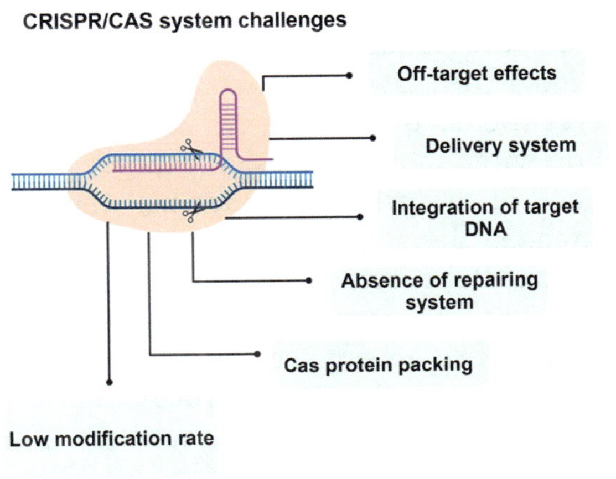

Figure 9.11. Challenges of the CRISPR-Cas system for genome editing purposes.

Source: https://www.researchgate.net/publication/367510204/figure/fig2/AS:11431281124933455@1678157704947/Challenges-of-the-CRISPR-Cas-system-for-genome-editing-purposes-Figure-created-with-the.png.

Ethical concerns surrounding gene editing also complicate its technical obstacles. The disruptive potential of gene editing in immunology necessitates careful scrutiny of inherent ethical considerations. Gene therapy issues revolve around the danger of creating long-lasting alterations that may be passed on through generations, raising questions regarding human enhancement, consent, and potential unexpected sociocultural impacts. As regulatory frameworks evolve, it is important to incorporate rigorous ethical assessments that are in harmony with technological advancement. An exchange of views on these ethical concerns will be of paramount significance not only towards enhancing public trust but also towards ensuring that gene editing methods are being used responsibly in the field of immunology (Zou, 2025) (Figure 9.11).

9.5.2. Off-target Effects and Safety Concerns

The development of gene editing technology, particularly CRISPR-Cas9, has drastically altered the landscape of immunology by providing variegated prospects for therapeutic interventions. Unfortunately, the technology is not without challenges. Off-target effects are one of the principal concerns, where the unintended alteration of the genome could lead to detrimental effects. Such unexpected changes can disrupt fundamental genes, which tends to cause negative effects such as oncogenesis or immune dysregulation. The rigorous examination of potential off-target sites is necessary in the evaluation of the overall safety of CRISPR-mediated use in immunological contexts, which highlights the requirement for precise methods to enhance specificity and mitigate dangers. By prioritizing thorough assessments and employing next-generation editing approaches, researchers can progress towards reducing such defects and ensuring the maximal therapeutic safety profile of gene editing drugs (Shaik et al., 2025). In addition to off-targeting effects, the broader themes of safety concerns surrounding CRISPR science include its delivery systems in therapeutic settings. Gene editing efficiency relies in part on the efficient delivery of CRISPR components into target cells, but current delivery methods have their own drawbacks. Viral vectors, nanoparticles, and electroporation all pose risks, such as potential immunogenicity or cytotoxicity, which may lead to undesirable immune responses or tissue damage. For instance, systemic viral vector delivery has the potential to cause harmful immune reactions, particularly in immunocompromised individuals. The complexity of managing such safety concerns underlines the importance of ongoing research in more effective and safer delivery systems, which would improve the therapeutic potential of gene editing in immunology while minimizing the risks associated with such treatment (Moses, 2025). The ethical implications of off-target consequences and safety considerations cannot be overlooked when talking of gene editing tools. With the prospect of advancing treatments to the clinical setting, full-scale moral analyses of these problems are now an urgency. The intrinsic uncertainty of off-target consequences and possible long-term effects demands frank disclosure of risks to patients of CRISPR-based treatments. Besides, firm regulatory guidelines must be established to regulate the use of gene editing on humans so that therapeutic processes are outlined by a preoccupation with efficacy and safety. It is also necessary to balance innovation against ethical sensibility to foster public trust and acceptance of gene editing technologies. By dealing with these ethical considerations, clinicians and scientists can help ensure that the gene editing technologies in immunology are responsibly developed and lay the foundations for groundbreaking advances in the field (Shaik et al., 2025).

9.5.3. Limitations in Current Research and Applications

When referring to gene editing shortcomings in immunology, the technical shortcomings inherent in the current gene editing technologies should be acknowledged. While technologies such as CRISPR-Cas9 have revolutionized the field with their precision and efficiency, concerns remain. Chief among them is that there could be off-target effects, whereby edits occur unintentionally at sites other than those expected, which can lead to deleterious consequences. Furthermore, the delivery vehicles employed to transfer these gene editing constructs to immune cells must be potent and precise so that they do not elicit immune reactions or fail entirely to edit target cells. Employment of viral vectors makes it even more challenging by posing risks of insertional mutagenesis and causing immune reactions against the vector itself. These limitations underscore the need for continuous upgrading of gene editing methods towards increased specificity and safety, vital in advancing therapeutic intervention in immunology. Another noteworthy limitation is the ethical dimension of gene editing used in immunology. With advances in this field gaining momentum, researchers must contend with complex ethics, particularly in light of germline edits and their potential effects on future generations. Furthermore, differences in access to such advanced treatments can create a sense of concern regarding balanced healthcare provisions. The possibility of creating designer immune systems or genetically modified traits raises public anxiety regarding eugenics and genetic disparities. Gene editing instruments must incorporate the art of balancing scientific progress and moral responsibility, thereby necessitating complex guidelines and regulating structures. Public consultation and dialogue are policies that play a vital role in attaining understanding and solving societal problems, such that the potential value of gene editing innovation in immunology can be attained without harm to ethical values. Lastly, there are significant gaps in the basic knowledge pertaining to the immune genetic foundation that continue to present a challenge to the realization of effective utilization of gene editing technologies. Difficult interactions between genes, epigenetic factors, and the environment complicate immune function and response to therapy. Current research often is not powered by large cohorts of data required to link some genetic alterations with expected immunological consequences, which limits gene editing's translation into the clinic. Laboratory techniques such as flow cytometry, though powerful, are handicapped by variability and standardization problems when applied to heterogeneous immune cell populations. Such heterogeneity can interfere with comparisons between studies, generating incoherent knowledge and unreliable outcomes. Filling the gaps is necessary to achieve the full potential of gene editing in immunology, leaving the opportunity for more efficient and directed therapy against immunological diseases and more robust vaccine development (Figure 9.12).

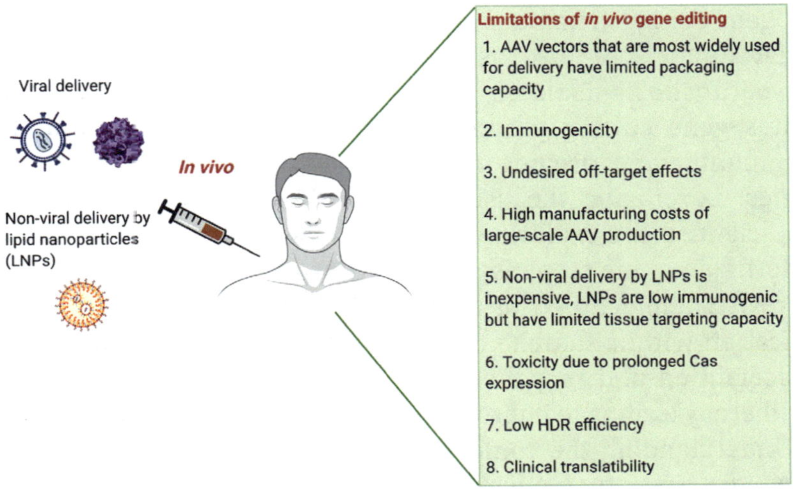

Figure 9.12. Schematic showing limitations of *in vivo* gene editing. *In vivo* gene therapy involves direct injection of the editing machinery into the patient by viral or nonviral delivery methods.

Source: https://www.researchgate.net/profile/Allison-Keeler-Klunk/publication/350296764/figure/fig1/AS:1004336809275393@1616463963222/Schematic-showing-limitations-of-in-vivo-gene-editing-In-vivo-gene-therapy-involves.png.

9.6. Future Directions

Future directions in immunology, with increasingly advanced gene editing technologies, are characterized by the exploration of new mechanisms that promise higher therapeutic efficacy with lower side effects. Some of the most promising directions are the engineering of adeno-associated viruses (AAVs) as safer and more effective tools for gene delivery. These vectors are favored because they are of low pathogenicity and have the ability to cause long-term gene expression in most tissue types, such that they can be the best vectors for the treatment of immunological disease. The establishment of rAAV also indicates the possibility of gene therapy improvement for autoimmune diseases and immunodeficiency. Although, as characterized in new research, manufacturing scalability issues and viral safety are controversial issues that must be solved to achieve maximum utility of these new technologies in the clinic (Wang et al., 2024). Along with vector engineering advancements, antibiotic-resistant pathogen development is an important issue that gene editing in immunology must resolve. The development of fluconazole-resistant Candida parapsilosis isolates, for instance, necessitates gene editing practices to enhance host immunity and provide new therapeutic strategies. Leveraging the use of CRISPR-based tools, scientists are exploring the potential for engineering immune responses to be effective against resistant infection. This may involve gene modification within immune cells to enhance their recognition and response to resistant pathogens, thereby leading to improved patient outcomes. Understanding the complex interactions between drug-resistant microbes and the immune system will be essential to designing effective gene editing technology that will not only address short-term therapeutic needs but also facilitate long-term immunity against microbes (Daneshnia et al., 2023). The future of gene editing in immunology will ultimately witness a blend of multi-mode strategies employing genetic engineering, immunotherapeutics, and new delivery systems. With increasing research, bridging the divide between clinical and laboratory discoveries will be the greatest step towards moving these therapies to the patients who can benefit from them. Interdisciplinary information exchanges between immunologists, geneticists, and bioengineers will allow for the development of multi-dimensional models of treatment that take advantage of gene editing technology to manipulate immune responses optimally. In addition, with changing regulatory scenarios, ensuring patient safety and embracing new gene therapy techniques will be the priority in defining the immunological therapy scenario. With joint collaboration, not only will the effectiveness of existing treatments increase, but it can also evolve responses to resist future immunological threats emerging in an ever-more heterogeneous medical field (Daneshnia et al., 2023; Wang et al., 2024).

9.6.1. Innovations in Gene Editing Technologies

The developments in the field of gene editing technology have utterly transformed the character of immunology. Among many techniques, there is one system that shines on its own merit: the CRISPR/Cas9 system. It is astonishing for the ease and accuracy with which this system has to offer. The technology itself has transformed the capability of editing single genes within the genome of an organism; thus, scientists can merely walk into the complex mechanisms of the immune responses. CRISPR/Cas9 has been found to be promising not just in the laboratory but also for therapy, i.e., the modification of immune cells to use in targeted cancer therapies. Research indicates that if CRISPR is used in hematopoietic stem/progenitor cells, then it can ablate genes that are known to be responsible for fetal hemoglobin production inhibition effectively, providing a means to cure selected hemoglobinopathies. In addition, the emerging new generation of CRISPR delivery systems is rendering it increasingly effective in a clinical setting and providing new possibilities for novel immunotherapy strategies (Bjurström et al., 2016). At the same time, gene delivery technologies have the potential to realize the full potential of gene editing in immunology. These technologies are designed to develop effective delivery systems for therapeutic agents such as gene-editing constructs, proteins, and medicines into target cells. Nanoscopic delivery vehicles, either chemically synthesized or naturally occurring, are robust potential options for the future effectiveness and specificity of gene-editing treatments. Harnessing the physical properties of these nanomaterials, in turn, enables researchers to modify their use in health care. Granularity of nanoparticle analysis includes size characterization, morphology, and agglomeration, each of which has a direct influence on its functionality within biological systems.

As the field continues to be on the ascent regarding academic and industry attention, it offers entrepreneurial potential, ultimately creating an active platform for strategic innovations in gene delivery (Savas et al., 2019). In addition, the integration of different gene editing technologies has ushered in a new era for precision medicine in immunology. Techniques like ZFNs and TALENs offer backup routes to modify the genome, in addition to CRISPR. ZFNs, for instance, have been very efficient in causing high degrees of gene disruption with specificity, particularly on targeted loci and those with immunofunctional associations. Comparative analyses of such technologies also exhibit their strengths; ZFNs and TALENs are expected to produce fewer off-target effects than CRISPR when appropriately engineered (Bjurström et al., 2016). With the enhancement of these methods by scientists, the possible synergistic benefit of using a combination of various systems of editing may lead to more effective therapeutic interventions that enhance the immune system's potential to fight disease, as the direction for gene editing technology is towards designing immunological therapies.

9.6.2. Potential Breakthroughs in Immunological Treatments

Innovations in immunotherapy milestones are significantly aided by the progress that has been observed in gene editing technology in recent years, namely the CRISPR-Cas9 system. The pioneering technology can allow for the cutting and rewriting of the genome with precision, thereby allowing researchers to edit and correct mutation-associated immune disorders. For instance, in hematologic diseases, gene editing has vowed to redesign hematopoietic stem cells not only to enhance their function and disease resistance but also their quality. Not only do they enhance the therapeutic efficacy in diseases like sickle cell disease, but they also open up new avenues to bypass the limitations of traditional therapies. With the advent of gene editing and personalized medicine, the future of immunotherapies can see a shift towards highly personalized modalities customized to the genetic makeup of an individual patient, ultimately leading to greater efficacy and reduced toxicity. Another potential subject of study is the cure for viral diseases, particularly the development of immunological therapy against diseases such as HIV-1. Recent studies have indicated that gene-editing instruments can successfully disrupt the viral genome and thus prevent the capacity of the virus to replicate and create reservoirs in the host. Based on recent overviews, integration of these gene editing tools with immunomodulatory therapy and novel antiretroviral drugs is progressing towards a foreseen cure for HIV-1. Such multifaceted approaches are designed not only to suppress but also to induce long-term remission regardless of continuous antiretroviral therapy. But translating these promising laboratory research into clinical use on the ground is with numerous challenges to be overcome in creating effective treatments for patients suffering from viral infections, underlining the need for ongoing study in this area (Borrajo, 2025). Moreover, synergistic integration of AI in immunotherapy is a classic example of another breathtaking accomplishment. Artificial intelligence technology is revolutionizing the history of bone marrow transplantation (BMT) by enhancing precision in the examination of data regarding patients. Recent updates on the developments of BMT suggest that AI has the potential to forecast the optimal donor-recipient match, significantly raising the success rate of treatment. Besides CRISPR-Cas9 gene editing, these technologies not only fix genetic defects but also improve the success rate of transplant operations themselves, which speaks volumes for an integrated approach to immunological therapy. However, application of these novel technologies is typically confronted with obstacles such as being expensive, less accessible, and more complex to use. Thus, ongoing research is necessary to develop these methods further and extend them so that a new generation of the treatment of immunological disease can be guaranteed (Zucon, 2024).

9.6.3. The Role of Gene Editing in Personalized Medicine

Advances in gene editing technologies, especially CRISPR-Cas9, have revolutionized the landscape of precision medicine, particularly immunology. With the ability to modify the genome, these technologies grant researchers and doctors a tool for building treatments as individual as a patient's gene set.

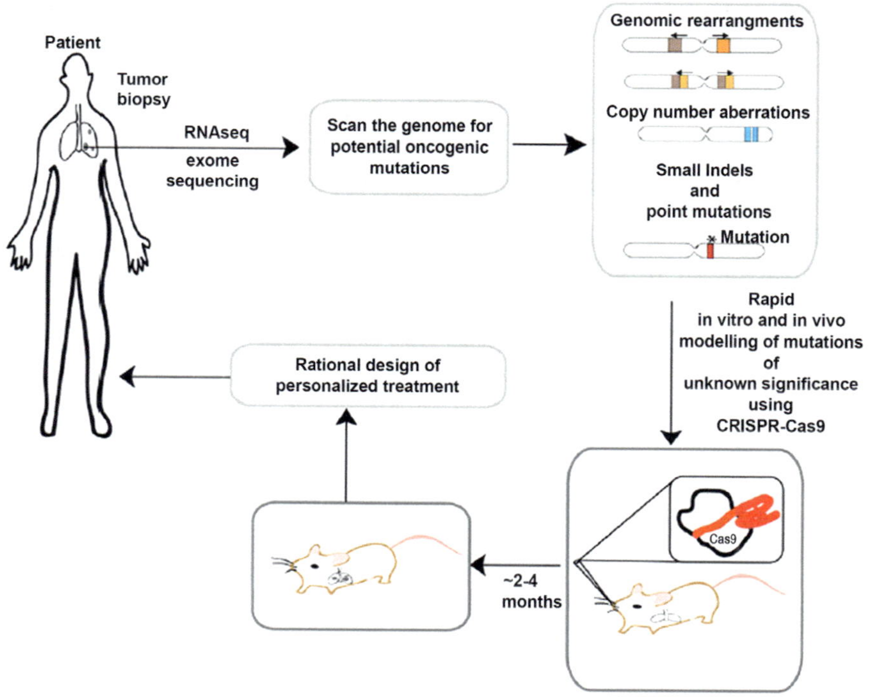

Figure 9.13. Applications of CRISPR-Cas9 in personalized medicine.

Source: https://www.researchgate.net/profile/Florin-Tripon-2/publication/313462381/figure/fig1/AS:459488789569536@1486562072688/Applications-of-CRISPR-Cas9-in-personalized-medicine-republished-with-the-permissions-of.png.

It's not about simplistic genetic code alteration but also about creating therapeutic interventions in an effort to elicit the best immune responses against cancers and other diseases. For instance, the interplay of gene editing and dietary practice may lead to more responsive immune profiles to enhance the efficiency of immunotherapies. Gene editing undertaken here not only advances the boundaries of therapeutic innovation but also tests the ethics of genetic manipulation, triggering ongoing debate among biomedical stakeholders. Moreover, gene editing is at the core of CAR T cell immunotherapy design, showing its potential to revolutionize cancer care. CAR T cells are made to target particular antigens on cancer cells, so that specifically the cancer cells would be destroyed without inducing much toxicity to normal tissue. Now, scientists can make CAR T cells more effectively using the CRISPR technology in such a manner that they become more effective and less toxic, thereby improving patient outcomes. The power to edit genes controlling immune checkpoints or to promote T cell survival is an order of magnitude advance in personalizing immunotherapies for the patient. Nevertheless, challenges abound, including overcoming severe side effects such as cytokine release syndrome for CAR T cell therapy. Scientists remain busy attempting to decrease risk and increase therapeutic benefit, and this highlights the intricacy that exists in personalized immunology. Finally, the integration of multi-omics approaches with gene editing is an exciting avenue for personalized medicine. By applying the combination of genomic, transcriptomic, and proteomic data, knowledge of personalized immune function is improved to allow for more targeted intervention. Single-cell sequencing technologies, for instance, are able to identify specific immune cell subpopulations which would be more responsive to a particular gene-edited therapy. Coupled with the potential of gene editing, clinical physicians are able to design personalized therapy taking into account genetic susceptibility and the patient's personal immune microenvironment. This coupling between high-throughput analysis and gene editing not only increases the precision of immunotherapies but also places at the center stage the potential of personalized medicine in combating complex diseases. Further research of these technologies is bound to uncover new modes of therapy and enhanced care for patients in the area of immunology (Figure 9.13).

SUMMARY

In concluding the revolutionizing potential of gene editing tools, particularly CRISPR-Cas9, it is not hard to recognize that the breakthroughs have profound implications for the practice of immunology. The capability to precisely edit genes has the potential to unlock avenues for path-breaking treatments for immune disorders, curing diseases that were previously believed to be incurable. With continuous research reflecting the promise of CRISPR in creating enhanced immune defenses and fixing genetic faults, the possibility of curing diseases like autoimmune diseases, allergies, and cancer in the future is immense. But using such strong technologies in hospitals must be carried out with utmost caution, considering not only the ethical dimension, but also long-term implications on human health and biodiversity. Besides this, while the clinical potential of gene editing is breathtaking, there is a felt need to address the ethics of using it in immunology. The ability to engineer genes that can cure genetic disorders poses questions of equity and consent as an ethical issue, particularly with its effects on future generations. It is such matters that necessitate fervent debate among scientists, ethicists, and policymakers to arrive at a framework of regulation that ensures appropriate application of this technology. Gene edits must not only be directed at efficacy but also at safety and fair distribution of benefit among diverse groups, in line with logic in the practice of general medicine and biotechnology. Ultimately, the future of gene editing in immunology is only beginning to unfold, with colossal success and formidable challenges. As researchers continue to advance these technologies, greater interdisciplinary coordination becomes an imperative. The intersection of information from multiple fields—genetics, immunology, ethics, and law—will be needed to manage the complexities built into gene editing. Additionally, in the interest of social concerns demonstrated in the present arguments, such as justice in the application of CRISPR technologies, it is imperative an attempt to gain public acceptability and trust. With ongoing research, keeping abreast of the technological revolution in terms of ethics will ensure that gene editing may be a boon in furthering human health and equity and justice in healthcare access (Sahin & Seli, 2025; Wheatley, 2025).

Technologies created using gene editing, in the case of the CRISPR-Cas9 system, have greatly enhanced the promise in immunology uses. Targeting is facilitated for the scientists by allowing them to edit genes with preternaturally high precision and the capability of specifically modulating immune responses. Enhancement of T cell function is one of the most reported applications, where gene editing can be employed to enhance anti-tumor immunity by editing the T cells to provide them with chimeric antigen receptors (CARs). With the ability to engineer immune cells, scientists are developing more effective cancer treatments and vaccines that have the potential to lead to greater survival rates among patients. Besides this, the use of gene editing technologies also makes it possible with greater therapeutic efficiency for personalized medicine in immunology through the tailoring of therapies on individual genetic information, thus leading to improved clinical outcomes. Another highly important field of gene editing in immunology is the control of extracellular vesicles (EVs) and their roles in intercellular communication. EVs, which are released by most cells, including immune cells, contain a complex mixture of different biomolecules, such as nucleic acids and proteins, that target adjacent cells and affect immune responses. The ability to precisely edit genes responsible for EV production and cargo content can facilitate an extension of immune process knowledge, including host-pathogen interactions. From the knowledge that has been created through EV research, researchers can develop new diagnostic and therapeutic strategies for infectious and chronic diseases with inappropriate immune responses. This new approach focuses on the potential of gene editing in advancing a more accurate understanding of immunological processes and improving patient outcomes in translational medicine (Gavinho et al., 2019). Furthermore, gene editing is likewise not a technological advancement within a silo; it overlaps with various disciplines, such as neuroimmunology, which has made clear how immune processes are integrated with neurological conditions. There is increasing evidence that immune mechanisms play a central part in a range of neurological conditions, from multiple sclerosis through to the neurodegenerative diseases. This cross-talk is potentially therapeutic for new therapeutic strategies for the modulation of neuroinflammation with targeted gene editing. With neuroimmunology expanding, there is also a requirement to embrace the progress in molecular biology and biomolecular research that are sure to increase our knowledge of immune-mediated modulation of the nervous system and temporal changes (Nutma et al., 2019). Such a paradigm shift has the potential to reveal novel therapeutic strategies that involve gene editing in combination with neuroimmunological information for better therapy.

A CLOSER LOOK

ZINC-FINGER NUCLEASES (ZFNS)

ZFNs are recombinant proteins that can be engineered to bind and cut specific DNA sequences, enabling targeted gene editing. They consist of a DNA-binding domain, which is typically constructed from zinc finger proteins, and a DNA cleavage domain, which is most often based on the FokI endonuclease. ZFNs are used to create site-specific double-strand breaks in DNA, which can then be repaired by the cell's own repair machinery, leading to gene knockout, gene correction, or gene addition (Figure 9.14).

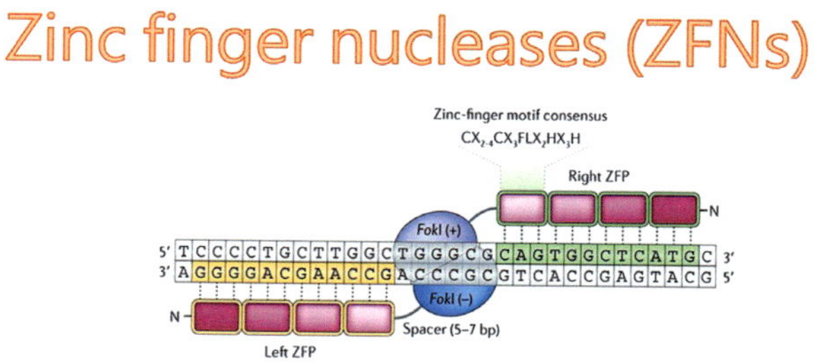

Figure 9.14. Illustration of Zinc-finger Nucleases (ZFNs).

Source: https://i.ytimg.com/vi/JArLDYv0Qw4/maxresdefault.jpg.

1. Structure and Function:

- a. **Zinc Finger Proteins (ZFPs):** The proteins are engineered to bind particular DNA sequences, typically 3–4 zinc fingers binding a 9–18 base pair sequence.
- b. **FokI Nuclease:** The enzyme domain cleaves the DNA, triggering a double-strand break in the target site.
- c. **Modular Design:** ZFNs are built by merging ZFPs and the FokI nuclease, which allows flexibility for targeting diverse DNA sequences by altering the ZFPs.

2. Applications:

- a. **Gene Disruption:** ZFNs can disrupt genes by causing a double-strand break, which has the consequence of causing insertions or deletions upon repair and makes the gene non-functional.
- b. **Gene Correction:** With a DNA homology template, the cell's repair mechanisms can utilize it to correct the gene sequence at the break site.
- c. **Gene Insertion:** ZFNs can also be used to insert a target DNA sequence into the genome at the target site, if a suitable template exists.

3. Benefits:

- a. **High Precision:** ZFNs can be designed to target specific DNA sequences, with minimal off-target effects.

b. **Flexibility:** ZFN technology can be used to target a wide range of organisms, from plants and animals to human cells.

c. **Very Efficient Gene Targeting:** ZFNs can make gene targeting much more efficient than existing methods.

4. Limitations:

a. **Design Difficulty:** Designing efficient ZFPs is time-consuming and could be challenging.

b. **Off-Target Effects:** ZFNs are designed to be specific, but off-target effects cannot be ruled out.

c. **Problems of Delivery:** Delivery of ZFNs into cells could be challenging, especially for some cell types or organisms.

5. Recent Developments:

a. **Improved FokI Variants:** Modifications of the FokI nuclease domain have led to increased activity as well as specificity.

b. **Alternative DNA Binding Domains:** Researchers have tried alternative applications of DNA binding domains, such as TALEs, as an alternative to zinc fingers.

c. **Clinical Application:** ZFNs are researched for the application of gene therapy in human beings for the treatment of HIV and other conditions.

REFERENCES

1. Nutma, E., Willison, H., Martino, G., & s, S. (2019). Neuroimmunology - the past, present and future. *Clinical and experimental immunology, 197*(3), 278–293. https://doi.org/10.1111/cei.13279(accessed on 27th June 2025).
2. Askeland, A., Botha, J., Rasmussen, R. W., & Handberg, A. (2019). ISEV2019 Abstract Book. *Journal of Extracellular Vesicles, 8*. https://www.semanticscholar.org/paper/a4c92b101ca17b1fe8f1ea2bc6808162744380e6 (accessed on 27th June 2025).
3. Roberts, A. W., Popov, L. M., Mitchell, G., Ching, K. L., Licht, D. J., Golovkine, G., Barton, G. M., & Cox, J. S. (2019). $Cas9^{+}$ conditionally-immortalized macrophages as a tool for bacterial pathogenesis and beyond. *eLife, 8*, e45957. https://doi.org/10.7554/eLife.45957 (accessed on 27th June 2025).
4. Bhattacharya, S., Dunn, P., Thomas, C. G., Smith, B., Schaefer, H., Chen, J., Hu, Z., et al. (2018). ImmPort, toward repurposing of open access immunological assay data for translational and clinical research. *Scientific Data, 5*. https://doi.org/10.1038/sdata.2018.15 (accessed on 27th June 2025).
5. Bjurström, C. F., Cooper, A., Hollis, R. P., Kaufman, M. L., et al. (2016). Reactivating fetal hemoglobin expression in human adult erythroblasts through BCL11A knockdown using targeted endonucleases. https://core.ac.uk/download/323076170.pdf (accessed on 27th June 2025).
6. Earle, K. E., Tang, Q., Zhou, X., Liu, W., Zhu, S., Bonyhadi, M. L., & Bluestone, J. A. (2005). In vitro expanded human CD4+CD25+ regulatory T cells suppress effector T cell proliferation. *Clinical immunology (Orlando, Fla.), 115*(1), 3–9. https://doi.org/10.1016/j.clim.2005.02.017(accessed on 27th June 2025).
7. Borrajo, A. (2025). Breaking barriers to an HIV-1 cure: Innovations in gene editing, immune modulation, and reservoir eradication. *Life, 15*. https://www.semanticscholar.org/paper/95ef2ca193a3d28c32ece0f1e3ea58d8f124414d (accessed on 27th June 2025).
8. Charrot, S., & Hallam, S. (2019). CAR-T cells: Future perspectives. *Hemisphere, 3*. https://doi.org/10.1097/hs9.0000000000000188 (accessed on 27th June 2025).
9. Ekser, B., Li, P., & Cooper, D. K. C. (2017). Xenotransplantation: past, present, and future. *Current opinion in organ transplantation, 22*(6), 513–521. https://doi.org/10.1097/MOT.0000000000000463 (accessed on 27th June 2025).
10. Daneshnia, F., de Almeida, J. N., İlkit, M., Lombardi, L., Perry, A. M., Gao, M., Nobile, C. J., et al. (2023). Worldwide emergence of fluconazole-resistant *Candida parapsilosis*: Current framework and future research roadmap. *The Lancet Microbe, 4*, e470–e480. https://doi.org/10.1016/s2666-5247(23)00067-8 (accessed on 27th June 2025).
11. Meiliana, A., Dewi, N. M., & Wijaya, A. (2017). Genome editing with CRISPR-Cas9 systems: Basic research and clinical applications. Genome Editing with CRISPR-Cas9 Systems (Meiliana A, et al.) https://core.ac.uk/download/229778116.pdf (accessed on 27th June 2025).
12. Dhar, S. (2025). Advances in clinical immunology. *Premier Journal of Immunology*. https://www.semanticscholar.org/paper/f02683d80692f51bda8086b9c7dc2533c19a00de (accessed on 27th June 2025).

13. Dunbar, C. E., High, K. A., Joung, J. K., Kohn, D. B., Ozawa, K., & Sadelain, M. (2018). Gene therapy comes of age. *Science, 359*. https://doi.org/10.1126/science.aan4672 (accessed on 27th June 2025).

14. Elkord, E. (2025). Preface. *Cancer Immunology Connect*. https://www.semanticscholar.org/paper/a62d6177daa8fde09fa73f6da5a5ca7fe4082ac8 (accessed on 27th June 2025).

15. Falus, A. (2006). Immunogenomics and human disease. https://www.semanticscholar.org/paper/14596a63cc183529fae4f67b1c33c0f4c1183280 (accessed on 27th June 2025).

16. Falzone, L., Salomone, S., & Libra, M. (2018). Evolution of cancer pharmacological treatments at the turn of the third millennium. *Frontiers in Pharmacology, 9*. https://doi.org/10.3389/fphar.2018.01300 (accessed on 27th June 2025).

17. Fang, Y. (2025). The role and impact of gene editing on vaccine development. *Theoretical and Natural Science*. https://www.semanticscholar.org/paper/95565577af140096e03fd90aaad1f59593c5f1f1 (accessed on 27th June 2025).

18. Feng, X., Li, Z., Liu, Y., Chen, D., & Zhou, Z. (2024). CRISPR/Cas9 technology for advancements in cancer immunotherapy: From uncovering regulatory mechanisms to therapeutic applications. *Experimental Hematology & Oncology, 13*. https://www.semanticscholar.org/paper/feea0d472ec0fea3694cb24c4486200a07abb1ba (accessed on 27th June 2025).

19. Forrest, A. (2020). The growing threat of agroterrorism and strategies for agricultural defense. https://core.ac.uk/download/322850909.pdf (accessed on 27th June 2025).

20. Galbraith, D. W., Loureiro, J., Antoniadi, I., Bainard, J. D., Bureš, P., Cápal, P., Castro, M., et al. (2021). Best practices in plant cytometry. *Cytometry Part A, 99*, 311–317. https://doi.org/10.1002/cyto.a.24295 (accessed on 27th June 2025).

21. Gavinho, B., Combes, V., Dlugonska, H., Hart, M. L., Evans-Osses, I., Rossi, I. V., Inal, J., et al. (2019). A new landscape of host–protozoa interactions involving the extracellular vesicles world. https://core.ac.uk/download/287580982.pdf (accessed on 27th June 2025).

22. Geuverink, W. P., Houtman, D., Retel Helmrich, I. R., Kist, J., Henneman, L., Cornel, M., & Riedijk, S. R. (2024). A decade of public engagement regarding human germline gene editing: A systematic scoping review. *European Journal of Human Genetics, 33*, 570–579. https://www.semanticscholar.org/paper/1e6a431ac5ccf8700b2813ca0c801ea8d033a2af (accessed on 27th June 2025).

23. Gupte, P., Dhingra, K., & Saloni. (2024). Precision gene editing strategies with CRISPR-Cas9 for advancing cancer immunotherapy and Alzheimer's disease. *Journal of Knowledge Learning and Science Technology*. https://www.semanticscholar.org/paper/0022d5a1dcbe7db7f0bd9b012fe358d45973badd (accessed on 27th June 2025).

24. He, S., Liu, Y., Zhang, Z., Cai, M., Hao, Y., & Hu, H. (2025). Gene editing in *Ganoderma lucidum*: Development, challenges, and future prospects. *Journal of Fungi, 11*. https://www.semanticscholar.org/paper/0e39f40a2a77c881994fcc883e7819f7613f7b05 (accessed on 27th June 2025).

25. Huang, H. (2024). Methodological exploration of using gene editing technology to study gene function and disease mechanism. *Transactions on Materials, Biotechnology and Life Sciences*. https://www.semanticscholar.org/paper/2d35de9c9154871bde5252e130f35eef7fd1e60e (accessed on 27th June 2025).

26. Keul, A., Farkas, A., Carpa, R., Dobrotă, C., & Iordache, D. (2022). Development of smart fruit crops by genome editing. *Turkish Journal of Agriculture and Forestry*. https://www.semanticscholar.org/paper/4ffdda87da09a5e450890a166ea632cabb3f7ea1 (accessed on 27th June 2025).

27. Khare, V. (2021). CRISPR, ZFNs, and TALENs for hemoglobinopathies: An analysis. *International Journal for Research in Applied Science and Engineering Technology*. https://www.semanticscholar.org/paper/b7e0f1441f6092539467427a87828e11299c519e (accessed on 27th June 2025).

28. Kumar, A., Kumar, A., McMichael, A. J., Das, A. T., Berkhout, B., Sponseller, B. A., Haynes, B. F., et al. (2013). Envelope determinants of equine lentiviral vaccine protection. https://core.ac.uk/download/12215485.pdf (accessed on 27th June 2025).

29. Lotfi, M., Tambuwala, M. M., Shahcheraghi, S. H., Ayatollahi, J., Aljabali, A. A. A., Al Zoubi, M. S., Panda, P. K., et al. (2022). Gene therapy for neuropsychiatric disorders: Potential targets and tools. *CNS & Neurological Disorders–Drug Targets, 22*, 51–65. https://doi.org/10.2174/1871527321666220304153719 (accessed on 27th June 2025).

30. McFadden, B. R., Rumble, J. N., Stofer, K., & Folta, K. M. (2024). U.S. public opinion about the safety of gene editing in the agriculture and medical fields and the amount of evidence needed to improve opinions. *Frontiers in Bioengineering and Biotechnology, 12*. https://www.semanticscholar.org/paper/cfe28a40c3777a604332051d4b97beed49a3e1e8 (accessed on 27th June 2025).

31. Menon, A., Song, B., Chao, L., Sriram, D., Chansky, P., Bakshi, I., Ulianova, J., et al. (2025). Unraveling the future of genomics: CRISPR, single-cell omics, and the applications in cancer and immunology. *Frontiers in Genome Editing, 7*. https://www.semanticscholar.org/paper/c507290af0e2ba4309109a058ca1b72e212ae70d (accessed on 27th June 2025).

32. Mitra, A., Barua, A., Huang, L., Ganguly, S., Feng, Q., & He, B. (2023). From bench to bedside: The history and progress of CAR T cell therapy. *Frontiers in Immunology, 14*. https://doi.org/10.3389/fimmu.2023.1188049 (accessed on 27th June 2025).

33. Moses, M. H. (2025). The role of CRISPR-based gene editing in eradicating latent HIV reservoirs in patients on antiretroviral therapy (ART): A scoping review. *Research Invention Journal of Scientific and Experimental Sciences*. https://www.semanticscholar.org/paper/928e0d725efe02a7417ea68b3d0ba02a05829344 (accessed on 27th June 2025).

34. s, S. A., & Pepper, M. S. (2016). CRISPR-Cas: Revolutionising genome engineering. *South African medical journal = Suid-Afrikaanse tydskrif vir geneeskunde, 106*(9), 870–871. https://doi.org/10.7196/SAMJ.2016.v106i9.11061(accessed on 27th June 2025).

35. Padaru, M., Shetty, P., Kini, A., & Bhat, R. (2025). CRISPR/Casmediated targeted gene editing of *Streptococcus mutans*: A promising approach for precision dentistry for the prevention and management of caries (Review). *World Academy of Sciences Journal*. https://www.semanticscholar.org/paper/872c61729a6c23ac1e6887d63c824ed03d8c793f (accessed on 27th June 2025).

36. Permyakova, N., & Deineko, E. V. (2024). Crop improvement: Comparison of transgenesis and gene editing. *Horticulture*. https://www.semanticscholar.org/paper/502403e36a163b234f0f8aeafaa05329c05d1d8f (accessed on 27th June 2025).

37. Powell, G. E., III. (2017). Embryos as patients? Medical provider duties in the age of CRISPR/Cas9. https://core.ac.uk/download/84098963.pdf (accessed on 27th June 2025).

38. Sahin, G. N., & Seli, E. (2025). Gene editing using CRISPR-Cas9 technology: Potential implications in assisted reproduction. *Current Opinion in Obstetrics and Gynecology, 37*, 141–148. https://www.semanticscholar.org/paper/1013bf1014632de45f27d6f58428ba3cd06f739c (accessed on 27th June 2025).

39. Salminen, S., Collado, M. C., Endo, A., Hill, C., Lebeer, S., Quigley, E. M. M., Sanders, M. E., et al. (2021). The International Scientific Association of Probiotics and Prebiotics (ISAPP) consensus statement on the definition and scope of postbiotics. *Nature Reviews Gastroenterology & Hepatology, 18*, 649–667. https://doi.org/10.1038/s41575-021-00440-6 (accessed on 27th June 2025).

40. Saul, M. C., Philip, V. M., Reinholdt, L. G., & Chesler, E. J. (2019). High-diversity mouse populations for complex traits. *Trends in Genetics, 35*, 501–514. https://doi.org/10.1016/j.tig.2019.04.003 (accessed on 27th June 2025).

41. Savas, P. E., Jr. (2019). Therapeutic delivery technology and its economic impact. https://core.ac.uk/download/213463611.pdf (accessed on 27th June 2025).

42. Shaik, F. T., & Yarra, S. (2025). Beyond the hype: A critical review of CRISPR-Cas9 gene editing therapies. *International Journal of Science and Research Archive*. https://www.semanticscholar.org/paper/bb77b9e0ce48213ec5bc29265bf3c3cfa0efaa8f (accessed on 27th June 2025).

43. Sies, H., Berndt, C., & Jones, D. P. (2017). Oxidative stress. *Annual Review of Biochemistry, 86*, 715–748. https://doi.org/10.1146/annurev-biochem-061516-045037 (accessed on 27th June 2025).

44. Steele, E. J. (2009). Lamarck and immunity: Somatic and germline evolution of antibody genes. https://core.ac.uk/download/11241786.pdf (accessed on 27th June 2025).

45. Tang, K., Zhou, X., Fang, S. Y., Vandenbulcke, E., Du, A., Shen, J., Cao, H., et al. (2024). High-fidelity enhanced AsCas12a knock-in mice for efficient multiplexed gene editing, disease modeling and orthogonal immunogenetics. *bioRxiv*. https://www.semanticscholar.org/paper/505c113bba418480e396c90a867004655d0f8a24e (accessed on 27th June 2025).

46. Wang, J. H., Gessler, D. J., Zhan, W., Gallagher, T. L., & Gao, G. (2024). Adeno-associated virus as a delivery vector for gene therapy of human diseases. *Signal Transduction and Targeted Therapy, 9*. https://doi.org/10.1038/s41392-024-01780-w (accessed on 27th June 2025).

47. Wheatley, M. C. (2025). Gene editing: CRISPR and beyond. *Premier Journal of Biomedical Science*. https://www.semanticscholar.org/paper/3d3edac3be6de29dcddbb09184c91781afbc8e3c (accessed on 27th June 2025).

48. Xie, N., Shen, G., Gao, W., Huang, Z., Huang, C., & Fu, L. (2023). Neoantigens: Promising targets for cancer therapy. *Signal Transduction and Targeted Therapy, 8*. https://doi.org/10.1038/s41392-022-01270-x (accessed on 27th June 2025).

49. Xue, M., & Jin, W. (2025). Editorial: Immunological precision therapeutics: Integrating multi-omics technologies and comprehensive approaches for personalized immune intervention. *Frontiers in Immunology, 16*. https://doi.org/10.3389/fimmu.2025.1581238 (accessed on 27th June 2025).

50. Yao, B., Yang, Q., Gonçalves, M. A. F. V., Schiffelers, R., Sluijter, J. P., & Lei, Z. (2025). Comparative analysis of methods for assessing on-target gene editing efficiencies. *Methods and Protocols, 8*. https://www.semanticscholar.org/paper/e247bc70958428459a75c4aeb6f07468560cfeee (accessed on 27th June 2025).
51. Zhao, Y. (2025). Application and prospect of gene editing technology in immunotherapy. *Highlights in Science, Engineering and Technology*. https://www.semanticscholar.org/paper/66b967d0fdf4ed6bfc1b5e284e255258c2c06284 (accessed on 27th June 2025).
52. Zou, J. (2025). The application progress, challenges, and future directions of gene editing technology in immunotherapy. *Highlights in Science, Engineering and Technology*. https://www.semanticscholar.org/paper/aef78936d35c11694159984e906cded82f540c47 (accessed on 27th June 2025).
53. Zucon, I. S. (2024). INOVAÇÕES BIOTECNOLÓGICAS: O papel das células–tronco e da engenharia genética no transplante de medula óssea. *Revita FT*. https://www.semanticscholar.org/paper/cab22428b5934782244b5289bcb9f3128f72e7fc (accessed on 27th June 2025).

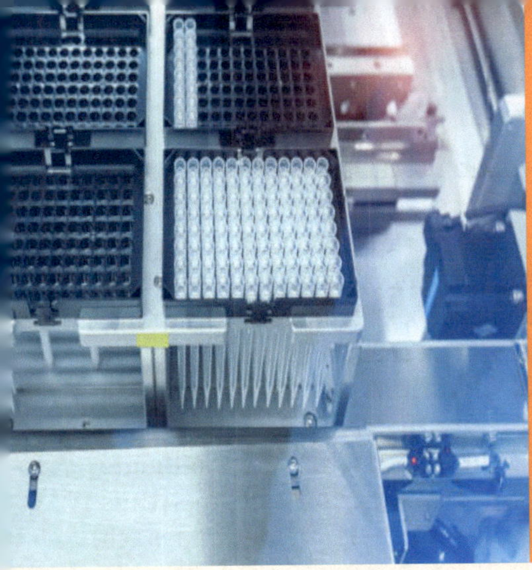

Chapter 10
HIGH-THROUGHPUT SCREENING IN IMMUNOLOGY

Contents

Introduction

High-throughput screening (HTS) has revolutionized immunology with its unparalleled prospects for investigating the complexity of the immune system. HTS technologies allow for concurrent analysis of thousands of samples, speeding up the research process in discovering new therapeutic targets, potential biomolecules, and information on immune responses. Classical approaches to immunology tended to require Herculean time and effort, making investigations narrow in scope and scope-limited. Yet, with HTS, scientists are now able to analyze the vast immune repertoire landscape more effectively. This ability is particularly important in the study of diseases like autoimmunity and cancer, in which the responses of the immune system can be complex and heterogeneous and therefore require sophisticated methodologies to make robust analysis possible. In immunology, HTS techniques play a particularly significant role since they can generate global data sets, which are necessary to decipher the adaptive immune system. The effector phase of the immune repertoire dissociates most B and

T cells from their antigen-specific receptors' diversity, which is quantitatively profiled with techniques such as adaptive immune receptor repertoire sequencing (AIRR-seq). By subjecting high-throughput sequencing information to computational and statistical analysis, researchers are able to uncover intricate immune receptor repertoire diversity patterns, which serve to clarify immune dynamics in health and pathological states. As hinted in recent summaries, understanding the architecture of the repertoire is key to immunotherapeutic, vaccine, and immunodiagnostic development and highlights the value of HTS in modern immunological research (Miho et al., 2018). Moreover, technological breakthroughs in droplet microfluidic technology have revealed novel opportunities for single-cell analysis in the high-throughput regime that is important in immunology. These technologies are applied in high-throughput screening to interrogate cellular behavior and metabolic profiles at record resolution. Noninvasive methods such as fluorescence lifetime imaging microscopy allow researchers to profile cell metabolism on a single-cell basis without sacrificing cell viability for subsequent analysis. This approach not only enables understanding of cell heterogeneity but also underscores the importance of metabolic states in immunology. As the complexity of immune reactions continues to be unraveled through HTS, the incorporation of such technologies becomes inevitable for the development of targeted treatments as well as better disease management strategies (Ma et al., 2019). Thus, HTS is an unparalleled bridge of technological advancement and groundbreaking research in immunology.

Definition of High-Throughput Screening (HTS)

HTS is an innovative method in immunology that is specifically founded on its ability to test thousands to millions of biological samples within a short period of time. It is achieved using advanced automation technologies, tiny assays, and informatics processing powers, all of which are integrated together to speed up the quest for lead therapeutic chemicals. HTS is being conducted in an orderly experimentation setting, making it easier for researchers to assess the biological effect of various agents on immune reactions. Consequently, this technology has become central in immunotherapeutic candidate development and optimization and has thus turned out to be the most significant approach in addressing complex immune-linked diseases such as cancer and autoimmunity. One of HTS's major strengths is to unravel the complexity of the adaptive immune system by interrogating immune repertoires. With the leverage of technologies such as AIRR-seq, researchers can quantitatively describe immune responses, resulting in high-dimensional data that reveals the complexity of immune receptor diversity and specificity.

This mass profiling is essential to identify how immune cells interact with tumor cells or pathogens and provide insights into the adaptive immunity behavior. The use of statistical tools and computational methods in the processing of this vast volume of data addresses immune repertoire complexity and enables better insight into immune mechanisms and how they are pertinent in therapy (Miho et al., 2018). In addition, HTS is not restricted to legacy high-expense equipment; development in digital imaging has made powerful screening processes widely accessible. To illustrate, affordable USB microscopes combined with open-source analysis software provide detailed cell motility assays and tracking experiments. This democratization enables more researchers to perform advanced analyses without paying exorbitant amounts of money. Therefore, these advancements enhance the throughput potential in immunology research, boosting the hopes of significant breakthroughs in vaccine discovery and immunodiagnostics (Lynch et al., 2014).

Overall, the integration of HTS into immunology accelerates the discovery process while also broadening the scope of candidate interventions for many immunological disorders (Figure 10.1).

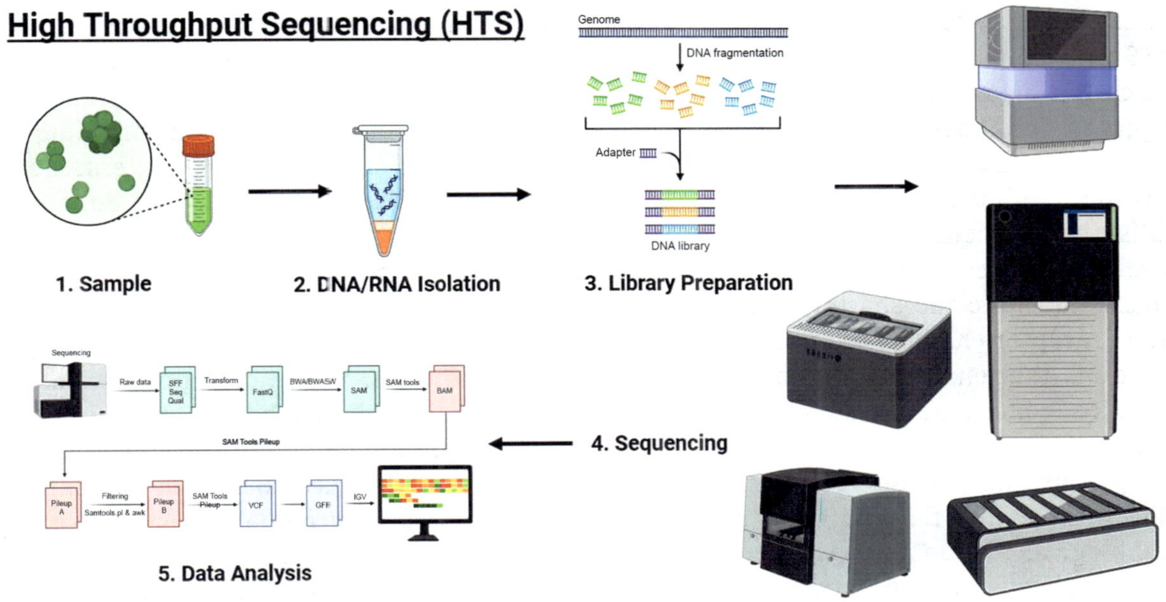

Figure 10.1. Illustration of high-throughput screening (HTS).

Source: https://microbenotes.com/wp-content/uploads/2024/09/High-Throughput-Sequencing-HTS.jpeg.

Importance of High-Throughput Screening (HTS) in Immunology

HTS greatly enhances immunological research by allowing scientists to rapidly test very large numbers of samples, thus accelerating the discovery of therapeutic targets and vaccines. The ability to run complex assays at an unprecedented scale has changed the manner in which scientists investigate immune responses For instance, HTS may be applied for the discovery of novel antibodies or T-cell receptors by interrogating the enormous diversity of the adaptive immune repertoire. This is central to the understanding of illnesses such as cancer and autoimmunity, whose composition of immune systems is altered or compromised. The computational methods devised to analyze data collected by means of AIRR-seq make this possible, as they can provide insight into the structure and specificity of the immune response, ultimately being used to inform rational immunotherapy and vaccine design that is more engaging for the immune system (Miho et al., 2018). Moreover, HTS has contributed to the dissection of pathogen interactions with the immune system and hence to valuable insights into infectious disease processes. Rapid identification of immune evasion strategies employed by viruses and bacteria allows researchers to devise vaccines and therapeutic interventions that can pre-emptively counter these strategies. As an example, studies on vampire bats have disclosed new hemotropic Mycoplasma species infecting blood hosts. By applying HTS methods, scientists may simultaneously screen large numbers of samples for identifying rapidly such interactions and their implications in host health. Such an ability not only allows enhanced knowledge in disease dynamics but also aids in predicting potential zoonotic transmissions, informing public health policy to pre-emptively mitigate risks associated with emerging infectious diseases (Volokhov et al., 2017). The integration of HTS into immunology not only accelerates research but also fosters collaboration across disciplines, enhancing the field's overall efficacy. The data generated through high-throughput methodologies can be leveraged to establish comprehensive databases that serve as resources for researchers worldwide. These databases facilitate the sharing of findings on immune receptor characteristics and pathogen interactions, thus enriching the global scientific community's collective understanding of immune dynamics. Moreover, HTS allows machine learning algorithms to be used, which makes predictive modeling feasible that can predict immunological responses, opening the doors for personalized medicine strategies tailored to individual immune profiles. The ongoing technological advancement of HTS will probably revolutionize immunology as a science able to inform new health care and disease prevention approaches using solid and high-dimensional data analysis (Miho et al., 2018).

10.1. Historical Background of High-Throughput Screening (HTS)

The origins of HTS date back to the need for efficient and successful methods in the post-genomic era in accordance with biotechnology and informatics development. HTS was originally used in pharmaceutical research, wherein drug research sought to accelerate drug discovery through screening huge compound libraries against target biological molecules. This strategy revolutionized the paradigm from traditional, manpower-based assays to automated platforms where it was now possible to analyze thousands to millions of samples simultaneously. Advances in robotics and microfluidics, along with new computational tools, were of critical significance in evolving HTS strategies. Consequently, this time has allowed not just the identification of new drug leads but also the probing of biomolecular interactions critical to the understanding of numerous diseases, opening the door towards their application in immunology. As scientists began to appreciate the usefulness of HTS in immunological research, the technique was applied to explore complex immune responses and pathways. Sensational progress has been made in the identification of cytokines and their role in immunological processes, which was highlighted in particular with the emergence of gene knockout models in mice. The models highlighted the capacity of cytokines to modulate immune responses, thereby providing avenues for wide-scale investigation into their therapeutic use. As the techniques for HTS advanced, researchers began employing them in order to uncover cytokine, immune cell, and disease connections, eventually finding key molecular targets for vaccines and medicines. Being able to quickly analyze HTS datasets has enabled the scientific community to learn more about cytokine networks, demonstrating how HTS has fortified modern immunology by providing a tool with which complex immune dynamics can be probed, deconstructed, and manipulated. Furthermore, the recent overlap of HTS with genomic and proteomic technologies has accelerated the progress of immunological science. The identification of avian homologs for the regulator molecules, such as interferons and interleukins, indicates how new technology has expanded the application of HTS from mammals to other organisms and advanced comparative studies in immunology. Low sequence conservation that originally limited conventional approaches has given way to high-throughput sequencing, which allows improved characterization of immune-related genes across species. This robust platform not only facilitates optimization of cytokine-targeted therapy but also optimizes the fundamental knowledge required for vaccine design. With increased enhancement of HTS, the technology has the potential to unlock novel immunological mechanisms and enhance the pace of therapeutic intervention discovery, an essential step toward precision-based method in immunology.

10.1.1. Development of High-Throughput Screening (HTS) Technologies

Breakthroughs in HTS technologies have transformed drug discovery and immunology as scientists are now able to conduct large-scale experiments that would otherwise be impossible. Established in the beginning in the area of small molecule screening, HTS has now come to utilize a variety of biological assays, including those aimed at targeting particular immune responses. The advent of robotic probes and advanced screening techniques has given the possibility of examining thousands of chemicals or biological probes in hours, as opposed to the conventional techniques. This pace has somehow bridged the gap between discovery and drug development, and it is now possible to find lead candidates that more effectively modulate immune responses, and in doing so, pave the way for new therapies for immune-related diseases. Secondly, combining HTS with systems biology approaches makes it more efficient by providing a holistic approach to explaining the vast amounts of data generated. Systems biology addresses connected biological systems rather than discrete components, and this is specifically true in the understanding of complex immune responses. The combination of HTS with advanced computational analysis facilitates easier identification of potential biomarkers and drug targets by looking at the dynamic interaction between genetic, proteomic, and metabolomic data. In doing so, scientists can develop sophisticated models that predict the behaviors of biological systems, hence more efficient and targeted drug discovery. This synergy between HTS and systems biology is a major advancement in the execution of immunological studies, where therapeutic interventions are informed by a systems-level understanding of immune processes (Woelders et al., 2011). The future of HTS technologies in immunology is further propelled by developments in bioprocessing, including the integration of microscale and nanoscale methodologies. Such advanced methods can revolutionize workflows through increased versatility and productivity in biologic screening, particularly for therapeutic antibodies and cell-based therapies. For instance, optical manipulation instruments enable precise control of single cells within a microenvironment, encouraging more sophisticated analysis of cellular reactions and interactions. As researchers increasingly draw on such advanced instruments, prospects for the discovery of breakthrough treatments for previously challenging diseases expand. Development of integrated platforms that mechanize a number of processes—ranging from cell culture to analytics—will broaden HTS capabilities, enabling a paradigm shift in immunological research and drug development (Jorgolli et al., 2019).

10.1.2. Early Applications in Drug Discovery

Early uses within drug discovery have established foundational building blocks for the intricate situation of modern pharmacology, above all in HTS. Historically, drug discovery initially rested on empirical methods and accidents. The accidents, for example, of Alexander Fleming's penicillin, demonstrated the infancy of a process that had taken much time and effort. Such a method generally entailed cumbersome separation and testing of natural products for healing properties. As advances were being made, the inclusion of biological knowledge and techniques in chemistry gave rise to the advent of systematic methodology. The advent of combinatorial chemistry and high-throughput screening is a revolutionary shift that has facilitated the screening of thousands of compounds at once. This upgraded the process of lead discovery in drug development, which paved the way for contemporary practices to optimize and accelerate drug discovery processes. High-throughput screening techniques also revolutionized initial drug discovery work by significantly enhancing the productivity of the drug development process. HTS made it possible for researchers to screen huge chemical libraries on a large scale, enabling rapid discovery of active compounds against specific biological targets. It facilitated much quicker analysis of enormous libraries, enabling a better systematic survey of drug candidates. Specifically, automation of assay formats, combined with advanced analyzing systems such as robotics, took the discovery process to a whole new level. HTS application has also been extended to the field of immunology, enabling scientists to discover new therapeutic antibodies and immunomodulators, hence expanding the range of therapeutics that can be applied in the management of immune-related diseases. The significance of these developments highlights the imperative interface between high-throughput methods and drug discovery. With the evolution of drug discovery over the years, the addition of systems biology as an auxiliary tool has greatly enhanced earlier usage, particularly through its ability to amalgamate massive amounts of HTS data into an effective biological narrative. Systems biology is focused on understanding the dynamic interaction of biological components, thereby enabling researchers to better see and understand the complexity of drug interactions in living organisms. This systems perspective is distinct from the reductionist methodologies of the past, offering a fuller understanding of drug effectiveness and safety. Systems biology in the field of immunology explains the multi-dimensional aspects of immune response and provides deeper insights into how new therapeutics may affect such response. The integration of early drug discovery techniques and systems biology principles allows researchers to transcend increasing therapeutics complexity, resulting in innovations that provide better and more specific treatment strategies in immunology, such as advances from optical manipulation technologies and workflow-integrated drug research (Woelders et al., 2011; Jorgolli et al., 2019).

10.1.3. Evolution of High-Throughput Screening (HTS) in Immunological Research

Development of HTS in immunological research has had a profound effect on the methods by which researchers learn about the immune system and create new drugs. HTS methods were initially mainly used in drug discovery, but advances in technology have allowed them to be widely applied in immunology. Through the capability to analyze many samples at the same time, HTS has enabled scientists to study intricate biological processes with more ease. This has been particularly useful in the immunoreceptor repertoire characterization. The ability to quantify and analyze heterotypic immune receptor sequences facilitates easier identification of mechanisms of autoimmune diseases, cancer, and infection, thereby gaining a better understanding of adaptive immunity and informing therapeutic uses (Miho et al., 2018). HTS has thus become a valuable resource, enabling the identification of potential vaccines and immunotherapeutics at unprecedented speed. With the increased capacity to create data, the importance of bioinformatics in immunology has also increased. Methods like adaptive immune receptor repertoire sequencing (AIRR-seq) have generated humongous amounts of immune receptor-associated data. However, the difficulty lies not in creating the data but in analyzing it later. The integration of new computational methods—like machine learning, clustering, and network analysis—is no longer optional when unraveling the complexity of immune repertoires (Miho et al., 2018). Computational methods not only allow the identification of specific immune responses but also increase our ability to predict patient outcomes and provide tailored therapies. By mapping immune response evolution and specificity, researchers are closer to perfecting immunotherapies and self-vaccination techniques. Also, the cooperative setting of current immunological research focuses on a shift towards data-driven approaches. Researchers increasingly realize the significance of an integration of computational and experimental approaches for adding value to the implications of research outcomes. This shift in dynamics reflects the shift away from putting weight on data generation towards placing focus on good data analysis and interpretation. As publicly accessible data have grown exponentially, computational biologists have become integral to shaping research initiatives that make use of the abundant resource. Ultimately, by making the intersection of experimental and computational efforts possible, the creation of HTS in immunological research elevates the overall knowledge of the immune system and lays the foundation for future innovations in the field.

10.2. Principles of High-Throughput Screening (HTS)

HTS is a central technology in modern immunology that allows scientists to screen large numbers of compounds in an efficient and effective manner to identify potential therapeutic agents. HTS relies on automation and miniaturization, which allow scientists to run assays in parallel with numerous samples and minimal hands-on time. These platforms leverage high-end robotic platforms and multimodal detection technology to greatly enhance throughput at the cost of reduced costs over traditional screening methods. This capacity not only accelerates the discovery of new immunotherapeutics but also provides data on the mechanisms of action of compounds in modulating immune responses. Through HTS, scientists can quantitatively determine the effects of individual compounds on immune cells and unlock the potential for more directed and effective treatments for diseases, such as autoimmune diseases and cancer. Perhaps the most significant development in HTS is the creation of diverse libraries that include small molecules, peptides, or even libraries of RNA, which are poised to be screened against an immunological target of interest. AIRR-seq is a model for the implementation of high-throughput approaches in immunology, with the capability to systematically interrogate immune cell function and diversity. With the vast amount of data generated through HTS, sophisticated computational tools must be employed to handle and analyze it. Application of clustering and machine learning approaches can further unleash the potential of HTS results, for such applications can be used to categorize immune repertoires and recognize patterns of immune cell activation or inhibition. The ideas of HTS, therefore, not only facilitate the rapid screenings but also help enhance our understanding of the dynamic interactions of the immune system, serving as the foundation of future breakthroughs in immunology. HTS also offers possibilities for generating immunodiagnostics and vaccines essential in managing emerging infectious diseases and public health concerns. By combining metabolic profiling techniques, such as those explained in droplet microfluidic technology and fluorescence lifetime imaging, researchers are able to profile the metabolism of single cells in high-throughput configurations. This method enables a label-free, noninvasive method to analyze the metabolic states of various types of immune cells in various experimental conditions. By correlating metabolic profiles with sequences of immune receptors, as highlighted in recent studies, scientists are able to ascertain the functional relevance of specific immune responses in real-time. Therefore, not only do high-throughput screening practices enable drug discovery, but they also provide essential knowledge on the elementary workings of the immune system, eventually taking immunological research to newer frontiers.

10.2.1. Automation and Robotics in High-Throughput Screening (HTS)

The application of automation and robotics in HTS has transformed the equation of immunology research. By streamlining experimental protocols, these technologies enable scientists to screen thousands of samples in a relatively brief time period. Automation provides accurate and reproducible liquid handling, and robotics permits rapid sample and reagent movement, eliminating human error and variability. This efficiency gain not only accelerates the discovery of therapeutic leads but also increases reproducibility, essential in immunological studies. As a result, the application of automatic systems has transformed HTS into a high-throughput and more flexible enterprise by turning it into a less hands-on, more time-consuming undertaking, which allows scientists to focus on their data interpretation and continued research development. New technologies have also introduced innovations that supplement current automatic systems, promoting HTS capabilities. For instance, advances in microfluidics and lab-on-a-chip technologies enable the miniaturization of biological assays, and this facilitates the study of cellular behaviors at dimensions never anticipated before. These new technologies are indispensable in the field of complex systems like immunology, where multiple-dimensional interactions must be assessed economically. An authentic integration of these methods can significantly accelerate drug discovery pipelines by enabling the screening of hundreds of compounds against an array of biological targets in parallel. As explained in recent publications, advanced technologies that enable accelerating growth in biologics drug discovery are needed. The requirement for new platforms capable of enabling complex workflows aligns perfectly with the latest attempts to optimize immunological research outcomes (Jorgolli et al., 2019). The future of HTS in immunology also depends on the ability to leverage data-driven insights for enhanced decision-making. With machine learning and AI, automated screening platforms can now be capable of analyzing big datasets that are generated through experiments, even patterns and correlations that are not evidently observed.

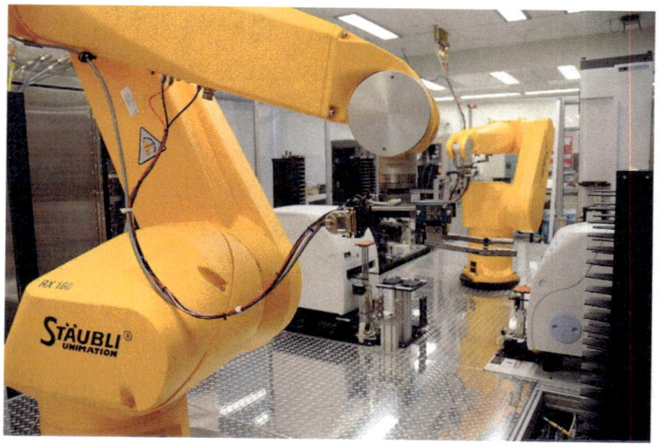

Figure 10.2. High-throughput screening (HTS) robots.

Source: https://upload.wikimedia.org/wikipedia/commons/thumb/2/27/Chemical_Genomics_Robot.jpg/1280px-Chemical_Genomics_Robot.jpg.

This analytical capability can inform researchers which drugs have the greatest potential for therapeutic application, thereby efficiently prioritizing resources. Nevertheless, the gap between what was originally expected of laboratory automation and what has indeed transpired in the development of technologies inspires a tentative optimism; while much of the prognostications has yet to come to pass, the rapidly unfolding integration of automation into scientific operations is indeed unlocking unprecedented performance potential in laboratory environments (Kricka et al., 2015). With advancing technology, ongoing investment in such transformational technologies promises to redefine the methods employed in immunological research, stimulating insights heretofore impossible (Figure 10.2).

10.2.2. Types of Assays Used in High-Throughput Screening (HTS)

Immunology HTS encompasses a variety of assays that allow for swift interrogation of biological processes. Among the dominant formats employed are enzyme-linked immunosorbent assays (ELISAs), which are critical in the quantification of proteins such as cytokines and antibodies in body fluids. ELISAs employ microplate formats that enable bulk samples to be assayed at the same time, thereby greatly enhancing throughput.

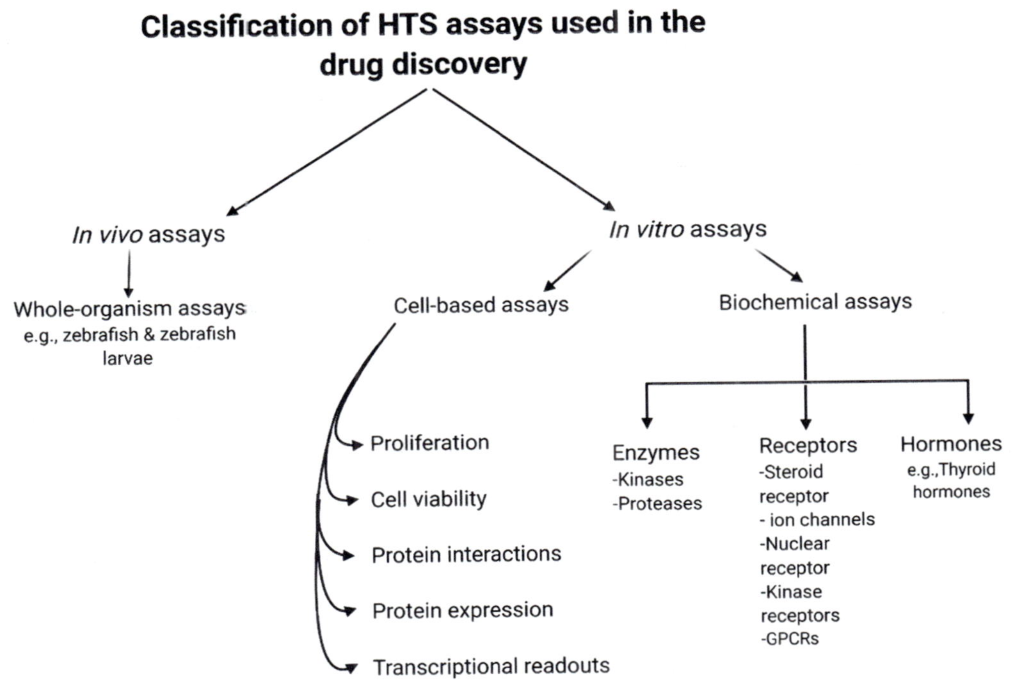

Figure 10.3. General classification of high-throughput screening (HTS) assays.

Source: https://www.researchgate.net/publication/349542133/figure/fig2/AS:114312813752047 67@1744636103421/General-classification-of-high-throughput-screening-HTS-assays.tif.

Furthermore, advancements in detection technology, such as fluorescence and luminescence, have enhanced the sensitivity and velocity of ELISAs, thereby being invaluable in immune response detection. Generally, the ease of use of ELISA in the quantitation of single immune markers demonstrates how old technologies are adapted to meet the needs of high-throughput environments in immunology research. Another extremely influential kind of assay used in HTS is the cell-based assay, in which cells are considered in the presence of varied compounds. These assays can quantify cellular responses such as proliferation, apoptosis, and differentiation and hold promise in the assessment of immune system function and disease processes. Technologies such as flow cytometry and imaging assays enable real-time quantification of cellular change with the possibility of processing numerous samples in parallel for high-throughput applications. Integration of these technologies with automated systems further enables workflow, with potential large-scale screening opportunities. Through the application of cell-based assays in HTS platforms, researchers can efficiently discover new drug targets and evaluate the immunogenicity of the candidate drugs, a critical aspect of drug development. Nucleic acid-based assays have also gained considerable attention within HTS, particularly vaccine discovery and pathogen identification. Techniques such as real-time PCR and next-generation sequencing have revolutionized how researchers can access genetic material from numerous pathogens and immune cells. Not only do these methods enable researchers to recognize and quantify specific genes, but they also allow researchers to examine genetic variation and its implications in the context of immunological response. For example, tests such as TypeSeq have been found to be extremely precise in detecting greater than one HPV genotype, allowing for research in cancer prevention (Wagner et al., 2019). The ability to perform large-scale sequencing in a high-throughput setting not only increases the pace of investigation but also advances the understanding of complex immunological interactions, eventually leading to more effective therapeutic intervention (Jorgolli et al., 2019) (Figure 10.3).

10.2.3. Data Management and Analysis Techniques

Data management and analysis in the case of HTS in immunology are of utmost significance to understand complex biological interactions. Omics technologies have created vast amounts of data, which need sophisticated data management techniques to facilitate analysis and interpretation. Systems biology is also a paradigm here, which focuses on an understanding of biological systems rather than individual components. With the help of statistical methods, bioinformatics, and mathematical models, scientists are able to extract reliable information from large datasets. This integrative approach provides a more comprehensive insight into immunological responses by revealing the dynamic interactions between various biological entities, critical for successfully applying HTS in immunology (Woelders et al., 2011). In addition, effective data management approaches should be employed in handling the sheer volume of data HTS generates. Issues such as storing, retrieving information and harmonizing datasets that come from different sources are significant hindrances to researchers. Effective use of robust databases and data processing pipelines can easily make such issues a breeze, such that retrieving data systematically can be a simple task and have it ready when needed. Through the utilization of robust computational tools and algorithms, researchers can effectively utilize data for identifying potential therapeutic targets or immunological research biomarkers. In addition, predictive modeling by high-throughput screening models with significant advancements in machine learning and artificial intelligence is becoming more efficient, and consequently, the accuracy of outcomes improves, and immunology is facilitated in terms of innovation (Seaman & Whitehouse, 2001). Furthermore, the collaborative nature of modern scientific research brings attention to networking and data sharing between disciplines for the formulation of immunological research. Establishing productive dialogue between educational institutions, as in the case of expansion into marine biotechnology, can make it easier to work together on developing databases that are tailor-made for use in immunology. A collective approach serves to integrate diverse expertise and ensures new evidence is rapidly disseminated and used effectively. Therefore, the availability of a wide range facilitates not only the discovery of funding sources but also enhances collaborative capability that is necessary for optimum comprehensive analysis of high-throughput screening data. Finally, the convergence of collaborative tactics, sophisticated data handling procedures, and state-of-the-art analytic techniques will significantly alter the face of immunology (Seaman & Whitehouse, 2001).

10.3. Applications of High-Throughput Screening (HTS) in Immunology

HTS has revolutionized immunology science by greatly accelerating the process of identifying candidate therapeutics and defining immune responses. One major use is in drug discovery, whereby HTS enables the quick screening of a thousand or more compounds to see if they may modulate immune functions. This is particularly useful to design novel immunotherapies against diseases such as cancer and autoimmunity, where traditional screening protocols were too time-intensive or burdensome. By enabling researchers to evaluate the efficacy of compound candidates at high throughput, these new techniques conserve enormous amounts of time and cost associated with drug discovery, paving the way for faster therapeutic interventions. Another significant application of HTS in immunology is its capacity for examining complex immune receptor repertoires through techniques like AIRR-seq. This can facilitate detailed profiling of B-cell and T-cell populations, and this is a critically essential prerequisite for the comprehension of the adaptive immune response to pathogens and tumor antigens. The ability to read the high-dimensional complexity of immune receptor sequences has transformed immunological research, allowing both immune diversity and specificity to be maximally understood. Computational methods of analyzing large AIRR-seq datasets have allowed researchers to intensively study immune repertoire dynamics, facilitating the identification of putative disease biomarkers and targets of new immunotherapies (Miho et al., 2018). Also, the integration of microfluidic technology into HTS platforms enhances the capabilities of immunological research through the facilitation of *in vivo*-like cellular interaction analysis. The technology allows for the simulation of the complex cellular environment of tissues, and this enhances improved cell culture systems that can more accurately model biological conditions. For example, microfluidic systems are able to generate controlled gradients of biochemical signals and provide dynamic cell culture conditions, which are crucial for immune cell interactions and behavior to be analyzed. These are particularly useful for immunology applications requiring prolonged cell studies, as they allow for continuous analysis and conditions to be changed in real-time (Tehranirokh et al., 2013). The confluence of microfluidics and HTS thus represents a thrilling new frontier in the quest to provide a better understanding of immunologic function and to develop new medicines.

10.3.1. Identification of Novel Immunotherapeutics

The identification of new immunotherapeutics has been greatly aided by HTS methodologies, which enable rapid assessment of a very large number of candidate therapeutic compounds. By employing these sophisticated techniques, researchers are able to systematically investigate the adaptive immune response, with emphasis on highly effective agents capable of activating immune system activities against cancers and infectious pathogens. Not only does this systematic approach accelerate the identification process, but it also facilitates extensive screening of potential candidate compounds with diverse modes of action. In this complexity of high-dimensional immune repertoires is hidden the explanation of being unraveled by AIRR-seq, capable of tracking the cellular interaction dynamics and response mechanisms. The integration of both HTS and AIRR-seq enhances the discovery of highly specific immunotherapeutics, leading to groundbreaking drugs that are capable of filling the gaps left by existing immunotherapy (Miho et al., 2018). Following the embracement of advanced technology, genetic engineering and phage display technologies have been instrumental in manipulating and designing antibodies for the identification of novel immunotherapeutic drugs. High-throughput technologies make it possible to create novel recombinant antibodies that are tailored for the precise targeting of specific antigens associated with cancers and infectious diseases. Engineered antibodies exhibit enhanced characteristics, including increased binding affinity, activation of immune effector functions, and maximum tissue penetration. The ongoing evolution of antibody engineering is crucial; not only does it broaden the scope of potential therapeutics, but it also overcomes the inherent limitations of traditional monoclonal or polyclonal antibodies. Therefore, studies that concentrate on such sophisticated techniques notably contribute to the list of immunotherapeutics available for use in clinical practice, thereby paving the way for more effective therapies in the context of immunology (Saeed et al., 2017).

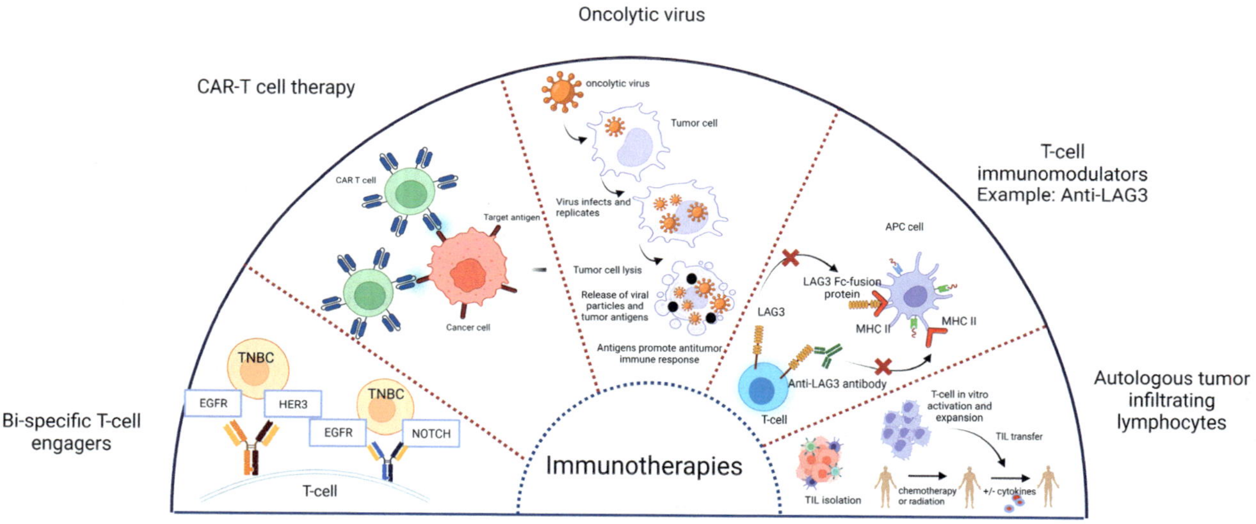

Figure 10.4. Novel immunotherapies with their mechanism of action.

Source: https://www.researchgate.net/publication/373236344/figure/fig2/AS:11431281182906754@1692618729586/Novel-immunotherapies-with-their-mechanism-of-action-Created-with-BioRendercom.ppm.

In addition, the convergence of machine learning methods with high-throughput screening data is reshaping the identification and optimization phases of novel immunotherapeutics. By utilizing computational approaches that decipher complex data sets, scientists are able to convert patterns and predict the efficacy of new candidates before commencing clinical trial phases. This type of convergence between experimental and computational information creates an overwhelming synergy that enhances the precision of immunotherapeutic innovation. The ability to quantify and compare immune repertoires with the help of advanced analytical tools is key to understanding how immunotherapies are going to act in real-world clinical scenarios. With ongoing interdisciplinary strategies, the stage for immunology is soon going to see gigantic strides and result in revolutionary treatments, making patient treatment personalized and boosting outcomes for diseases ranging from diverse disease areas (Miho et al., 2018) (Figure 10.4).

10.3.2. Screening for Immune Modulators

Immune modulator screening is an essential aspect of immunological investigation, the aim being to identify compounds that have the ability to activate or suppress specific immune response. It plays a vital role in the formation of therapeutic approaches to numerous conditions, such as autoimmune disorders and cancer, where immune modulation could play a pivotal role. HTS methods allow this to be achieved by allowing researchers to screen thousands of compounds with great efficiency and speed. The automated strategies are able to quantify biochemical interactions and cellular responses, thereby accelerating the discovery of new immune modulators. By this means, the use of HTS has revolutionized drug discovery within the immunology community by providing information that was previously unattainable using traditional methods. The immunocomplexity requires a broad understanding of the target mechanism and pathways. For instance, work on the human cytomegalovirus (HCMV) has revealed the complexity of immune evasion mechanisms employed by the pathogen. Deletion of specific viral genes has been shown to impact the function of natural killer (NK) cells profoundly, illustrating how cell-specific immune modulation can be achieved. Scientists have also discovered several viral genes that inhibit NK cell activation and function, hence signaling the importance of screening for compounds that can reverse such immune evasion mechanisms. By identifying these mechanisms, screenings can lead to directed therapies that allow for immune recognition and response against cancerous or infected cells, signifying the groundbreaking potential of this research area (Patel et al., 2018). Besides, the applicability of HTS extends beyond research in the early phases to the realm of personalized medicine. As has been emphasized in recent reviews, HTS is a robust platform for the immunological validation of immune modulators that would be tailored to individual patient profiles. The ability to screen compound libraries of large size against cells derived from patients is opening the doors towards precision therapies for specific immune dysfunctions. This is in accordance with a new trend in immunotherapy, whereby the therapies are attuned to the unique immunological environment of the individual patient. Through the integration of high-throughput techniques and clinical insight, researchers are capable of establishing the groundwork for new therapies that not only address the underlying cause of immune diseases but also effectively harness the premise of precision medicine (Saxena, 2022) (Figure 10.5).

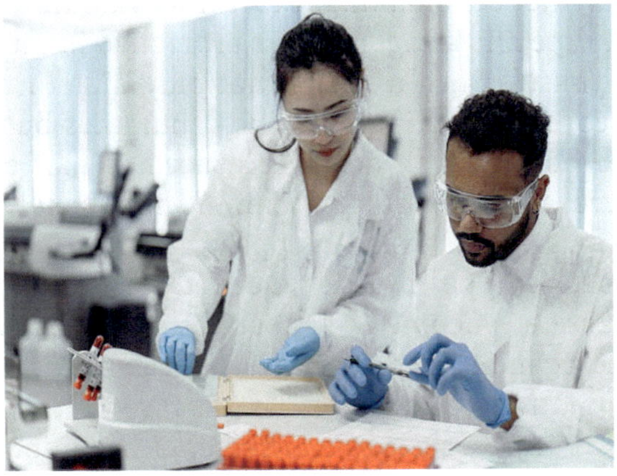

Figure 10.5. Screening for immune modulators is a fundamental aspect of immunological research, aiming to identify compounds that can enhance or suppress specific immune responses.

Source: https://static.theprint.in/wp-content/uploads/2023/09/ANI-20230905121343.jpg.

10.3.3. Role in Vaccine Development

HTS has transformed vaccine development in its very essence with the ability to screen and evaluate rapidly large quantities of candidate immunogens. The traditional methods of vaccine creation were long, cyclical processes that imposed limitations on how quickly new vaccines could be created and tested. HTS allows one to comprehensively search a multitude of antigens to find highly reactive candidates from different libraries. This aspect is particularly important during outbreaks of infectious diseases, when the need for speed of vaccine production predominates. By applying HTS efficiencies, researchers are able to significantly reduce discovery-to-product time and eventually deliver more potent countermeasures against emerging pathogens, enhancing global health security. With new techniques, HTS enables the detailed immune repertoire dynamics analysis essential in vaccine development. AIRR-seq has elucidated the complexity of immune responses and provided insights into the specificity and variability of adaptive immune receptors. The integration of computational strategies enables researchers to evaluate large-scale immunology data, hence enabling the understanding of how specific antigens elicit protective immune responses. Such a design not only aids in the discovery of optimal vaccine candidates but is also beneficial in designing vaccines that can successfully modulate immune responses in various populations. An appropriate knowledge of such a type is greatly needed for designing effective vaccines, especially in handling heterogeneity of immune responses in various populations and states of disease (Miho et al., 2018). Besides, advancements in antibody engineering, aided by HTS, have led to the design of more effective therapeutic and vaccine modalities. The identification of gene-designed antibodies and phage display technologies has ushered in a new era of vaccine design that allows scientists to create highly specific recombinant antibodies. Engineered antibodies perform critical functions, including enhancing immune responses and attacking some pathogens with gigantic precision. By integrating these advanced approaches into vaccine development pipelines, researchers are not only maximizing immunogenicity but also maximizing the therapeutic potential of vaccine approaches to combat infectious diseases and cancer. This union of high-throughput technologies with innovative antibody production constitutes a paradigm shift in the field of immunology and ultimately envisions a healthier future through effective vaccination campaigns (Saeed et al., 2017) (Figure 10.6).

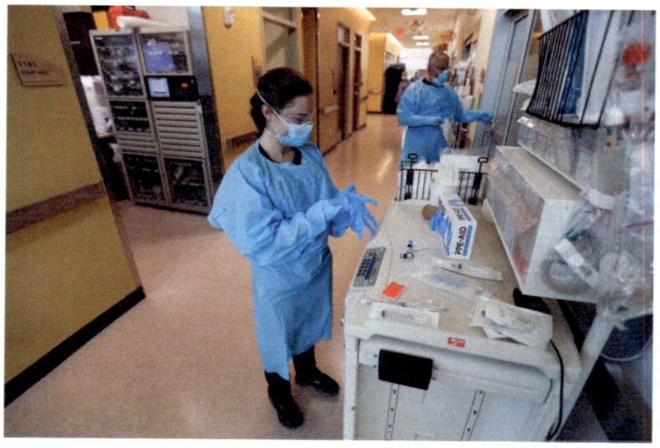

Figure 10.6. High-throughput screening (HTS) has fundamentally transformed vaccine development.

Source: https://nypost.com/wp-content/uploads/sites/2/2021/07/AP21197648496865.jpg?quality=90&strip=all&w=1024.

10.4. Advantages of High-Throughput Screening (HTS)

HTS is a new technology in the field of immunology that holds colossal advantages in the identification of novel drugs and therapeutic targets. HTS has one of its greatest strengths in that it can screen huge numbers of compounds at a very high rate and level of efficiency. Traditional screening methods are slow and time-consuming and require extensive manual effort. Conversely, HTS is propelled by automation and advanced robotics to filter thousands of samples at once, hence accelerating the identification of possible immunomodulatory compounds. Apart from efficiency, saving valuable research time, it also allows researchers to focus on optimizing the best candidates towards development. As such, HTS results in a better drug discovery pipeline crucial in the treatment of complex immunological disorders (Woelders et al., 2011). Another significant advantage of HTS in immunology is that it can obtain high-resolution information, which enhances the description of biological systems. The integration of HTS and systems biology methods makes it possible to assess interactions among and within various biological components. The general strategy enables researchers to grasp how complex immune responses arise from the dynamic interactions between pathways, molecules, and cells, as opposed to studying each component separately. Using bioinformatics software to process the data generated from HTS, scientists are able to uncover revealing information regarding the mechanisms of immune responses and diseases. From this, more effective therapeutics are likely to be designed on an individualized immunological basis, which could translate to improved patient care in the clinic (Woelders et al., 2011). HTS also has the potential to significantly lower drug discovery costs in immunology. With high throughput and rapid screening pace, it becomes feasible for researchers to detect failing candidates early and reallocate resources to better ones. This aspect is particularly vital in an era where pharma research too frequently experiences lengthy timelines and high failure rates, committing funding and human resources in vain. HTS not just maximizes the early stages of discovery but also stimulates innovation because it makes possible the probing of diverse compound libraries, including those specialized in new discoveries in the immunology field. With this approach, the innovative method can produce novel therapeutic approaches at a much quicker rate than conventional ways, potentially addressing long-overdue medical requirements in the field.

10.4.1. Increased Efficiency in Research

Within the domain of immunological research, greater efficiency is a bulwark of progress, especially through the application of HTS techniques. These methods allow scientists to execute many experiments at the same time, greatly speeding up the process of therapeutics and biomarker discovery. As per the strategy in current research, the application of emerging technologies such as lab-on-a-chip systems is pivotal in simplifying processes for increased automation of advanced procedures that previously took much time and resources. Such advances enable the possibility of studying interactions on a microscale level and gaining insights into biological systems, ultimately boosting the general yield of drug discovery. By cutting down experiment time and increasing numbers of data acquisitions, HTS enhances the capability to overcome previously insurmountable challenges in immunology, eventually uncovering novel targets and therapeutic compounds required to treat disease in a variety of pathologies. Research tool development is critical in the enhanced efficiency seen in applications of high-throughput screening. Recent developments in proteomics have facilitated the generation of a broad range of biomarkers, and therefore demands are especially required for precise probes to effectively use these discoveries. Antibody engineering technologies, as per recent publications, have overcome universal problems of traditional antibody architectures, such as steric obstruction and specificity loss. The design of antibody constructs into smaller sizes—such as Fab and scFv—has been shown to increase binding affinities and, concurrently, address the issue of stability and directional immobilization. Employing these designed antibodies, researchers can perform biosensing assays more effectively, thereby making screening easier. This not only maximizes the research output but also fosters a more lively platform for innovative therapeutic inventions in the field of immunology. Lastly, the revolutionary potential of high-throughput screening in immunology is more than just technical advancement, as it enables researchers to cultivate a culture of fast experimentation and constant learning. The shift towards integrated platforms combining optics and microfluidics is harmonious with the demand for scalable solutions in biopharmaceutical development. By facilitating the manipulation and analysis of thousands of single cells in a relevant nanoenvironment, according to recent reviews, the interfacing systems can help revolutionize fundamental and applied biological research. Further advancement of such strategies will increasingly mitigate issues due to shattered and low-throughput workflows. Increased research effectiveness in no small way pushes the frontiers of immunological understanding but also leads to the timely development of breakthrough therapies, ultimately addressing key global health challenges at a time when speed and precision in research are most important (Figure 10.7).

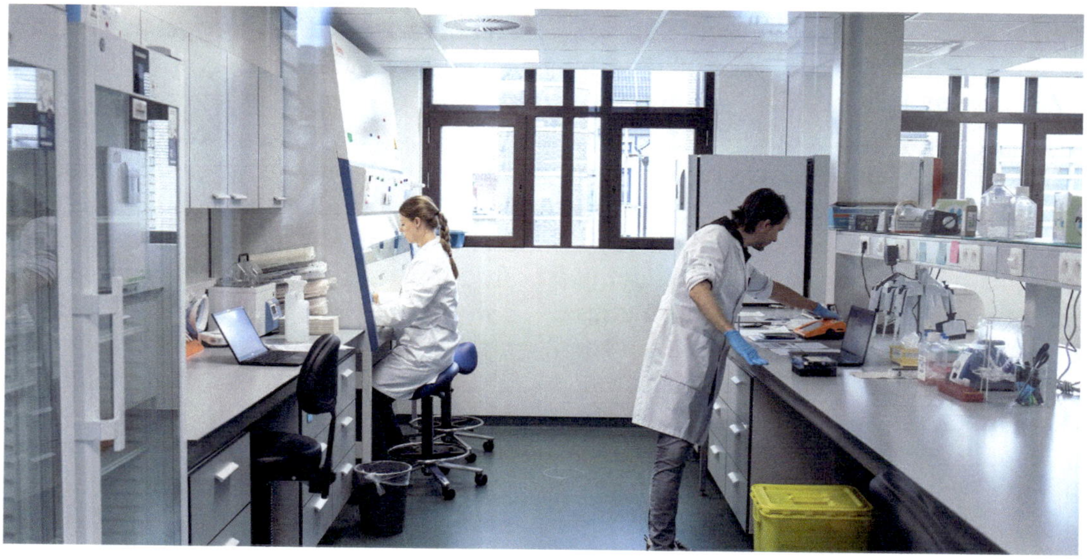

Figure 10.7. Immunological research with high-throughput screening (HTS).

Source: https://www.itg.be/storage/files/58d61634-6ac8-4479-b41d-aed60c0ae217/full_width__new-immunology-labs-header.jpg.

10.4.2. Cost-Effectiveness Compared to Traditional Methods

Cost-effectiveness of HTS in immunology becomes a significant advantage over conventional methods. Conventional approaches to making antibodies, such as hybridoma technology, typically suffer significant setbacks in that they are high-cost operations, with long development periods for obtaining desired antibodies. HTS, by contrast, allows researchers to screen thousands of compounds or biological samples simultaneously, saving the time and expense of drug discovery and antibody production. In addition, this cost-effectiveness not only means saving in terms of material and labor costs but also means that faster responses to emerging health crises can be provided.

With the globe calling for quicker immunological assessments, the need for cost-effective screening tools becomes increasingly dominant in the creation of therapeutic approaches in immunology. Apart from optimizing the cost-effectiveness of HTS, it can include advanced technologies such as genetic engineering and phage display technology. Such technologies have revolutionized the production of highly specific recombinant antibodies, which play a key role in combating infectious pathogens and complex diseases. Unlike traditional polyclonal and monoclonal antibody production using techniques that are typically time-consuming and resource-intensive, HTS enables the rapid design and selection of antibodies with superior efficacy and specificity. The ability to successfully design targeted treatments not only puts less of a strain on research facilities in terms of costs but also improves the quality of immunological research as a whole. This groundbreaking shift towards high-throughput approaches thus amounts to a benchmark for the field, calling for sustainable approaches to scientific investigation and treatment design. Additionally, the effects of HTS are not just monetary but also entail the broader effect on research and clinical outcomes. The potential of HTS to produce worthwhile candidates reduces not just the time to market for new medicines but also the probability of new treatments. As illustrated by progress in antibody engineering, whereby the introduction of HTS has facilitated the discovery of novel immunotherapeutics, cost-effectiveness exceeds monetary considerations. The ability to produce high-affinity antibodies at high efficiency and to rapidly adjust to changing research conditions speaks to the significance of HTS in modern immunology. Through the facilitation of an active reply to antibody discovery and new drug candidate hunting, HTS not only makes research affordable but also provides entry to groundbreaking interventions that will dramatically improve patient outcomes in the future.

10.4.3. Ability to Analyze Large Datasets

The present climate of immunology is heavily dictated by the ability to interrogate large data sets, a need raised with the advent of high-throughput screening platforms. These methodologies enable researchers to generate astronomical amounts of data, particularly pertinent to the adaptive immune system, e.g., analysis of antibody and T-cell receptor repertoires. High-dimensional data from AIRR-seq capture the complexity of the immune landscape, uncovering mechanisms of disease like autoimmunity and cancer. The analytical tools employed here not only enable comparison of the immune repertoires but detail the multidimensional dynamics of adaptive immunity itself. Therefore, the building of robust computational infrastructures for the analysis of such large sets of data is essential in the transformation of raw data into valuable biological understanding, ultimately translating to innovation in vaccine and immunotherapeutic design that is fundamental in addressing health challenges of the day. Concomitant with the evolution of high-throughput technologies, computational methods have evolved, enabling immunologists with access to tools for analysis of intricate biology. Machine learning algorithms and statistical models are now at the forefront of deciphering the intricacies of data generated through massive-scale sequencing, such as with AIRR-seq. With these sophisticated tools, investigators can conduct a number of analyses, from diversity analysis to clustering, phylogenetic reconstructions, and network analysis. Combining these computational strategies supports a further understanding of adaptive immune system structure and diversity, and enhanced predictive models of immune response in disease and health. Improved data analysis speeds allow immunologists to identify defining patterns and relationships that direct therapeutic strategies, illustrative of the essential role of data analysis capabilities for advancing immunological research and its clinical translatability. In addition, as our appreciation for immunology increases, the investigation of non-coding RNA, especially long noncoding RNAs (lncRNAs), represents yet another aspect of data complexity in the immune arena. The advent of next-generation sequencing technologies has enabled a more thorough analysis of the human transcriptome, uncovering levels of regulatory strategies that have not been acknowledged before. LncRNAs engage dynamically with proteins and other nucleic acids, with profound effects on immune responses. However, their work is often hindered by the agonies of data analysis and the non-conserved nature of these sequences. To overcome these obstacles, innovative analytical paradigms that can cope with the high dimensionality and heterogeneity of lncRNA data are needed. These advancements not only will unlock the biological significance of non-coding transcripts but also enhance our ability to therapeutically engineer immune pathways, and the critical role of data analysis in high-throughput immunology is further supported (Miho et al., 2018; Robinson et al., 2020) (Figure 10.8).

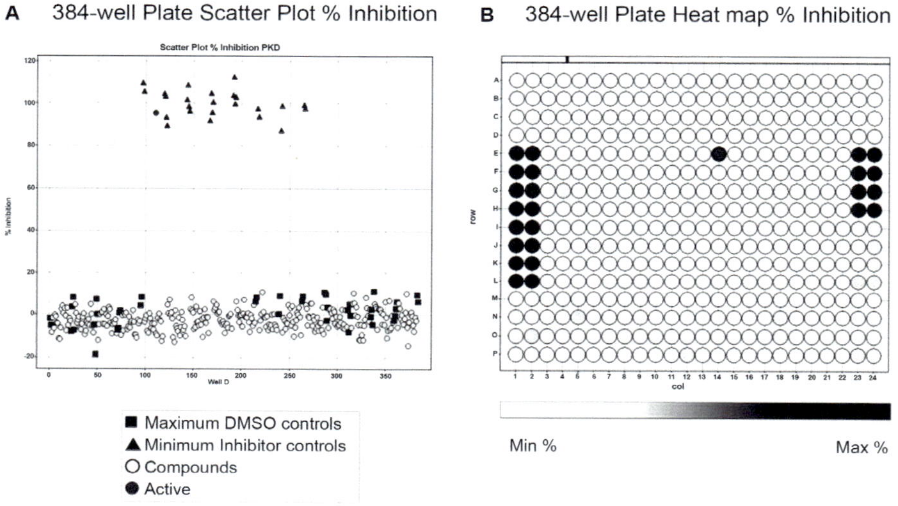

Figure 10.8. Primary high-throughput screening (HTS) data quality control review. (A) Percent inhibition single-plate scatter plot and (B) Percent inhibition data single-plate heat map from the pKd hts campaign.

Source: https://www.researchgate.net/profile/Elizabeth-Sharlow/publication/49685147/figure/fig1/AS:341495132508183@1458430192889/primary-high-throughput-screening-hts-data-quality-control-review-A-percent.png.

10.5. Challenges and Limitations of High-Throughput Screening (HTS)

The application of HTS in immunology has numerous challenges that could jeopardize the efficiency and reliability of this useful tool. One of the critical problems is the vastness of data generated by HTS, which overloads scientists and makes it difficult to interpret data. With increasing assays, variability and opportunities for false positives also increase, and it becomes increasingly difficult to identify genuinely useful biological signals. The complexity of the immune response also generally necessitates contextual information that is not drawn from HTS data in itself. This limitation emphasizes the need for the integration of HTS findings with other biological data and methods to create a better understanding of immune responses and their contribution to therapeutic development. The technology constraints in assay design and operation are another significant limitation of HTS in immunology. Most traditional high-throughput approaches struggle to replicate the subtleties of living biological systems, particularly regarding cell-cell interaction and fine behavior of immune cells. HTS thus accelerates screening, while the physiological validity of results is generally compromised. New answers, such as miniaturized lab-on-a-chip technology, could enhance these weaknesses by being capable of providing more biologically representative assay contexts. But even such tend not to have the cross-reactivity required for general use across a wide variety of immune responses, limiting their applications as generalized tools in drug discovery and development (Jorgolli et al., 2019). Moreover, issues associated with the translational aspect of HTS in immunology cannot be overlooked. While HTS also shows promise in screening potential therapeutics, the bench-to-bedside transition involves rigorous validation and characterization in more complex systems. The reliance on known available drugs through repurposing strategies may at best receive some advantage through the leverage of existing safety profiles, but it introduces other issues to the immune system where intricate responses are activated (Rodrigues & Thomaz, 2020). Therefore, researchers must contend with not just the problem of requiring accurate and relevant HTS outcomes but also the broader field of biological complexities that influence drug efficacy *in vivo*. This interplay of factors ultimately defines the trajectory of HTS in immunology and refers to its limitations during the process of making therapeutic breakthroughs.

10.5.1. Technical Limitations and Assay Variability

Technical limitations and assay variability are important issues in the field of HTS in immunology that affect the dependability and interpretability of results. One of the primary limitations arises from differences inherent in assay design and execution that lead to variability of data. Variability may stem from several factors, including reagent quality, equipment calibration, and environmental conditions during the assay. Such discrepancies can affect assay sensitivity and specificity, ultimately compromising the conclusions drawn from serological evaluations. For instance, discordant findings in neutralizing antibody responses are observed when different screening platforms are used, and emphasis on standardization is therefore called for to enhance assay robustness and reproducibility, particularly in low-resource laboratories, given that the dynamic nature of evolving viral strains necessitates frequent adaptation and verification of testing platforms (Molesti et al., 2014). Moreover, the drawbacks of detection methodologies applied in HTS are some of the contributing factors for assay variation. While innovations such as multiplex assays have been at the forefront of enhancing data gathering, the underlying technology must be stable to produce credible results. Retroviral pseudotype platforms, for example, have been employed to measure antibody response to influenza serotypes while maintaining sensitivity and the requirement for a stable testing platform. Nonetheless, clinical utility may be thwarted by the complexity of assay setup and performance, necessitating rigorous training and protocol compliance (Molesti et al., 2014). Overriding these technical challenges is critical in order to maintain data integrity, especially when testing responses in heterogeneous populations or across laboratories, as this variability can have important implications for public health surveillance and vaccine efficacy research. The application of next-generation sequencing (NGS) technology in immunology is the quintessential example of the potential as well as the pitfalls of contemporary assay technologies. While NGS supports integrative genetic analysis for the possible inclusion of pharmacogenetic considerations in informing therapy, its application is beset with both data quality and interpretational issues. The volume of data generated can overwhelm available analytics to produce variable data that makes clinical utility difficult. Additionally, ethical considerations regarding patient data handling contribute to the complexity, as implementation of pharmacogenetics in routine practice continues to be heterogeneous. Therefore, as HTS technology advances, the technical limitations must be addressed along with adherence to rigorous quality control regulations to enhance assay robustness and facilitate clinical application of immunology results.

10.5.2. Data Interpretation Complexities

The process of interpretation of data in HTS within the field of immunology creates enormous complexities that need to be tackled by scientists. While the quantity of generated data continues to grow exponentially, the process of sense-making becomes more complicated. High-throughput technologies can create vast quantities of data regarding immune responses, but variation in both technical and biological senses makes it more difficult to ascertain the quality of the data. Excessive noise, such as signal distortions caused by automated systems or sample heterogeneity, can lead to spurious conclusions if they are not eliminated. Hence, the establishment of strong analytical frameworks becomes very critical so that the underlying biological implication of findings is emphasized and possible artifacts, which can skew the results, are kept a minimum. Furthermore, application of NGS technologies has revolutionized data interpretation in immunology to enable extensive profiling at the genomic level. Although this development is a welcome one, it poses problems of sequence data quality and interpretation, and hence there is a stringent need for establishing clinical guidelines for its effective use. Pharmacogenetic data analysis, as seen in the case of immunological responses, can provide discordant results for some genetic variants, limiting the application of personalized medicine techniques. As scientists grapple with complexity in data, evidence-based concordance between experts irrevocably shines to surpass the discordances. Such collaboration may favor the development of open standards that not only maintain data integrity but also facilitate smoother transition from the bench to the bedside in immunology. Lastly, the high-dimensionality associated with immune repertoire analysis accentuates another level of interpretation complexity in HTS. AIRR-seq underlies the intricacies of immune reactions, revealing diverse antigen-binding capabilities that reflect an organism's adaptive immunity. Nevertheless, the huge volumes of data produced by AIRR-seq demand advanced computational and statistical methods to decode intricate interactions between immune repertoires. Techniques such as clustering, phylogenetic analysis, and machine learning have been trendy in this regard, enabling scientists to manage and disassemble the very intricacies inherent within the data. The efficacy of such methods does not merely enable quantification and comparison of immune responses but also the identification of potential immunotherapeutics. An in-depth understanding of these analytical methods is important to move ahead with immunology research and optimize therapeutic potential in the wake of immune disorders to ultimately enhance patient care based on evidence-based advice.

10.5.3. Ethical Considerations in Immunological Research

The immunology research field, and particularly high-throughput screening, is beholden to immense ethical concerns that require detailed consideration. As researchers try to chart immune responses and develop treatments, the use of human samples poses questions around autonomy and consent. Not only must informed consent educate participants about risks, but also inform them about what they know about how their biological samples are treated in research. Ethical review procedures, like Institutional Review Boards (IRBs), play a critical role in reviewing studies so that participants' rights are preserved. Transparency in these processes is paramount; scientists have to indicate how their findings can impact society, particularly in developing drugs that can influence public health. In addition, the application of emerging technologies such as NGS in immunology has unique ethical issues with respect to genomic data.

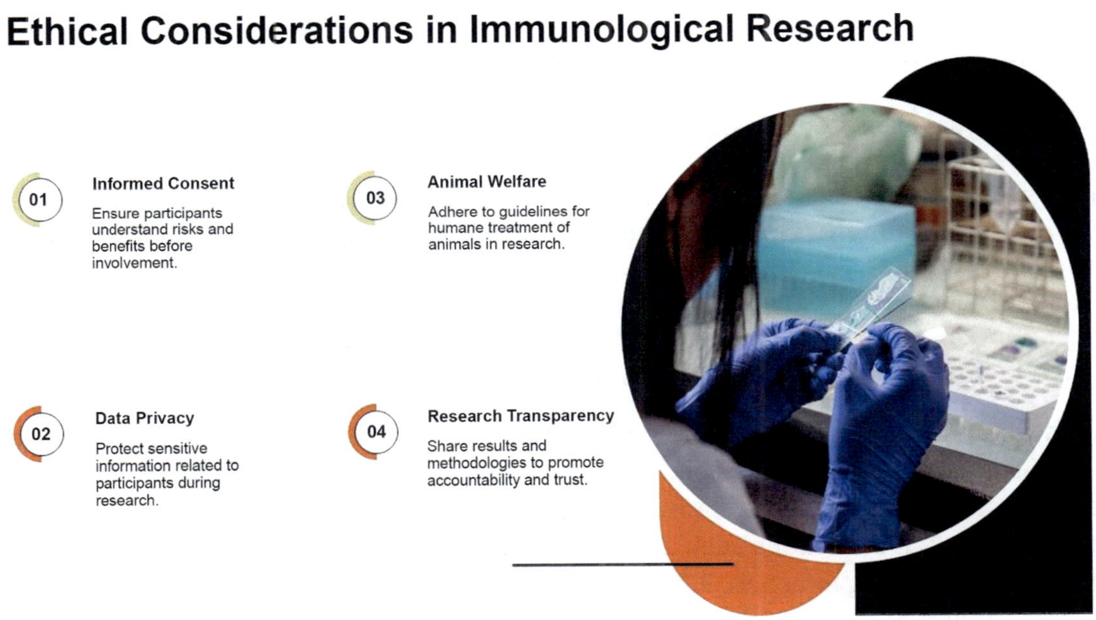

Figure 10.9. Ethical considerations in immunological research.

Source: https://www.slideteam.net/media/catalog/product/cache/560x315/e/t/ethical_considerations_in_immunological_research_cd4_cells_ppt_presentation_st_ai_ss_slide01.jpg.

While these technologies allow for the investigation of vast quantities of genetic information, they also create concerns about ownership of the data and privacy. The complexity of genetic information makes its abuse a cause of discrimination or stigmatization of the individual on the basis of his or her genetic inclination. Ethical standards must ensure that data protection is in line with progress in pharmacogenomics, allowing for responsible outcome communication. This balance is particularly necessary in light of the rapid progress with which biotechnology has evolved as a discipline in pharmaceutical sciences, as proposed in literature on integrating biotechnology within curricula (Stoimenova et al., 2011). Finally, the intersection of research ethics and pharmacogenetic use in immunology underscores the necessity to define evidence-based principles. As pharmacogenetics gains increasing relevance in personalized medicine, the ethical implications of similar practices must be examined intently. The variation in patient responses to treatments based on gene differences calls for a comprehensive understanding of how such variables impact clinical practice. Research that seeks to address these differences needs to be guided by strong ethical standards in order to facilitate equity and justice in the delivery of healthcare. The evolution of high-throughput screening technology must go hand in hand with a vigilant perspective toward ethical concerns, so that a culture is established where scientific progress would never compromise moral responsibility and social justice (Vanakker & De Paepe, 2013) (Figure 10.9).

10.6. Future Directions in High-Throughput Screening (HTS)

The advance in HTS technology is steering the future of immunological research towards more efficient and productive approaches. One of the areas in which advance is being witnessed is via the synergy of droplet microfluidics with high-end imaging techniques. Synergizing allows researchers to perform noninvasive, label-free single-cell analysis, an enormous leap from the legacy assays that are based on the use of fluorescent labels and extended cell handling. The technique's ability to recognize metabolic conditions in diverse populations of cells creates new avenues for the examination of diverse immunological reactions, particularly in cancer research. The technology can potentially allow researchers to acquire the critical information regarding cell discrimination between proliferating and resting cells and contribute in a superior manner to the understanding of the kinetics and viability of immune cells in diverse situations, thus resulting in novel therapeutic interventions (Ma et al., 2019).

Furthermore, HTS's future in immunology relies more on probing immune repertoires using new sequencing tools. AIRR-seq is becoming increasingly core and enables scientists to map the intricate landscape of immune receptor diversity. The technique not only exposes the complexity of immune responses in conditions such as cancer and autoimmunity but also enables the probing of immune dynamics during infection. Future directions can involve the merging of AIRR-seq data with advanced computational tools, including machine learning and phylogenetic analysis, to obtain deeper insights into the architecture and evolution of immunity. These combined approaches can eventually provide deeper insight into personal immune profiles and guide personalized immunotherapy and vaccine design for individual patient needs (Miho et al., 2018). Cooperative strategies that integrate high-throughput screening with emerging fields such as systems immunology are set to redefine immunological research paradigms. The synergistic cooperation of HTS technologies with computational biology has the prospect of transforming therapeutic and diagnostic innovations. Through the application of the powerful data analytics tools available, scientists can leverage and exploit meaningful patterns and correlations from the large datasets generated by HTS strategies. Such integration can make it possible to uncover novel immunogenic targets and more accurate predictions of immunity. As the field continues to advance, the integration of these technological advances will be crucial in translating laboratory findings into the clinic, so that high-throughput screening continues to be a revolutionary tool in immunology as it becomes more data-driven and personalized.

10.6.1. Integration of Artificial Intelligence (AI) and Machine Learning

The integration of machine learning and AI in HTS has had a transformational effect on immunology research. Through the utilization of large sets of data that are generated from experimental screens, these technologies enable researchers to identify potential candidates for therapy with greater effectiveness and accuracy than traditional methods. For instance, AI systems can take complex biological data into account, identifying patterns and correlations not immediately apparent to human scientists. This ability is particularly important in immunology, where immune responses are complex and multi-dimensional. Apart from accelerating the identification of drug targets, machine learning also optimizes the entire screening process to reduce both the time and expense involved in the research pipeline. As such, AI incorporation has the ability to further boost HTS predictive power, fueling innovation in immunological therapies. Within drug discovery, the use of AI and machine learning presents special benefits in the interpretation of high-throughput screening data, especially in the creation of new immunotherapies. As recent research has pointed out, AI methods can optimize the selection process for compounds by forecasting their interactions with immune targets based on various biological parameters. The ability to model and simulate complex immune interactions allows researchers to shortlist the compounds that possess maximum efficacy potential within the clinical context. Moreover, merging AI-driven strategies negates typical issues in the form of data quality and interpretability, being the key to the success of therapeutic innovation. With technology continually advancing computationally, the integration of machine learning and immunology research opens a new horizon for unraveling strong therapeutic strategies. Despite the promising potential of AI and machine learning in immunology, various challenges still exist that must be addressed to enable their complete potential to be realized. Data heterogeneity challenges, explainability of algorithms, and the regulatory framework continue to feature prominently as barriers to implementation. Quality and representativeness of data employed to train machine learning models are critical, as biased or inadequate data may lead to unreliable predictions and compromise the screening process.

Moreover, ensuring that researchers can interpret and validate AI-generated results remains a pressing concern, particularly in clinical applications. As indicated in the literature, overcoming these challenges is essential for harnessing the transformative impact of AI in drug discovery and vaccine development. Collaborative work between computational scientists, immunologists, and regulatory agencies is important in developing stable paradigms that facilitate the practical application of AI-based approaches in high-throughput screening, thereby expanding the reach of immunological investigation and therapeutic development (Figure 10.10).

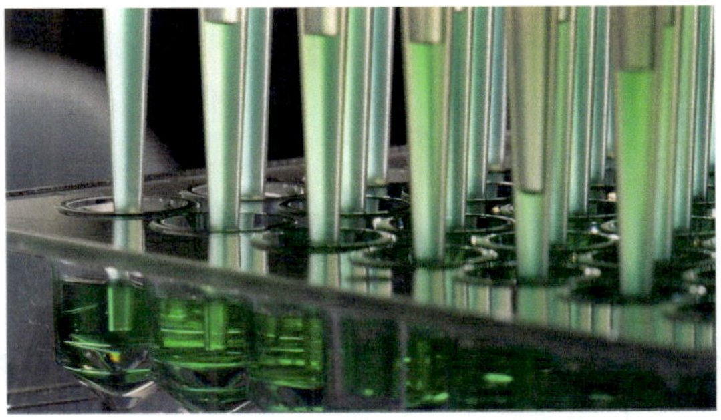

Figure 10.10. Revolutionizing high-throughput drug screening with artificial intelligence (AI).

Source: https://assets.technologynetworks.com/production/dynamic/images/content/381697/revolutionizing-high-throughput-drug-screening-with-ai-and-organoids-381697-960x540.jpg?cb=12587702.

10.6.2. Advances in Miniaturization and Multiplexing

Recent advances in miniaturization and multiplexing technologies are revolutionizing the practice of high-throughput screening in immunology. Such a transition is largely owing to the need for better ways of handling sophisticated biological interactions in dimensions not previously possible. By applying lab-on-a-chip technology, researchers are able to conduct numerous experiments simultaneously from a single small platform, drastically reducing the time and expense in relation to traditional tests. This integration of microscale technologies not only increases the throughput but also allows for more comprehensive data acquisition, allowing scientists to examine interactions in a more biologically relevant setting. As highlighted by recent literature, an integrally complete nanoscale approach that enables manipulation and analysis of thousands of individual cells in a pertinent nanoenvironment can potentially bypass many issues prevalent in current biopharmaceutical workflows and even in advanced drug discovery procedures (Jorgolli et al., 2019).

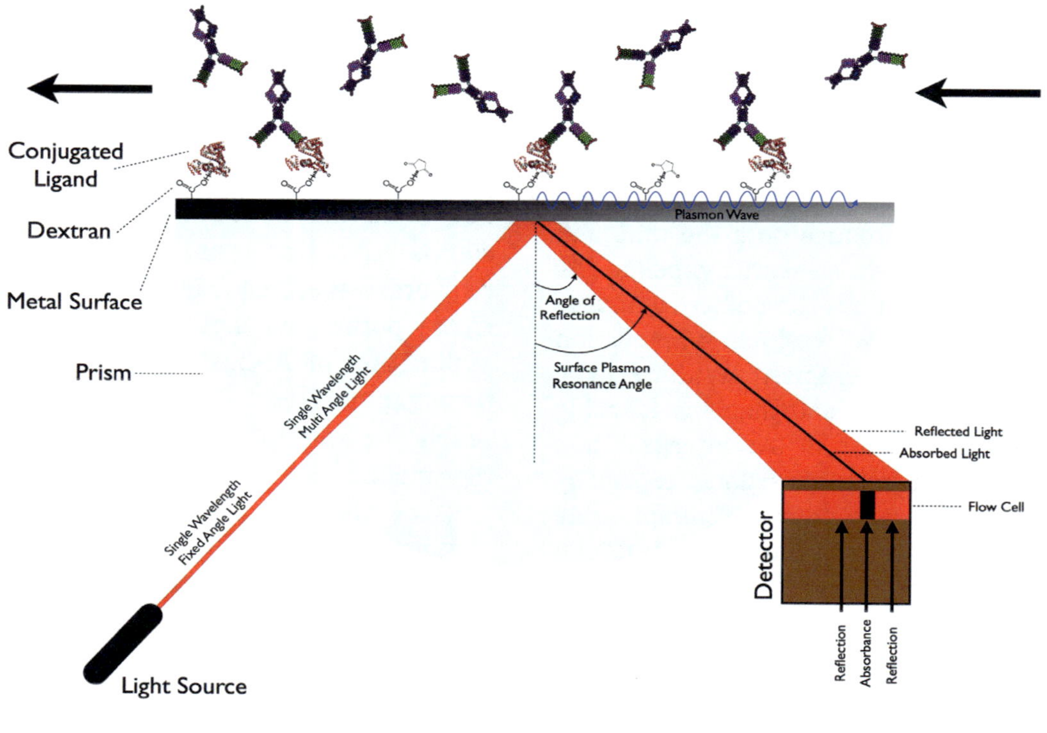

Figure 10.11. Illustration of surface plasmon resonance (SPR).

Source: https://upload.wikimedia.org/wikipedia/commons/thumb/d/d5/Surface_Plasmon_Resonance_%28SPR%29.jpg/1280px-Surface_Plasmon_Resonance_%28SPR%29.jpg.

Moreover, the advancement of optical biosensors has significantly added to the quest for high-throughput screening methods in immunology. Surface plasmon resonance (SPR) technology, conventionally a gold standard for label-free analysis of biomolecular interactions, is being revolutionized by miniaturization and innovative designs. Current developments in nanopatterned interferometric SPR sensors allow highly sensitive optical techniques to be incorporated into simple, yet more compact formats. This revolution not only allows simpler experimental configurations but also enables multipoint detection to be achieved on a single chip. These capabilities are valuable for immunological applications, facilitating in-depth characterization of immune response and identification of putative therapeutic targets. With successful conversions from traditional older SPR systems to more advanced plasmonic platforms having been completed, the potential implications for point-of-care diagnostics and general immunological research are all the more promising (Gao, 2014) (Figure 10.11). By detecting multiple analytes simultaneously, researchers can better comprehend the sophistication of the immune system. These advances facilitate antibody discovery and bioassay development productivity, resulting in candidate fast track validation for immunotherapeutics. Furthermore, the inclusion of sophisticated imaging and analytical tools optimizes the capability of viewing the *in vivo* interactions of immune cells in real-time, enabling better comprehension of their functional dynamics. With labs increasingly employing these new technologies, the hope for groundbreaking discoveries in the area of immunology is significantly increased because it facilitates investigating new treatments and diagnostic strategies in the era of precision medicine (Jorgolli et al., 2019) (Figure 10.12).

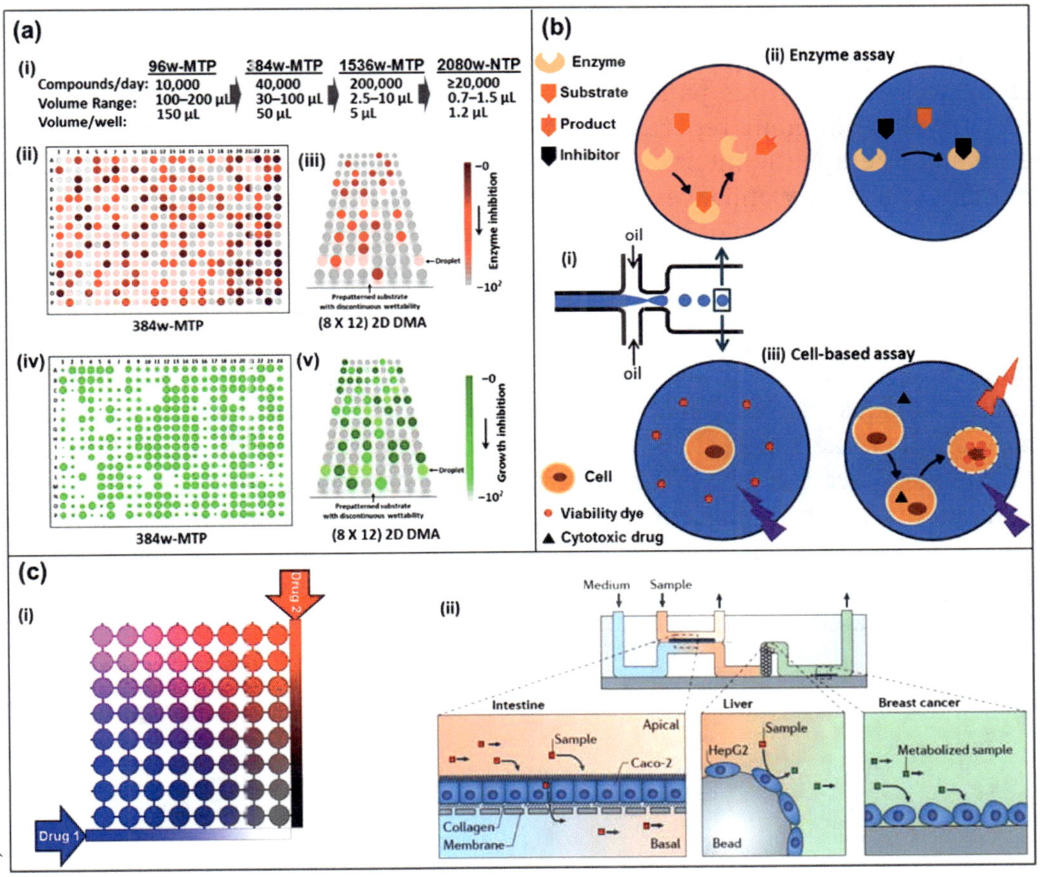

Figure 10.12. (a) Miniaturization of high-throughput screening in array formats. (i) Miniaturization of well-plate screening formats. (ii) Schematics of high-throughput screening using a colorimetric assay.

Source: https://www.researchgate.net/profile/Dharmendra_Dheeman/publication/325891542/figure/fig2/AS:639776420012032@1529545993368/a-Miniaturization-of-high-throughput-screening-in-array-formats-i-Miniaturization-of.png.

10.6.3. Potential for Personalized Medicine Applications

The use of HTS in immunology has exceptional potential to advance the prospects of personalized medicine applications, particularly in the field of pharmacogenetics. Personalized medicine seeks to individualize therapeutic interventions based on personal genetic profiles to maximize the effectiveness of treatment. However, the clinical use of pharmacogenetics has been hampered by limitations such as inconsistency between multiple genetic variants and without universally accepted clinical guidelines. As this chapter emphasizes, the introduction of NGS has revolutionized the ability to analyze pharmacogenetic profiles rapidly and accurately. This breakthrough allows for the simultaneous sequencing of multiple genes and may enhance therapeutic regimens, particularly for drugs whose efficacy is unpredictable across various individuals (Vanakker & De Paepe, 2013). High-throughput technology allows researchers to streamline the hunt for genetic influences that shape drug response, opening up the possibility of more effective, patient-specific therapies. Moreover, the discovery of immune repertoire sequencing adds another dimension to the future use of personalized medicine, in the form of tailoring immunotherapy treatments. The adaptive immune system is designed to recognize a vast universe of antigens through the general antigen-binding capabilities of antibodies and T-cell receptors. High-throughput technologies, such as AIRR-seq, allow for thorough profiling of these immune repertoires, thereby revealing intricate features of immune responses in various pathological disorders, e.g., cancer and autoimmunity (Miho et al., 2018). Quantitative immune repertoire diversity analysis permits clinicians and researchers to customize immunotherapeutic interventions based on individual immune profiles. Thus, immune repertoire analysis not only enhances the precision of immunotherapies but further promotes a more integrated comprehension of adaptive immunity, allowing for new strategies of personalized medicine. As high-throughput screening techniques continue to advance, they possess enormous capability in closing the gap between clinical application and fundamental immunological research. The large datasets produced by NGS and AIRR-seq can be processed by advanced computational algorithms, leading to improved insight into complex immune dynamics. For instance, machine learning methodologies can decipher vast immune repertoire datasets, allowing for improved identification of biomarkers capable of predicting treatment response or disease outcomes. These computer strategies pave the way for the integration of high-throughput screen data into clinical decision-making, ultimately transforming the approach to personalized medicine in immunology. Through synchronizing technological advancements with clinical understanding, vast opportunities exist to devise personalized therapeutic regimens that intimately associate with patient-specific profiles in order to maximize overall healthcare outcomes.

SUMMARY

Briefly, the integration of HTS technologies within immunology has tremendously transformed the therapeutic discovery and understanding of the disease landscape. These novel methods enable the investigation of large-scale biological interactions to solve complex immune responses in unmatched depth. Fast analysis and management of heterogeneous biological samples give a better picture of immune systems under various conditions, whether health or disease. As emphasized through systems biology approaches that capitalize on computational simulation and data integration, the synergy between HTS and statistical as well as bioinformatics capabilities is paramount to extracting meaningful information from massive data sets generated in immunology, ultimately providing a gateway to novel therapeutic paradigms in vaccine development and immunodiagnostics (Woelders et al., 2011). Furthermore, high-throughput analysis of adaptive immune receptor repertoires is a crucial advance in the immunological complexity of response. AIRR-seq technologies, for example, provide deep mapping of immune diversity with groundbreaking insights into the mechanisms of action of several immunotherapies. The capacity to measure and dissect the complex architecture of immune receptor sequences further our knowledge of pathologies like cancer and autoimmunity and directs clinical approaches to how to leverage the immune system for therapeutic benefit. With ongoing advances in computational analysis and machine learning, future research will likely give us improved insights into immune dynamics, thus opening doors to the development of targeted strategies that might further refine patient outcomes (Miho et al., 2018). Lastly, the convergence of high-throughput screening and powerful computational tools represents a new era in immunology that will refine our understanding of immune functionality and drive therapeutic interventions. By embracing a systems biology mindset, researchers are able to move beyond traditional reductionist approaches to investigate the interplay between different elements of the immune system as an overall system. Not only does this change in mindset allow us a better comprehension of complex immune processes, but it also encourages innovative solutions to vaccine development and immunotherapeutic design. Since the field continues to evolve, the concept of high-throughput strategies in immunology will undoubtedly bring about unprecedented innovation and a deeper understanding of immune-mediated diseases, bringing us closer to more efficient treatments for patients worldwide (Woelders et al., 2011). In immunology, HTS has been a landmark technology accelerating the discovery and development of novel therapeutic products.

By enabling the simultaneous screening of thousands of compounds, HTS enables the determination of candidate modulators of immune responses. Mechanistic insights, at least as much, cannot be exaggerated within the drug discovery framework. Current literature points out that intricate interactions between cancer cells and their environment, e.g., the activity of the sympathetic nervous system (SNS), are the most important concerns in the development of successful therapies. This intersection of cancer biology and immune modulation highlights the need to explore new therapeutic strategies that are capable of targeting cellular signaling pathways and immune cell activity, with the ultimate aim of improving the outcome of the patient in oncology (Kim et al., 2016). Besides oncology, implementation of HTS extends to the realm of infectious diseases as well, where it plays a vital role in the detection of agents for diagnostics and therapeutics. For instance, soil-transmitted helminths are a global public health concern, infecting over 1 billion people. The limitations of traditional methods bring forth the urgency for new screening methods to increase detection and surveillance of such infections. With continuously evolving areas of immunological research, the synergy of molecular diagnosis and HTS can be used to better understand complex host-parasite interactions. The development of new assays will not only translate into better disease control but will also disclose important information on the immune mechanisms used in infectious diseases, paving the way to the discovery of targeted therapies and interventions (Lamberton & Jourdan, 2015). The incorporation of HTS technology into immunology fosters an integrative view of therapeutic and diagnostic advancement. Emphasizing the need for further investment in research, particularly mechanobiology of cancer and infectious diseases, is essential for bridging knowledge gaps. The comprehension of immune cell interactions with the surrounding environment, such as the extracellular matrix, presents a multidisciplinary explanation for disease formation and treatments. Besides, continued advances in adapting HTS technology to address different classes of pathogens and immune challenges will significantly enhance our capacity to address global health risks. Thus, the convergence of the approaches of cancer biology and infectious disease investigation via high-throughput screening holds the potential to inaugurate a new era of immunological investigation and treatment (Lamberton & Jourdan, 2015; Kim et al., 2016).

A CLOSER LOOK

THE IMPACT OF HIGH-THROUGHPUT SCREENING (HTS) ON THE FUTURE OF IMMUNOLOGY

The advent of HTS has revolutionized the landscape of immunology by enabling researchers to rapidly screen large libraries of compounds or biological reagents. This increased efficiency allows the identification of therapeutic targets at unparalleled speed and accuracy. Among the most thrilling areas affected by HTS is the investigation of neoantigens for cancer immunotherapy. As tumor-specific antigens generated through single mutations in cancer cells, these neoantigens represent a compelling target for personalized therapies. HTS allows the comprehensive characterization needed to identify and profile these neoantigens and thereby facilitate the development of personalized cancer immunotherapies that can enhance patient outcomes, namely in the case of solid tumors, where traditional treatment modalities might fall through. The use of HTS in immunology does not only speed up discovery; it also streamlines the path to clinical use (Figure 10.13).

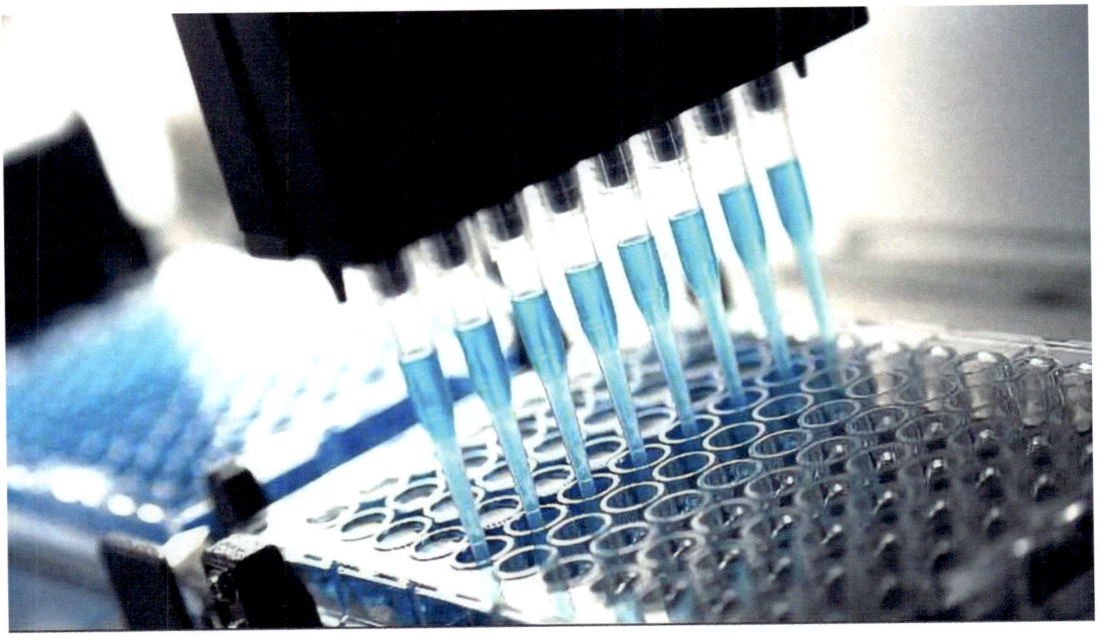

Figure 10.13. High-throughput screening accelerating drug discovery efforts.

Source: https://assets.technologynetworks.com/production/dynamic/images/content/288926/high-throughput-screening-accelerating-drug-discovery-efforts-288926-960x540.jpg?cb=11727967.

By screening large numbers of therapeutic compounds against biologically relevant systems, researchers are able to pick up those most likely to bypass inherent and acquired mechanisms of drug resistance. For instance, understanding how cancer cells develop to be resistant to treatments enables new strategies that can circumvent MDR to be established, with promise for resistant patients with cancer. High-throughput strategies allow for the screening of numerous compounds and their effects on immune pathways, unveiling the mechanism through which certain drugs can modulate the immune response effectively. As a result, the results of HTS may have the potential to develop novel therapeutic regimes aimed at both the tumor and its resistant nature, thereby maximizing treatment efficacy and patients' survival. The future of immunology will stand to benefit significantly from the existing technologies in HTS, particularly in the context of neoantigen discovery and the circumvention of MDR.

With an increasing number of researchers utilizing these methodologies, they will inevitably discover new targets and pathways that can be targeted by immunotherapy, giving rise to new therapeutic paradigms. Besides, the combination of bioinformatics and machine learning with HTS data could potentially allow the identification of biomarkers to treatment responses for numerous immunotherapies, as has been the case with the recent interest in the association of neoantigens and immune checkpoint blockade responses. Therefore, the overlap of HTS with cutting-edge genomic and proteomic technologies has the potential to revolutionize the field of immunology, opening the windows of opportunity for the identification of precision medicine strategies that may be utilized for the management of a variety of diseases, such as cancer and autoimmune diseases.

REFERENCES

1. Abedalthagafi, M., Alqahtani, S., Brazma, A., Butte, A., et al. (2024). The evolution of computational research in a data-centric world. https://core.ac.uk/download/650677750.pdf (accessed on 27th June 2025).
2. Miho E, Yermanos A, Weber CR, Berger CT, Reddy ST, Greiff V. Computational Strategies for Dissecting the High-Dimensional Complexity of Adaptive Immune Repertoires. *Front Immunol.* 2018;9:224. Published 2018 Feb 21. doi:10.3389/fimmu.2018.00224(accessed on 27th June 2025).
3. Ma, N., Kamalakshakurup, G., Aghaamoo, M., Lee, A. P., & Digman, M. A. (2019). Label-Free Metabolic Classification of Single Cells in Droplets Using the Phasor Approach to Fluorescence Lifetime Imaging Microscopy. *Cytometry. Part A : the journal of the International Society for Analytical Cytology, 95*(1), 93–100. https://doi.org/10.1002/cyto.a.23673(accessed on 27th June 2025).
4. Volokhov, D. V., Becker, D. J., Bergner, L. M., Camus, M. S., Orton, R. J., Chizhikov, V. E., Altizer, S. M., & Streicker, D. G. (2017). Novel hemotropic mycoplasmas are widespread and genetically diverse in vampire bats. *Epidemiology and infection, 145*(15), 3154–3167. https://doi.org/10.1017/S095026881700231X (accessed on 27th June 2025).
5. Stoimenova, A., Savova, A., Manova, M., Angelovska, B., & Petrova, G. (2011). Pharmaceutical Biotechnology in Pharmacy Education: USA Pharmacy Schools. *Biotechnology & Biotechnological Equipment, 25*(3), 2533–2537. https://doi.org/10.5504/BBEQ.2011.0074(accessed on 27th June 2025).
6. Antoine-Moussiaux, N., Do Duc, L., Farnir, F., Kafidi, A., et al. (2013). Évaluation morphométrique des chevaux pur-sang Arabe en Algérie: mensurations corporelles et proposition d'équations barymétriques. http://orbi.ulg.ac.be/bitstream/2268/157229/1/proceedings2013.pdf (accessed on 27th June 2025).
7. Arbyn, M., Benoy, I., Bogers, J., Poljak, M., et al. (2019). Using the VALGENT-3 framework to assess the clinical and analytical performance of the RIATOL qPCR HPV genotyping assay. https://core.ac.uk/download/322828811.pdf (accessed on 27th June 2025).
8. Woelders, H., Te Pas, M. F., Bannink, A., Veerkamp, R. F., & Smits, M. A. (2011). Systems biology in animal sciences. *Animal : an international journal of animal bioscience, 5*(7), 1036–1047. https://doi.org/10.1017/S1751731111000036(accessed on 27th June 2025).
9. Bhuyan, R., Kumari, P., Prakash, A., Tyagi, R., et al. (2024). Revolutionizing anti-cancer drug discovery: The role of artificial intelligence. https://core.ac.uk/download/646080774.pdf (accessed on 27th June 2025).
10. Bishop, N., Gillet, V. J., Holliday, J. D., Willett, P., et al. (2003). Chemoinformatic research at the University of Sheffield: A history and citation analysis. https://core.ac.uk/download/59871.pdf (accessed on 27th June 2025).
11. Wagner, S., Roberson, D., Boland, J., Kreimer, A. R., Yeager, M., Cullen, M., Mirabello, L., Dunn, S. T., Walker, J., Zuna, R., Porras, C., Cortes, B., Sampson, J., Herrero, R., Rodriguez, A. C., Quint, W., Van Doorn, L. J., CVT Group, Hildesheim, A., Schiffman, M., ... Wentzensen, N. (2019). Evaluation of TypeSeq, a Novel High-Throughput, Low-Cost, Next-Generation Sequencing-Based Assay for Detection of 51 Human Papillomavirus Genotypes. *The Journal*

of infectious diseases, 220(10), 1609–1619. https://doi.org/10.1093/infdis/jiz324(accessed on 27th June 2025).

12. Robinson EK, Covarrubias S, Carpenter S. The how and why of lncRNA function: An innate immune perspective. *Biochim Biophys Acta Gene Regul Mech*. 2020;1863(4):194419. doi:10.1016/j.bbagrm.2019.194419 (accessed on 27th June 2025).
13. Molesti, E., Wright, E., Terregino, C., Rahman, R., Cattoli, G., & Temperton, N. J. (2014). Multiplex evaluation of influenza neutralizing antibodies with potential applicability to in-field serological studies. *Journal of immunology research, 2014*, 457932. https://doi.org/10.1155/2014/457932(accessed on 27th June 2025).
14. Jorgolli M, Nevill T, Winters A, et al. Nanoscale integration of single cell biologics discovery processes using optofluidic manipulation and monitoring. *Biotechnol Bioeng*. 2019;116(9):2393-2411. doi:10.1002/bit.27024(accessed on 27th June 2025).
15. David-Olawade, A. C., Fapohunda, O., et al. (2024). Leveraging artificial intelligence in vaccine development: A narrative review. https://core.ac.uk/download/615274647.pdf (accessed on 27th June 2025).
16. Vanakker, O. M., & De Paepe, A. (2013). Pharmacogenomics in children: advantages and challenges of next generation sequencing applications. *International journal of pediatrics, 2013*, 136524. https://doi.org/10.1155/2013/136524(accessed on 27th June 2025).
17. Patel, M., Vlahava, V. M., Forbes, S. K., Fielding, C. A., Stanton, R. J., & Wang, E. C. Y. (2018). HCMV-Encoded NK Modulators: Lessons From *in vitro* and *in vivo* Genetic Variation. *Frontiers in immunology, 9*, 2214. https://doi.org/10.3389/fimmu.2018.02214(accessed on 27th June 2025).
18. Kricka LJ, Polsky TG, Park JY, Fortina P. The future of laboratory medicine - a 2014 perspective. *Clin Chim Acta*. 2015;438:284-303. doi:10.1016/j.cca.2014.09.005(accessed on 27th June 2025).
19. Tehranirokh M, Kouzani AZ, Francis PS, Kanwar JR. Microfluidic devices for cell cultivation and proliferation. *Biomicrofluidics*. 2013;7(5):51502. Published 2013 Oct 29. doi:10.1063/1.4826935 (accessed on 27th June 2025).
20. s, Y. (2014). *Nanostructured Plasmonic Interferometers for Ultrasensitive Label-Free Biosensing*. Presented to the Graduate and Research Committee of Lehigh University in Candidacy for the Degree of Doctor of Philosophy in Electrical Engineering Lehigh University https://core.ac.uk/download/pdf/228638231.pdf (accessed on 27th June 2025).
21. Lamberton, P. H., & Jourdan, P. M. (2015). Human Ascariasis: Diagnostics Update. *Current tropical medicine reports, 2*(4), 189–200. https://doi.org/10.1007/s40475-015-0064-9(accessed on 27th June 2025).
22. Kim, T. H., Rowat, A. C., & Sloan, E. K. (2016). Neural regulation of cancer: From mechanobiology to inflammation. https://core.ac.uk/download/323080309.pdf (accessed on 27th June 2025).
23. Lynch, A. E., Triajianto, J., & Routledge, E. (2014). Low-cost motility tracking system (LOCOMOTIS) for time-lapse microscopy applications and cell visualisation. *PloS one, 9*(8), e103547. https://doi.org/10.1371/journal.pone.0103547(accessed on 27th June 2025).
24. K. Saxena, S. (Ed.). (2022). High-Throughput Screening for Drug Discovery. IntechOpen. doi: 10.5772/intechopen.91075(accessed on 27th June 2025).

25. Rodrigues, P. da F. S., & Thomaz, D. V. (2020). A brief overview of current drug repurposing approaches for COVID-19 management. https://core.ac.uk/download/323185228.pdf (accessed on 27th June 2025).

26. Saeed, A. F. U. H., Wang, R., Wang, S., & Ling, S. (2017). Antibody engineering for pursuing a healthier future. https://core.ac.uk/download/pdf/82883279.pdf (accessed on 27th June 2025).

27. Seaman, W., & Whitehouse, J. H. (2001). Florida marine biotechnology: Research, development and training capabilities to advance science and commerce. https://core.ac.uk/download/11016354.pdf (accessed on 27th June 2025).

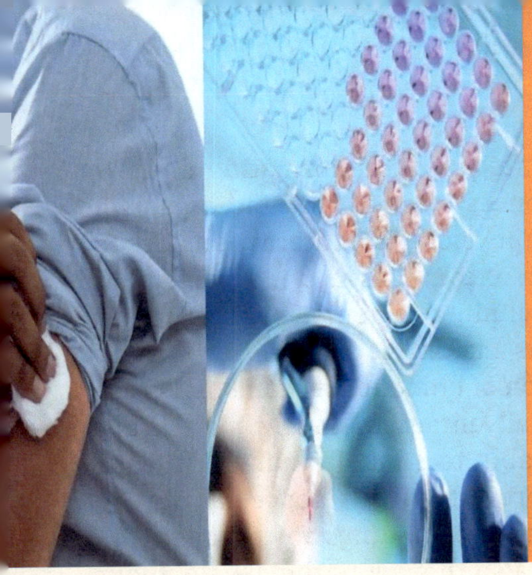

Chapter 11

IN VIVO MODELS IN IMMUNOLOGY

Contents

Introduction

The study of *in vivo* models of immunology has progressively become central, with scientists desiring to demystify complicated immune responses as well as create efficacious therapeutic interventions. *In vivo* models, which involve the study of biological processes in intact living beings, provide a holistic understanding of immune interactions compared to *in vitro* work, which often misses the intricate dynamics involved in the immune system. These models allow for the examination of various factors, such as cellular dynamics, pathogen/pathogen interactions, and immune system regulatory mechanisms in a way that mimics human physiology. Hence, the ability to mimic disease or immune processes within a living organism allows for risk assessment of an entire kind as well as the detection of potential therapeutic targets, thereby enhancing the predictive validity of immunology research. The creation of frameworks like the adverse outcome pathway (AOP) concept represents a significant advance in structuring our understanding of the molecular mechanisms of immune processes. By positioning the mechanisms underlying processes like IgE-mediated food allergy into context, the AOP framework structures the current *in vitro* methods, explaining why they are helpful and their shortcomings. Notably, this model enables the systematic identification of key events to immune sensitization and guides the development of novel strategies that can reduce reliance on animal models in safety assessments. Particularly, the realization of innate and adaptive immune response mechanisms via the highly developed pathways will lead researchers to realize the balance between allergy development and the need for adequate immune functionality, hence the prime means of intervening effectively in food allergy complications (Lozano-Ojalvo et al., 2019). Further, the importance of *in vivo* models extends to the study of conditions for chronic inflammation, such as depicted by Rheumatoid Arthritis (RA). The pathophysiology of RA highlights the complexity of immune dysregulation, where inflammatory processes become autoamplifying and cause tissue damage. Of note, recent data highlight the role of myeloid cells in chronicity and inflammation by several regulatory pathways, which mandates models that closely reflect chronic disease states. By investigating these mechanisms in *in vivo* environments, scientists can discover possible therapeutic targets that initiate pro-resolving mechanisms, thus providing pathways towards new interventions. Continued advancements in the development of such models will definitely provide more understanding into immune interactions, thus enhancing the efficacy of therapeutic interventions for chronic inflammatory diseases (Alivernini et al., 2018).

Definition of In Vivo Models

In vivo models are crucial reagents in immunology that allow scientists to study complicated biological processes within a living organism. As opposed to *in vitro* experiments, which are conducted using cells or tissues in a biological context external to the body, *in vivo* experiments provide information on how immune responses work in a whole organism where several physiological interactions occur. These models encompass a wide variety of organisms, including rodents, primates, and mammals, thus making it possible to expand the investigation of immune mechanisms across species. Some advantages of *in vivo* models are that they are able to simulate human disease conditions more effectively, hence improving the translatability of findings to the clinic. As such, they are also the key to the development of vaccines and therapies by providing vital information on immune system pathology and function, leading to enhanced understanding of immunological responses in disease and health. The application of *in vivo* models is necessary in order to untangle complex immune cell interactions and behaviors that cannot be traced in less complex model systems. One of the key fields of research involves T cell fate and dynamics. Recent studies reveal that T cell activity, including division and apoptosis, may be regulated by cell age as well as by other factors, influencing immunotherapy. For instance, experiments demonstrate that *in vivo* models can reveal age-independent dynamics of T cell responses, which goes against previous assumptions derived from *in vitro* data. These findings have implications for the development of age-related immunotherapies. Using *in vivo* models, researchers are able to quantify the impact of various factors on immune responses, refining intervention strategies for better performance in clinical applications, which underscores the key position of such models to advance immunological science (Del Amo et al., 2020). Secondly, *in vivo* models offer the option to explore disease states that involve the immune system, such as chorioamnionitis during pregnancy. This disease exemplifies the intricate interaction of immune cells at the maternal-fetal interface, in which inflammation will have significant implications for maternal and fetal well-being. Using various animal models, researchers have been able to determine the pathophysiology of this disease, and valuable information regarding the role of immune responses has been gleaned. *In vivo* models have illustrated a correlation between microbial infection and maternal inflammation. In doing so, they have better explained how maternal tolerance towards allografts of fetal origin can be disrupted. These findings are crucial in the development of therapeutic regimens to counteract poor outcomes related to infection during pregnancy. The models thus remain a vital tool in immunology, acting as the missing link between fundamental research and clinical translation (Cappelletti et al., 2020) (Figure 11.1).

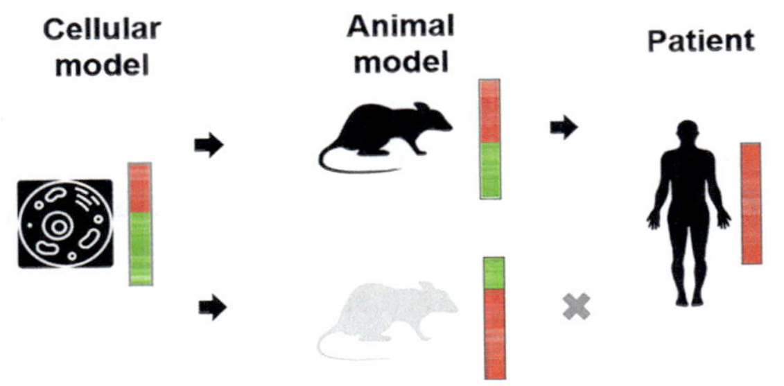

Figure 11.1. Choosing an appropriate *in vivo* model for hit and MoA validation.

Source: https://www.researchgate.net/profile/Fabien-Vincent-3/publication/344139711/figure/fig7/AS:933820975026181@1599651678641/Choosing-an-appropriate-in-vivo-model-for-hit-and-MoA-validation-An-in-vivo-model.jpg.

Importance of Immunology in Health and Disease

Immunology is key to health and the understanding of disease, as it is the basis of the body's defense strategies against infectious pathogens. Through the highly organized network of immune cells, tissues, and signaling molecules, the immune system recognizes and removes invading foreign pathogens, including bacteria, viruses, and parasites. *In vivo* studies of such responses are crucial in immunology research; *in vivo* models enable researchers to study the complex interactions under infection, inflammation, and autoimmunity. These observations have profound implications for vaccine and therapeutic strategy design, particularly for immunologically demanding diseases with strong immune evasion, e.g., those by African trypanosomes. On this score, failure to generate effective vaccines, as borne out by the persistence in the use of chemotherapy and its resultant toxicity, is an added testament to the need for research into higher immunology (Stijlemans et al., 2017). Helminth infections have also taught us about the duality of the immune system in both health and disease. Surprisingly, the immune response modulation by the parasitic worms is connected to the decrease in autoimmune diseases in developing countries. According to the Hygiene Hypothesis, increases in autoimmune illnesses in industrialized nations are believed to be due to improved sanitation, and the subsequent decline in helminth infections. Exploring these systems in *in vivo* models allows for the immunomodulatory function of helminths, such as that of ES-62, a renowned immunomodulator, to be dissected. Such investigations have revealed the potential treatment methods by employing such naturally occurring processes to control immune reactions without affecting overall host immunity and thus offering promising treatments for autoimmune illnesses (Pineda et al., 2014). Continued advances in *in vivo* models in immunology both enhance our knowledge of immune function and establish the therapeutic significance of findings. The knowledge gained from the study of host defenses and pathogen evasion strategies directs the design of new interventions, including vaccines and immunotherapies. For emerging infections and antibiotic resistance, the need for research cannot be overstated. While immunology keeps pace with advances in models, such as the use of nanobodies to diagnose and treat disease, e.g., African trypanosomiasis, this is strong evidence of the cutting-edge thinking in the discipline. Generally, however, the convergence of immunology and health emphasizes the necessity for continuing research and development for the purpose of fostering better disease control and public health in general.

11.1. Historical Background of In Vivo Models

The progression in the application of *in vivo* models has largely shaped the field of immunology. At first, science was carried out using mainly rudimentary animal models that provided very limited insights into human pathophysiology. However, as veterinary medicine enhanced and genetics became a more practical aid, scientists came to understand the necessity of working with more sophisticated models, such as genetically altered organisms, which better mimic human immune reactions. The production of such models has enabled researchers to investigate complex immunological mechanisms. This advancement is important as it will allow researchers to evaluate therapeutic interventions in a biologically relevant environment with the aim of sharpening our understanding of disease and treatment. Infectious diseases have historically motivated the generation of *in vivo* models. For instance, the therapy of malaria and vaccine development necessitated the use of non-human primates to investigate Plasmodium species. Of particular importance are investigations of the multidrug-resistant *P. falciparum* Thai C2A strain in Aotus primates, which highlight the need for special models in understanding drug resistance patterns and treatment failures. The data accessed via these investigations underscore that potent *in vivo* models are critical for investigating the pharmacological profile of infectious disease and developing novel therapeutic strategies, thus bringing to light the symbiotic relationship between veterinary practices and immunology in biomedical research (Obaldía et al., 2016).

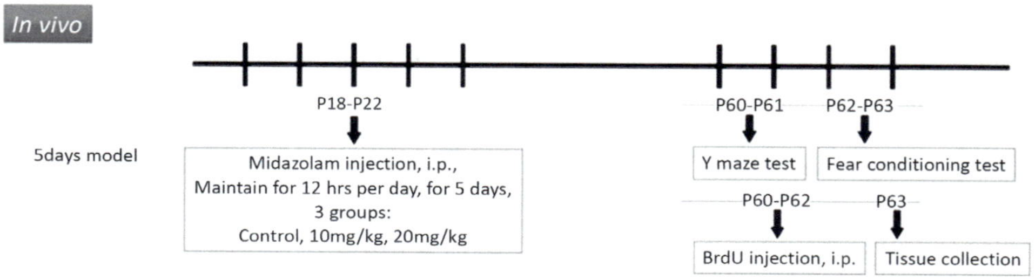

Figure 11.2. Schematic representation of the experimental timeline *in vivo*.

Source: https://www.researchgate.net/profile/Jing-Xu-75/publication/330060472/figure/fig1/AS:713543586414594@1547133456704/Schematic-representation-of-the-experimental-timeline-in-vivo-and-in-vitro-A-In-vivo.png.

At the same time, the advent of zoonotic pathogens has underscored the need for *in vivo* models to reflect human disease phenotypes. A prime example is the research on *Campylobacter jejuni* infections in IL-10-/- mice, which replicates an acute presentation of campylobacteriosis that resembles human disease. Such models have facilitated researchers in exploring potential therapeutic agents like vitamin C, which exhibited encouraging anti-inflammatory effects. Such findings not only broaden the range of applications for *in vivo* models but also validate their utility in addressing public health issues posed by newly arising infectious diseases. The time frame context of these investigations indicates that *in vivo* models are critical tools in immunology, bridging research in the laboratory and the clinic, ultimately resulting in new therapies and prevention methods (Mousavi et al., 2020) (Figure 11.2).

11.1.1. Early Experiments in Immunology

The initial foundations of immunology were laid during the 19th century, through classic experiments examining the body's defense mechanisms against infectious pathogens. A case in point is Louis Pasteur, whose vaccination experiments revolutionized acquired immunity knowledge. Pasteur's experiments demonstrated that inoculating subjects with attenuated forms of the infectious agents responsible for anthrax and rabies elicited protective immune responses. This study not only made vaccination a key tool for the prevention of infectious diseases but also emphasized the promise of *in vivo* models, as animals treated with such vaccines were found to be highly resistant upon subsequent exposure to the virulent strains. Such observations placed particular emphasis on the role of *in vivo* systems in the investigation of immune responses and paved the way for subsequent studies and clinical applications in immunology. Another important breakthrough in the early immune studies involved the discovery of antibodies as a fundamental component of the immune system. Emil von Behring and Kitasato Shibasaburo made significant contributions to this area in their experiments on serum therapy, which illustrated how animal serum containing antibodies could be used to confer immunity against infectious diseases like diphtheria and tetanus. Their experiments employed animal models, primarily rabbits and guinea pigs, to demonstrate the curative efficacy of immunoglobulins obtained from infected animals. Their method provided them with useful insights into humoral immunity, which demonstrated the dynamic interaction between pathogens and immune system components. The success of serum therapy pointed to the significance of *in vivo* models for revealing mechanisms of the immune response, presaging the discovery of and isolation of monoclonal antibodies for application in modern immunotherapy. Initial research into the immune system also continued to explore inflammation and its role in defense mechanisms. Scientists ventured into the cellular reactions to infection and found a variety of immune cells, including macrophages and lymphocytes, that are actively involved in inflammation.

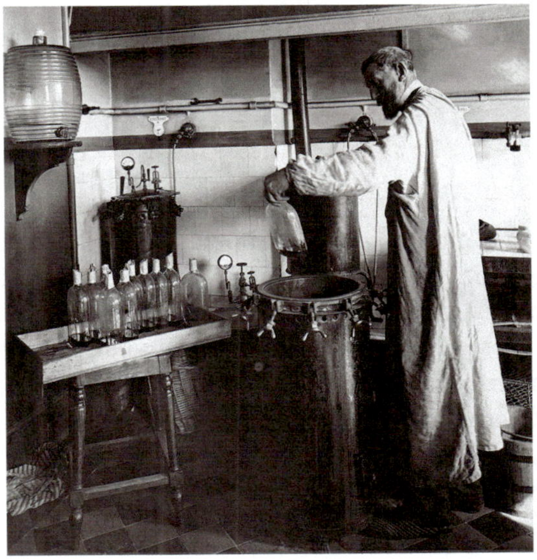

Figure 11.3. Louis Pasteur, whose work on vaccination revolutionized the understanding of acquired immunity.

Source: https://upload.wikimedia.org/wikipedia/commons/thumb/4/44/Louis_Pasteur_experiment.jpg/800px-Louis_Pasteur_experiment.jpg.

The development of *in vivo* models to assess such processes proved to be crucial, as this allowed scientists to observe the behavior of immune cells surrounding pathogens and between themselves in living organisms in real-time, a glimpse of the complexity of immune dynamics. Most prominently, scientific studies with acute inflammation models in animal models illustrated how the factors such as cytokines and biological lipids influence immune cell behavior.

For instance, one study indicated the role of sphingosine-1-phosphate (S1P) in maintaining activated CD4 T cells at sites of inflammation, showing that the biochemical environment determines cellular convergence in immune responses (Jaigirdar et al., 2017). Early immunological studies have greatly enriched our understanding of immune response, placing emphasis on the importance of *in vivo* models in describing how the immune system functions (Figure 11.3).

11.1.2. Development of Animal Models

Development of animal models plays a key role in expanding our understanding of immunological processes and disease mechanisms. Such models allow scientists to investigate the complex interactions between disease agents and the immune system in a controlled setting, information that would otherwise often not be obtainable through other methods. Previously, numerous studies have utilized animal models, such as mice, rabbits, and non-human primates, to examine immune responses to infectious disease and cancer.

Model choice is often a function of the specific immune reactions being studied and the relevance of the model to human physiology. Accordingly, researchers are continually refining these models to provide them with greater predictive capability in relation to human response, so that they can adequately portray the biological nuances of human health and disease. A pertinent example of the necessity to develop animal models is in hepatitis C virus (HCV) research. With more than 71 million people globally who are chronically infected, HCV is a significant public health issue. While there have been improvements in antiviral therapies, such that treatment currently has much better outcomes, the absence of an effective protective vaccine is an indicator of the necessity for ongoing research. In order to clarify HCV biology and virus-host interactions, and to evaluate potential antiviral strategies, in this context, the right animal models play an essential role. Chimpanzees were once the model of choice based on their susceptibility to HCV infection, but ethical and practical constraints have led researchers to look for alternatives. They include a variety of transgenic and humanized mice, which have proven very valuable in the research of immune responses against HCV infection, thus delineating the necessity for new model development in immunological research (Burm et al., 2018).

Within the context of cancer, the generation of animal models has also been instrumental in the evaluation of new therapeutic strategies, such as vaccines based on dendritic cells. These models allow the examination of complex tumor microenvironments and interactions between tumor cells and immune responses. Despite the therapeutic potential of dendritic cell treatments to enhance anti-tumor immunity, their clinical effectiveness has been underwhelming. Experimental models allow for the mass screening of tumor-associated antigens (TAAs) and how tumors evade immune surveillance. By applying various animal platforms, scientists strive to maximize vaccine strategies and the efficacy of immunotherapy. This ongoing pursuit demonstrates the promise and challenges in developing effective animal models that can inform knowledge key to cancer control and confirm the importance of animal models in unraveling immune functions (Koido et al., 2010) (Figure 11.4).

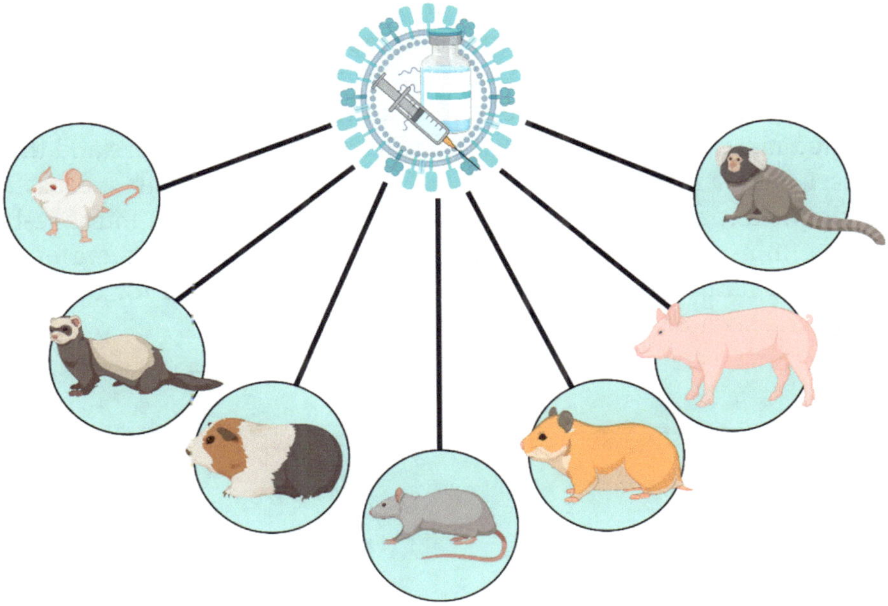

Figure 11.4. Animal models for virus vaccine development.

Source: https://www.mdpi.com/vaccines/vaccines-09-00787/article_deploy/html/images/vaccines-09-00787-g001.png.

11.1.3. Milestones in Immunological Research

Immunological research landmarks are intricately linked to advances in *in vivo* models, which are critical reagents for the understanding of immune responses and the development of effective therapies. Such a landmark is the creation of patient-derived xenograft (PDX) models, which allow researchers to study the interaction between human immune cells and tumors under conditions closely resembling human physiology. This is important since traditional murine models have been found wanting in simulating human immune response. The use of MHC class I and class II-deficient NOG mice in research, for example, against lung adenocarcinoma, exemplifies how these new models guarantee the evaluation of immune checkpoint inhibitors (ICIs). By enabling chronic engraftment of human peripheral blood mononuclear cells (PBMCs), researchers can make valuable observations on therapeutic effect and on the mechanisms of tumor-immune interaction (Hanazawa et al., 2025). Progress in immunology is also marked by advances in understanding immune-mediated disease through the use of advanced *in vivo* techniques. For instance, recent meetings have highlighted the application of animal models as a means of neurodegenerative disease research, specifically their application to decipher pathogenesis and therapeutic possibilities for diseases like multiple sclerosis and Alzheimer's disease. These *in vivo* models enable a close examination of immunological self-tolerance, hence creating new therapeutic remedies aimed at modulating immune responses. The data acquired through such research highlight the pressing need for models capable of simulating the complexity of human neuroimmunology, which creates the doors for the creation of actionable strategies to combat autoimmune diseases (Fusaro et al., 2025). This intersection of immunology and neurobiology marks the dual application of *in vivo* models and their applicability in cutting-edge therapeutic research. As ongoing advancement in immunological research continues to open new windows of opportunities, the integration of cutting-edge *in vivo* models is an essential strategy for accelerating the discovery of novel immunotherapies. The establishment of novel models recapitulating human-tumor interaction not only enhances our understanding of immune escape mechanisms but also facilitates real-time assessment of therapeutic compounds like ICIs. Findings of studies using modified mouse models show remarkable shrinking of tumors and the engagement of T cell populations crucial for further elucidating the immune landscape in successful therapy. Such advances mark a significant step towards more tailored and efficacious immune-based therapies. Briefly, milestones in immunology research increasingly rely on sophisticated *in vivo* models that replicate human disease pathways, and, therefore, emphasize the need for constant innovation in this area of study (Hanazawa et al., 2025) (Figure 11.5).

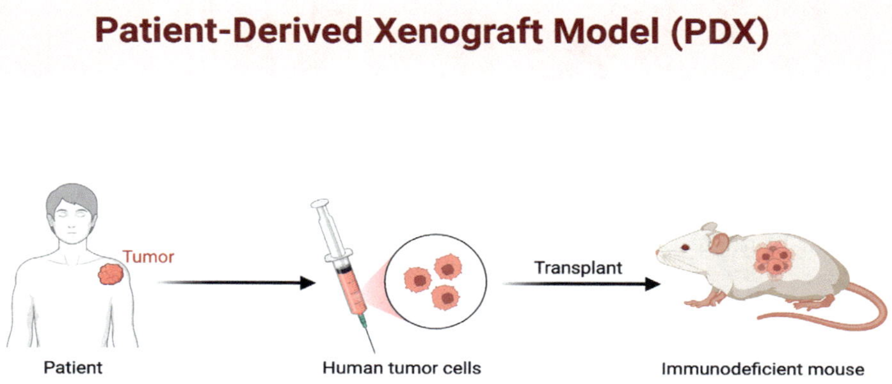

Figure 11.5. Patient-derived xenograft (PDX) model.

Source: https://cdn.prod.website-files.com/621e95f9ac30687a56e4297e/64adcb449e7c21c6bc4fca5b_V2_1679496909177_3b3a66ef-afed-4b18-acc1-86a84647644d_HIGH_RES.png.

11.2. Types of *In Vivo* Models

In vivo systems are critical for creating our understanding of immunological mechanisms and disease pathogenesis and remain precious instruments both for investigation and therapeutic design. Murine models, specifically, have been extensively used because they are similar to humans on genetic, biological, and anatomical levels. The use of C57BL/6 and BALB/c mice, among many widely used strains, offers controlled experimentation, which is the basis for the evaluation of immune responses under conditions that can be manipulated. These models allow researchers to model inflammation, autoimmune reactions, and infection and thereby shed light on the functions of certain immune cell types and cytokines during pathogenesis. In addition, the controlled genetic backgrounds of these models serve to minimize variability experienced in immunology studies and hence enhance the validity of the information gathered, which can then be used to inform and tailor therapeutic approaches for various diseases. Exploratory *in vivo* models can also be larger mammals, including non-human primates and pigs, since they share more of a similar physiology to the human immune response. These provide the unique advantage when looking at specific human diseases, such as those with heavy genetic components or complex multi-system interactions. For instance, big animal models of disease are likely to mirror better the cardiovascular and metabolic derangements associated with atherosclerosis, in which both innate and adaptive immune responses play a primary role, highlighted by the contribution of T lymphocytes and their costimulatory receptors (Antunes et al., 2012). The clinical applicability of information gained from the bigger models is enormous as they offer the means to bridge basic immunological research with the clinic. By the same token, although traditionally accompanied by ethical concerns and logistical challenges, large animal models can offer valuable information that will be sacrificed in reduced models. *In vitro* strategies have been supplemented increasingly by *in vivo* models quantifying immune responses in a more authentic biological environment. The use of the adverse outcome pathway (AOP) framework has facilitated scientists in making the mechanisms of immune sensitization more precise using food protein analysis and interaction with immune systems (Lozano-Ojalvo et al., 2019). This approach focuses on the use of integrated testing approaches by merging *in vitro* and *in vivo* strategies with the ultimate goal of minimizing the application of animal tests. By doing so, the scientific community not only offers more robust biological rationale for immunology research but also resolves concomitant ethical dilemmas of animal welfare. By connecting traditional *in vivo* methods to new test paradigms, researchers can achieve improved treatments without risk and with efficacy for novel therapies against immune-mediated disorders.

11.2.1. Rodent Models (Mice and Rats)

Rodent models, such as mice and rats, are invaluable in the study of immunology as they are surrogates for human biological response because of their genetic, biological, and behavioral resemblance. Rodent models provide a controlled system to examine the complex immune system, permitting researchers to examine different immunological phenomena, including cell signaling, pathogen interaction, and vaccine efficacy. The genetic manipulations that can be conducted in these animals, including the generation of knockout and transgenic mice, enable a better understanding of specific immune mechanisms and disease processes. The models also provide for therapeutic strategies to be investigated *in vivo* since immune responses can be analyzed in real time, giving valuable insight into the effectiveness and safety of potential treatments (Cook et al., 2024). One of the most significant advantages of using rodent models in immunological research is that they can simulate human disease and conditions. Some mouse strains are genetically engineered to develop autoimmune diseases, lymphomas, or infectious diseases for specialized research on disease onset and reaction to medication. Having the ability to reproduce these conditions in a lab is of extreme importance in judging both disease pathophysiology and the effect of different immunotherapies. Furthermore, rodent models allow for the investigation of genetic and environmental influences that affect immune responses, providing an overall image of how a combination of elements is responsible for disease outcomes. Although immunology science is still evolving, these models remain at the forefront of translation research because they help to connect discoveries from the laboratory with translating them into clinical applications (Grannonico et al., 2024). In addition to application in immune response research, rodent models are effective platforms for the testing of new therapeutic methodologies. The development of lentiviral gene therapies is one of the outstanding examples of applying these models in the evaluation of new treatments for immunological disorders. For instance, in rodent models, it has been demonstrated that a lentivirus vector with the feline erythropoietin (EPO) gene is effective. In such research, viral vectors have been administered by researchers to determine the therapeutic effectiveness and safety of such vectors, illustrating the use of rodent models to new biotechnological modalities (Cook et al., 2024). Upon confirmation of findings from such models, scientists can optimize strategies before advancing to higher-order systems so that emerging immunological therapy is both effective and safe for final application to human populations. The contribution of rodents and rats to this continuum of research cannot be overemphasized, as they yield extremely valuable insight that drives the innovation in immunotherapy (Figure 11.6).

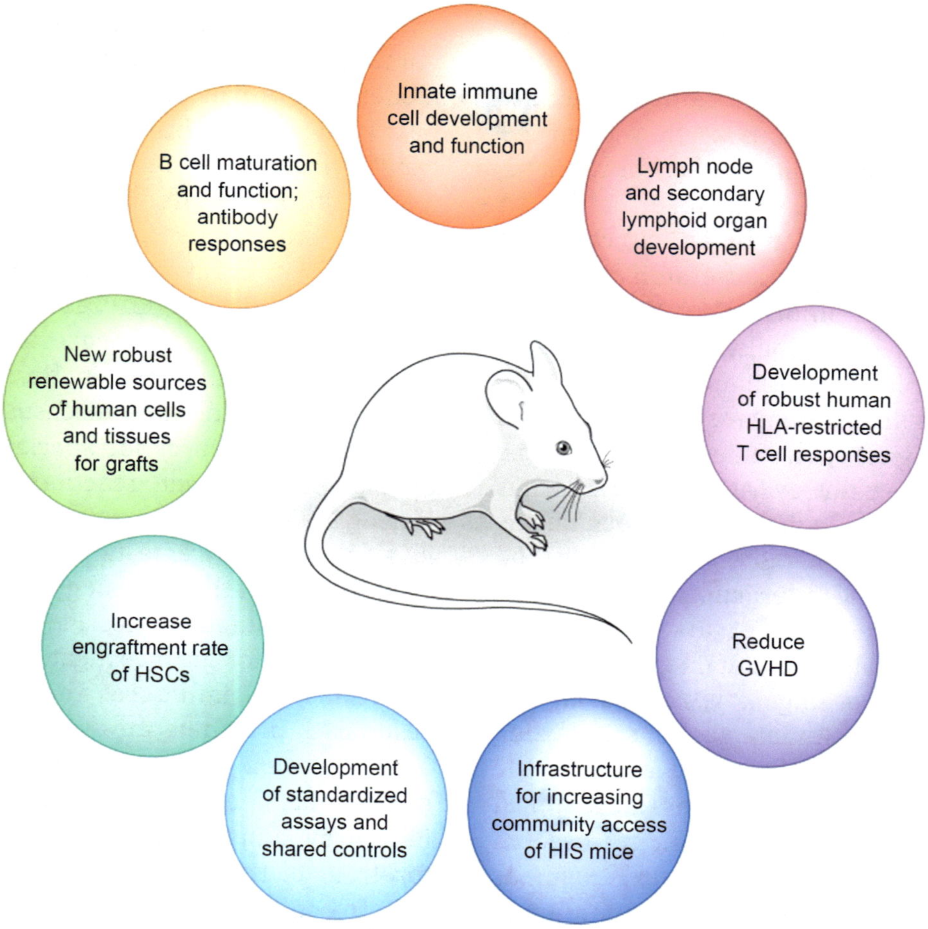

Figure 11.6. Rodent models are indispensable in the field of immunology, serving as surrogates for human biological responses due to their genetic, biological, and behavioral similarities.

Source: https://media.springernature.com/lw685/springer-static/image/art%3A10.1038%2Fs41590-019-0416-z/MediaObjects/41590_2019_416_Fig2_HTML.png.

11.2.2. Non-human Primate Models

Non-human primate models have been extremely valuable for the study of immunology as a model system that bridges basic research and clinical application. The models, particularly macaques, closely resemble human immune systems both genetically, physiologically, and immunologically. Their ability to acquire spontaneous diseases similar to those in humans makes them of greater interest in studies of infectious diseases, autoimmune diseases, and transplantation. Most importantly, xenotransplantation in non-human primates makes it possible to investigate human-specific immune reactions to grafts from gene-modified donor animals and gain information on rejection and tolerance mechanisms. Such research is at the core of optimizing the rates of organ transplant success, currently depending on human donors and can inform the development of transgenic models using new immune modulation protocols (Schmalkuche et al., 2024). Beyond their utility in transplantation studies, non-human primate models are also critical for exploring complex diseases, including type 2 diabetes (T2D).

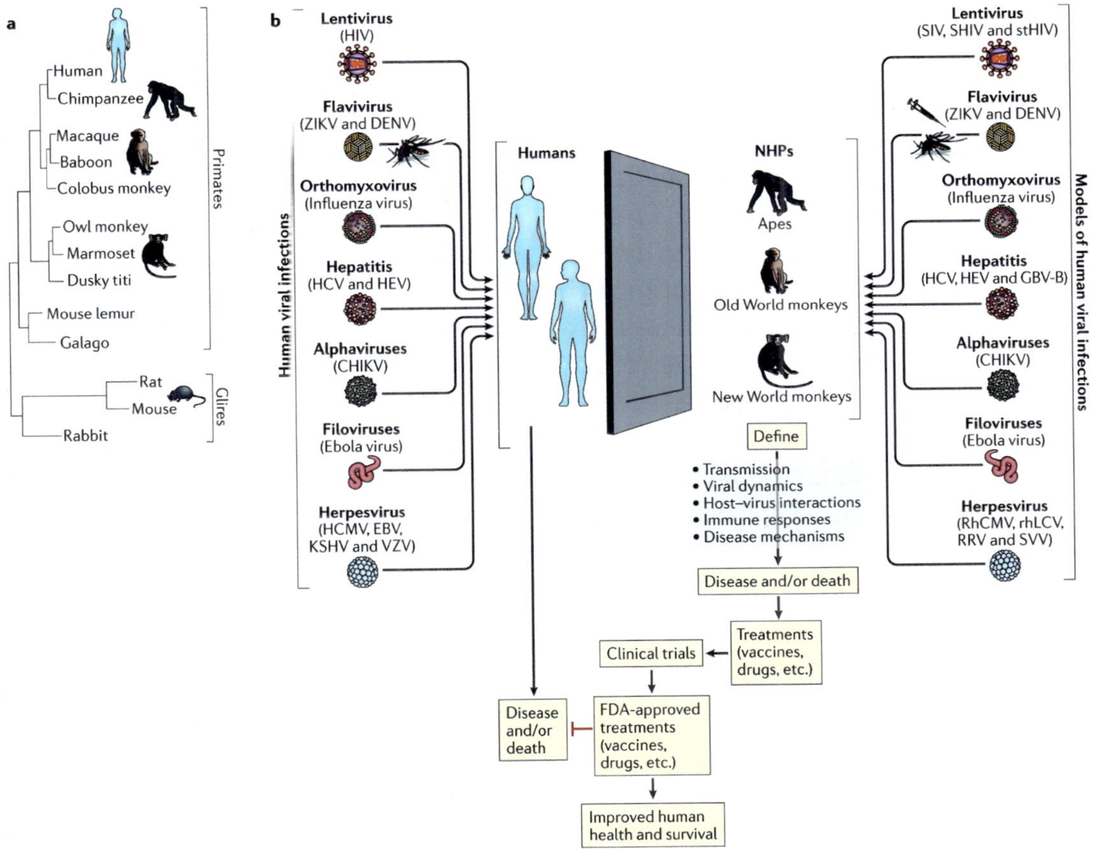

Figure 11.7. Nonhuman primate models of human viral infections.

Source: https://media.springernature.com/full/springer-static/image/art%3A10.1038%2Fs41577-018-0005-7/MediaObjects/41577_2018_5_Fig1_HTML.jpg.

Research in these primate models facilitates longitudinal examination of metabolic alterations consistent with those in humans. Of specific value, experiments with paradigms such as *in vivo* magnetic resonance spectroscopy have revealed global alterations in brain metabolism to hyperglycemia in diabetic primates. Modeling the human disease progression, these models are essential to elucidating the neurochemical profiles and cellular responses characterizing T2D.

The similarities between primate models and human conditions that are noted highlight the significance of non-human primates to the study of immunology because they enable enhanced understanding of disease mechanisms and potential therapeutic interventions (Choi et al., 2023). With the continued need for advanced immunological research protocols, the ethical concerns regarding the use of non-human primates are subject to increasing scrutiny. While these models offer significant experimental advantages, researchers must contend with a complex framework of ethical guidelines to maintain humane care and justified utilization. Sustained efforts at maximizing protocols and improving animal welfare strategy are of the greatest significance to research integrity in non-human primates. Furthermore, utilizing alternative *in vitro* systems and humanized mouse models might ultimately mitigate some of the ethical implications of primate research. But the unique immunological properties of non-human primates remain essential for applying findings to the clinic, emphasizing their continued relevance in the evolving universe of immunology research (Figure 11.7).

11.2.3. Other Species Used in Immunological Studies

Other animal models have, in recent years, become increasingly prominent in immunological research as valuable tools for the investigation of various infectious diseases. Among them, transgenic mice have contributed significantly to studying virus-host interactions. Especially, immunodeficient strains of these mice, e.g., those with human hepatocytes, offer insights into human-specific HCV infection. The traditional models, e.g., the use of chimpanzees, are limited by cost, practicality, and ethical considerations in their use for experimental infection. Thus, researchers today prefer transgenic mice that mimic the human response, thus making it simpler to interpret innate and adaptive immunity during infection with HCV. These models provide a vital stepping stone in designing therapeutic interventions and constructing prophylactic vaccines, proving their worth in advancing immunological research towards the fight against global disease challenges related to HCV (Burm et al., 2018). Zebrafish have also become a valuable model organism in immunological studies, helping particularly in aquaculture and fish disease evaluation. Aquatic conditions and optimal genetic manipulation techniques of zebrafish facilitate unprecedented *in vivo* imaging and analysis of immune responses. Immunological studies with zebrafish have shed much light on the immunological process underlying a variety of bacterial, viral, and parasitic infections in aquaculture species. Not only do these studies further the understanding of fish immunology, but they also inform prophylactic interventions into preventing disease breakouts in aquaculture production. Also, being able to generate transgenic lines of zebrafish for specific research questions further enhances their use as a model for the examination of innate and adaptive immune responses, highlighting their uses in both basic and translational immunological studies (von Jørgensen, 2020). Other than mice and zebrafish, non-human primates (NHPs) are still an essential part of immunological studies, particularly for conditions that have a strong correlation with human pathophysiology. Though ethical concerns usually limit their use, NHPs such as macaques present a sophisticated means of defining complex immune functions against pathogens like the human immunodeficiency virus (HIV). The intricate interaction between the immune system and pathogens in such models offers invaluable insights into disease development and treatment pathways. In addition, the use of such species poses concerns regarding the ethical aspect and the necessity for the development of alternative models with the ability to reproduce NHP immunity without associated ethical expense. While scientists struggle with these issues, continuous research of diverse species in immunology is essential to the advancement of knowledge and treatment in the area (Burm et al., 2018).

11.3. Applications of In Vivo Models in Immunology

In vivo models are central to enhancing our understanding of immune response, especially in comprehending the complexity of allergic responses and other immune dysfunctions. These models provide a biologically pertinent environment that cannot be replicated with *in vitro* methods alone, allowing researchers to observe the complex interaction between various types of immune cells and their microenvironment. For instance, some of the latest studies using these models have provided insight into the mechanisms of IgE-mediated food allergy. With the use of the AOP strategy, researchers can logically evaluate the sensitization potential of novel dietary proteins well before their release into the market, ensuring safety before they can be brought in. In this holistic method, it is essential to incorporate *in vivo* models in the process of risk assessment of food allergy because traditional *in vitro* methods may not detect significant adaptive immune reactions (Lozano-Ojalvo et al., 2019). Additionally, models *in vivo* are essential for the study of chronic inflammatory diseases, such as atherosclerosis, that incorporate both innate and adaptive immune mechanisms. Research has established T lymphocytes and B cells as central to the disease process, demonstrating the central importance of immune cell interaction to atherosclerosis development. With the application of *in vivo* models, researchers are able to investigate the functions of diverse immune modulators, such as the costimulatory receptors of the tumor necrosis factor receptor (TNFR) family, that play an important role in the regulation of T cell activation. Such observations can be useful for developing future therapies that would specifically target pathogenic T cells, which can eventually lead to improved treatments for patients with atherosclerosis and related conditions. Consequently, *in vivo* models are not only fundamental to unraveling disease processes but also to creating focused immunotherapies (Antunes et al., 2012). In addition, *in vivo* models are even used to extend to vaccine design, where they are also crucial to determining the safety and effectiveness of new immunizations. Preclinical studies using animal models give researchers a chance to test immunological responses, determine optimal levels of dosages, and observe potential side effects prior to conducting human trials. This is important in ensuring vaccines stimulate robust and protective immune responses and avoid adverse effects. Finally, *in vivo* models give scientists a chance to study the long-term effects of vaccination and the duration of immunity elicited. By incorporation of such models in vaccine research, scientists can maximize vaccine formulations and delivery systems, ultimately culminating in the best control of infectious disease. Essentially, *in vivo* models are an important link between basic immunological research and clinical practice, thus reaffirming the significance of *in vivo* models in immunology.

11.3.1. Vaccine Development and Testing

The design and testing of vaccines demand a delicate approach with the use of *in vivo* models to accurately recapitulate human immune responses. These models are critical in the initial phases of vaccine development so that screening of immune responses is made possible before launching into costly and time-consuming human clinical trials. With animals whose immune systems more closely mimic those of humans, scientists are able to track the efficiency of adjuvants and delivery systems in various vaccine formulations. This stage is critical as it identifies the dosage and regimen that most effectively stimulates the immune system with minimal side effects. Notably, new findings in personalized medicine, such as in the design of therapeutic cancer vaccines, demonstrate the potential for tailor-made interventions in enhancing anti-tumor immunity and consequently positioning animal models at the forefront of the new paradigm of immunotherapy in the clinic (Shemesh et al., 2020). *In vivo* models are also central to regulatory and safety evaluations of new vaccines. When scaling up from preclinical testing to human trials, these models allow the therapeutic agents not to produce unexpected adverse effects. As a case in point, humanized mouse models with human immune system components have been highly valuable in evaluating immune reactions to vaccines against some pathogens or tumors. This allows researchers to track potential site-specific immune reactions and systemic influence in a more relevant biological system. In addition, these models make it possible to study the pharmacokinetics and biodistribution of vaccine components, which are crucial in determining what is done with vaccines once they have been administered in the human body (Stripecke et al., 2020).

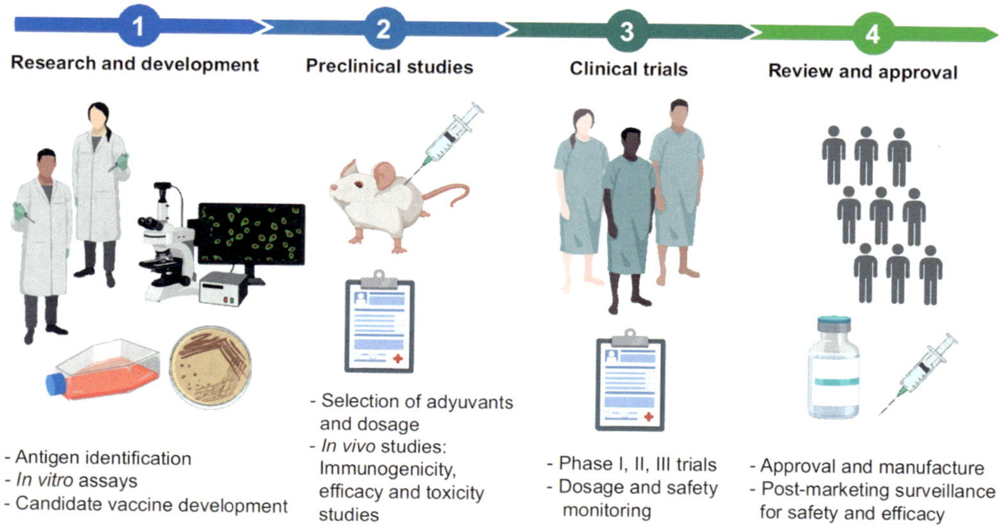

Figure 11.8. General description of the vaccine development pipeline.

Source: https://www.researchgate.net/publication/377239610/figure/fig2/AS:11431281242278900@1715427917849/General-description-of-the-vaccine-development-pipeline-The-process-of-designing.tif.

The ability to track immune responses through time using these models ultimately leads to speeding up vaccine design and regulatory procedures. Also, continued refinement in *in vivo* models keeps enhancing the predictive value of vaccine response in human trials. New technology, such as genetically modified mice, has enabled researchers to probe the unique functions of various immune cells and mechanisms involved in vaccine response. Such models can model diverse conditions in man, such as immune senescence with increasing age or comorbidities, not included in traditional vaccine trials. This not only facilitates a greater insight into the mechanisms of vaccines but also highlights the requirement of personalized vaccination strategies. In summary, the synergy of new *in vivo* models and vaccine development is crucial in creating effective and safe immunizations that, subsequently, enhance public health initiatives (Shemesh et al., 2020; Stripecke et al., 2020) (Figure 11.8).

11.3.2. Understanding Disease Mechanisms

Awareness of disease mechanisms is key to designing therapeutic principles in immunology, particularly where host immunity and pathogens meet. Models *in vivo* give valuable information on how organisms can respond to infection, injury, and autoimmunity. *In vivo* models enable researchers to trace complex interactions of biology within a live organism, hence producing vital information on the progression of disease and immune behavior. For instance, helminth infections have been found to have interesting dynamics under which these parasites are able to modulate the immune response. Their immunomodulatory products may be the basis for autoimmune disease treatments and, hence, studies on host-pathogen interactions within disease mechanisms that may offer new therapeutic avenues, as seen in the Hygiene Hypothesis in Pineda et al. (2014). In the context of neurodegenerative disease, an understanding of the mechanisms by which amyloid β-protein (Aβ42) oligomers cause cognitive impairment in Alzheimer's disease is a dramatic example of the mechanism of disease investigation. The synaptotoxic action of Aβ42 oligomers offers an understanding of cellular processes involved in neuronal dysfunction and degeneration. *In vivo* studies using transgenic mouse models have provided insight into the comparative toxicity of oligomers versus fibrils, with complex synaptic dysfunction mechanisms. Besides, the ability of macrophages to protect synapses from Aβ42 oligomers pinpoints the immune system's contribution towards neuroprotection. These are extensions of our understanding of immunological responses in the central nervous system and open up the doors for selective treatments taking advantage of the innate immune system in alleviating synaptic loss, as shown in the paper on macrophage interactions in Li et al. (2020). Ultimately, the incorporation of *in vivo* models in immunology brings forth a complicated comprehension of disease processes. These models not only describe the disease's biological mechanisms but also direct the development of new immunotherapies. Through demonstrations of immune modulation's dual roles—where it promotes protective immunity while contributing to pathology—scientists can design therapies that leverage the body's natural response without compromising overall health. The discovery of helminth-derived immunomodulators as therapeutic agents against autoimmune diseases is evidence of this delicate balance. Similarly, an understanding of the protective action of activated macrophages against neurodegenerative events provides a promising direction for future Alzheimer's therapy. Ultimately, these findings demonstrate the value of *in vivo* models in ongoing efforts to dissect the complexity of disease processes in immunology.

11.3.3. Evaluating Therapeutic Interventions

Therapeutic intervention assessment is critical in immunology as it allows the safety and efficacy of novel therapies for immune modulation to be assessed. *In vivo* models form the core of this assessment as they give information on the complex interactions that occur in biological systems. These models enable the study of the impact of therapeutic drugs upon immune cell subsets and how these, in turn, influence disease progression. Of specific interest to cancer immunotherapy is knowing how the immune infiltrate within the tumor microenvironment can determine patient outcome. In-depth characterization of such immune cells, as emphasized by recent reports, can reveal immune evasion mechanisms, directing the design of targeted therapies that maximize patient outcomes (Zhang et al., 2020). In the context of infectious diseases, particularly those caused by emergent pathogens such as SARS-CoV-2, therapeutic strategies need to be cautiously assessed for potency in preclinical models. The critical requirement during the COVID-19 pandemic accelerated the development of neutralizing antibodies (nAbs) that target distinct viral proteins. Not only their neutralization activity, but also their impact on the host immune system, in particular, for inducing unwanted effects such as antibody-dependent enhancement (ADE), should be assessed. Studies on previous coronaviruses, i.e., SARS-CoV and MERS-CoV, highlight the need for rigorous *in vivo* testing to understand the therapeutic value and safety profiles of these novel interventions (Jiang et al., 2020). Intensive testing ultimately informs clinical decisions and lays the foundation for successful and safe therapies. Moreover, the integration of state-of-the-art technologies in evaluating therapeutic interventions has significantly transformed the field of immunology research. Techniques such as single-cell RNA sequencing and mass cytometry enable a high-resolution analysis of immune cell populations after therapy. Such data granularity enables one to quantify the heterogeneity of the immune response, which is necessary in order to titrate the right therapy to a particular patient. As treatment choices increase, particularly in cancer and infectious diseases, regular evaluations of their efficacy based on models *in vivo* guarantee that interventions with maximal efficiency are discovered. By systematic analysis of how these treatments change immune cell dynamics and influence the course of disease, researchers can better plan therapeutic strategies in the future to bring the most benefit to patients with minimal risks (Zhang et al., 2020). The critical assessment of these interventions will definitely open the way for new approaches that optimize clinical results in immunology (Figure 11.9).

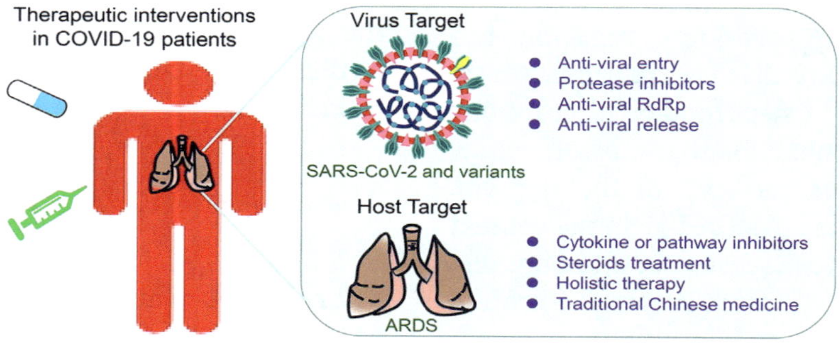

Figure 11.9. Therapeutic interventions in COVID-19 patients.

Source: https://ars.els-cdn.com/content/image/1-s2.0-S2001037022000344-ga1.jpg.

11.4. Ethical Considerations in Using In Vivo Models

The ethical concerns in the use of *in vivo* models in immunology cannot be overemphasized, particularly given the fact that the use of these models contributes immensely to expanding the knowledge of complex immunological events. Such concerns extend beyond mere regulatory compliance and entail a fundamental responsibility for humane treatment of animal subjects. A philosophy of the 3Rs—Replacement, Reduction, and Refinement—is one of guiding philosophy. Replacement encourages the exploitation of alternative models to animal models where available, reduction advocates for minimizing the number of animals used in studies, and refinement seeks to enhance the welfare of animals and reduce pain and distress. In this case, scientists must constantly check for the necessity of *in vivo* studies and come up with new technologies that would minimize animal use without compromising scientific research quality. Empirical research tends to require models from animals to investigate intricate immune responses as well as disease processes, and therefore, these investigations must be carried out ethically. For instance, studies grounded on *Plasmodium knowlesi* infections in macaques provide important data on malaria antigenic variation and raise the potential benefits of *in vivo* studies in humane settings. However, scientists must also consider the welfare of animal subjects, determining whether experimental goals are compatible with animal well-being. Ethical models require rigorous approval processes, including institutional review board evaluations and adherence to tight standards for animal welfare, to ensure that the worth of research is greater than the ethical cost of animal testing. In addition, ongoing controversy regarding the ethical importance of *in vivo* models demonstrates the public's growing concern over animal research. While scientists aim for a breakthrough in immunology, ethical accountability and transparency are most important. The guarantee of adherence to shared values is necessary in order to maintain public trust and sustained support. Such central revelations as regarding the efficacy of various anthelminthic medicines that have been tested by rigorous trials are an example of how ethical issues are employed in the verification of research. To this effect, taking up ethical processes not only enhances the scientific integrity of research but also promotes advocacy for continued enhancement in practices to ensure the welfare of the animal subjects is a top concern alongside scientific advancement (Belew et al., 2015; Galinski et al., 2018).

11.4.1. Animal Welfare Regulations

The interaction between legislation on animal welfare and the use of *in vivo* models in immunology is complex and integral to ethical practice in research. Regulatory frameworks are established to determine humane treatment of animals during scientific research, particularly where research is conducted on expected pain, distress, or damage. *In vivo* models are important in immunological response research as well as for the assessment of vaccine efficacy, yet scientists have to contend with rigorous legal and ethical demands. Complying with animal welfare legislation not only guarantees excellent care for the animals but also enhances the validity and replicability of research findings. Research must adhere to guidelines by various regulatory bodies, which manage parameters such as housing, transportation, and reducing stressors (Younis et al., 2018). Moreover, the efficacy of vaccination regimens also largely relies on the quality of preclinical assessment in animal models. Adhering to established animal welfare regulations can allow scientists to reduce parameters that can interfere with findings. For instance, the immunogenicity of vaccine formulations can be assessed through measurement of specific immune responses, including the stimulation of cytokine production and antibody titers in various animal models (Earley et al., 2007). Such testing is important because it informs the final application of human vaccines. Researchers should hence ensure that their procedures are not only scientifically justified but also ethically justified, fostering public trust and acceptance of immunological investigations. Also, the ethical implications of such research dictate the constant refinement of welfare policies to keep up with the advancements in immunological science. With the continued advancement of immunological science, emphasis is increasingly given to the development of new alternative *in vivo* models that reduce the use of traditional animal testing while remaining in compliance with animal welfare law. Technologies such as advanced cell culture techniques and computer simulations have been created, which may replace or complement animal tests in certain cases. These fall within the goals of the 3Rs—Replacement, Reduction, and Refinement—at the center of animal welfare law (Earley et al., 2007). By integrating these innovative approaches, researchers can contribute to more humane practices for immunological research that could revolutionize our understanding of immune responses without compromising the welfare of animals. This step, beyond simple ethical concerns, enhances the effectiveness and accuracy of immunological research and has researchers poised to uncover new frontiers while keeping their commitment to humane treatment of research animals (Figure 11.10).

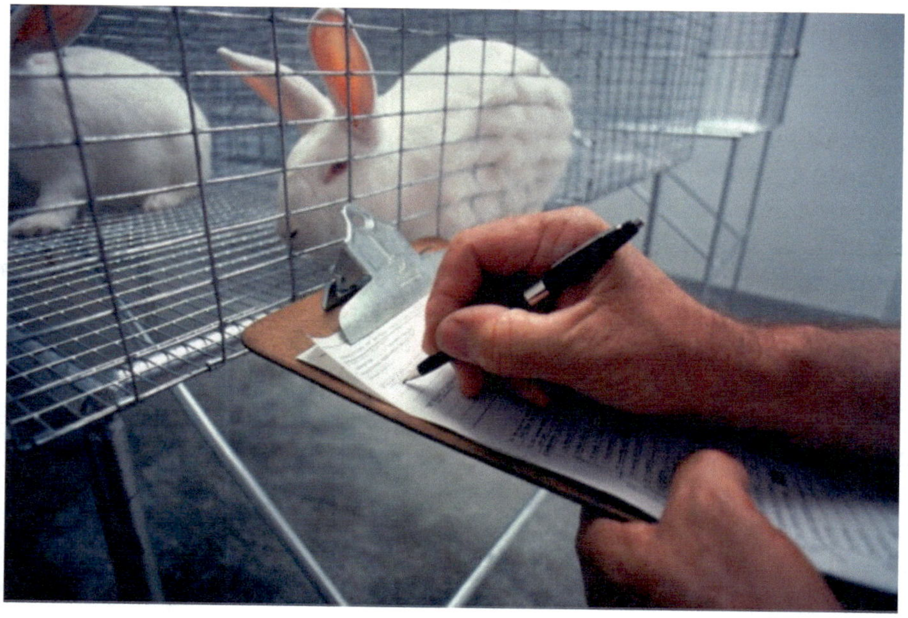

Figure 11.10. The use of animals in laboratories remains controversial. Animal welfare advocates push for enforced standards to ensure the health and safety of those animals used for tests.

Source: https://upload.wikimedia.org/wikipedia/commons/b/b7/Lab_animal_care.jpg.

11.4.2. Alternatives to Animal Testing

Increased demands for ethical research approaches have spearheaded the pursuit of alternatives to traditional animal testing, particularly in immunology. Animal models have been used centrally in understanding immune responses and disease mechanisms; yet, ethical limitations and rising costs necessitate the introduction of novel approaches. Emerging technologies, like *in vitro* cell culture and computer simulation, are becoming increasingly popular, as they give researchers the chance to investigate immunological processes without employing animal models. These alternatives not only reflect the tenets of the 3Rs—Replacement, Reduction, and Refinement—but also promise to yield valid data that can inform therapeutic interventions. The worth of creating these alternatives is their ability to provide information regarding immune function and disease onset at the expense of ethical breaches in research procedures. One such alternative is the employment of stimulated co-cultures in the assessment of cytokine profiles. Traditional procedures tend to use animal models to track immune responses in real-time, but the process tends to cause undue stress and suffering to the animals. Recent advancements have identified that if T cells, splenocytes, and fibroblast-like synoviocytes are cultured together, it is possible to obtain useful data on cytokine production without sacrificing animals. This method was recently validated using multicolor panel optimization and provided a sophisticated environment to mimic complex immune interactions. Such developments have rendered the option of generating similar, if not superior, data with a near elimination of the ethical concerns of animal testing possible, hence opening the door for further research into immunological diseases employing cutting-edge *in vitro* models (Aleith et al., 2025). Furthermore, research on biocompatible materials for medical applications introduces yet another dimension of alternative testing. For instance, polymeric heart valves (PHVs) have been under heavy research and have been found to possess potential for substituting conventional mechanical and bioprosthetic valves. The material characteristics of materials such as poly(styrene-block-ethylene/butylene-block-styrene) (SEBS) reflect the advancements in material science that are entangled with immunological research. Tests have shown these materials possess positive characteristics, including durability and minimal adverse immune reactions, which are essential while using novel biomaterials in human health. *In vivo* testing, although necessary to validate function, can be enhanced by such developments, with focus given to reconciling materials science with immune testing. As scientists continue to work on developing these alternative approaches, they can seek to innovate while addressing ethics issues in immunology (Wang et al., 2025) (Figure 11.11).

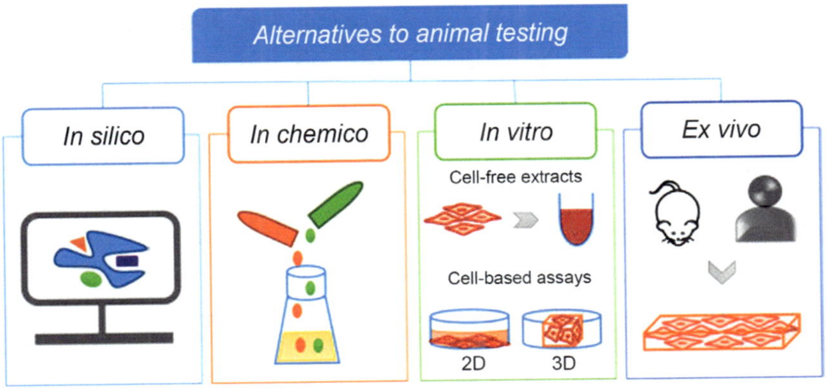

Figure 11.11. Exploration of alternatives to traditional animal testing.

Source: https://ars.els-cdn.com/content/image/3-s2.0-B9780128239667000013-f20-01-9780128239667.jpg.

11.4.3. Ethical Implications of Research Findings

Ethical concerns are given utmost consideration when evaluating the results of research, especially those derived from *in vivo* models of immunology. These models, when they often involve using animals as objects of experiments, pose high hurdles towards animal welfare and rationale behind such experimentation. Researchers are required to work within a multi-level institution of ethical standards that regulate humane handling of animals and balance the needs of scientific advancement. For instance, the data collected by *in vivo* studies can potentially be utilized to overturn our understanding of immune reactions and the discovery of new drugs. The moral implications of risking animal life for human benefit, nonetheless, lead scientists to challenge their actions and whether or not they are needed. Thus, ethical concern becomes an essential part of the research process that initiates continuous debate on the acceptability of methods used in immunological studies. In the example of recent findings on the roles of tumor-associated macrophages (TAMs) in the prostate cancer tumor microenvironment, ethical issues extend beyond animal welfare to societal values. With researchers showing us targets such as TREM2 to be potential targets for therapeutic intervention, the public responsibility for ensuring that such information is used ethically becomes apparent. The intersection of biomedical advancement and clinical translation generates challenges to access to care as well as vulnerability of vulnerable populations to exploitation. It is up to the scientific community to ensure that research translates to equitable healthcare practice. As per the latest definition in research, more emphasis is placed on integrating ethics education into research endeavors to ensure awareness of the social implications of scientific advancement, which also places emphasis on the importance of ethical considerations in immunological studies (Choi et al., 2024). Additionally, the evolving environment of ethical norms in biomedical studies necessitates continued reflection on the meanings of research findings. As developing procedures for ethical oversight emerge, researchers are invited to consider ethical issues not merely within the research endeavor but also within the sharing and utilization of their results. The focus on ethical concerns is shared with the idea that research must ultimately be for the public good, bringing scientific inquiry into conformance with ethical standards. This alignment is particularly pertinent in the backdrop of the way discoveries in *in vivo* models inform treatment modalities and public health policy. By being cognizant of the ethical dimensions involved in their endeavor, researchers establish an environment where innovation accompanies accountable stewardship of information such that advances in immunology serve both scientific inquiry and the common good (Villa-Pulgarín et al., 2024). Thus, the ethical consequences of research findings should always be a primary focus of scientific research in immunology.

11.5. Limitations of *In Vivo* Models

The excessive dependency on *in vivo* models in immunology has crucial drawbacks that can hinder the translation of findings to human applications. A significant drawback is biological variability in living organisms and the resulting erratic findings when findings are being compared between studies. Genetic background, setting, and underlying health status are some of the variables likely to impact immune functions in animal models. As an example, strain-specific differences in immuneresponses can shape interpretation of therapeutic effect, potentially casting doubt on the potential relevance of observations to the human clinical context. Such inconsistencies are a cause for concern regarding experiment design and data interpretation because they could impact the perceived efficacy of candidate immunotherapeutic strategies. A second major limitation comes from ethical considerations for animal testing. The modern ethical climate increasingly disfavors the use of animals in tests, particularly when there may be potential *in vitro* alternatives that would provide comparable insight into immune function without killing live animals. As scientific communities strive to achieve ethical requirements, researchers are invited to minimize the use of *in vivo* models. This shift to other methods also raises the issue of consistency and integrity of information. While *in vivo* responses can generate new information about systemic interactions, the dilemma is how to maintain ethical standards versus the need for important scientific advances as precise as possible in representing human immunological responses. Also, the limitations of presently available *in vivo* models often prevent scientists from completely at the intricacy of complex human diseases. For example, certain immune mechanisms and disease processes are uniquely human and cannot be accurately represented by existing animal models. Other problems may arise as a result of extrapolation from small animal experiments to humans, as illustrated in therapeutic oligonucleotide experiments. Although progress such as the use of extracellular vesicle (EV)-based delivery platforms holds a lot of promise for targeted therapy, their effectiveness in animal models can prove not to hold when applied to human subjects with variations in physiology and with varying immune responses (Jo et al., 2025). Further, early detection of disease progression using serum biomarkers is also difficult, as has been observed in lung injury models and imaging techniques (Boswinkel et al., 2023). Thus, the restriction of *in vivo* models necessitates continuous evolution of complementary experimental approaches in order to ensure that findings are relevant and translatable to human health.

11.5.1. Differences Between Species

It is of the utmost significance in immunology to identify species differences to be able to choose appropriate *in vivo* models for study. Various species possess varied immune system characteristics that can greatly influence disease development and treatment response. For instance, the adaptive immune response of humans differs notably from that of mice due to variation in cytokine concentrations and receptor expression. These variations must be accommodated when findings from animal models are translated to the human condition. Variation in genes across species is also the basis of variation in disease susceptibility and drug metabolism, as it mirrors the requirement of personalized approaches in experimental designs with heterogeneous *in vivo* models. The relevance of such models resonates in submissions that eventually seek to develop effective therapeutic interventions, pointing to the relevance of species-specific differences in immunology studies. Specific animal models, particularly non-human primates and rodents, have also been indispensable in comprehending the complexities of immune responses. Non-human primates, such as chimpanzees, have played the most crucial roles in virus-host interaction research, particularly in the case of the HCV (Burm et al., 2018). While their potential for mimicking human immune responses cannot be eclipsed, ethical and practical concerns have pushed researchers to seek alternatives. Rodent models, including transgenic and immunodeficient mice, are decent candidates, though these have shortcomings of not exactly duplicating human immune physiology.

These differences necessitate being cautious when interpreting the results of such models, especially considering that researchers are evaluating new antiviral approaches, prophylactic vaccines, and immune-targeted treatments in order to combat infectious disease. Greater access to sophisticated methodological methodologies, such as real-time monitoring technology, also enables researchers to investigate species variation in immunology with greater precision. Developments like bioluminescence imaging, as demonstrated through pulmonary fibrosis studies, enable non-invasive *in vivo* monitoring of the disease process and gaining a better understanding of the response of different species to therapies over time (Stellari et al., 2017). These strategies highlight the potential for cross-species result translation, allowing for therapeutic strategy formulation and testing. Nonetheless, differences in underlying physiology and immunology represent a limitation that must be overcome by investigators. Utilization of such advanced techniques for comparative studies fosters a greater overall understanding of immunological phenomena and directly affects therapeutic effectiveness as well as influences future research priorities across species boundaries.

11.5.2. Complexity of Immune Responses

The complexity of immunological responses is a result of the intricate interaction between innate and adaptive immune systems, both of which are essential when responding to pathogens. Innate immune response is an immediate first line of defense that consists of various cell types, such as macrophages, dendritic cells, and natural killer cells, that recognize and kill intruders. However, this initial response is typically nondiscriminatory in nature, thus giving rise to the need for the adaptive immune system, one that is antigen specific.

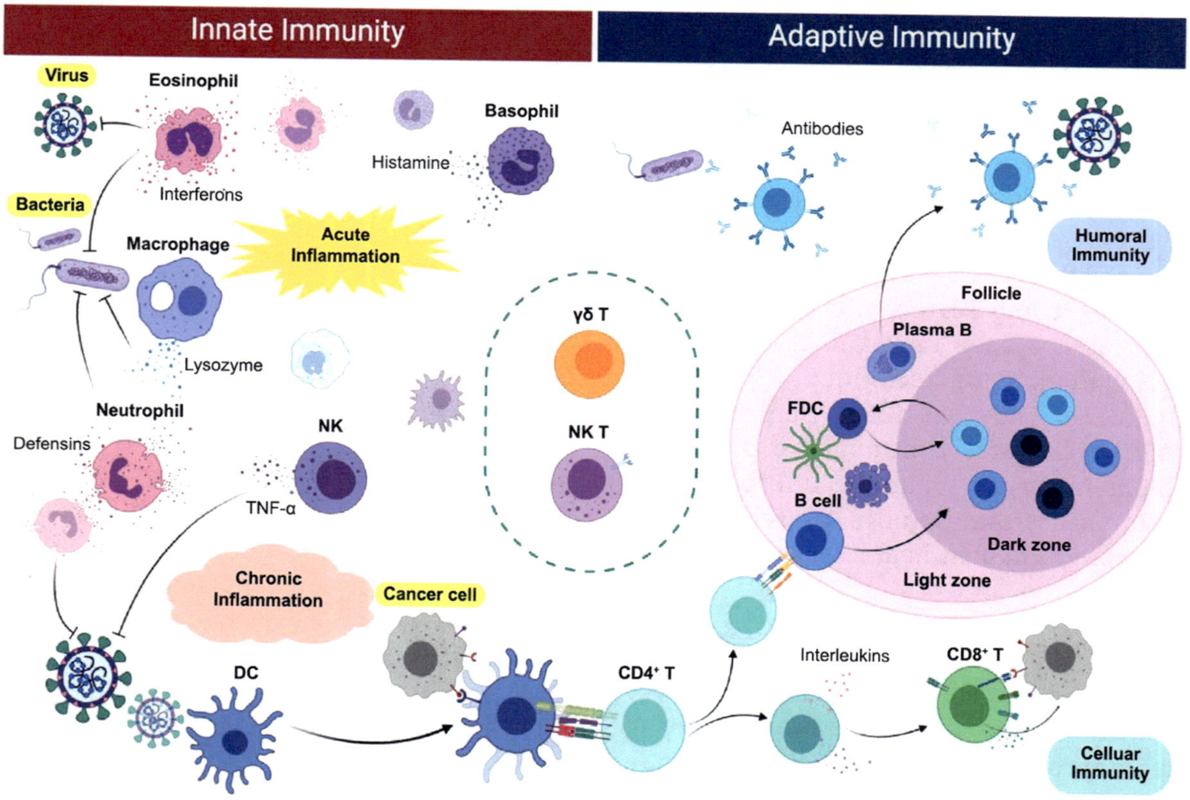

Figure 11.12. Schematic of the complex network of the host immune system, comprising innate and adaptive immunity, to recognize and target non-self-pathogens, including viruses, bacteria, and cancer cells.

Source: https://www.researchgate.net/publication/343898081/figure/fig2/AS:1143128117335 1846@1688825946546/Schematic-of-the-complex-network-of-host-immune-system-comprising-innate-and-adaptive.png.

This complexity is also accentuated by the need for precise signaling pathways, the T and B cell differentiation being influenced by the cytokine environment as well as the nature of the antigenic stimulus. Understanding this multicomponent interaction between immune factors is pivotal to developing effective immunotherapies and vaccines, particularly *in vivo* models that reflect the complexity of human immune responses within a significant biological context. Research on the complexity of immune responses demands robust *in vivo* models that can simulate human physiology and immune responses to a considerable degree. One such direction is the use of large animal models, such as pigs, whose immune systems are closer to those of humans compared to other rodent-based models. Recent studies using pigs identified specific markers, such as CD154, to help explain antigen-reactive T cell behavior. This approach enhances the understanding of how these cells respond to pathogens and can completely revolutionize knowledge on host-pathogen interactions. These models facilitate a more detailed exploration of T cell responses, including the dynamics of immune regulation and activation that might be challenging to model in lower organisms. The application of large animal models thus provides an opportunity to augment the translational value of immunological research. Besides, the theoretical AOP framework is central to comprehending intricate pathways mediating immune responses, especially in food allergens. Through integration with *in vitro* and *ex vivo* strategies, this framework can assist in categorically assessing the sensitizing ability of different food proteins before going to market. By structuring existing test protocols against specific key events in the AOP, researchers can identify holes in the current evaluation strategy and pave the way for more effective and safer sources of protein. Such integrative approaches, if implemented, not only speed up the risk assessment but can also decrease reliance on traditional animal tests. This development is important in deriving an informed understanding of immune complexity, finally resulting in more secure diet choices and therapeutics in immunology, as emphasized in current research efforts (Ebner et al., 2017; Lozano-Ojalvo et al., 2019) (Figure 11.12).

11.5.3. Challenges in Data Interpretation

Data interpretation for gene expression data using *in vivo* models of immunology is bedeviled by several issues that can make a considerable difference to the validity and utility of research findings. One of the problems is the complexity of biological systems that respond in different ways, commonly multifactorially, to experimental manipulations. This makes it challenging to differentiate discrete mechanistic pathways that are accountable for the effects obtained. For instance, the dynamics of interaction between the tumor cells and immune components can introduce variability in immune responses that are difficult to discern. These complexities necessitate that researchers adopt robust analytical paradigms that can support variability in biological responses, so that inferences made from the data are not artifacts of the experimental model itself. In addition, the use of genetically engineered organisms in immunological studies, and more so those that utilize CRISPR technologies, introduces additional nuances in the interpretation of data. While CRISPR *in vivo* screens have been very promising to unveil tumor-immune interactions and uncover therapeutic targets, concerns arise from the immunogenicity of CRISPR reagents themselves. Off-target risk and undesirable immune responses need meticulous experimental planning and rigorous post-hoc analysis of the resulting data. For example, findings in syngeneic models where CRISPR platforms are differentially immunogenic have the potential to skew the interpretation of the data and thereby create inaccurate conclusions regarding the efficacy of novel immunotherapeutic treatments (He et al., 2024). Thus, scientists need to make careful choices regarding the implications of their model choice according to the interpretation of results. Lastly, data from numerous sources, including *in vitro* experiments and computational models, make data interpretation even more difficult in immunology studies. The quest to predict drug-induced liver injury (DILI), for instance, requires the development of sound computational models that can effectively draw data from various studies. The DILIPredictor model is one such strategy that combines structural features along with *in vitro* and *in vivo* data to enhance the predictive accuracy (Seal et al., 2024). Difficulty, however, can be faced in preserving the fidelity and utility of the model output across different biological contexts. Animal models to human response variations produce confusion in data interpretation, and rigorous validation and cross-species comparisons are necessary to achieve meaningful insights in immunology studies.

11.6. Future Directions in *In Vivo* Immunology Research

The future of *in vivo* immunology studies is poised to take revolutionary steps forward with the pace of advances in artificial intelligence (AI) and machine learning (ML). Blending these technologies with research techniques allows for improved analysis and interpretation of complex biological data. For example, using ML models to distinguish between pediatric lung sounds has been found with high accuracy, which also has the potential for non-invasive immunology diagnosis. While these technologies become increasingly entrenched in biomedical research, they may have the potential to allow for the detection of targeted immune responses in various disease states, thereby enlarging our understanding of immunological processes. Standardization of techniques in this area of research should be noted, though, so that data from multiple sources could be harmonized and validated across laboratories, thus enhancing the validity of research findings in immunology. Future *in vivo* models must also consider environmental and genetic determinants influencing immune responses. Recent advances in genomics and epigenomics allow researchers to examine the interactions of host genetics and microbial exposure, which are crucial to ascertaining immune system function. With the integration of classical and novel *in vivo* models, scientists can realize the intricacy of immune responses under various conditions. For instance, the integration of genetic engineering techniques with existing animal models provides informative insights into the roles of some genes in mediating immunity. Furthermore, microbiome effects studied using *in vivo* approaches can reveal opportunities for therapeutic modulation of host immunity to avert allergic reactions or autoimmune disorders. Continuing this research may lead to an ever-more individualized approach to immunotherapy founded on individual genetic profiles and environmental exposure. The study of *in vivo* models is not limited to basic research alone; it also has significant impacts on therapeutic development and clinical use. The future holds promise in terms of the application of large-scale multicenter clinical trials that employ *in vivo* modeling with the purpose of verifying potential immunotherapies more reliably. Such experiments can also utilize advanced monitoring technologies, such as telehealth platforms or wearable sensors, to collect real-time data on immune responses in different populations across different settings. Using the predictive abilities of AI, these strategies can streamline drug discovery by quickly identifying effective treatment regimens for individual patient profiles. In addition, by addressing the challenges of dataset heterogeneity and comprehensive validation that have been brought to light by more recent works, researchers can play a pivotal role in bringing transformative immunotherapies into mainstream practice, advancing the science of immunology into more effective, patient-centered solutions.

11.6.1. Advances in Genetic Engineering

Genetic engineering science has advanced far from where it was, particularly when wielded as a tool for the science of immunology with *in vivo* models. Perhaps the most exciting development is the production of genetically engineered T-cells in the form of chimeric antigen receptor (CAR) T-cells. These are designed to recognize malignancies such as gliomas, previously fiendishly difficult due to their infiltrative growth pattern and the anatomy of the brain. The specificity of CAR T-cells for recognizing and eliminating tumor cells provides a new therapeutic option, potentially with the ability to alter patient outcomes. However, several challenges remain in applying these therapies, particularly T-cell homing to the brain and glioma's immunosuppressive microenvironment. Research and clinical trials are necessary to overcome such challenges and maximize treatment effectiveness (Chuntova et al., 2018).

Meanwhile, the combination of genetic engineering with *in vivo* models has triggered further innovation in the clarification of immune reactions towards allergens, including food proteins. The AOP approach is a technique that has come into application as a method to assess the sensitization potential of new dietary proteins. By structuring existing *in vitro* methods according to AOP, researchers can improve the comprehension of the most essential molecular and cellular pathways that play roles in IgE-mediated food allergic disorders. This approach allows for a better evaluation of proteins before they enter the market and, as a consequence, the likelihood of fewer allergic responses in consumers. Genetic alteration to modify allergenic proteins or increase immune reactivity by employing engineered therapies can lead to more effective interventions in treating food allergy (Lozano-Ojalvo et al., 2019). Furthermore, as genetic engineering advances, its impact on *in vivo* immunology research is very significant. It is now possible for scientists to engineer not only cellular response but also to manipulate whole organisms for the purpose of studying complex immune interactions.

Fine-tuning models of animals, which have been engineered to have human-specific genes, enhances the ability to foresee human immune responses. This is very much emphasized in the ethical standards of researching with animals, aiming to minimize pain and increase awareness of human-relevant immune processes as much as possible. The use of sophisticated *in vivo* models enables researchers to study immuneresponses in the context of a background, making more accurate and refined treatments. With such developments, the future of genetic engineering has the potential to revolutionize therapeutic modalities in immunology (Chuntova et al., 2018; Lozano-Ojalvo et al., 2019) (Figure 11.13).

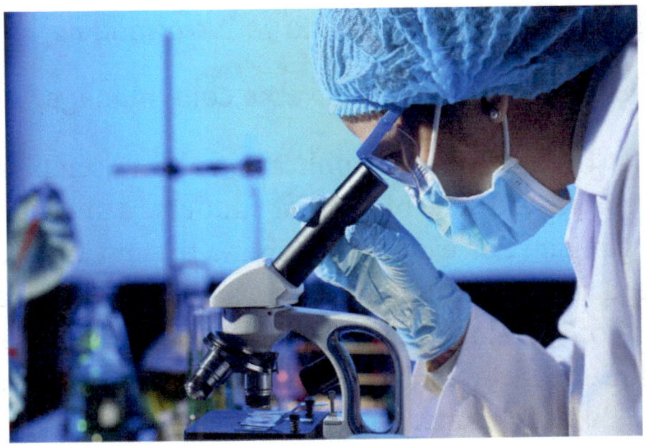

Figure 11.13. Examining a sample with a microscope.

Source: https://leanership.org/wp-content/uploads/sites/10/2024/07/examining-sample-with-microscope.jpg.

11.6.2. Integration of In Vitro And In Vivo Approaches

The integration of *in vitro* and *in vivo* approaches is a revolutionary method in immunological studies, offering a comprehensive view of immune responses during health and disease. *In vitro* experiments enable manipulation of cellular milieus under controlled conditions, which enable scientists to isolate molecular interactions and elucidate mechanisms of immune function. By using various types of cells—T cells, B cells, and dendritic cells—scientists can examine specific areas of immune system behavior, thus developing elementary insights that direct future *in vivo* studies. However, extrapolation of the findings from these results to the whole organism is fraught with challenges, as cellular-level responses in a laboratory setting are bound to be starkly different from cellular responses within a higher-order biological system. Thus, the use of combined *in vitro* models and *in vivo* research enhances the predictive validity of study outcomes by bridging the gap between cellular mechanisms and systemic physiological responses. It is within the area of immunology that it cannot be overstressed that *in vitro* and *in vivo* methodologies need to be amalgamated, particularly in therapeutic strategy.

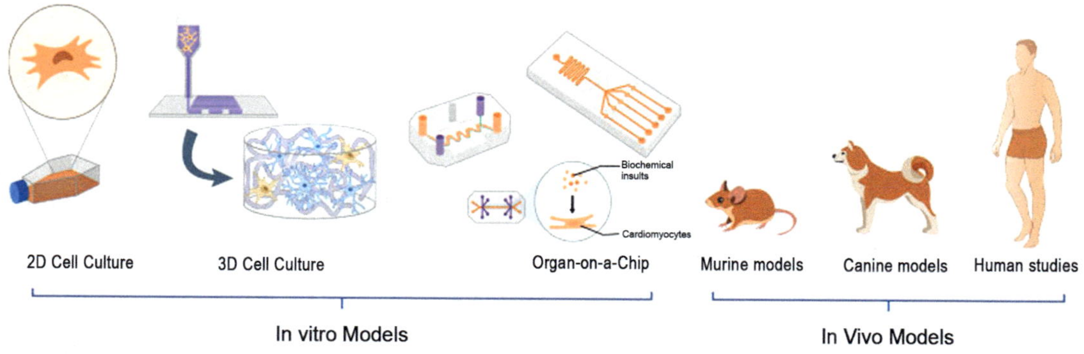

Figure 11.14. *In vivo* and *in vitro* models.

Source: https://www.cusabio.com/manage/upload/202403/In-vivo-and-in-vitro-models.jpg.

Their combined application allows scientists to try out hypotheses based on *in vitro* experiments through the use of animal models, a mimicry of the intricate interactions occurring in a living organism. For example, systems biology applied to vaccine development has been beneficial in this regard. As has been noted at the Global HIV Vaccine Enterprise workshop, new methods that make use of systems biology have the potential to provide insights into the dynamism and intricacies of immune systems beyond that which can be achieved through *in vitro* science alone (Pulendran et al., 2010). Further, *in vivo* models allow for the examination of immune response in its physiological environment, communicating the multifactorial character of immune challenge in a way that can direct more effective vaccine development and therapeutic intervention. The marriage of *in vitro* and *in vivo* work not only strengthens an understanding of immunological phenomena but also avoids practical problems in drug development and evaluation. Regulatory authorities favor increasingly preclinical models most closely mimicking human physiology, and this necessitates an effective synergy of different experimental strategies. It is particularly important in evaluating the safety and effectiveness of new immunotherapeutics before clinical trials. Discussions during the Global HIV Vaccine Enterprise workshop highlighted the imperative for interdisciplinary teamwork to meet challenges in emerging sciences in vaccine development and advance immunological knowledge (Pulendran et al., 2010). Through synergizing *in vitro* data with *in vivo* data, scientists can improve predictive models and develop more effective strategies for the war against infectious diseases and the harnessing of immune responses for therapeutic gain, setting the stage for new developments in personalized medicine and immunotherapy (Figure 11.14).

11.6.3. Potential for Personalized Medicine

Personalized medicine has received much attention in the recent past, especially under the umbrella of immunology. The addition of *in vivo* models allows researchers to quantify individual patient reactions to various treatments more precisely. This is important since traditional one-size-fits-all treatment protocols are increasingly recognized as not adequate to handle the complexity of human diseases, like cancer and autoimmune disease. Personalized medicine aims to tailor therapies based on the unique genetic, environmental, and lifestyle factors of each patient, which is exemplified in immunotherapy advances. By the employment of *in vivo* models, scientists can more accurately mimic human physiological responses, hence making better predictions of therapies and outcomes. This shift toward personalization has the promise of not only better therapies but also fewer side effects, ultimately resulting in more effective healthcare. Despite the apparent breakthroughs, the route to fully realized personalized medicine is fraught with challenges. One significant drawback is the reliance on a small number of preclinical models that may not reflect the intertumor heterogeneity or intratumor diversity among patients. Such limitations restrict the optimisation of therapeutic probes necessary for effective treatment. Innovators thus need to develop several probes derived from diverse molecular pathways, possibly mimicking those employed in molecular pathology. Such an approach would enhance our understanding of disease mechanisms and improve the translational aspects of personalized medicine. Second, the inclusion of ultrahigh-resolution imaging technology offers more finely detailed data capture so key biological differences are not overlooked. Overcoming these challenges is vital to translating the promise of personalized medicine into actual clinical use in immunology. Economic issues and regulatory barriers are the major impetus driving the development of personalized approaches in medicine as well. With advancing advancement, understanding the advanced balance between cost-effectiveness reduction of manufacturing and the promising revenue generated through innovative therapies becomes increasingly important. Developments like fluorescent labeling of commercial antibodies and early-phase microdosing with small molecules indicate that viable methods are being searched for to integrate personalized methodologies into mainstream medicine. But the necessity of robust systems that can react to emerging technologies without trading off patient safety cannot be stressed too much. Mentioned in visions for the future of laboratory medicine, the incessant rate of emerging technologies and techniques will shape the future of personalized medicine (Kricka et al., 2015). The recognition of such challenges despite tapping into the potential of useful tools like *in vivo* models is a way forward for developing the practice of personalized medicine in immunology (Pogue et al., 2018).

SUMMARY

The use of *in vivo* models in immunology has delivered essential knowledge required for the progression of therapeutic approaches against a number of diseases. These models have, by nature, allowed for the understanding of immune function and disease pathogenesis, such as autoimmune disease and viral infection. With improving science, reliance on these *in vivo* experiments underscores their pivotal role in overcoming basic to clinical translation. An example is given, for example, with research into regulatory T cells (Tregs), where new strategies for their expansion have been investigated to optimize their therapeutic potential. These *in vivo* experiments are essential in probing the treatment avenues for diseases such as autoimmune disorders and graft-versus-host disease because they constituted the foundational knowledge that propels the quest for effective interventions in the clinic (Earle et al., 2005). Additionally, there remain very significant challenges in the discipline, particularly with respect to the need for more ethical and effective models. Historically employed animal models, for example, the chimpanzees, have been integral to studies of viral infection, including that of the HCV. Ethical and pragmatic constraints have necessitated an investigation into alternative models. The development of transgenic and humanized mice has emerged as a viable option since it fulfills the requirement of being relevant while reducing the ethical concerns associated with employing more traditional methods. With their use, researchers can efficiently investigate virus-host interactions and immune responses, which are crucial to vaccine development and antiviral therapies (Burm et al., 2018). The advancement proves the necessity for a balance between scientific excellence and ethical standards in biomedical research. The future of *in vivo* models in immunology hinges on the progression towards more advanced, ethically justifiable alternatives that ensure the advancement of immunological investigation. Continued innovation in new models that can mimic human physiological responses will be necessary. These developments not only will further the study of complicated immune reactions, but they will also heighten results validity that can be applied to clinical use. The unrelenting progress of these models is a point of intersection between ethical considerations and scientific progress that offers the promise of a better understanding of diseases and treatments. This commitment to the development of the scientific environment underpins the crucial importance of *in vivo* models to surmount current and future challenges in the field of immunology (Earle et al., 2005; Burm et al., 2018).

From a review of *in vivo* models within immunology, there are numerous bedrock points that attest to the importance of these systems to define immune reactions. First of all, the ability to build such models facilitates their evaluation of complex interactions between heterogeneous immune cells, as well as their response to pathogens or therapies. As shown by evidence, *in vivo* strategies allow researchers to investigate immune modulation processes and thus discover and maximize vaccine candidates. This is particularly relevant for such diseases as HIV, where the rational design of vaccine components takes a central position to trigger robust immune responses. The conclusions drawn after the discourses by the Global HIV Vaccine Enterprise Working Group on the subject of vaccine components and antigen processing are a classic demonstration of the efficacy of *in vivo* models to elicit the dynamics of good immunological responses (Mascola et al., 2010). Moreover, the role of specific receptors and their intracellular signaling mechanisms within *in vivo* contexts cannot be overstressed. To illustrate, recent findings have highlighted the role of CXCR2, an important mediator of neutrophil recruitment to sites of inflammation. Regulation of this pathway within *in vivo* models illustrates how inflammatory responses are controlled by

CXCR2, either enhancing or inhibiting recruitment of a range of leukocyte populations. Through a series of experiments using CXCR2-knockout mice, researchers observed counterintuitive outcomes demonstrating an exaggerated inflammatory response due to reduced expression of resolution-related cytokines (Dyer et al., 2017). These findings underscore the value of *in vivo* models in unraveling the complexities of inflammatory signaling and cell-cell interaction and thereby enabling the therapeutic targeting of immunology studies. Finally, consolidating findings from many *in vivo* experiments provides a general overview that guides further work toward the development of therapeutic and vaccine interventions. Such models are necessary platforms for not only examining immune processes but also for the translation of laboratory findings into medical applications. The findings obtained in immunology with *in vivo* research underscore the importance of understanding the intricate dynamics at play, particularly in chronic inflammation and cancer. With scientists employing these models increasingly, they will discover novel paradigms in disease mechanisms and immune regulation and make future therapies and vaccine constructs more effective against a wide array of immunological challenges (Mascola et al., 2010; Dyer et al., 2017).

A CLOSER LOOK

PATIENT-DERIVED XENOGRAFT (PDX) MODELS

PDX models are a pre-clinical model in which tumor tissue derived from human patients is transplanted to immunocompromised mice. PDX models are used for the study of cancer biology, evaluation of new drugs, and the prediction of clinical outcomes in cancer patients (Figure 11.15).

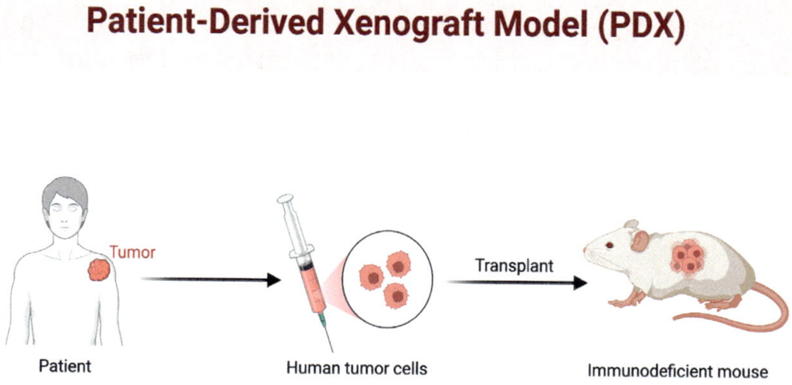

Figure 11.15. Patient-derived Xenograft model (PDX).

Source: https://cdn.prod.website-files.com/621e95f9ac30687a56e4297e/64adcb449e7c21c6bc4fca5b_V2_1679496909177_3b3a66ef-afed-4b18-acc1-86a84647644d_HIGH_RES.png.

Key Features of PDX Models:

a. **Patient-Derived:** PDX models are created from the tumor tissue of the patient directly, hence, they represent the complex biology of the patient's cancer more accurately than cell line models.

b. **Immunodeficient Hosts:** The tumors are implanted into immunodeficient mice to prevent rejection of the human tissue by the host.

c. **Maintenance of Tumor Heterogeneity:** PDX models can maintain the intratumor heterogeneity of the original patient's tumor, which is critical for drug resistance and predicting responses to treatment.

d. **Microenvironment of the Tumor:** PDX models can replicate the microenvironment of the tumor, including the stroma and vasculature associated with the tumor, and these can affect tumor growth and drug sensitivity.

Benefits of PDX Models:

a. **Higher Predictive Value:** PDX models have been shown to be more predictive of clinical responses compared to traditional cell line models and genetically modified mouse models.

b. **Personalized Medicine:** PDX models can be used to study the individual characteristics of patient tumors, which can be used to plan individualized treatments.

c. **Drug Development:** PDX models can be used to evaluate the efficacy of new drugs and measure drug resistance pathways in a more physiologically relevant setting than the traditional models.

Limitations of PDX Models:

a. **Cost and Time:** It is expensive and time-consuming to develop PDX models.

b. **Engraftment Challenges:** Not all patient tumor samples will successfully engraft in mice, and the engraftment rate can also vary with tumor type as well as the strain of mouse.

c. **Strain Variation:** The specific strain of mouse used to create the PDX model can influence tumor growth and drug response.

Applications of PDX Models:

a. **Drug Screening:** PDX models are used to screen potential therapeutic drugs and identify the most effective treatments for a specific form of cancer.

b. **Mechanistic Studies:** PDX models are used to study the mechanisms of drug resistance, tumor heterogeneity, and the role of the tumor microenvironment in cancer formation.

c. **Precision Medicine:** PDX models are used to personalize cancer treatment by matching patients to the best treatments against the nature of their tumors.

REFERENCES

1. Pogue, B. W., Rosenthal, E. L., Achilefu, S., & van Dam, G. M. (2018). Perspective review of what is needed for molecular-specific fluorescence-guided surgery. *Journal of biomedical optics, 23*(10), 1–9. https://doi.org/10.1117/1.JBO.23.10.100601(accessed on 27th June 2025).
2. Alivernini, S., Tolusso, B., Ferraccioli, G., Gremese, E., Kurowska-Stolarska, M., & McInnes, I. B. (2018). Driving chronicity in rheumatoid arthritis: perpetuating role of myeloid cells. *Clinical and experimental immunology, 193*(1), 13–23. https://doi.org/10.1111/cei.13098(accessed on 27th June 2025).
3. Pulendran, B., Rappuoli, R., Aderem, A. *et al.* Novel approaches, including systems biology, to HIV vaccine research and development: Report from a Global HIV Vaccine Enterprise Working Group. *Nat Prec* (2010). https://doi.org/10.1038/npre.2010.4798.1(accessed on 27th June 2025).
4. Ebner, F., Schwiertz, P., Steinfelder, S., Pieper, R., Zentek, J., Schütze, N., Baums, C. G., Alber, G., Geldhof, P., & Hartmann, S. (2017). Pathogen-Reactive T Helper Cell Analysis in the Pig. *Frontiers in immunology, 8,* 565. https://doi.org/10.3389/fimmu.2017.00565 (accessed on 27th June 2025).
5. Aleith, J., Bergmann-Ewert, W., & Müller-Hilke, B. (2025). Maximizing insights, minimizing animal testing: A framework for validating multiparametric single-cell cytokine analysis panels. *European Journal of Immunology, 55.* https://www.semanticscholar.org/paper/048728f487ba63837087f6841943c93b15e7cb5d (accessed on 27th June 2025).
6. Chuntova, P., Downey, K. M., Hegde, B., Almeida, N. D., & Okada, H. (2019). Genetically Engineered T-Cells for Malignant Glioma: Overcoming the Barriers to Effective Immunotherapy. *Frontiers in immunology, 9,* 3062. https://doi.org/10.3389/fimmu.2018.03062(accessed on 27th June 2025).
7. Pineda, M. A., Al-Riyami, L., Harnett, W., & Harnett, M. M. (2014). Lessons from helminth infections: ES-62 highlights new interventional approaches in rheumatoid arthritis. *Clinical and experimental immunology, 177*(1), 13–23. https://doi.org/10.1111/cei.12252(accessed on 27th June 2025).
8. Jaigirdar, S. A., Benson, R. A., Elmesmari, A., Kurowska-Stolarska, M. S., McInnes, I. B., Garside, P., & MacLeod, M. K. L. (2017). Sphingosine-1-Phosphate Promotes the Persistence of Activated CD4 T Cells in Inflamed Sites. *Frontiers in immunology, 8,* 1627. https://doi.org/10.3389/fimmu.2017.01627(accessed on 27th June 2025).
9. Antunes, R. F., Kaski, J. C., & Dumitriu, I. E. (2012). The role of costimulatory receptors of the tumour necrosis factor receptor family in atherosclerosis. *Journal of biomedicine & biotechnology, 2012,* 464532. https://doi.org/10.1155/2012/464532(accessed on 27th June 2025).
10. Costa Del Amo, P., Debebe, B., Razavi-Mohseni, M., Nakaoka, S., Worth, A., Wallace, D., Beverley, P., Macallan, D., & Asquith, B. (2020). The Rules of Human T Cell Fate *in vivo. Frontiers in immunology, 11,* 573. https://doi.org/10.3389/fimmu.2020.00573(accessed on 27th June 2025).
11. Galinski, M. R., Lapp, S. A., Peterson, M. S., Ay, F., Joyner, C. J., LE Roch, K. G., Fonseca, L. L., Voit, E. O., & MAHPIC CONSORTIUM (2018). Plasmodium knowlesi: a superb in vivo nonhuman

primate model of antigenic variation in malaria. *Parasitology, 145*(1), 85–100. https://doi.org/10.1017/S0031182017001135(accessed on 27th June 2025).

12. Obaldía, N., 3rd, Dow, G. S., Gerena, L., Kyle, D., Otero, W., Mantel, P. Y., Baro, N., Daniels, R., Mukherjee, A., Childs, L. M., Buckee, C., Duraisingh, M. T., Volkman, S. K., Wirth, D. F., & Marti, M. (2016). Altered drug susceptibility during host adaptation of a Plasmodium falciparum strain in a non-human primate model. *Scientific reports, 6*, 21216. https://doi.org/10.1038/srep21216(accessed on 27th June 2025).
13. Daniel Lozano-Ojalvo, Sara Benede, Celia M. Antunes, Simona L. Bavaro, Grégory Bouchaud, et al.. Applying the adverse outcome pathway (AOP) for food sensitization to support in vitro testing strategies. Trends in Food Science and Technology, 2019, 85, pp.307-319. ⟨10.1016/j.tifs.2019.01.014⟩. ⟨hal-02623081⟩(accessed on 27th June 2025).
14. Mousavi, S., Escher, U., Thunhorst, E., Kittler, S., Kehrenberg, C., Bereswill, S., & Heimesaat, M. M. (2020). Vitamin C alleviates acute enterocolitis in Campylobacter jejuni infected mice. *Scientific reports, 10*(1), 2921. https://doi.org/10.1038/s41598-020-59890-8(accessed on 27th June 2025).
15. Li, S., Hayden, E. Y., Garcia, V. J., Fuchs, D. T., Sheyn, J., Daley, D. A., Rentsendorj, A., Torbati, T., Black, K. L., Rutishauser, U., Teplow, D. B., Koronyo, Y., & Koronyo-Hamaoui, M. (2020). Activated Bone Marrow-Derived Macrophages Eradicate Alzheimer's-Related $A\beta_{42}$ Oligomers and Protect Synapses. *Frontiers in immunology, 11*, 49. https://doi.org/10.3389/fimmu.2020.00049(accessed on 27th June 2025).
16. Earle, K. E., Tang, Q., Zhou, X., Liu, W., Zhu, S., Bonyhadi, M. L., & Bluestone, J. A. (2005). In vitro expanded human CD4+CD25+ regulatory T cells suppress effector T cell proliferation. *Clinical immunology (Orlando, Fla.), 115*(1), 3–9. https://doi.org/10.1016/j.clim.2005.02.017f (accessed on 27th June 2025).
17. Boswinkel, M., Raavé, R., Veltien, A., Scheenen, T., Fransén Petterson, N., In 't Zandt, R., Olsson, L. E., et al. (2023). Utilizing MRI, [18F]FDG-PET and [89Zr]Zr-DFO-28H1 FAP-PET tracer to assess inflammation and fibrogenesis in a reproducible lung injury rat model: A multimodal imaging study. *Frontiers in Nuclear Medicine, 3*. https://www.semanticscholar.org/paper/a59402a88646c7684764ae424a392e8919c7cd88 (accessed on 27th June 2025).
18. Stijlemans B, De Baetselier P, Caljon G, Van Den Abbeele J, Van Ginderachter JA, Magez S. Nanobodies As Tools to Understand, Diagnose, and Treat African Trypanosomiasis. *Front Immunol*. 2017;8:724. Published 2017 Jun 30. doi:10.3389/fimmu.2017.00724(accessed on 27th June 2025).
19. Cappelletti, M., Kallapur, S. G., & Presicce, P. (2020). Immunobiology of acute chorioamnionitis. https://core.ac.uk/download/323062691.pdf (accessed on 27th June 2025).
20. Choi, I. Y., Wang, W. T., Kim, B., Hur, J., Robbins, D. C., Jang, D. G., Savelieff, M. G., et al. (2023). Non-invasive *in vivo* measurements of metabolic alterations in the type 2 diabetic brain by 1H magnetic resonance spectroscopy. *Journal of Neurochemistry, 168*, 765–780. https://www.semanticscholar.org/paper/41acbaf96670246257b9c44ae8c00cb211a4ec58 (accessed on 27th June 2025).
21. Choi, J. I., Yang, E., & Goo, E. H. (2024). The effects of an ethics education program on artificial intelligence among middle school students: Analysis of perception and attitude changes.

Applied Sciences. https://www.semanticscholar.org/paper/2632a3877612271accf1970e617abd368e96b187 (accessed on 27th June 2025).

22. Cook, S. E., Castillo, D., Wolf, T., Hillman, C., Bauer, K., Williams, S., & Murphy, B. G. (2024). A lentivirus-vectored feline erythropoietin gene therapy strategy in tissue culture and rodent models for the potential treatment of chronic renal disease-associated anemia. *American Journal of Veterinary Research*. https://www.semanticscholar.org/paper/a3d40315d76a1f7ebaf442e5c0ce8edae89a88a4 (accessed on 27th June 2025).

23. Belew, S., Getachew, M., Suleman, S., Mohammed, T., Deti, H., D'Hondt, M., Wynendaele, E., Mekonnen, Z., Vercruysse, J., Duchateau, L., De Spiegeleer, B., & Levecke, B. (2015). Assessment of Efficacy and Quality of Two Albendazole Brands Commonly Used against Soil-Transmitted Helminth Infections in School Children in Jimma Town, Ethiopia. *PLoS neglected tropical diseases*, *9*(9), e0004057. https://doi.org/10.1371/journal.pntd.0004057(accessed on 27th June 2025).

24. Stellari, F. F., Ruscitti, F., Pompilio, D., Ravanetti, F., Tebaldi, G., Macchi, F., Verna, A. E., Villetti, G., & Donofrio, G. (2017). Heterologous Matrix Metalloproteinase Gene Promoter Activity Allows *In Vivo* Real-time Imaging of Bleomycin-Induced Lung Fibrosis in Transiently Transgenized Mice. *Frontiers in immunology*, *8*, 199. https://doi.org/10.3389/fimmu.2017.00199(accessed on 27th June 2025).

25. Earley, B., Murray, M., & Prendiville, D. J. (2007). Animal transport: Developing optimum animal handling procedures and effective transport strategies in the food production chain to improve animal welfare and food quality. https://core.ac.uk/download/45656676.pdf (accessed on 27th June 2025).

26. Kricka LJ, Polsky TG, Park JY, Fortina P. The future of laboratory medicine - a 2014 perspective. *Clin Chim Acta*. 2015;438:284-303. doi:10.1016/j.cca.2014.09.005(accessed on 27th June 2025).

27. Fusaro, L., Bangari, D. S., Pasterkamp, R., Fernández-Ruiz, J., Youssef, S. A., & Sharma, A. K. (2025). Neurodegenerative diseases: Pathogenesis and preclinical models for translational drug discovery. *Toxicologic Pathology*. https://www.semanticscholar.org/paper/48842144437e3692d4af4c03bc432f8a5f79c8a7 (accessed on 27th June 2025).

28. Koido, S., Homma, S., Hara, E., Namiki, Y., Takahara, A., Komita, H., Nagasaki, E., Ito, M., Ohkusa, T., Gong, J., & Tajiri, H. (2010). Regulation of tumor immunity by tumor/dendritic cell fusions. *Clinical & developmental immunology*, *2010*, 516768. https://doi.org/10.1155/2010/516768(accessed on 27th June 2025).

29. Grannonico, M., Miller, D. A., Liu, M., Krause, M. A., Savier, E., Erisir, A., Netland, P. A., et al. (2024). Comparative *in vivo* imaging of retinal structures in tree shrews, humans, and mice. *eNeuro, 11*. https://www.semanticscholar.org/paper/4741d460e0261f0141e459ea477719c723bf664e (accessed on 27th June 2025).

30. Hanazawa, A., Sakai, S., Nishime, C., Ogo, N., Suzuki, M., Hata, J. I., Asai, A., et al. (2025). Abstract LB122: Establishment of an *in vivo* ICI evaluation system using lung adenocarcinoma-derived PDX inoculated PBMC-huNOG-ΔMHC mice. *Cancer Research*. https://www.semanticscholar.org/paper/75a9c95b14c3a4c75c7a390334000063184b2698 (accessed on 27th June 2025).

31. He, Y., Liu, Y., Wang, X., Li, X., Dong, W., Hao, T., Zhu, C., et al. (2024). Abstract 2634: CRISPR *in vivo* screen utilizing removable Cas9 system to identify epigenetic immune response

modulators in antigen-sensitive mouse syngeneic models. *Cancer Research*. https://www.semanticscholar.org/paper/95689e04c1d502881b2ea55d2600528967ac10e7 (accessed on 27th June 2025).

32. Jiang, S., Hillyer, C. D., & Du, L. (2020). Neutralizing antibodies against SARS-CoV-2 and other human coronaviruses. *Trends in Immunology, 41*, 355–359. https://doi.org/10.1016/j.it.2020.03.007 (accessed on 27th June 2025).

33. Jo, M., Jeong, Y., Kim, Y. K., Song, S. H., Joo, H., Choi, Y., Lee, I., et al. (2025). Abstract 476: *In vivo* CD47-mediated targeted oligonucleotide delivery for Endo lysosomal escape in cancer treatment. *Cancer Research*. https://www.semanticscholar.org/paper/371b8611a41d3f55f8a5e85374b4bf278ab93304 (accessed on 27th June 2025).

34. Dyer, D. P., Pallas, K., Medina-Ruiz, L., Schuette, F., Wilson, G. J., & Graham, G. J. (2017). CXCR2 deficient mice display macrophage-dependent exaggerated acute inflammatory responses. *Scientific reports, 7*, 42681. https://doi.org/10.1038/srep42681 (accessed on 27th June 2025).

35. Mascola, J., King, R., Steinman, R. *et al.* Immunogens and Antigen Processing: Report from a Global HIV Vaccine Enterprise Working Group. *Nat Prec* (2010). https://doi.org/10.1038/npre.2010.4796.2(accessed on 27th June 2025).

36. Burm R, Collignon L, Mesalam AA, Meuleman P. Animal Models to Study Hepatitis C Virus Infection. *Front Immunol*. 2018;9:1032. Published 2018 May 14. doi:10.3389/fimmu.2018.01032(accessed on 27th June 2025).

37. Park, J. S., Park, S. Y., Moon, J. W., Kim, K., & Suh, D. (2025). Artificial intelligence models for pediatric lung sound analysis: Systematic review and meta-analysis. *Journal of Medical Internet Research, 27*. https://www.semanticscholar.org/paper/3d124d272c80f7dbc9c731751c696fc0f7f8255c (accessed on 27th June 2025).

38. Schmalkuche, K., Rother, T., Besli, S., Schwinzer, R., Blasczyk, R., Petersen, B., Figueiredo, C., et al. (2024). Human PD-L1 overexpression decreases xenogeneic human T-cell immune responses towards porcine kidneys. *Frontiers in Immunology, 15*. https://www.semanticscholar.org/paper/34d858769f77a993623224281f28b403e9fe9fac (accessed on 27th June 2025).

39. Seal, S., Williams, D. P., Hosseini-Gerami, L., Mahale, M., Carpenter, A., Spjuth, O., & Bender, A. (2024). Improved detection of drug-induced liver injury by integrating predicted *in vivo* and *in vitro* data. *Chemical Research in Toxicology, 37*, 1290–1305. https://www.semanticscholar.org/paper/f074bac4dc28b648b8e21aea43e75b9dacc4e064 (accessed on 27th June 2025).

40. Shemesh, C. S., Hsu, J., Hosseini, I., Shen, B. Q., Rotte, A., Twomey, P., Girish, S., et al. (2020). Personalized cancer vaccines: Clinical landscape, challenges, and opportunities. *Molecular Therapy, 29*, 555–570. https://doi.org/10.1016/j.ymthe.2020.09.038 (accessed on 27th June 2025).

41. Stripecke, R., Münz, C., Schuringa, J. J., Bissig, K. D., Soper, B. W., Meeham, T., Yao, L. C., et al. (2020). Innovations, challenges, and minimal information for standardization of humanized mice. *EMBO Molecular Medicine, 12*. https://doi.org/10.15252/emmm.201708662 (accessed on 27th June 2025).

42. Younis, S. Y., Barnier-Quer, C., Heuking, S., Sommandas, V., Brunner, L., Vd Werff, N., Dubois, P., Friede, M., Kocken, C., Collin, N., & Remarque, E. (2018). Down selecting adjuvanted vaccine formulations: a comparative method for harmonized evaluation. *BMC immunology, 19*(1), 6. https://doi.org/10.1186/s12865-018-0245-0(accessed on 27th June 2025).

43. Tian, S., Zhang, T., Liu, J., Wang, J., Wu, X., Zhu, X., Zhang, R., et al. (2025). Exploring the role of large language models in cybersecurity: A systematic survey. *ArXiv, abs/2504.15622*. https://www.semanticscholar.org/paper/2590a8e157d4ed0eb9741e11fa4eb3725539b506 (accessed on 27th June 2025).

44. Villa-Pulgarín, J. A., Chan, U. I., Khani, F., Socciarelli, F., Wu, J., Carelli, R., Kraynak, J., et al. (2024). Abstract 4987: TREM2 is a radiation-induced target for immunomodulation of tumor-associated macrophages in the prostate cancer tumor microenvironment. *Cancer Research*. https://www.semanticscholar.org/paper/4bc67d8f1922eb4638050f1958b7be21935fea05 (accessed on 27th June 2025).

45. von Jørgensen, L. G. (2020). Zebrafish as a model for fish diseases in aquaculture. https://core.ac.uk/download/333604678.pdf (accessed on 27th June 2025).

46. Wang, W., Cao, J., Yan, X., Yu, Z., Qiao, F., Ning, X. P., Yu, M., et al. (2025). Design a novel polymeric heart valve PHV-SH and test the feasibility using *in vivo* pre-clinical non-inferiority trial. *Macromolecular Bioscience*. https://www.semanticscholar.org/paper/35ae04d92bacce32a074a1c91a776098e3269710 (accessed on 27th June 2025).

47. Zhang, Y., & Zhang, Z. (2020). The history and advances in cancer immunotherapy: Understanding the characteristics of tumor-infiltrating immune cells and their therapeutic implications. *Cellular and Molecular Immunology, 17*, 807–821. https://doi.org/10.1038/s41423-020-0488-6 (accessed on 27th June 2025).

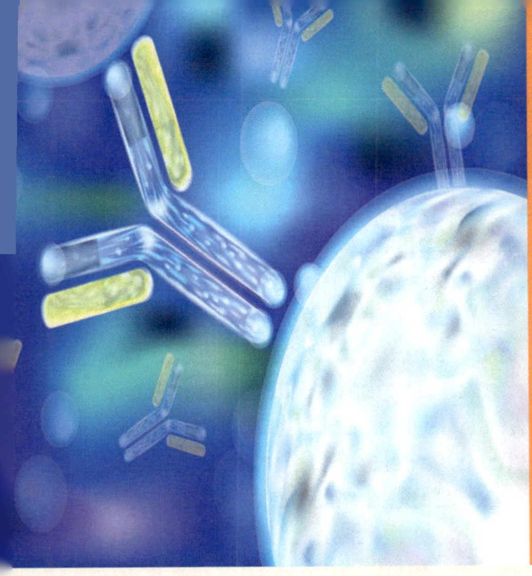

Chapter 12

STRUCTURAL IMMUNOLOGY TECHNIQUES

Contents

Introduction

The subject of structural immunology has developed as a cornerstone area of the overall field of immunology research, enabling a more profound comprehension of the molecular mechanisms of immune responses. Through the assistance of advanced techniques to visualize and describe immune molecule structures, researchers are capable of outlining the way antibodies recognize antigens and initiate subsequent immune processes. These results are crucial, particularly in the development of novel therapeutic methods to combat infectious diseases and autoimmune disorders. In addition, structural immunology serves as an interdisciplinary bridge, thus enabling interdisciplinary collaboration and innovation. The use of techniques such as X-ray crystallography, nuclear magnetic resonance spectroscopy, and cryo-electron microscopy is a testament to the field's maturity and its capacity to answer difficult biological questions that have eluded solution for decades. Structural immunology's progress also has a critical role to play in the solution of major global health problems, among them those presented by parasitic infections such as African trypanosomiasis. The intricate interaction of the Trypanosoma parasite with the host highlights the need for new vaccine and treatment strategies. Current methods, which are highly toxic and are reaching a stage of increasing drug resistance, necessitate a reappraisal of therapy modalities to achieve maximal efficacy and reduce the disease burden. To this end, nanobodies present a promising tool for diagnosis and therapy in accordance with the strengths of high affinity and selectivity toward targets. With the description provided in literature, their application in disease fight underscores the promise of structural immunology approaches to inform and revolutionize response to chronic medical challenges (Stijlemans et al., 2017). The second major advantage of structural immunology is that it can expand the map of scientific inquiry, wherein exchanges between multiple academic domains can illuminate novel avenues of research. Recent efforts at spanning disciplinary divides through citation networks have provided valuable data on the collaborative research potential of research units. Yet, the validity of these associations can be improved by studying the research area pertaining to a particular individual or organization, as is supported by more recent findings in the area. This underscores the need to rely on empirical facts regarding career paths when planning future research work (Guevara et al., 2016). Consequently, structural immunology not only expands our understanding of immune mechanisms but also facilitates a team spirit that can lead to revolutionary breakthroughs in the various fields of science.

Definition of Structural Immunology

The field of structural immunology is a stringent confluence of immunology and structural biology, focusing on the three-dimensional organization of biomolecules involved in immune processes. Structural immunology strives to grasp how the three-dimensional shape of various proteins, such as antibodies and antigens, determines their function and interaction within the immune system. Applying techniques such as X-ray crystallography, nuclear magnetic resonance (NMR) spectroscopy, and cryo-electron microscopy, scientists can visualize the fine shape of immunological molecules at the atomic level, which is critical to comprehend their mechanism of action. This is a subtle understanding of molecular structure that not only expands our information about immune system dynamics but also invites the creation of new therapeutic strategies, including vaccines and monoclonal antibodies, to control immune responses more effectively. The use of structural immunology is even more critical in vaccine design, where the structural rationale for antigen recognition plays a central role. By following the conformational changes as an antigen to a specific antibody, scientists can identify major epitopes, areas of antigens that the immune system recognizes. This knowledge is used to create more targeted vaccine formulations that will induce a robust immune response. Besides, integration of structural data with bioinformatics resources allows prediction of immune recognition effects of antigen structure variations and guides the creation of next-generation vaccines. Through such structural data, immunology can be pushed toward personal medicine approaches, rendering immunotherapies sensitive to patient individual profiles, thus improving clinical outcomes in cancer and autoimmune diseases. Along with it, the synthesis of computational modeling and structural immunology has opened up new avenues for the understanding of immune interaction dynamics at the molecular level. It is possible to model immune agents' behavior dynamics and their interaction environment using high-level algorithms, which yield valuable information about reaction kinetics as well as thermodynamics. This convergence of computational and experimental approaches enables one to have a more advanced idea of how structural properties influence function, eventually leading to improved predictive models of immune responses. The ability to simulate complex biological systems in silico is an adjunct to traditional laboratory techniques and the spirit of cooperation of modern biomedical research. These advances not only enhance our knowledge of the immune system but are also essential to developing effective means of combating new pathogens, demonstrating the significance of structural immunology to contemporary biomedical science (Guevara et al., 2016; Saxena, 2022) (Figure 12.1).

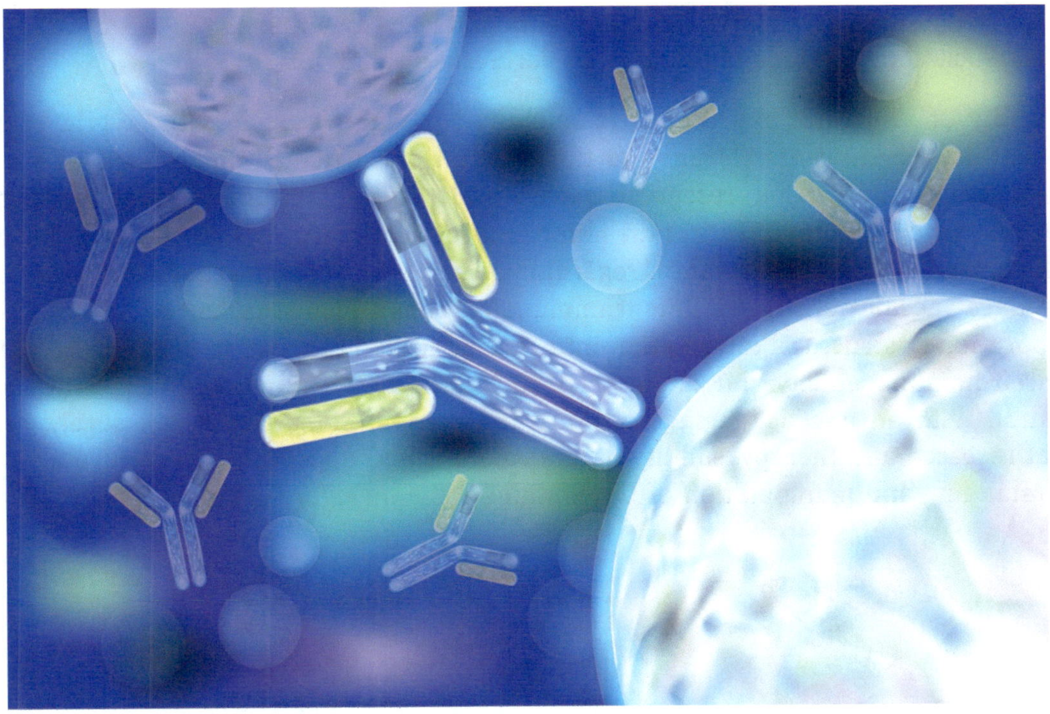

Figure 12.1. Illustration of structural immunology.

Source: https://www.icgeb.org/wp-content/uploads/2018/12/Salunke-AdobeStock_228290620-Converted.jpg.

Importance of Structural Techniques in Immunology

The intricate nature of the immune system necessitates the application of structural techniques to decipher the immune response and interaction complexities. Structural immunology techniques, such as X-ray crystallography and cryo-electron microscopy, provide high-resolution data on the three-dimensional protein and complex structures involved in immunity. The determination of these structures provides the ability to locate key binding sites and conformational changes upon immune activation. Also, adding conceptual theories, such as systems theory and cybernetics, greatly enhances teaching immunology since these structural findings are placed within broader biological processes. As has been discovered through recent findings, underrated theoretical paradigms result in the ignorance of students relating to the communication and regulatory process of the immune system, necessitating sound pedagogical interventions that incorporate these findings to develop learning and comprehension in immunology (Ouhtit et al., 2025). Structural approaches are particularly important in the interpretation of the roles of glycosylation in immune recognition and signaling. Gangliosides, a group of glycosphingolipids, have also emerged as prominent modulators in immunological processes. The engagement of immune receptors, i.e., Siglec-7, with the glycosylated ligands underscores the importance of structural studies to explain how dysregulated expression of gangliosides can affect immune evasion in neoplastic and autoimmune diseases. Techniques like NMR and computer modeling allow researchers to trace the binding energies and energetic landscapes of such interactions and reveal how conformational transitions of ligands can impact immune responses. Structural strategies, thus, not only increase our insight into immune processes but also reveal potential diagnostic and therapeutic interventions that can take advantage of these molecular associations to manage disease (Di Carluccio et al., 2025).

The utility of structural approaches in immunology extends beyond the world of scientific studies; they hold significant relevance to the creation of particular therapies and vaccines. By applying structural information, researchers are able to design immunotherapeutics that will act selectively on particular components of the immune system, minimizing side effects and maximizing efficacy. As a case in point, information regarding structures of tumor-associated antigens allows one to produce vaccines eliciting a potent immune response against tumor cells. Along with this, the incorporation of structural information into vaccine design can lead to optimized formulations for enhanced immunogenicity and safety profiles. As structural immunology continues to evolve, incorporation with advanced imaging methods and computational tools will surely bring new avenues of research and therapy, solidifying the role of these approaches even further in guiding our understanding and manipulation of the immune system (Figure 12.2).

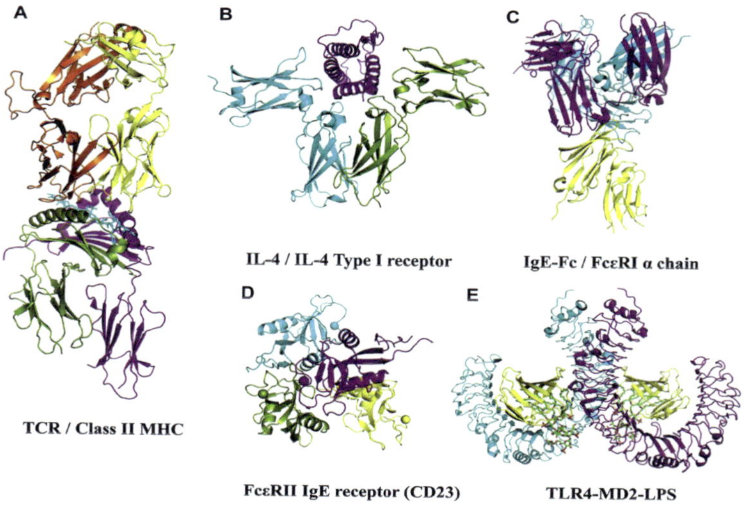

Figure 12.2. X-ray crystal structures of human molecules involved in immunology and allergic disease.

Source: https://www.researchgate.net/profile/Martin-Chapman-5/publication/279808196/figure/fig2/AS:284629023117318@1444872255658/ray-crystal-structures-of-human-molecules-involved-in-immunology-and-allergic-disease-A.png.

12.1. X-ray Crystallography

X-ray crystallography is a cornerstone of structural biology, providing insights unmatched to the three-dimensional structure of biological macromolecules such as proteins and nucleic acids. This technique is a process of applying X-ray beams onto a crystallized sample, which creates treatable mathematical diffraction patterns to reveal the atomic structure of the crystal. The accurate determination of molecular architectures enables researchers to make sense of the mechanisms behind certain biological processes, including immune processes. For instance, structural determination of proteins in the immune system can lead to the identification of significant antigens. This is essential for designing targeted therapies and novel vaccine constructions, which are pivotal to the control of infectious diseases. Synergy between X-ray crystallography and related methods significantly enhances resolution and accuracy for structural work. For example, while X-ray diffraction provides static structures, methods like small-angle X-ray scattering (SAXS) provide information on protein dynamics and conformational change in solution. These hybrid approaches facilitate a broad understanding of protein function under physiological milieus, in contrast to isolated crystalline environments. Structural findings from X-ray crystallography, specifically, have immediate application to the vaccine research area. Epitope mapping at high resolution facilitates vaccine design capable of effectively eliciting immune responses, as attested to by ongoing research targeting antigens of interest for a variety of pathogens. These methods collectively contribute to public health by providing the basis for designing safe and efficient vaccines. Applications of X-ray crystallography also come through in the field of pharmaceutical development, where structural data is utilized to guide the design of inhibitors against particular proteins. In the determination of FolX of Pseudomonas aeruginosa, for instance, it has been revealed as being octameric in structure and with implications for drug design against this opportunistic pathogen. By defining the binding sites and molecular interactions in proteins, scientists can synthesize inhibitors that can effectively disrupt important biological processes of disease-causing microorganisms. Moreover, the knowledge accumulated from the development of vaccines, including that arising from Bordetella pertussis research, demonstrates the mutual dependence of immunology and structural biology. The ability to utilize X-ray crystallography not only increases the understanding of molecular structures but also increases developments in methods of approach to the battle against immunological disorders and infectious diseases and therefore highlights its pivotal role in structural immunology techniques.

12.1.1. Principles of X-ray Crystallography

The principles of X-ray crystallography constitute the foundation of understanding of biological macromolecules, particularly in structural immunology. This technique involves directing X-ray beams onto a crystallized sample of the target molecule, and this gives a diffraction pattern that one can investigate to reveal detailed three-dimensional structures. The atomic structure within the crystal lattice has a wealth of information about molecular interaction, dynamics, and conformational states. Structural immunology provides insights into the protein structure, for instance, of antibodies or of T-cell receptors, so that scientists can comprehend through which mechanisms the proteins recognize and bind antigens. The knowledge about these interactions is critical to be able to generate targeted immunotherapies since it is possible to design drugs that are capable of either activating or suppressing immune responses against specific pathogenic dangers or tumor-associated antigens. The significance of X-ray crystallography to structural immunology is brought out by its ability to inform about the finer details of antigen-antibody interactions and T-cell receptor (TCR) recognition processes. For example, by probing how TCRs recognize peptide–human leukocyte antigen (pHLA) complexes, X-ray crystallography can provide insight into the specificities of such interactions that would usually be sub-optimal in a natural context. Explaining these interactions at the molecular level is critical in developing engineered TCRs with enhanced binding affinities for tumor antigens and, consequently, enhancing cancer treatment outcomes in patients. The majority of laboratories employ the integration of X-ray crystallography with other biophysical strategies to explain these interactions, which de-mystifies the structural motifs that dictate T-cell function and guides rational design of TCR modifications (MacLachlan et al., 2017). Besides that, recent developments in X-ray crystallographic techniques have brought deep innovation in drug-delivery systems in the field of structural immunology. For instance, ferritin-based nanocarrier engineering has targeted cancer cells by demonstrating high affinity for the transferrin receptor. With the use of X-ray crystallography, researchers have determined the structural conformation of the nanocarriers, learning about their assembly and function at the molecular level. The ability to visualize the incorporation of new properties, such as fluorescence imaging, is more informative about the optimization of these systems for effective drug delivery. As has been demonstrated in recent studies, the determination of ferritin-homopolymers allows defining other binding sites, thus further enlarging the applicability of X-ray crystallography for the creation of more advanced immunotherapeutic strategies (Calisti et al., 2018). Thus, X-ray crystallography remains at the forefront of structural immunology and proves significant in the design and efficacy of modern therapies (Figure 12.3).

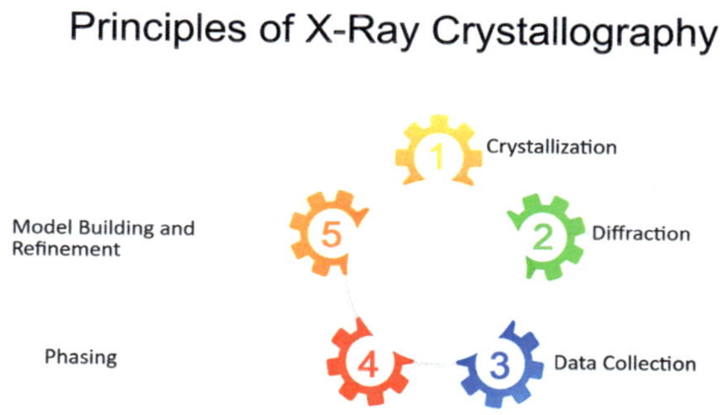

Figure 12.3. Principles of X-ray Crystallography.

Source: https://fastercapital.co/i/X-Ray-Crystallography--Decoding-Molecular-Structures--Principles-of-X-Ray-Crystallography.webp.

12.1.2. Applications in Protein Structure Determination

Protein structure is essential in structural immunology as it directly influences designing diagnostic and therapeutic strategies against many diseases. Powerful techniques for determining protein structure, such as X-ray crystallography and nuclear magnetic resonance (NMR) spectroscopy, have become central instruments in the discovery of the three-dimensional macromolecular structures of biomolecules. These techniques have been responsible for revealing the structural details of many proteins, such as immune response proteins. Through providing data in relation to protein folding, conformational changes, and binding sites for ligands, such techniques enhance our understanding of protein function in the immune system. Ultimately, understanding protein structures can allow researchers to create more effective vaccines and drugs, thus advancing the field of structural immunology. Furthermore, advances in cryo-electron microscopy (cryo-EM) have revolutionized protein structure determination, making it possible to image large complexes as well as membrane proteins that often present challenges for study by traditional methods. Cryo-EM enables the study of proteins at near-native conditions, yielding valuable information concerning their functional states.

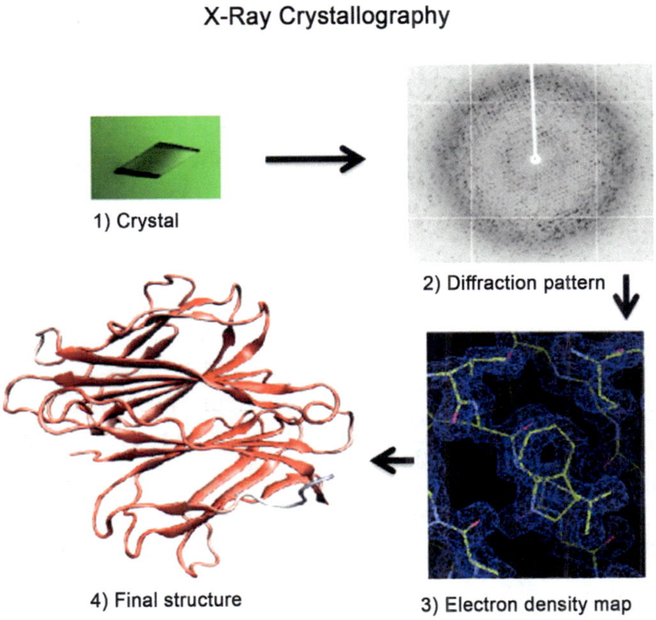

Figure 12.4. Four steps are important to solve a protein structure by X-ray crystallography: (1) to crystallize the protein, (2) to collect diffraction patterns, (3) to calculate the electron density map, and (4) to refine and validate the model of the structure of the protein.

Source: https://www.researchgate.net/profile/Sushil-Mishra-3/publication/221925550/figure/fig2/AS:304724969574401@1449663502773/Four-steps-are-important-to-solve-a-protein-structure-by-X-ray-crystallography-1-to.png.

This approach has garnered considerable attention in structural immunology, as it allows the study of antibody–antigen interactions critical to vaccine design and therapy. Structural data acquired from cryo-EM not only permits enhanced insight into the immune process but also aids in the identification of potential targets for drug discovery. Consequently, through the integration of cryo-EM in structural analysis, researchers can maximize their approach to combat infectious diseases better. Additionally, the integration of proteomics and bioinformatics tools has further promoted protein structure determination as a discipline. Through the utilization of techniques such as mass spectrometry, researchers can liken protein modifications against pathogens, including *A.ocellatum*, as documented in the context of gilthead sea bream plasma proteome. This approach provides robust correlations between changes in protein expression and various physiological reactions, for example, inflammation and immune regulation (Moreira et al., 2017). Similarly, in the case of African trypanosomiasis, the identification of nanobodies (Nbs) has also been an optimistic avenue with high specificity and stability for therapy against trypanosomes (Stijlemans et al., 2017). Cumulatively, these multiscale methods of protein structure analysis enable comprehensive insight into immune processes, and this results in structural immunology innovations in diagnostics and therapies (Figure 12.4).

12.1.3. Limitations and Challenges

In the area of structural immunology methods, there are some limitations and challenges that impede their broader application and effectiveness. Of particular concern is the complexity of biological systems. Immune cells' complex interactions and the wide range of antigens require having advanced methods in place to be able to monitor these dynamics effectively. However, all these structural immunology methods, such as X-ray crystallography and cryo-electron microscopy, are prone to resolution problems and native structure stability during sample preparation. The outcomes may be partial or incorrect snapshots of molecular interactions. Consequently, while these approaches are crucial to determining protein structure, their built-in constraints necessitate continued optimization and improvement of support methodologies toward complete insight into immune responses and future therapeutic targets (Saxena, 2022). Another daunting challenge is presented by the pace of genetics and molecular biology outpacing current structural immunology methods. Next-generation sequencing (NGS) has transformed our knowledge regarding genetic variations and their consequences in immunological reactions. Nevertheless, it has become a challenging problem to translate this immense genetic information into functional knowledge regarding proteins and immune interactions. In most cases, the interpretations of genetic variants yield conflicting results, hence making it more difficult for the application of findings to be adopted in personalized medicine. These limitations highlight the need for standard protocols and clinical guidelines to bridge the gap between genetic data and structural investigation, whereby researchers and clinicians can utilize such information appropriately for targeted treatment regimens (Vanakker & De Paepe, 2013). Furthermore, the high financial and resource-level expenses of advanced structural techniques add another plane of sophistication to the field. Techniques with high resolution, such as cryo-EM, are extremely complex and require advanced equipment, experienced personnel, and enormous investment, and thus are accessible only to well-funded research laboratories. Such unequal access hinders cooperation and information exchange, particularly in resource-constrained settings. In addition, the ethical concerns of handling biological specimens and interpreting genetic data become increasingly important. The solution of these ethical challenges is crucial to foster ethics in research and to ensure equitable access to developing technologies. In general, overcoming these limitations and drawbacks is critical to advance the science of structural immunology and to enhance its contribution to understanding immune mechanisms and developing new therapeutics (Saxena, 2022).

12.2. Nuclear Magnetic Resonance (NMR) Spectroscopy

In structural immunology, NMR spectroscopy is a key tool for studying the molecular organization of biomolecules, including proteins mediating immune processes. With the help of magnetic moments of atomic nuclei, NMR provides a high-resolution view of conformational mobility and protein-protein interactions at the atomic level. This is particularly worth understanding in the comprehension of intricate structures, such as nematode polyprotein allergens (NPAs), as found in recent studies. These allergens, which play the pivotal role in initiating immune responses, possess unique binding characteristics with lipids that can influence inflammatory pathways. By making use of NMR, researchers can trace the three-dimensional structures of NPAs, thereby revealing how they modulate immune functions and possibly exploit the mechanisms for therapeutic advancement (Ekser et al., 2011). Moreover, NMR spectroscopy possesses unparalleled advantages in monitoring metabolic processes key to shedding light on immune responses. As an example, in cancer immunology, understanding the metabolic pathways of tumors can reveal their weak points metabolically that affect immune evasion. Dynamic Nuclear Polarization (DNP) enhances NMR sensitivity, which enables real-time tracking of metabolic conversions, such as pyruvate conversion to lactate in tumor cells, as indicated in studies on pancreatic tumors. This capability provides the possibility of detecting metabolic biomarkers with which the susceptibility of tumors to immunotherapy can be determined as a significant predictor. Researchers, by integrating NMR techniques with metabolomics, are capable of quantifying the way in which different immunocompetent and immunocompromised situations impact the biology of tumors for more tailored therapeutic interventions (Weygand, 2017). The inclusion of NMR spectroscopy in structural immunology not only deepens our knowledge of immune-associated proteins but also bridges the gap between structural information and functional implication. Having the ability to study protein-lipid interactions at a molecular level provides much-needed context to the understanding of allergenicity, particularly for NPA that aim at host immune responses. Moreover, the use of high-resolution NMR metabolomics in immunology research allows scientists to map the metabolic topology of cancers and communicate with the immune system. The global perspectives create a multistep view of immune responses, which opens doors to innovative therapeutic approaches considering both structural and metabolic properties of cellular interactions. Through the ability to better understand these interrelated factors, NMR spectroscopy is at the forefront of structural immunology technique development (Cooper et al., 2011; Weygand, 2017).

12.2.1. Fundamentals of Nuclear Magnetic Resonance (NMR) Spectroscopy

NMR spectroscopy is a key analytical tool in structural immunology, facilitating detailed analysis of biomolecules, particularly proteins and nucleic acids. This sensitive method makes use of the magnetic properties of atomic nuclei, such as hydrogen or carbon, to provide information concerning the molecular structure, dynamics, and interactions of biological macromolecules with very high precision. By using a magnetic field and radiofrequency radiation, NMR enables researchers to describe the three-dimensional conformations of proteins in solution, which provides information on their mechanism of function. These structural findings are crucial when one considers immune responses since proteins' states of conformation play an important role in determining whether they get recognized by other molecules, i.e., antibodies and antigens, thus controlling immune signaling pathways. Application of NMR spectroscopy to the investigation of mesenchymal stem cells (MSCs) and their secretome further justifies its significance in immunology. MSCs possess the unique ability to differentiate into various forms of cells and secrete a variety of bioactive molecules affecting surrounding cells, an aspect that is increasingly being recognized for its therapeutic potential. Through advanced NMR technologies, researchers can decipher the complex composition of secretomes of MSCs, which include cytokines, growth factors, and extracellular vesicles. The detailed description of these secretomes using NMR can reveal critical mechanisms of MSC therapeutic effects in inflammatory and regenerative processes. Furthermore, the correlation of these findings with biophysical properties can enhance insights into molecular reasons behind MSC therapeutic effect in treating intricate diseases like autoimmune diseases and tissue injury, as indicated in current research (Ivanova et al., 2016).

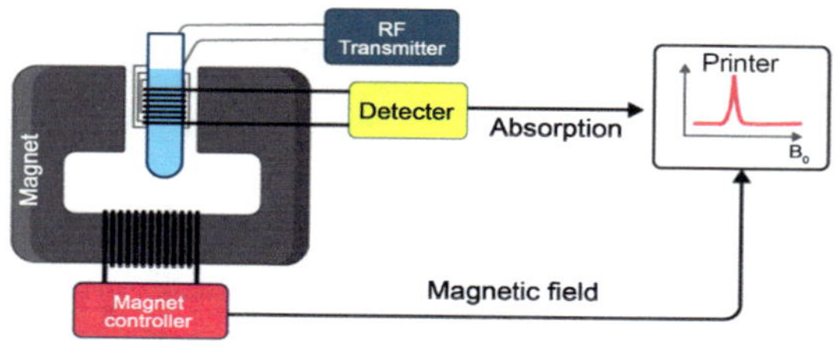

Figure 12.5. Nuclear magnetic resonance (NMR) spectroscopy instrumentation.

Source: https://cdn1.byjus.com/wp-content/uploads/2017/10/NMR-Spectroscopy-700x385.png.

Advances in NMR spectroscopy have been revolutionary in the investigation of molecular interactions relevant to structural immunology. Dynamic observation of protein structural changes that accompany interactions with ligands or biological partners provides unparalleled insight into mechanisms of immune recognition. Dynamic assessment is critical in defining sites of binding and understanding allosteric effects in protein structures. Using NMR data alongside other types of analysis, such as mass spectrometry and chromatography, researchers can construct comprehensive models describing immune molecule interactions. This type of integrated approach helps construct targeted therapy and vaccines by providing precise information regarding structural requisites for effective immune responses (Cornell University, 1998). As such, NMR not only supports basic scientific understanding but also counsels practical use in the field of therapeutic development for structural immunology (Figure 12.5).

12.2.2. Role in Studying Protein Dynamics

Protein dynamics are significant to comprehend in structural immunology since the activity and behavior of proteins exert a significant influence on immune responses. Protein conformational changes upon various stimuli are of basic significance to their functional roles in the immune response. Techniques such as X-ray crystallography, NMR spectroscopy, and cryo-electron microscopy provide information about the dynamic process at a molecular level. By comparing structures in various states, researchers are able to decipher the mechanism of protein interaction and its relevance in signaling cascades or antigen recognition. With scientists refining these methods, visualization of real-time protein dynamics will offer greater insights into the way immune proteins function at both the structural and functional levels, which in their turn will reduce the gap between activity and structure in immunological contexts. The latest breakthroughs in imaging technology have allowed researchers to probe protein dynamics at unprecedented resolution, facilitating a better understanding of molecular interactions within cellular microdomains. Techniques like electron tomography and immuno-electron microscopy permit proteins to be visualized *in situ*, and they provide insights into their organization in space and their interaction networks. For instance, studies have shown how synaptic plasticity, a main mechanism for learning and memory, is enabled by the semi-ordered structure of the neurotransmitter receptors in synapses. These results are not unique to neuroscience but extend to immunology, as structural organization and immune receptor migration can regulate cellular response to pathogens. Application of such high-resolution imaging modalities derives insight into the complex interaction between structural organization and protein dynamics, necessitating interdisciplinary approaches to studying immune function. The given implications of protein dynamics transcend the abstract sphere of knowledge; they have practical uses in developing therapy interventions against various diseases. Protein interaction mechanism and conformational change characterization enable scientists to propose possible drug development candidates. For example, protein-protein interaction modulation can be employed to develop novel therapies for immune-related disorders or enhance vaccines. Also, the collaboration of academe and industry, as documented in marine biotechnology initiatives reports, highlights the networking imperative in advancing research. Interconnecting scientists from different disciplines is meant to stimulate innovation and introduce new sources of funding, hence accelerating the pace of structural immunology as a discipline. Lastly, the study of protein dynamics not only advances our fundamental knowledge of biological systems but also ushers in the possibility of practical use in medicine and biotechnology (Figure 12.6).

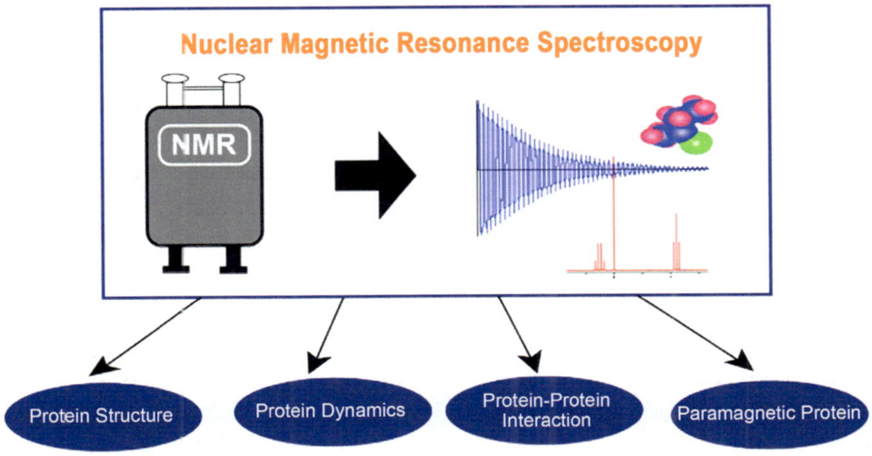

Figure 12.6. Nuclear magnetic resonance (NMR) spectroscopy for protein research.

Source: https://www.profacgen.com/wp-content/themes/profacgen/img/Nuclear-Magnetic-Resonance-NMR-1.png.

12.2.3. Advantages and Disadvantages

Methods of structural immunology confer substantial advantages to the study of immune responses and the planning of immunotherapeutics. By the three-dimensional structures in high-resolution images of antigens, antibodies, and their complexes, these techniques—such as X-ray crystallography and cryo-electron microscopy—are capable of visualizing the specificity and affinities of such biomolecules. Such structural information is paramount for the rational design of vaccines and monoclonal antibodies that can be translated into more effective therapeutic interventions. For instance, gelatin material affinity for fibronectin, as revealed by various analysis techniques, illustrates how structure-function interactions dictate materials design in the case of immunological applications

(Vos et al., 2009). This knowledge can facilitate the design of personalized medicine approaches with enhanced therapeutic effectiveness and fewer adverse effects in treatments. However, alongside their positives, there exist significant disadvantages in structural immunology techniques that are important to consider. There is a single major challenge, which is the time-consuming and complex nature of such methods. It tends to decelerate the pace of research and development. Trained experts, specialized equipment, and high investment costs are sometimes necessary, which makes it available in fewer locations, particularly in under-equipped environments. Structural data can also be difficult to interpret and can make false representations if not handled carefully. For example, while advances in pharmacogenetics are promising for personalized medicine, heterogeneity of genotyping results necessitates tight regulations for clinical use (Vanakker & De Paepe, 2013).

This complexity not only affects the reproducibility of findings but also raises ethical concerns regarding the application of such technologies in the clinic. In all, a balance of knowledge of the strengths and weaknesses of structural immunology methods is required to proceed in the field. These methods clearly refine what is known about immune mechanisms and the development of new therapeutics. Scientists simply need to exercise caution about the limitations and drawbacks of these techniques. Bridging the resource challenges and optimizing protocols will be critical to maximizing the utility of structural immunology while minimizing potential adverse effects. With advancements continuing, ongoing dialogue among scientists, clinicians, and policy experts will be necessary to refine these methods and ensure proper translation into the clinic, towards increasingly sophisticated and customized treatment regimens.

12.3. Cryo-Electron Microscopy (Cryo-EM)

Cryo-EM has risen to the top in structural immunology due to its ability to image biological macromolecules and complexes at near-atomic resolution. Cryo-EM preserves the native conformation of samples by rapidly freezing samples to cryogenic temperatures and, thereby, preventing the introduction of ice crystals that could suppress finer details. As a result, Cryo-EM enables researchers to obtain high-resolution views of proteins, viruses, and other cellular structures and gain useful insights into their relationship between structure and function. Of specific interest in immunology is the accurate composition of antigens and antibodies, which plays a key role in vaccine development and therapeutic treatment. Cryo-EM's ability to uncover complex molecular machines that are involved in immune responses brings a valuable dimension to the study of pathogenic interactions and immune mechanisms of recognition. Cryo-EM plays a key role in the study of viruses in viral science, as it uncovers the viruses' complex structure, something that is normally challenging to study due to their tiny size and complexity. By taking pictures of viruses in their native structure, researchers can show information such as viral capsid structure, envelope protein structure, and how they bind to host cell receptors. This level of detail is important when studying viral infection mechanisms and how immune systems bypass them. For instance, as indicated in research, viruses exist in diverse structural forms with varying levels of complexity, e.g., those encapsulated in lipid structures derived from the host cell membrane, whose characterization is more complicated (Orlova et al., 2012). The insight achieved through Cryo-EM provides a foundation for the creation of antiviral drugs and vaccines tailored to specific viral components. Additionally, the advancement of Cryo-EM technology has led to improved imaging techniques, such as cryo-electron tomography, for three-dimensional visualization of biological samples. This capability is particularly advantageous in the study of synaptic structures in the nervous system, where molecular organization plays a pivotal role in synaptic function and plasticity. Through such high-resolution approaches, researchers are able to qualitatively investigate synaptic structures crucial to learning and memory (Liu et al., 2019). Moreover, the combination of cryo-EM with other imaging modalities facilitates the immune complex analysis to reveal interactions at the nanoscale. Such collaborative methodologies enhance our understanding of immune processes, paving the way for novel therapeutic modalities for immune modulation.

12.3.1. Overview of Cryo-Electron Microscopy (Cryo-EM) Techniques

In structural immunology, techniques by cryo-EM have revolutionized how scientists perceive and understand macromolecular complexes. The techniques of cryo-EM are marked by the ability to capture specimens at near-native conditions, freezing in their liquid state without crystallization, which is traditionally a drawback for other structural biology methods like X-ray crystallography. This approach facilitates structural analysis of big protein complexes and integral membrane proteins that take part in immune processes, allowing for the examination of conformational dynamics and heterogeneous populations in biological systems. With the use of advanced electron detectors and intricate image processing computer codes, cryo-EM produces high-resolution 3D reconstructions that enhance the understanding of molecular interactions in the immune system. Cryo-EM data processing has improved substantially, with novel computational approaches being developed.

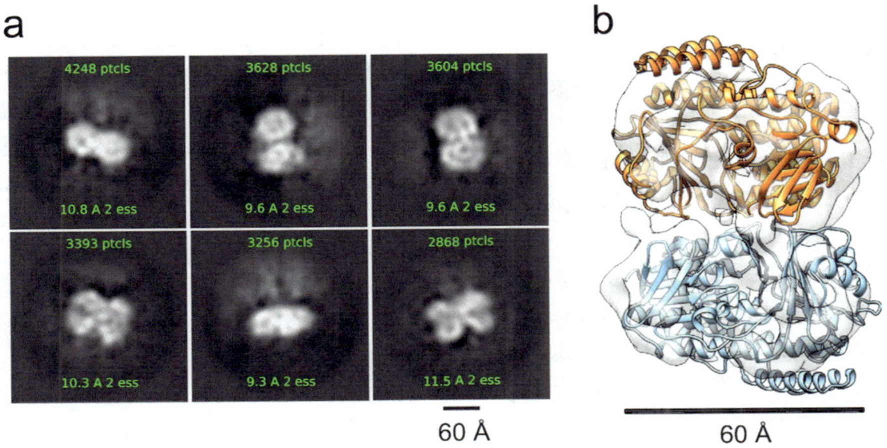

Figure 12.7. Cryo-electron microscopy for the empirical structural elucidation of PrnC. Single-particle cryo-EM analysis of PrnC reveals that the protein exists as dimers in solution, as seen from both the 2D class averages and b docking of the homology model into the 3D reconstruction.

Source: https://www.researchgate.net/publication/377186952/figure/fig4/AS:11431281216001370@1704514611205/Cryo-electron-microscopy-for-the-empirical-structural-elucidation-of-PrnC-Single-particle.png.

Traditional refinement techniques found it difficult to strike a balance between data fit and physico-chemical reasonableness of structures. Novel contributions such as EMMIVox, with its foundation in Bayesian inference, have emerged to fill such voids. By correcting for data noise and correlation automatically, EMMIVox can generate single-structure models or structural ensembles with both high fit to experimental data and excellent stereochemical quality. Therefore, such progress not only increases the accuracy of immune complex descriptions but also enables greater insight into the molecular mechanisms of immune function and dysfunction, thereby making the discipline of structural immunology richer (Hoff et al., 2024). Furthermore, the integration of cryo-EM into structure-based drug design (SBDD) pipelines underscores its essential contribution to biomedical research. The method offers a backup when conventional approaches, including X-ray crystallography, are inadequate, particularly with respect to difficult targets. Now that cryo-EM produces high-resolution reconstructions daily, it is opening the door to an optimized SBDD procedure that will enable scientists to make more efficient therapeutic agents. Becoming aware of the advantages and weaknesses of cryo-EM is crucial to realizing its full potential in the development of drugs. Advances in cryo-EM in recent times pointed to its growing relevance in drug discovery, as it illustrates how the technique not only explains fundamental immune processes but also assists in shaping solutions to combat disease (Cebi et al., 2024). This union of cryo-EM with structural immunology propels the field towards new therapeutic methods, indicating tremendous progress in addressing complex health challenges (Figure 12.7).

12.3.2. Impact on Visualizing Large Complexes

The visualization of large complexes in structural immunology plays a crucial role in enhancing our knowledge on molecular interactions. Techniques such as electron microscopy (EM) have revolutionized the ability to observe subcellular structures at never-before-seen resolutions. By facilitating the detailed study of such complexes as antigen-bound antibodies or three-dimensional immune synapses, EM enables the observation of structural hierarchies and their ensuing functions. By utilizing high-resolution imaging methods, it is now possible to quantitatively interrogate nanoscale structures, giving insights into dynamic immune response changes. As described in experiments with synaptic plasticity, the structural arrangement of protein complexes can be mapped in detail with different EM methods, thereby enhancing our understanding of their function in immunity and forming the basis for therapeutic intervention (Liu et al., 2019). Live-cell imaging is supplementary to static imaging approaches by providing a dynamic snapshot of large complexes in real-time. This technique is particularly valuable in the field of structural immunology, where spatial location and timing of molecular interactions can critically influence immune outcome. Fluorescent marking techniques, especially on nucleic acids such as mRNA and plasmid DNA, allow researchers to observe signaling pathways and complex forms as they occur. These techniques give researchers not only such detailed pictures, but data on kinetics and localization of assemblies related to the immune system as well. Weighing the advantages and disadvantages of various labeling strategies allows researchers to identify bespoke strategies for particular requirements, maximizing visualization of the large complexes that are involved in immune signaling pathways (Rombouts et al., 2016). The ability to track these processes *in vivo* is a significant advancement in structural immunology. Linking advanced computational methods with traditional structural biology approaches further maximizes our capacity for visualizing large complexes. For example, cryo-electron tomography enables the reconstruction of three-dimensional structures from two-dimensional images, effectively surpassing some of the limitations on sample heterogeneity and thickness. Integrating these techniques with machine learning algorithms can improve complex visualization accuracy and efficiency towards the detection of new structural motifs that are pivotal in immune response. As these technologies converge, researchers have the potential to discover previously unknown properties of large complexes, central to the construction of targeted immunotherapies. The potential for interdisciplinary synergy in this field promises a rosy outlook where the marriage of imaging and computational sciences continues to propel the science of structural immunology forward.

12.3.3. Comparison with Other Structural Techniques

In structural immunology, a number of approaches possess specific strengths and limitations in de-mystifying the intricate structure of immune molecules. X-ray crystallography has long remained the gold standard, providing high-resolution atomic images of protein structures. However, this method usually requires proteins to be crystallized, which may induce them to deviate from their native conformations and may mask functional conformations. On the other hand, NMR spectroscopy is feasible in solution, hence preserving the native conformation of the molecules being studied. Unfortunately, NMR typically cannot be applied to large proteins because the larger complexes are hard to analyze due to spectral congestion. A study of a range of methods for structure determination is imperative, as each of them has something unique towards the understanding of the dynamic and flexible character of immune proteins and their complexes. Of the more recent structural techniques, cryo-EM has proven to be a useful alternative, especially for large macromolecular complexes. Cryo-EM permits observation of samples in almost native form without crystallization, avoiding some of the restrictions of X-ray crystallography and NMR. The method is better suited to describe those complexes difficult to crystallize by virtue of their size or inherent conformational mobility. Recent progress in cryo-EM has enhanced its resolution capability to a considerable extent, and scientists can now explain the organization of proteins in the immune system more accurately. For instance, understanding the structural attributes of multifunctional immune-regulatory proteins has been advanced through the reactivity of cryo-EM by prioritizing consideration of multiple structural approaches in establishing the correlation between structure and protein function. The relative comparison of structural immunology techniques, as applied within the context of complement regulators, highlights their relative merits. For instance, the explanation of segmental flexibility is indispensable for understanding human factor H and other such proteins' interaction with other molecules within the immune cascade. Use of residual dipolar couplings derived from NMR can potentially retrieve information regarding interdomain motions, as in the example of three N-terminal domains of human factor H. Flexibility can enhance the functional dynamics of the proteins, for example, in the processing of complement proteins like C3b. The blending of information from multiple structural methods ultimately results in a greater overall insight into molecular interactions in immunology, highlighting the value of combining several approaches with each other for large-scale interpretation of structural data in this complex field (Zachau, 2000; Maciejewski et al., 2011).

12.4. Mass Spectrometry (MS)

MS is now a key resource for structural immunology, enabling scientists to describe the complex interactions between antibodies and antigens at the molecular level. The technique involves ionizing chemical species and analyzing the resulting ions in terms of mass-to-charge ratios. This is a critical capability in the determination of protein function and structure, as it allows detection of post-translational modifications, which have a significant impact on biological activity. Besides, the sensitivity and accuracy of mass spectrometry allow the identification of low-abundance proteins, thereby providing a complete immunological view.

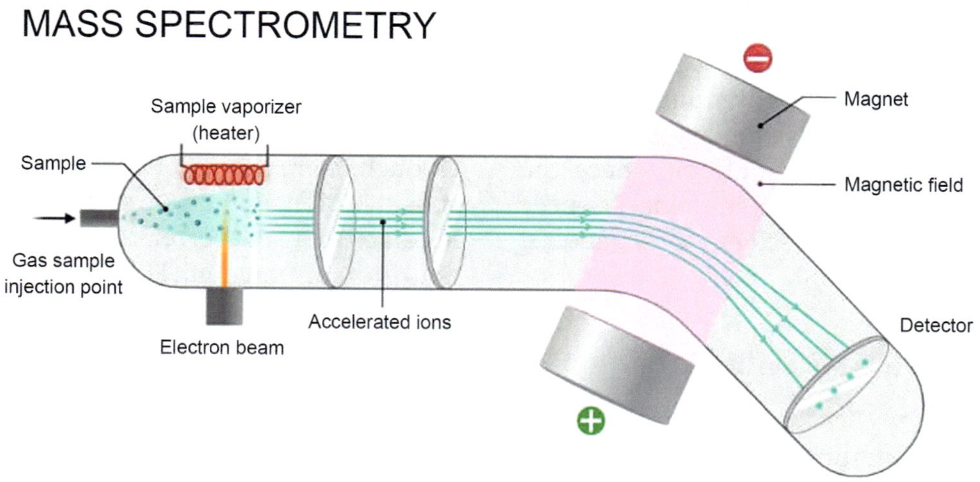

Figure 12.8. Illustration of mass spectrometry (MS).

Source: https://microbenotes.com/wp-content/uploads/2018/12/Mass-Spectrometry-MS.jpeg.

Through the integration of data obtained from mass spectrometry with other structural techniques, such as X-ray crystallography and NMR, researchers can generate a more detailed image of protein dynamics and interactions behind immune responses and enhance the field of structural immunology. The value of mass spectrometry extends beyond identification alone; it is also key to the quantitation of biomolecules, a critical element of structural immunology. Tools such as multiple reaction monitoring (MRM) allow for the targeted measurement of specific proteins in mixed populations, thereby enabling the examination of immune responses under conditions of interest. This quantification becomes extremely relevant in studies to correlate the concentration of a particular biomarker with disease states, such as autoimmune diseases or cancers. Mass spectrometry imaging also provides spatial information on protein distribution in tissues, which facilitates the interpretation of the functional importance of protein interactions under physiological conditions. As the field advances, the development of these approaches has the potential to uncover new knowledge regarding the complexity of the immune system. Apart from its numerous advantages, application of mass spectrometry to structural immunology does pose challenges, namely issues of methodological bias and reproducibility of results. The intrinsic tendency of biological samples towards heterogeneity introduces variability in measurements, and hence stringent validation protocols for mass spectrometric approaches. To address such dilemmas, researchers have advocated for the application of standard procedures and reproducible analytical protocols to ensure data credibility. Further, inclusion of oxidative stress biomarkers has been emphasized, as evident in ongoing controversies regarding their role in clinical use to determine health. This underscores the necessity for an integrated approach with the use of more than one analytical technique, for example, mass spectrometry, in order to not only quantify immune function but also assess overall redox status across various disease states (Marrocco et al., 2017). As a result of critical evaluation and optimization of mass spectrometric methods, the potential for structural immunology's future boost is increasing day by day (Figure 12.8).

12.4.1. Basics of Mass Spectrometry (MS) in Immunology

MS has emerged as a key methodology in the science of immunology, greatly contributing to the unraveling of biological systems. With precise measurement of biomolecular masses, MS allows scientists to detect and detail proteins, peptides, and other immune response-efficacious biomolecules. Its analytical capability is particularly applicable to the study of post-translational modifications, protein folding, and interactions that are critical to immune function. Also, mass spectrometry sensitivity and specificity facilitate the detection of low-abundance proteins, which offer hints at their functions in diseases such as cancer and autoimmune disease. With these applications, the integration of mass spectrometry in structural immunology techniques is a precious milestone, unifying molecular biology and clinical diagnostics and enabling a deeper insight into immune processes. Mass spectrometry in immunology is complemented by techniques such as liquid chromatography (LC), which offers an initial separation of biomolecules before mass analysis. This complementarity contributes to resolution and accuracy in protein characterization toward holistic profiling of immune proteins and protein complexes. Such breakthroughs, coupled with advances in mass spectrometry technologies through high-resolution instrumentation, have enabled researchers to carry out quantitative measurements with spookily high accuracy. For example, the ability to detect isoforms of protein molecules involved in immune signaling pathways has the potential to reveal significant insight into immune regulation. As a result, synergistic integration of MS and LC both supports the data obtained and broadens the scope of studies for uncovering the complex immunodynamics. Moreover, the advent of nanobody technology opens up new hopeful directions for mass spectrometry utilization in the area of immunology. Nanobodies are small single-domain antibodies produced in camelid animals and possess remarkable features responsible for their promise as research reagents. Their antigen-binding specificity improves the selectivity of mass spectrometric analysis, particularly in complex biological samples. In addition, nanobodies have proven useful in explaining protein-protein interactions and their role in immune processes, thus being precious in the world of mass spectrometry. As noted in recent literature, the trailblazing engineering of nanobodies positions them as powerful tools in structural immunology, paving the way for their broader application in mass spectrometry and expanding their utility across many areas of immunological study, thus narrowing the gap between theoretical understanding and practical application in research on immunology (Beghein & Gettemans, 2017).

12.4.2. Use in Analyzing Protein Interactions

In structural immunology, the study of protein interactions is crucial in understanding advanced biological processes. Techniques such as NMR spectroscopy provide one with glimpses of protein dynamics and conformations, which are crucial to decipher their interactions. NMR provides researchers with the ability to evaluate interdomain motions in protein structures, which reveal how proteins act as collaborators. For example, research into the human factor H (FH1–3) revealed segmental mobility essential for complement regulation. Segmental mobility is crucial, since it enables binding and recognition of complement components like C3b, showcasing the importance of conformational change in influencing protein interactions involving immune response, thus proving the importance of residual dipolar couplings measured by NMR in immunological structure (Maciejewski et al., 2011). Although the power of NMR cannot be overstated, other techniques have been just as important in exploring protein interactions in structural immunology. Another technique is through examination of tertiary lymphoid organs (TLOs) in autoimmune diseases such as multiple sclerosis (MS). These structures, situated within the central nervous system, are localized sites of immune response, highlighting B cell and T cell interaction. Understand how these interactions result in chronic inflammation and neuronal injury will be important in working towards developing specific therapies. Experimental models of disease, including experimental autoimmune encephalomyelitis (EAE), have shed light on how TLOs can impact the course of disease and the mechanism of autoreactive cell differentiation. With the assistance of these models, researchers can explore the particular role of protein interactions within the immune system that can offer insight into future therapeutic intervention in MS (Mitsdoerffer & Peters 2016). Structural biology is also enabling us to investigate protein interactions with greater specificity. Techniques such as X-ray crystallography and cryo-electron microscopy enable researchers to observe protein complexes at high resolution, revealing the intricate web of interactions that underpin cellular processes. These methods complement NMR and provide robust structures from which to infer how protein conformations change upon binding. By combining such structural insights, researchers can formulate hypotheses for the mechanistic underpinnings of immunity, paving the way for new avenues of intervention in disease. The conjunction of several techniques in structural immunology demonstrates the holistic approach necessary to dispel the mysticism of protein interactions, with a perspective towards guiding the design of more effective therapeutic approaches under disease states (Maciejewski et al., 2011; Mitsdoerffer & Peters, 2016) (Figure 12.9).

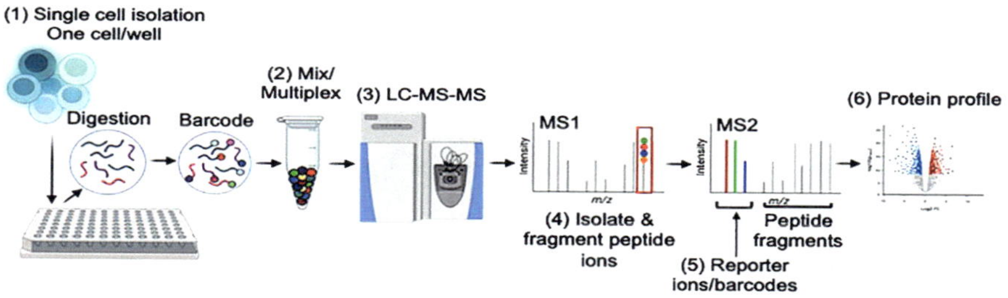

Figure 12.9. Basic overview of single-cell mass spectrometry workflow. Single-cell proteomics tends to use a "bottom-up" approach.

Source: https://www.researchgate.net/publication/365429725/figure/fig1/AS:11431281254477662@1719198273783/Basic-overview-of-single-cell-mass-spectrometry-workflow-Single-cell-proteomics-tends-to.tif.

12.4.3. Technological Advances in Mass Spectrometry (MS)

The evolution of MS has significantly transformed the science of structural immunology through enhanced analytical capabilities for the characterization of biomolecules. Enhanced sensitivity, resolution, and velocity in equipment have enabled researchers to subject proteins, peptides, and glycoproteins that are essential in the immune response to advanced structural analysis. Modern forms of MS technology allow for high-throughput analysis, which makes it possible to delineate intricate biological interactions and modifications at the molecular level. Of particular note, techniques such as tandem MS/MS and matrix-assisted laser desorption/ionization (MALDI) have revolutionized the identification of new immunogenic epitopes.

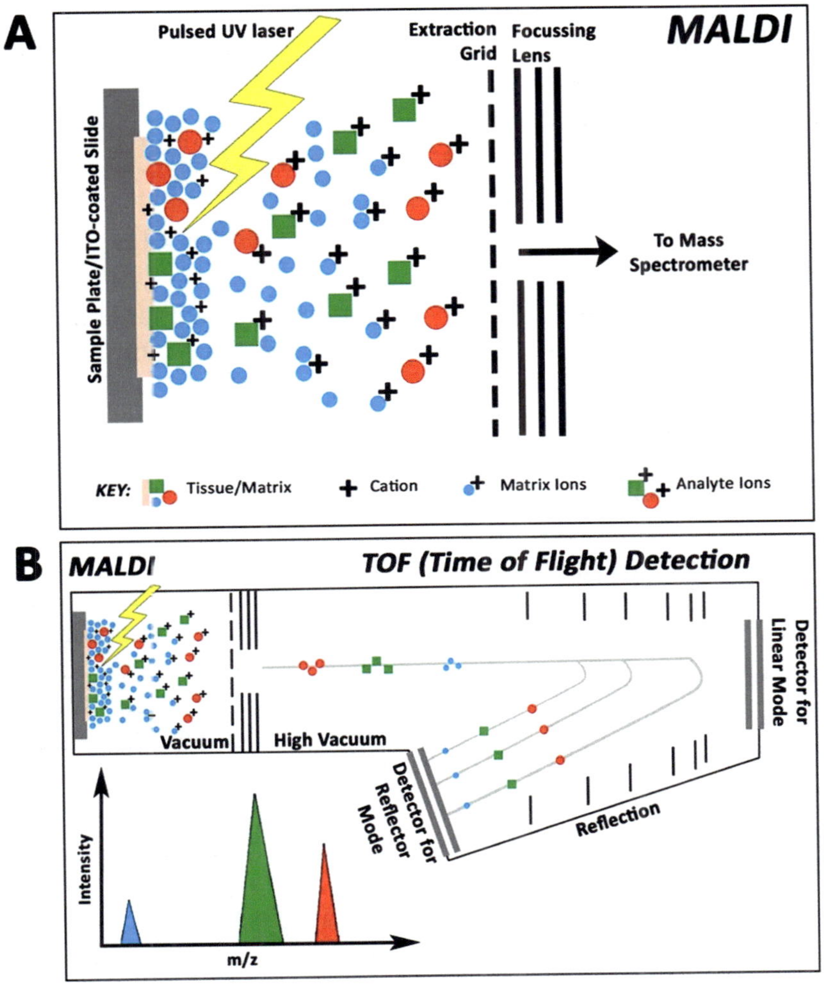

Figure 12.10. Principle of matrix-assisted laser desorption/ionisation (MALDI)-time of flight (TOF) mass spectrometry. (A) The matrix creates a mixture with analyte molecules of the fresh, frozen brain tissue. When placed in the instrument, brief UV laser pulses hit the mixture, desorbing and ionising molecules. (B) The ionised molecules (denoted by the + sign) are accelerated through the electrostatic field in the ion source and directed to the flight tube.

Source: https://www.researchgate.net/profile/Lakshini-Mendis/publication/315792953/figure/fig5/AS:613448060784658@1523268823455/Principle-of-matrix-assisted-laser-desorption-ionisation-MALDI-time-of-flight-TOF.png.

In structural immunology, it is necessary to understand how proteins interact with antibodies and immune cells. Moreover, the integration of MS with other analytical instruments is establishing new directions for immunogenicity investigation and illuminating therapeutic protein design, thereby promoting the synthesis of targeted immunotherapies (Sánchez-Vidaña et al., 2017). Utilization of advanced mass spectrometry techniques is critical in order to overcome obstacles presented by food allergens and their interactions at the molecular level in humans. For instance, MS developments have demonstrated their promise in the analysis of allergenic proteins, the identification of their epitopes, and the determination of the mechanisms involved in allergy. The accuracy and sensitivity of modern MS techniques allow for the identification of low-abundance allergens that could not be easily examined before. By enhancing our understanding of the structural features that are associated with allergenicity, scientists can devise better diagnostic and therapeutic methods (Lozano-Ojalvo et al., 2019). These improvements in analysis not only refine allergenic protein identification in food products but also help in understanding the molecular properties causing food intolerance, which ultimately leads to food safety and consumers' well-being. Furthermore, ongoing developments in mass spectrometry instruments have the ability to reveal even greater horizons for investigation in structural immunology. The introduction of new methodologies such as ion mobility spectrometry (IMS) enables the examination of protein conformational dynamics in real time, enabling scientists to learn more deeply about their functional conformations and interactions. The ability to visualize protein folding and conformational changes in the context of immune response gives insights into how such biomolecules are engaged in disease states. Moreover, the possibility of mixing MS with bioinformatics and computational modeling is opening the door to predictive structural analysis of immunological responses. As these technologies evolve, they will undoubtedly discover new applications in biomedical research as well as aid in the design of new immunotherapeutics that can target specific molecular pathways, thus improving patient outcomes (Lozano-Ojalvo et al., 2019) (Figure 12.10).

12.5. Computational Modeling

Computational modeling is an essential part of structural immunology and serves as a good predictor and describer of complex molecular interactions in the immune response. By combining highly strong algorithms with computational capacity, researchers are capable of simulating the movement of proteins, antibodies, and pathogens, providing extremely valuable information on their structural dynamics. The reliability of such models is relevant to extending our existing knowledge of immune responses and the development of targeted vaccines. Computational modeling can be utilized to examine conformational changes in antigen-antibody complexes, which can reveal the chief mechanisms of immune recognition. It is not only complementary to experimental methods but also facilitates hypothesis generation, i.e., computational modeling can also assist in accelerating discovery in structural immunology. One of those areas where computational modeling has greatly assisted is in the domain of immunotherapeutic design. Through high-throughput computational techniques, scientists are able to predict how modifications in protein structures would render them more stable or more effective. For instance, structural models can design novel antibodies with improved binding affinities to specific epitopes, which would make them more therapeutic in character. Furthermore, the application of such methods as molecular dynamics simulations helps researchers assess the long-term functioning of these biomolecules in a simulated controlled space. The computational design process of iterative refinement of structures by simulated feedback permits researchers to remake their ideas and move towards more helpful immunotherapeutic agents that could eventually be applied clinically. Furthermore, the application of computational modeling to structural immunology extends far beyond even this modest aim of engineering immune-based therapies. It encompasses broader systems biology approaches to elucidating the dynamic networks regulating immune response. Workshops, such as the one that was run by The Global HIV Vaccine Enterprise, have also emphasized the importance of implementing computational methods in making predictions on how the immune system responds to a variety of stimuli, including pathogens and vaccines (Pulendran et al., 2010). Systems-based approaches allow identification of key pathways and regulatory processes that may affect vaccine effectiveness. Therefore, as computational power continues to evolve, they will naturally become ever more central to the information informing structural immunology approaches, eventually contributing to the development of novel therapeutic strategies and advancing our overall understanding of the immune landscape.

12.5.1. Introduction to Computational Techniques

The introduction of computational approaches to structural immunology represents a paradigm shift in the description of immune system dynamics. Computational methods are able to model complex biological systems and enable one to simulate immune interactions at the molecular level. Tools such as molecular dynamics simulations and protein structure prediction enable researchers to visualize and forecast how antibodies will work against pathogens and thus help in the design of vaccines and therapeutics. These computational approaches not only reduce experimental time and expense but also refine the search for new immunotherapeutics by concluding unattainable prior to their application. They, therefore, serve as a powerful bridge between theoretical immunology and practical methods, an era in which data-driven decision-making guides immunological advancement and therapeutic intervention, ultimately resulting in better health outcomes in various immunological disorders. A good example of the utility of computational approaches can be found in diseases like Common Variable Immunodeficiency (CVID). CVID is a heterogeneous, complex disorder with several immunological defects that complicate timely and accurate diagnosis. The application of machine learning pipelines, such as those described in recent research, demonstrates how computational approaches can critically investigate flow cytometric immunophenotyping data. Through offering a computer-aided identification of B cell populations, such pipelines not only eliminate subjective prejudices inherent in the human analysis but also enhance diagnosis. Such advancements again underscore the significance of computational techniques in structural immunology, where precise identification of immune profiles is crucial to differentiate between different antibody deficiencies and implement the appropriate treatment protocols, as in Emmaneel et al. (2019). Also, the increase of computational techniques in structural immunology promises more efficient research methods and therapeutic advances. With advancing computational powers, researchers can employ large datasets to search for patterns and correlations that inform their interpretation of immune responses. This is particularly evident through high-throughput sequencing and biostatistical analysis, which enhance researchers' ability to observe the complexity of the immune system. With machine learning and artificial intelligence, the potential to predict outcomes from immunotherapy has increased dramatically. These methods supplement traditional experimental approaches, setting computational methods at the center of new immunology research and paving the way for more effective, targeted medical therapies. The integration of computational and structural approaches is the future direction of immunology, in harmony with the emergent need for advanced diagnostic and therapeutic techniques in diverse immune disorders, as discussed in Pappalardo et al. (2015) (Figure 12.11).

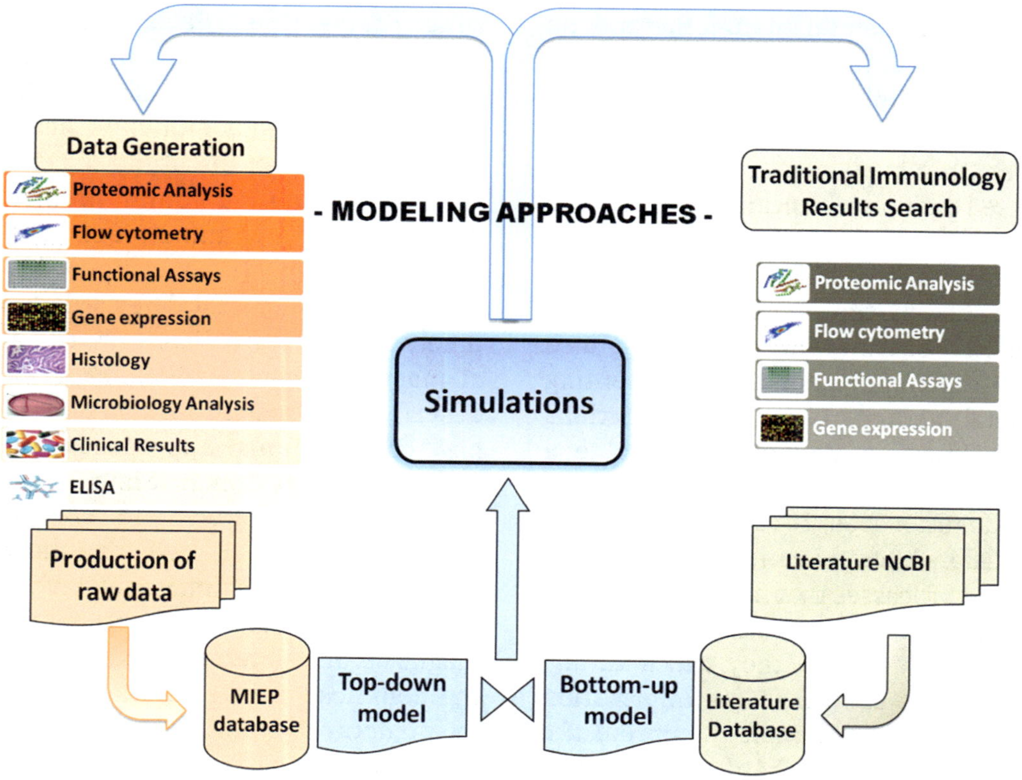

Figure 12.11. The integration of computational techniques into structural immunology represents a paradigm shift that enhances our understanding of immune system dynamics.

Source: https://www.nimml.org/images/figures/Modeling-figure-white-background-1024x758.png.

12.5.2. Role in Predicting Protein Structures

In the discipline of structural immunology, protein structure predictive modeling is increasingly significant. With highly advanced computational techniques, scientists can model and visualize proteins' three-dimensional structures, which is crucial in understanding their functions in the immune system. For example, in-silico B-cell epitope prediction tools demonstrate how molecular mechanics can enhance the classification and analysis of protein structures. With the use of such sophisticated algorithms, researchers are not only enhancing the accuracy of structural predictions but also opening the way to more efficient vaccines and therapeutics. These advances are a testament to the synergy between protein structure information and its potential application in immunology, particularly in making targeted therapies reliant on correct molecular interaction (Reitmaier, 2007). Protein structure prediction is also at the heart of understanding the mechanism of many immunological diseases. A very good example of such a case could be CVIDs. With the help of advanced techniques such as whole genome sequencing coupled with transcriptomic profiling, researchers can identify genetic variants responsible for causing CVIDs, which usually have a heterogeneous presentation.

This form of analysis not only suggests disease-associated pathways, such as T cell regulation and B-cell receptor signaling, but also provides insight into individual-specific aetiologies that can be used to inform personalized treatment strategies. Therefore, the integration of structural predictions and genetic data allows deeper insights into immune system disorders to be attained, guiding the search for targeted and effective therapies (van Schouwenburg et al., 2015). Besides, the progress of computational methods in structural prediction sheds light on interdisciplinary collaboration in structural immunology. The complementation of data derived from molecular dynamics simulations and experimental approaches, e.g., X-ray crystallography or NMR spectroscopy, refines the predictive system, whereby computer models can be tested. Such collaboration increases resolution at the level of protein structure required for immune perception and response. Although scientists are constantly refining these predictive approaches, implications for vaccine development, antibody manufacture, and therapeutic treatments become increasingly profound. By merging this computational prediction with empirical data, not only are significant advances in structural immunology made, but also the potential to cure complex immune-related diseases effectively is improved (Reitmaier, 2007; van Schouwenburg et al., 2015) (Figure 12.12).

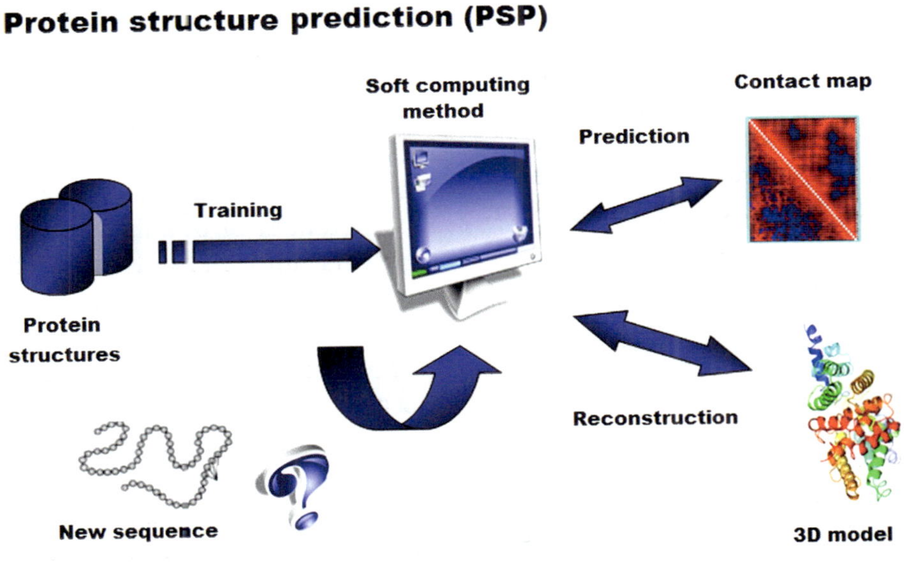

Figure 12.12. Protein structures prediction (PSP).

Source: https://ars.els-cdn.com/content/image/1-s2.0-S1568494615003737-fx1_lrg.jpg.

12.5.3. Integration with Experimental Data

The integration of experimental data with structural immunology techniques is a central crossroads of immune complexity understanding. Using techniques such as X-ray crystallography and cryo-electron microscopy, researchers are able to reveal the three-dimensional structure of macromolecules involved in immune activity. This structural insight enables the identification of interaction interfaces so that specific research on how diverse immunological entities, such as antibodies and antigens, interact can be undertaken. Moreover, merging experimental findings allows structural hypotheses to be confirmed, which ensures that models represent biological realities. Such integration not only enhances our initial knowledge but also provides access to the development of novel therapeutic interventions and vaccine design, whose effects directly influence clinical results. For EAE as an MS model, however, the necessity of integrating experimental data with structural information is perhaps even more vital. The presence of TLOs within the central nervous system, as in MS patients, underscores the necessity of combined information at multiple scales of biological organization. Experimental data from EAE models also reveal crucial aspects of TLO formation and operation that are at the heart of explaining the disease's pathological characteristics. As outlined in more recent studies, the finding that B cells potentially have a significant role to play in chronic inflammation and their involvement in relation to TLOs further complicates the immune response landscape. This intricate dance necessitates the meeting of structural and experimental paradigms to dissect underlying mechanisms and facilitate the design of targeted interventions (Mitsdoerffer & Peters, 2016). Moreover, the ramifications of uniting structural data with experimental observation extend beyond mere research to inform clinical applications. Explaining the unique roles of B cells and T cells in the TLOs can be used to uncover disease-progression biomarkers and treatment targets. Although scientists progress toward seeing immune architecture at high resolution, it becomes essential that these observations be correlated with clinical data. TLO cell-cell interactions are so intricate that they require the application of sophisticated computational models that agree with structural information as well as experimental results. This integrative approach not only enhances hypothesis testing but also provides an interactive platform for predicting how changes in immune structure may influence disease outcome. Through the collaboration of structural immunologists and experimental biologists, the future becomes promising paths towards identifying successful solutions in autoimmune condition management (Pappalardo et al., 2015).

12.6. Hybrid Techniques

The discipline of structural immunology has increasingly embraced hybrid approaches to probe and regulate protein structures with increasing precision and versatility. One such major advance is the design of hybrid proteins, wherein segments of one protein or peptide are incorporated into one system. It is reported that the deployment of class A -A-lactamases as universal scaffolds is one illustration of the potential of building bifunctional proteins by this approach. Hybrid proteins allow researchers to carry out various functions, such as the expression of proteins that would otherwise be structurally unstable or difficult to characterize. By the insertion of exogenous peptides at permissive locations, researchers are able not only to better comprehend protein structure-function correlation but also to generate antibodies against otherwise nonimmunogenic epitopes, thereby increasing the repertoire available for the performance of immunological research (Huynen et al., 2013). Furthermore, the establishment of nanobodies, which are derived from Camelid heavy-chain-only antibodies, has revolutionized the application of hybrid approaches in structural immunology. These single-domain antibodies possess various advantageous characteristics, making them preferable over traditional antibodies, particularly in a laboratory setting. Because of their small size and stability, nanobodies can penetrate tissues more readily and bind to epitopes that would be inaccessible to large antibody formats. Recent debate highlights the role of nanobodies in various applications, including reagents in detection in fluorescence microscopy and in protein-protein interaction studies, particularly in mass spectrometry. Their ability to be engineered to enhance their versatility gives them significance as analytical tools for studying protein function and dynamics within complex biological systems, hence their validity in hybrid strategies to understand immunological processes (Beghein & Gettemans, 2017). The use of hybrid methods in structural immunology not only increases experimental modes but also provides more precision for immunological studies. By combining various components from different protein sources, researchers can create new, innovative reagents to get past specific challenges in structural description. Hybrid nanobodies and proteins are perfect examples, with prospects to develop specific reagents that can be used across a variety of study applications. Since we move ahead to grow protein engineering, integrating these hybrid approaches together brings challenging opportunities to recognize new therapeutic options and understand immune response mechanisms at the molecular level. Such a union of hybrid approaches and structural immunology thus holds revolutionary potential for biomedical research in the future (Huynen et al., 2013; Beghein & Gettemans, 2017).

12.6.1. Definition and Importance of Hybrid Approaches

Structural immunology hybrid approaches integrate disparate techniques to better understand complex biological systems. Through integration of traditional experimental techniques and advanced computational frameworks, researchers are better able to characterize the multiple-dimensional nature of immune responses. For instance, experimental data from animal models, cell-based assays, or tissue cultures can systematically be evaluated via machine learning algorithms. Such convergence facilitates the identification of novel therapeutic targets and biomarkers for drug response prediction. Such kind of approaches are critical in immunology when the pathophysiologies of diseases like atopic dermatitis (AD) are not well known. A combined strategy yields more precise data about disease mechanisms that are often overlooked by individual-study research, hence illuminating the basal cutaneous biology, molecular mechanisms, and therapeutic advances (Eyerich et al., 2018). Moreover, the structure of hybrid proteins itself shows the utilitarian application of hybrid approaches in structural immunology. By manipulating protein scaffolds through protein engineering techniques, researchers are in a position to engineer bifunctional proteins, which have basic roles in drug discovery and disease modeling. Specifically, the ligation of exogenous peptides or protein pieces into exogenous scaffolds, such as class A -lactamases, is responsible for generating structures that are not naturally occurring. This technique not only provides a better understanding of structure-function interactions but also propels the creative design of antibodies against nonimmunogenic epitopes (Huynen et al., 2013). Thus, through circumventing limitations inherent to traditional protein expression and characterization techniques by hybrid approaches, researchers can markedly increase the scope of immunological studies. The worth of hybrid approaches lies not in their direct application but in inducing an era of innovation in treatment planning. Blending different models and approaches applies even to precision medicine, where customized treatments are sought through patient-specific profiles. As an illustration, integrating predictive computational models with *in vivo* and *in vitro* studies unravels specific AD subtypes and thereby informs specific treatment protocols. With increasing research, these integrative methods will indeed be crucial in bridging gaps in our knowledge of immune-related diseases. Such an integrated method equips researchers with the means to tackle the intricateness of immunological responses and gives impetus to the achievement of efficient, personalized therapeutic regimens, particularly in scenarios where existing models fall short (Eyerich et al., 2018) (Figure 12.13).

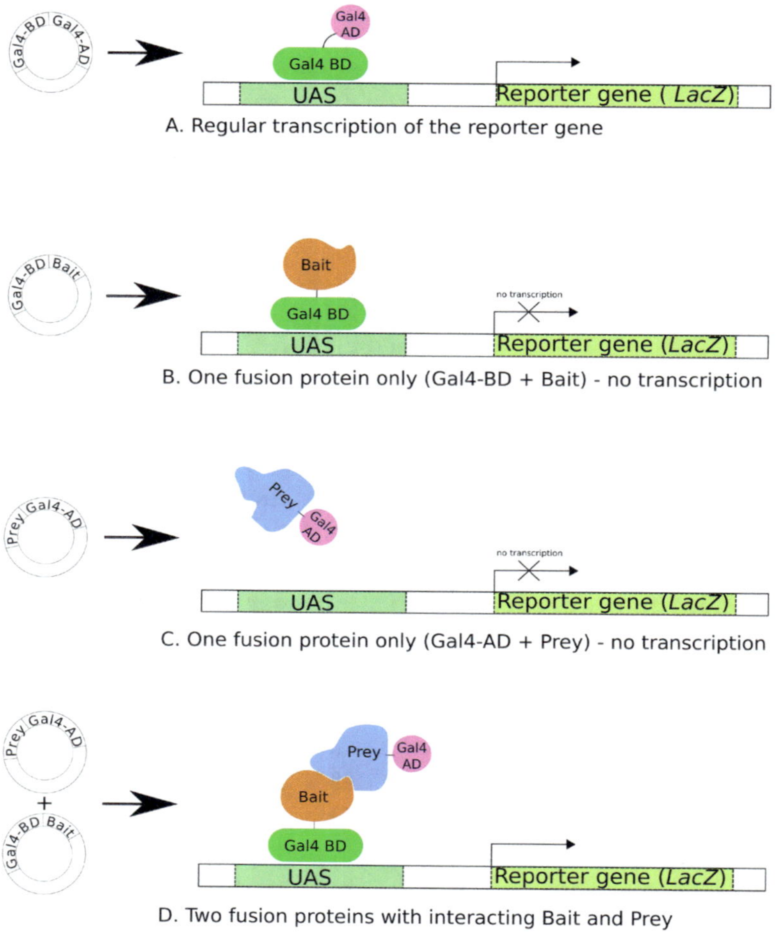

Figure 12.13. Overview of two-hybrid assay, checking for interactions between two proteins, called here Bait and Prey. A. The Gal4 transcription factor gene produces a two-domain protein (BD and AD) essential for transcription of the reporter gene (LacZ). B, C. Two fusion proteins are prepared: Gal4BD+Bait and Gal4AD+Prey. Neither of them is usually sufficient to initiate transcription (of the reporter gene) alone. D. When both fusion proteins are produced and the Bait part of the first fusion protein interacts with the Prey part of the second, transcription of the reporter gene occurs.

Source: https://upload.wikimedia.org/wikipedia/commons/thumb/6/61/Two_hybrid_assay.svg/800px-Two_hybrid_assay.svg.png.

12.6.2. Examples of Hybrid Techniques in Use

The use of hybrid methods in structural immunology indicates the onward convergence of computational and experimental methods. A good example is data mining in the analysis of medical data sets, i.e., dermatology. Using classification, clustering, and association mining procedures, researchers can obtain crucial information that helps in the diagnosis of erythemato-squamous disease. These methods enable the identification of patterns among large volumes of data from cases of skin disease, enhancing diagnostic reliability and leading to targeted therapy. These evidence-based approaches emphasize how computational resources need to be integrated into routine biological research, ultimately leading to improved patient care through informed decisions and successful diagnosis (Barati et al., 2011).

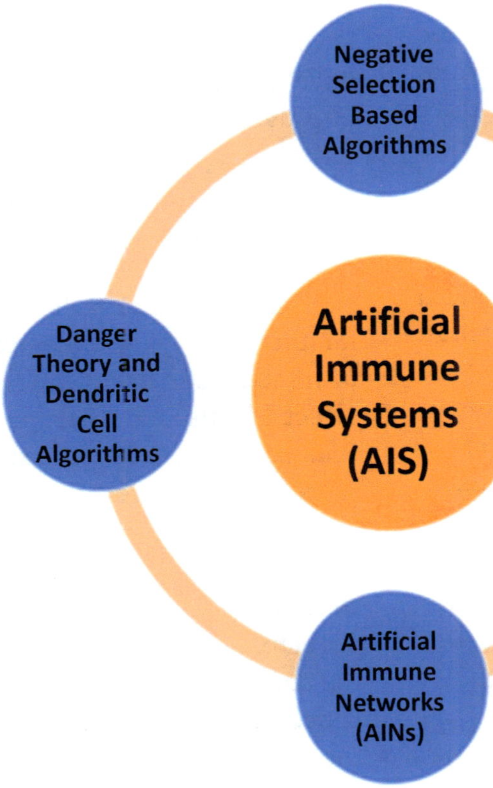

Figure 12.14. Artificial immune systems (AIS).

Source: https://www.researchgate.net/profile/Raed-Zitar/publication/339666692/figure/fig4/AS:1038233781665800@1624545631792/Artificial-immune-systems-AIS.png.

Moreover, Artificial Immune Systems (AIS) are currently in development as a new hybrid approach that combines computational intelligence and immunology principles. AIS simulate the human immune system to address multi-computational issues. Recent advancements have proved that AIS can optimise algorithms for many applications, including image classification and anomaly detection in medical images. By mimicking the adaptive immunity response, AIS can be employed to enhance data analysis in structural immunology and thereby facilitate the development of new therapeutic strategies. The hybrid approach emphasizes the importance of interdisciplinary research towards establishing the field (Al-Enezi et al., 2010). In addition to data mining and AIS, another prominent hybrid approach is the integration of structural biology with computational modeling and simulation. Such a strategy allows researchers to see and predict immune molecule behavior at the atomic scale. Methods like X-ray crystallography and cryo-electron microscopy, complemented with simulation approaches, offer important information regarding immune response mechanism dynamics. By combining empirical observations with computationally derived predictions, scientists are able to build better models of immune interactions, laying the groundwork for novel vaccine designs and treatments. This confluence of experimental and computational approaches is typical of the evolving new face of structural immunology, which promises improved treatments and a deeper understanding of immune dynamics (Figure 12.14).

12.6.3. Future Directions for Hybrid Methodologies

In the ongoing evolution of structural immunology, future directions in hybrid methodologies are essential in answering the sophisticated questions of the field. One of the most important challenges remains the need for a robust framework capable of accommodating the synthesis of heterogeneous methods and technologies. This leads to the challenge of formalization, and it becomes more imperative to have a generic model that not only defines the intricate details of hybrid structures but also facilitates comparative studies for differing hybrid systems. The evolution of hybrid methods will require concerted activity in system design to make sure that structural immunology embraces an integrated process which brings together disparate disciplines so as to foster cooperation and creativity in theory and practice (Hamann et al., 2016). In addition, the interdisciplinarity of structural immunology creates the imperative for effective synthesis of methodologies across various fields.

This combination of immunology, computational modeling, and biotechnology necessitates a hybrid strategy that allows researchers to capitalize on insights from several different fields. Recent investigations have highlighted the advantages of integration of proven techniques and advanced technology, e.g., AI-based analytics, that can potentially be applied to enhance our understanding of immunological responses at the molecular level. These activities are needed not only to improve experimental approaches but also to account for the underlying biological rules, which will ultimately benefit the development of more effective disease therapeutic interventions (Valente et al., 2013). Lastly, embracing these future possibilities for hybrid methods can potentially make structural immunology a more generalized and integrated science. By identifying times of increased significance within biological development—such as the research described in the aquaculture setting—scientists can establish concentrated strategies that bolster insight into the comprehension of immune reactions and the effectiveness of vaccines. By establishing working platforms that allow for knowledge to be exchanged across disciplines, hybrid approaches can be significantly maximized. As boundaries between natural and artificial systems become more blurred, the advancement of this interdisciplinary conversation will be pivotal to the innovative structural immunology methods, ultimately reaching improved global health results (Hamann et al., 2016).

SUMMARY

The advancement in structural immunology methods has enabled us to grasp the intricacy of immune systems to a large degree. Technologies such as crystallography and cryo-electron microscopy have enabled us to determine the three-dimensional structures of complex immune molecules. In addition to this advance in knowledge about how antibodies and antigens interact, it paves the way for new therapeutic approaches against a large number of diseases. As highlighted by recent studies, the application of new computational methods can further improve epitope prediction and classification, emphasizing the integrative process characteristic of contemporary immunology research (Reitmaier, 2007). The continuous evolution of such methods underscores the necessity of combining traditional experimental approaches with cutting-edge technology to propel this field. Furthermore, the impact of such structural approaches extends beyond basic research to guide applied purposes in drug and vaccine design. For example, understanding the structural dynamics of immunity has led to more effective vaccine preparations that induce robust immunological reactions. The interactions between the structural properties of antigens and the consequent immune system responses validate the importance of a detailed approach towards developing immunotherapy methods in compliance with specific patient needs. As also observed in the case of the problem generated by pathogens such as Amyloodinium ocellatum, it is essential to perform ongoing research involving proteomic and immunological studies. Appreciation of the roles played by these pathogens on host responses illustrates the value of state-of-the-art structural approaches in unmasking the pathogenic mechanisms and immunoevasion strategies employed (Moreira et al., 2017).

Ultimately, the future of structural immunology methods awaits further advancement, coinciding with the request for interdisciplinarity between researchers. With the evolving tools, the focus should be on integrating genetic, biochemical, and clinical data to effectively address immune responses to diseases. This multi-pronged approach will not only reveal deeper insights but also enable the creation of personalized therapies and vaccines so that they can evolve with evolving pathogens. By embracing the worth of various methodologies, the field can continue to make significant advances in combating disease and ultimately improve human health outcomes. The integration of these advanced methods promises a new future for immunology, one in which thoughtful decision-making through the availability of structural knowledge is the basis of inquiry and clinical practice. In structural immunology, there is a variety of fundamental techniques crucial to the understanding of the complex interactions between antigens and antibodies. Among the best-known is X-ray crystallography, through which scientists can study the atomic structure of immunological complexes at high resolution. The technique has enabled researchers to visualize significant binding sites and understand how specific conformational changes drive immune response. In addition to X-ray crystallography, NMR spectroscopy provides a dynamic view of the inherent mobility of proteins in solution and illuminates the way conformational states can affect antigen recognition. Together, these methods provide more insight into the molecular mechanisms of immune responses and pave the way for the rational design of vaccines and therapeutic antibodies. Cryo-EM has become a critical technique in structural immunology, particularly for large and complex macromolecular complexes that cannot easily be crystallized. Cryo-EM rapidly freezes samples, and as they do so, they stabilize proteins and assemblies of proteins in their native conformations and provide valuable information on their structures and motions. This is particularly useful when analyzing multi-subunit immune complexes, where standard methods might not be sufficient. Additionally, the ability to examine proteins in a quasi-physiological environment also places cryo-EM as a powerful tool in unveiling how different conditions regulate antigen-antibody interactions. These observations are critically significant in the development of new immunotherapies and for attaining an appreciation of the intricate processes involved in antigen processing and presentation. Cryo-EM hence, considerably enriches the armory at the hands of immunologists, bridging the structure-function gap. Another key structural immunology method is that of bioinformatics, which operates parallel to experimental procedures through the provision of computational models and simulations to anticipate the molecular interaction. Bioinformatics uses algorithms to probe large sets of data and assists in identifying candidate epitopes and antigenic determinants that are not immediately obvious from studies of the structure alone. Machine learning is further refining the predictive power of such models so that good targets for vaccine development and antibody development can be rapidly established. By combining bioinformatics with experimental results, researchers are able to narrow down what they expect to happen and streamline the process of discovery. The combination of computational prediction and experimental confirmation ultimately propels the efficiency and efficacy of research in structural immunology, facilitating the creation of novel therapeutics as well as enhancing our understanding of immune responses (Seaman & Whitehouse, 2001; Smits et al., 2006).

A CLOSER LOOK

PROTEIN STRUCTURE DETERMINATION

Proteins are a major component in the research community and their structures are of great concern to the researcher.

Various techniques and methods have been used to determine this, but one of the most influential has been the development and identification of X-ray crystallography.

The tertiary structure of a protein determines its properties and behavior. The primary methods used to study this are:

X-Ray Crystallography:

- This method provides maximum information regarding the tertiary structure of a protein. X-rays are passed through a rotating crystal and diffracted rays are focused on a target and recorded by computerized systems.
- Crystal quality is critical; thus, it generates highly high-resolution data for atomic structure within a strongly held protein with other neighboring ions, ligands and molecules, but will perhaps not be so successful with proteins with large flexible domains and thus don't yield highly ordered crystalline forms. It requires relatively large amounts of the protein.
- As this reason, recombinant proteins are typically produced in the specified quantity and then purified of contaminants, protein refolding and crystallization studies. It can provide very high resolution.

Electron Microscopy and Cryo-Electron Microscopy:

- These methods are suitable for the study of large macromolecule complexes or even organelles from within cells, which are relatively larger on the molecular scale, and can be employed to reconstruct the tertiary structure of a single particle. This has the huge advantage of circumventing the challenging need for protein crystallization.
- Cryoelectron microscopy is a temperature form at or below liquid nitrogen and can observe protein structures of very high resolution, though lower than that of methods like NMR spectroscopy or crystallography.
- It also accepts minute protein amounts and reduces the artefacts due to radiation damage.

Nuclear Magnetic Resonance (NMR) Spectroscopy:

- This method depends on the effect of varying radiofrequency waves on the nuclear resonance of various atoms in the protein.
- It needs increased protein quantities in a stable soluble form at room temperature, and stable for the long duration of data accumulation.
- The proteins also need to be small in size to avoid overlapping peaks.

- Even so, it offers a better resolution. It is ideal if protein crystallization is impossible, such as in the case of flexible proteins or where system dynamics need to be explained in detail.

Small-Angle X-Ray Scattering and Small-Angle Neutron Scattering:

- Both methods are suitable for protein structure analysis, where limited resolution will suffice. Experimental conditions can be better controlled because the protein is usually in solution.

Homology Modeling:

- This enables researchers to achieve a three-dimensional view of a protein. It makes use of knowledge of the close homologue or template, which has a very high proportion of identical amino acid sequence to the analyte.
- Protein modeling from this template is dependent on the aspect that protein structure is conserved in the majority of cases.

Partial Structural Study Methods:

- They include ultracentrifugation, mass spectrometry and fluorescence spectrometry, which can be used to complement other approaches (Figure 12.15).

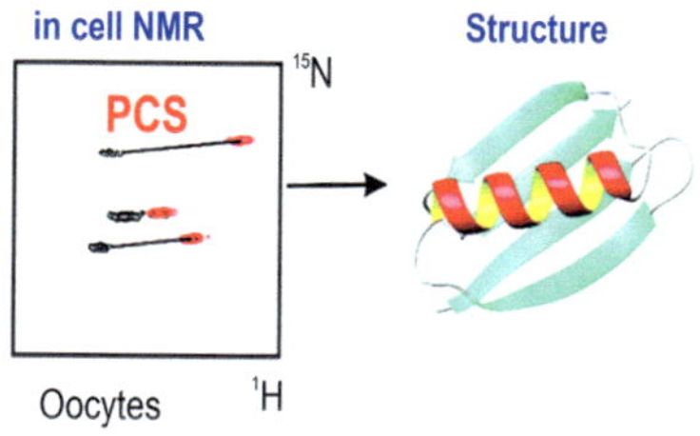

Figure 12.15. 3D structure determination of a protein in living cells using paramagnetic NMR spectroscopy.

Source: https://pubs.rsc.org/en/Content/Image/GA/C6CC05490K.

REFERENCES

1. Al-Enezi, J. R., Abbod, M. F., & Alsharhan, S. (2010). Artificial immune systems–Models, algorithms and applications. IJRRAS 3 (2) ● May 2010. https://core.ac.uk/download/8010.pdf (accessed on 27th June 2025).
2. Moreira, M., Schrama, D., Soares, F., Wulff, T., Pousão-Ferreira, P., & Rodrigues, P. (2017). Physiological responses of reared sea bream (Sparus aurata Linnaeus, 1758) to an Amyloodinium ocellatum outbreak. *Journal of fish diseases*, *40*(11), 1545–1560. https://doi.org/10.1111/jfd.12623(accessed on 27th June 2025).
3. Achari, A. J. R., Barton, G., Bond, P., Davis, R., Emsley, P., Evans, J., et al. (2012). FolX from *Pseudomonas aeruginosa* is octameric in both crystal and solution. https://core.ac.uk/download/1439067.pdf (accessed on 27th June 2025).
4. Pulendran, B., Rappuoli, R., Aderem, A. *et al.* Novel approaches, including systems biology, to HIV vaccine research and development: Report from a Global HIV Vaccine Enterprise Working Group. *Nat Prec* (2010). https://doi.org/10.1038/npre.2010.4798.1(accessed on 27th June 2025).
5. Barati, E., Mohammadi, A., Adibi, N., Ahmadzadeh, M. R., et al. (2011). A survey on utilization of data mining approaches for dermatological (skin) diseases prediction. https://core.ac.uk/download/1667194.pdf (accessed on 27th June 2025).
6. Valente, L.M.P., Moutou, K.A., Conceição, L.E.C., Engrola, S., Fernandes, J.M.O. and Johnston, I.A. (2013), What determines growth potential and juvenile quality of farmed fish species?. Rev Aquacult, 5: S168-S193. https://doi.org/10.1111/raq.12020(accessed on 27th June 2025).
7. Marrocco I, Altieri F, Peluso I. Measurement and Clinical Significance of Biomarkers of Oxidative Stress in Humans. *Oxid Med Cell Longev*. 2017;2017:6501046. doi:10.1155/2017/6501046(accessed on 27th June 2025).
8. Maciejewski, M., Tjandra, N., & Barlow, P. N. (2011). Estimation of interdomain flexibility of N-terminus of factor H using residual dipolar couplings. *Biochemistry*, *50*(38), 8138–8149. https://doi.org/10.1021/bi200575b(accessed on 27th June 2025).
9. Miguel R. Guevara, Dominik Hartmann, Manuel Aristarán, Marcelo Mendoza, and César A. Hidalgo. 2016. The research space: using career paths to predict the evolution of the research output of individuals, institutions, and nations. Scientometrics 109, 3 (Dec 2016), 1695–1709. https://doi.org/10.1007/s11192-016-2125-9(accessed on 27th June 2025).
10. Calisti, L., Trabuco, M. C., Boffi, A., Testi, C., Montemiglio, L. C., des Georges, A., Benni, I., Ilari, A., Taciak, B., Białasek, M., Rygiel, T., Król, M., Baiocco, P., & Bonamore, A. (2018). Engineered ferritin for lanthanide binding. *PloS one*, *13*(8), e0201859. https://doi.org/10.1371/journal.pone.0201859(accessed on 27th June 2025).
11. Beghein, E., & Gettemans, J. (2017). Nanobody Technology: A Versatile Toolkit for Microscopic Imaging, Protein-Protein Interaction Analysis, and Protein Function Exploration. *Frontiers in immunology*, *8*, 771. https://doi.org/10.3389/fimmu.2017.00771(accessed on 27th June 2025).
12. Liu, Y. T., Tao, C. L., Lau, P. M., Zhou, Z. H., & Bi, G. Q. (2019). Postsynaptic protein organization revealed by electron microscopy. *Current opinion in structural biology*, *54*, 152–160. https://doi.org/10.1016/j.sbi.2019.02.012(accessed on 27th June 2025).

13. MacLachlan, B. J., Greenshields-Watson, A., Mason, G. H., Schauenburg, A. J., Bianchi, V., Rizkallah, P. J., Sewell, A. K., Fuller, A., & Cole, D. K. (2017). Using X-ray Crystallography, Biophysics, and Functional Assays to Determine the Mechanisms Governing T-cell Receptor Recognition of Cancer Antigens. *Journal of visualized experiments : JoVE*, (120), 54991. https://doi.org/10.3791/54991(accessed on 27th June 2025).

14. Eyerich, K., Brown, S. J., Perez White, B. E., Tanaka, R. J., Bissonette, R., Dhar, S., Bieber, T., Hijnen, D. J., Guttman-Yassky, E., Irvine, A., Thyssen, J. P., Vestergaard, C., Werfel, T., Wollenberg, A., Paller, A. S., & Reynolds, N. J. (2019). Human and computational models of atopic dermatitis: A review and perspectives by an expert panel of the International Eczema Council. *The Journal of allergy and clinical immunology, 143*(1), 36–45. https://doi.org/10.1016/j.jaci.2018.10.033(accessed on 27th June 2025).

15. Emmaneel, A., Bogaert, D. J., Van Gassen, S., Tavernier, S. J., Dullaers, M., Haerynck, F., & Saeys, Y. (2019). A Computational Pipeline for the Diagnosis of CVID Patients. *Frontiers in immunology, 10*, 2009. https://doi.org/10.3389/fimmu.2019.02009(accessed on 27th June 2025).

16. Hamann H, Khaluf Y, Botev J, Divband Soorati M, Ferrante E, Kosak O, Montanier J-M, Mostaghim S, Redpath R, Timmis J, Veenstra F, Wahby M and Zamuda A (2016) Hybrid Societies: Challenges and Perspectives in the Design of Collective Behavior in Self-organizing Systems. Front. Robot. AI 3:14. doi: 10.3389/frobt.2016.00014(accessed on 27th June 2025).

17. Pappalardo, F., Brusic, V., Pennisi, M., & Zhang, G. (2015). Advances in Computational Immunology. *Journal of immunology research, 2015*, 170920. https://doi.org/10.1155/2015/170920(accessed on 27th June 2025).

18. Stijlemans B, De Baetselier P, Caljon G, Van Den Abbeele J, Van Ginderachter JA, Magez S. Nanobodies As Tools to Understand, Diagnose, and Treat African Trypanosomiasis. *Front Immunol.* 2017;8:724. Published 2017 Jun 30. doi:10.3389/fimmu.2017.00724(accessed on 27th June 2025).

19. Ekser, B., Li, P., & Cooper, D. K. C. (2017). Xenotransplantation: past, present, and future. *Current opinion in organ transplantation, 22*(6), 513–521. https://doi.org/10.1097/MOT.0000000000000463

20. Ivanova, G., Pereira, T., Caseiro, A. R., Georgieva, P., & Maurício, A. C. (2016). Metabolomic and Proteomic Analysis of the Mesenchymal Stem Cells' Secretome. InTech. doi: 10.5772/66101 (accessed on 27th June 2025).

21. van Schouwenburg, P. A., Davenport, E. E., Kienzler, A. K., Marwah, I., Wright, B., Lucas, M., Malinauskas, T., Martin, H. C., WGS500 Consortium, Lockstone, H. E., Cazier, J. B., Chapel, H. M., Knight, J. C., & Patel, S. Y. (2015). Application of whole genome and RNA sequencing to investigate the genomic landscape of common variable immunodeficiency disorders. *Clinical immunology (Orlando, Fla.), 160*(2), 301–314. https://doi.org/10.1016/j.clim.2015.05.020(accessed on 27th June 2025).

22. Cebi, E., Lee, J., Subramani, V. K., Bak, N., Oh, C., & Kim, K. K. (2024). Cryo-electron microscopy-based drug design. *Frontiers in Molecular Biosciences, 11*. https://www.semanticscholar.org/paper/96e1eff9ea182c39c6287827fef66bd55a065373 (accessed on 27th June 2025).

23. Cooper, A., Garofalo, A., Cooper, A., Buschiazzo, A., Brunger, A. T., Kragelund, B. B., Smith, B.

O., et al. (2011). Solution structure of a repeated unit of the ABA-1 nematode polyprotein allergen of *Ascaris* reveals a novel fold and two discrete lipid-binding sites. https://core.ac.uk/download/110380.pdf (accessed on 27th June 2025).

24. Daniel Lozano-Ojalvo, Sara Benede, Celia M. Antunes, Simona L. Bavaro, Grégory Bouchaud, et al.. Applying the adverse outcome pathway (AOP) for food sensitization to support in vitro testing strategies. Trends in Food Science and Technology, 2019, 85, pp.307-319. ⟨10.1016/j.tifs.2019.01.014⟩. ⟨hal-02623081⟩

25. Cornell University. (1998). *College of Veterinary Medicine*. https://ecommons.cornell.edu/bitstream/handle/1813/38441/COS_v89_1997_98_16.pdf?sequence=1&isAllowed=y (accessed on 27th June 2025).

26. Vanakker, O. M., & De Paepe, A. (2013). Pharmacogenomics in children: advantages and challenges of next generation sequencing applications. *International journal of pediatrics, 2013*, 136524. https://doi.org/10.1155/2013/136524(accessed on 27th June 2025).

27. De Vos, F., Dubruel, P., Schacht, E., Van Vlierberghe, D., et al. (2009). Affinity study of novel gelatin cell carriers for fibronectin. https://core.ac.uk/download/55759270.pdf (accessed on 27th June 2025).

28. Elke Smits, Elie Ratinckx, Vincent Thoen o.l.v. prof. Koenraad Debackere, Elisabeth Monard, Danielle Raspoet (2006). *Technologie en innovatie in Vlaanderen: Prioriteiten*. https://core.ac.uk/download/pdf/6468460.pdf (accessed on 27th June 2025).

29. Di Carluccio, C., Padilla-Cortés, L., Tiemblo-Martín, M., Gheorghita, G. R., Oliva, R., Cerofolini, L., Masi, A. A., et al. (2025). Insights into Siglec-7 binding to gangliosides: NMR protein assignment and the impact of ligand flexibility. *Advanced Science, 12*. https://www.semanticscholar.org/paper/f9af6a01cd4b07964ff9f1b00e49a3979d742c50 (accessed on 27th June 2025).

30. Huynen, C., Filée, P., Matagne, A., Galleni, M., & Dumoulin, M. (2013). Class A β-lactamases as versatile scaffolds to create hybrid enzymes: applications from basic research to medicine. *BioMed research international, 2013*, 827621. https://doi.org/10.1155/2013/827621 (accessed on 27th June 2025).

31. Hoff, S. E., Thomasen, F. E., Lindorff-Larsen, K., & Bonomi, M. (2024). Accurate model and ensemble refinement using cryo-electron microscopy maps and Bayesian inference. *PLOS Computational Biology, 20*. https://www.semanticscholar.org/paper/13cb254aefef892d2b876b37f1edf0d5ec926ebb (accessed on 27th June 2025).

32. Kornahrens, W. J. (2014). Recent advances and challenges in antigen engineering & vaccine development. https://core.ac.uk/download/211337211.pdf (accessed on 27th June 2025).

33. Mitsdoerffer, M., & Peters, A. (2016). Tertiary Lymphoid Organs in Central Nervous System Autoimmunity. *Frontiers in immunology, 7*, 451. https://doi.org/10.3389/fimmu.2016.00451(accessed on 27th June 2025).

34. K. Saxena, S. (Ed.). (2022). High-Throughput Screening for Drug Discovery. IntechOpen. doi: 10.5772/intechopen.91075(accessed on 27th June 2025).

35. Orlova, E. (2012). Bacteriophages and their structural organization. https://core.ac.uk/download/19509491.pdf (accessed on 27th June 2025).

36. Ouhtit, A., Zerhane, R., & Janati-Idrissi, R. (2025). How do theoretical frameworks influence immunology teaching? Insights from case studies in Morocco. *Multidisciplinary Science*

Journal. https://www.semanticscholar.org/paper/264768cd47c8eff8c32ec7a84593788e4a4615f5 (accessed on 27th June 2025).

37. Sánchez-Vidaña DI, s R, Wong MS. The Use of Omic Technologies Applied to Traditional Chinese Medicine Research. *Evid Based Complement Alternat Med.* 2017;2017:6359730. doi :10.1155/2017/6359730(accessed on 27th June 2025).
38. Reitmaier, R. (2007). Review of immunoinformatic approaches to *in-silico* B-cell epitope prediction. https://core.ac.uk/download/pdf/287415.pdf (accessed on 27th June 2025).
39. Rombouts, K., Braeckmans, K., & Remaut, K. (2016). Fluorescent labeling of plasmid DNA and mRNA: Gains and losses of current labeling strategies. https://core.ac.uk/download/55851519.pdf (accessed on 27th June 2025).
40. Seaman, W., & Whitehouse, J. H. (2001). Florida marine biotechnology: Research, development and training capabilities to advance science and commerce. https://core.ac.uk/download/11016354.pdf (accessed on 27th June 2025).
41. Weygand, J. (2017). Identifying the immune related metabolic properties of pancreatic cancer using nuclear magnetic resonance spectroscopy and dynamic magnetic resonance spectroscopic imaging with hyperpolarized pyruvate. https://core.ac.uk/download/130044971.pdf (accessed on 27th June 2025).
42. Zachau, H. G. (2000). The immunoglobulin κ gene families of human and mouse: A cottage industry approach. https://core.ac.uk/download/19418517.pdf (accessed on 27th June 2025).

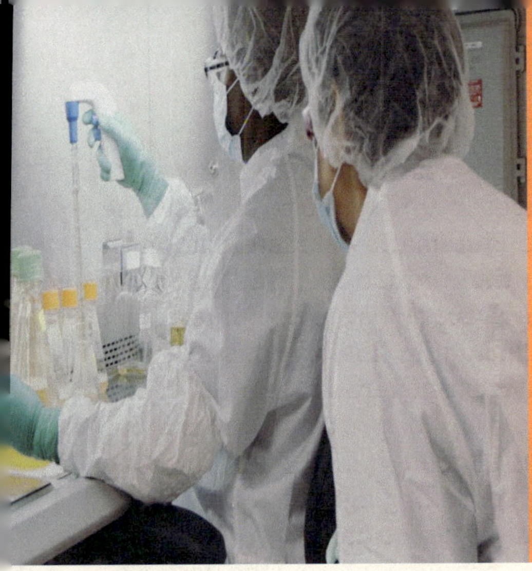

Chapter 13

IMMUNE PROFILING AND OMICS APPROACHES

Contents

Introduction

Omics technologies have revolutionized the field of immunology to enable the precise definition of immune responses based on the analysis of large amounts of data. Omics approaches like genomics, transcriptomics, proteomics, and metabolomics offer researchers the tools to investigate the intricate networks involved in immune functions at the biological level. Through the application of these methodologies, researchers can identify novel biomarkers and therapeutic targets, particularly in complex diseases wherein dysregulation of the immune system is the determining feature. For instance, by means of proteomic analysis, scientists have begun to unravel the physiological impact of parasitic infections, as reported in investigations of Amyloodinium ocellatum infestations of gilthead sea bream, illustrating how immune profiling can provide insight into host-pathogen interaction (Moreira et al., 2017). Thus, I.P., when integrated with omics approaches, can significantly enhance our understanding of immune mechanisms. Moreover, the interaction of the immune system with a multifaceted microbiome also further emphasizes the need to integrate omics technologies with I.P. The human metabolome and microbiome reveal an array of complexity far greater than our current fund of knowledge in human genomics. Emerging evidence indicates that specific microbial communities and the resultant metabolic byproducts play a profound role in influencing immune responses, hence the necessity for an interdisciplinary examination of immunity. With continued discoveries of new associations between microbes, metabolites, and immune processes, an organized research model is necessary to analyze and exploit such interactions effectively (Dorrestein et al., 2014). By extensively examining these networks, investigators can gain better insights into the function of the microbiome in disease and health and, in turn, develop novel approaches for immunotherapeutic interventions. In total, the union of immune profiling with omics technology represents a paradigmatic revolution in immunology that enables the full understanding of immune dynamics in health and disease. With the development of the discipline, continuous refinement of analytical techniques and computational methods will facilitate the extraction of meaningful conclusions from extremely complex datasets generated through omics analysis. Moreover, overcoming the challenges posed by the complexity of immune responses, particularly in diverse groups and under varied environmental conditions, remains an urgent agenda. With the overcoming of these obstacles, scientists can leverage the synergy between immune profiling and omics to develop more effective diagnostic and therapeutic interventions, enhancing disease control and better health outcomes in different settings. Through this, the possibility of an in-depth understanding of immune mechanisms seems more within reach.

Definition of Immune Profiling

Immune profiling is a vital principle underlying the complex association of the immune system with disease, especially in the context of personalized medicine. In simple terms, immune profiling is the systematic characterization of immune cells, their functions, and secreted molecules. This process makes use of an array of techniques, including flow cytometry, mass cytometry, and next-generation genomic and proteomic analysis to provide researchers with a snapshot of an individual's immune profile. Through shedding light on the personal immune signatures associated with health or disease, immune profiling informs the design of precision therapies aimed at targeted immune pathways for enhanced efficacy and decreased side effects. The integration of immune profiling and omics approaches is a conceptual shift in immunology research. Omics technologies, such as genomics, transcriptomics, and proteomics, yield vast data sets that, when combined with immune profiling, can delineate the intricate molecular mechanisms responsible for immune responses. As an illustration, the use of transcriptomic information in combination with immune profiling can define how particular gene expressions correlate to immune cell activation or damage. Furthermore, the use of multimodal omics strategy facilitates researchers to construct detailed models of immune system responses to various circumstances, such as disease or autoimmune disease. Not only do such an understanding increase our awareness of immunological processes but also facilitate identification of personalized biomarkers that might usher in improved disease management approaches. In the context of chronic disease, immune profiling is of particular interest because it allows for the identification of distinct immune signatures that may have the potential to influence the development of diseases and responsiveness to therapies. As an example, in cardiometabolic conditions, understanding immune dysregulation may reveal informative biomarkers for assessing one's predisposition to such disease. As delineated in a recent review, the integration of multi-omics approaches with immune profiling has the potential to unveil intricate perspectives of disease mechanisms and therapeutic targets (Scola et al., 2019). Moreover, the expansion of immune profiling to other populations with regard to gender differences enhances our ability to customize interventions to individual-specific immunological profiles and, further, towards better healthcare outcomes (Fels et al., 2017). In short, immune profiling, integrated with omics science, is an emerging edge of immunological research that holds the potential to give rise to individualized therapeutic advances (Figure 13.1).

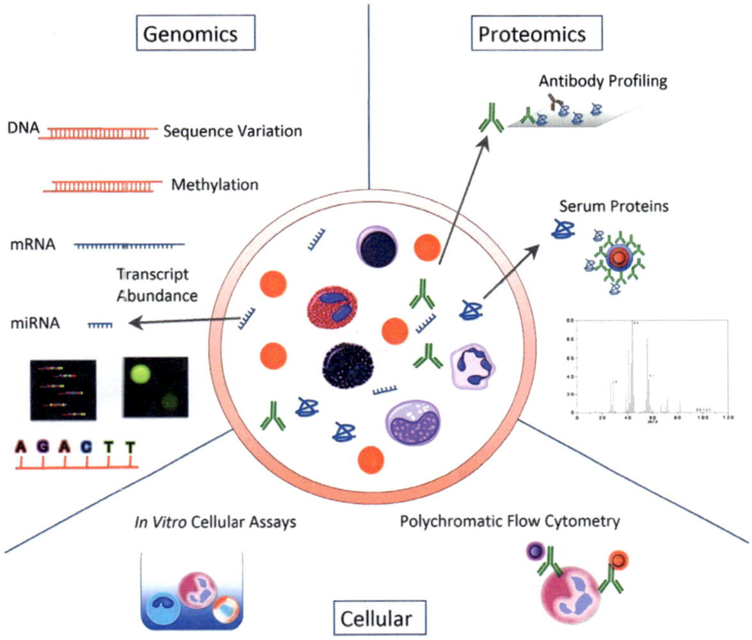

Figure 13.1. The immune profiling armamentarium. The number of high-throughput molecular and cellular profiling tools available for the assessment of the human immune system from blood is increasing rapidly.

Source: https://www.researchgate.net/profile/Nicole-Baldwin-3/publication/226732848/figure/fig1/AS:340299915251718@1458145230841/The-immune-profiling-armamentarium-The-number-of-high-throughput-molecular-and-cellular.png.

Overview of Omics Approaches

The omics term denotes a group of scientific disciplines that aim to extensively study biological molecules in various systems. The involved methodologies include genomics, proteomics, transcriptomics, and metabolomics, focusing on various molecular components and their functional importance. Genomics provides insights into genetic differences and inherited diseases, while transcriptomics looks into patterns of gene expression. Proteomics extends this assessment by studying the structure, function, and interactions of proteins. Together, these approaches enable scientists to construct an integrative view of cellular function and its derangement in disease. This global profiling is used to define biomarkers and therapeutic targets, particularly in immunology, where immune responses can be monitored and modulated readily. Metabolomics has emerged as a significant field here with emphasis on metabolite research, i.e., small molecules that reflect the biochemical status of cells. This profiling captures cellular metabolism and activity in real time, illuminating disease-related pathways. For instance, recent metabolomics research has elucidated the derangements in metabolism for multifactorial disorders like psoriasis and its comorbidities and revealed potential biomolecular signatures to guide clinical diagnosis and treatment (Yan et al., 2017). By charting the transformations in metabolic pathways, researchers are in a position to expose new therapeutic opportunities and biomarkers for enhancing the validity of immune profiling. Furthermore, advances in high-throughput technologies have significantly redefined the omics landscape. Next-generation sequencing and advanced proteomics allow for swift and accurate detection of pathogens and resistance profiles, particularly in infectious diseases. The increasing incidence of opportunistic infections necessitates the description of sensitive and specific diagnostic methods in an effort to effectively address therapeutic issues. Traditional methods lag behind because of attention to sensitivity and specificity, coupled with the need for pre-cultivation of pathogens. Conversely, new omics technologies pave the way for quicker diagnoses, such as yeast pathogen detection, showing that they have an essential role to play in clinical microbiology (Consortium OPATHY & Gabaldón, 2019). The transition towards the adoption of these technologies into practice in the healthcare sector shows they are capable of revolutionizing the management of disease and therapeutic precision (Figure 13.2).

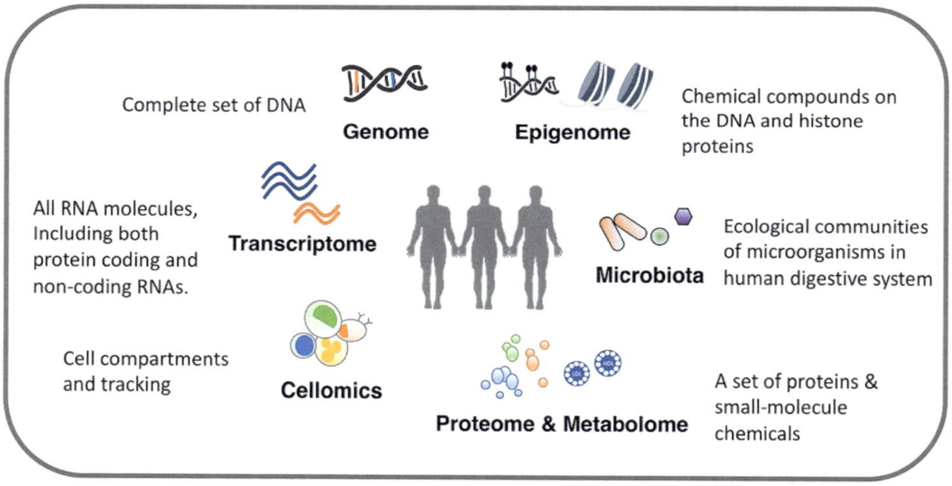

Figure 13.2. Overview of omics data.

Source: https://www.frontiersin.org/files/Articles/668045/fimmu-12-668045-HTML/image_m/fimmu-12-668045-g001.jpg.

Importance of Integrating Immune Profiling with Omics

The synergy between immune profiling and omics technologies is a breakthrough in the field of understanding the complexity of intricate biological systems. By combining information from various omics layers—genomics, transcriptomics, proteomics, and metabolomics—a scientist can get a holistic view of immune responses. The multiaxial approach allows for the detection of disease biomarkers, particularly in oncology. Through systems biology, which deals with the understanding of intricate interactions within biological entities, scientists can develop better predictive models of immune behavior and its implications on disease and health. Proper application of large datasets, as highlighted in recent studies, would be capable of pushing the body of knowledge in animal sciences and other biological sciences to personalized therapies that lean towards improved patient outcomes over conventional methods (Woelders et al., 2011). For cancer research, the combination of immune profiling data with omics has proven to have a great deal of potential in constructing more accurate treatment approaches. Immune processes are at the root of tumor development, and detailed immunoprofiling can potentially reveal clues about tumor biology and elucidate cancer cell-microenvironment interactions. It is now possible with new digital pathology and machine learning technologies to analyze extensive histological information, which can potentially better outline the immune tumor landscape. This could potentially enhance the risk stratification process and therapeutic decision-making, as observed through studies looking into the relation between immune markers and outcome (Frei, 2024). The repetitive process of combining immune profiling with omic information can create a feedback loop that continuously refines treatment modalities to trend toward the creation of precision medicine. Additionally, the revolutionary potential of combining immune profiling with omics extends into greater use cases beyond cancer, such as multiple disease applications, such as autoimmune diseases and infectious diseases. Omics technologies allow high-throughput analysis, which, together with immune data, can generate advanced networks reflecting interactions between genetic, environmental, and immunologic parameters. Such a combined platform allows not only disease-specific biomarker detection but also understanding the pathogenesis mechanisms. Such a holistic vision enables researchers and clinicians to adopt a systems biology approach, revealing new therapeutic targets and interventions. Hence, its significance is underscored by its potential to enhance multifactorial illness comprehension, ultimately benefiting public health initiatives and custom-fitted therapeutic plans (Woelders et al., 2011).

13.1. Fundamentals of Immune Profiling

Immune profiling has emerged to symbolize a significant part in the appreciation of the intricate dynamics between host immune responses and most pathogens. This field includes the scientific investigation of cellular and molecular components of immune response, typically using omics technologies to provide a detailed insight into immune function. Immune cells such as T-cells and B-cells, or cytokines and antibodies, can be profiled or tracked by scientists in order to define signatures that indicate the condition of immune systems in disease and health. The dynamic nature of immune profiling allows us to establish biomarkers that are pivotal for disease prognosis, monitoring the response to therapies, and personalizing treatments. Immune profiling is thus at the boundary of traditional immunology and modern genomics, opening the way for advanced computational and technological diagnostic and therapeutic strategies that have a significant beneficial effect on patient care. Omics approaches, including genomics, proteomics, and metabolomics, have revolutionized immune profiling by allowing researchers to examine large data sets associated with immune responses in unprecedented detail. These approaches enable researchers to not only investigate the components of the immune system but also their interactions and roles within the broader biological context. For instance, proteomics can determine how single proteins involved in immune response are regulated under certain conditions, and metabolomics gives an insight into the metabolic pathways responsible for immune activation and regulation. Integration of these multi-omics datasets will lead to the identification of new immunological patterns concealed in monomodal analyses. Therefore, synergistic application of omics technologies enhances immune response knowledge and emphasizes the worth of developing more sophisticated, specific immunotherapies for the treatment of diseases such as cancer and autoimmune disorders and reveals the intricacy of immune system performance and mechanisms. Despite the encouraging potential in immune profiling provided by the application of omics technologies, there are several challenges still present requiring additional study and development. Host-pathogen complexity, for instance, may mislead interpretation of profiling data, as recently depicted by the SARS-CoV-2 pandemic globally. The incident showed the limitation of information being solely generated from known pathogen agents and conveyed the need for an agnostic approach to biodefense, as seen in current research. Whereas there are robust assays to measure the different aspects of immune response, there are no analytical tools and computational software needed to measure the results in an integrated fashion. Bridging these gaps is crucial in optimizing the potential of immune profiling. Investment needs to be made in integrative analysis pipeline development to be able to harness new technologies to their complete potential, thereby making researchers learn to appreciate the complexity in immune profiling and aiding the creation of effective therapeutic regimens (Labuda et al., 2018; Lin et al., 2024).

13.1.1. Techniques Used in Immune Profiling

The immune profiling branch has undergone tremendous transformation due to the advances in omics methodologies that now allow for a holistic exploration of the complexity of the immune system. Of the most striking among these is mass cytometry, which allows for multiparametric measurement of numerous parameters at the single-cell level. The technology utilizes metal-tagged antibodies and allows researchers to quantify a wide range of immune cell types and functional states across the scope of various biological contexts. Mass cytometry's ability to deliver high-dimensional data allows for a better understanding of immune dynamics, particularly in cancer immunology, in which the identification of particular cell populations is directly translatable into therapeutic intervention. With all these new techniques being embraced by scientists, there is an added need to learn the mathematical models and computational systems underlying data analysis to obtain reliable consistency of outcomes (Wang & Sarwal, 2015). Single-cell RNA sequencing (scRNA-seq) is yet another essential technique for immune profiling. This strategy provides not just a snapshot, but a dynamic picture of gene expression patterns within single cells, and it uncovers the heterogeneity of immune cell populations. Through the examination of transcriptomic landscapes of immune cells, scientists can determine discrete gene signatures that relate to various states of activation or differentiation, and these can be linked with disease progression and treatment outcomes. This approach is especially beneficial in cancer biology, where immune mapping could lead to the identification of novel biomarkers and targets for therapy. The scRNA-seq data complexity requires sophisticated computational techniques for the best analysis and interpretation. It is associated with visualization and selection of crucial biological information, underlining the importance of unifying immunological insights with sophisticated computational approaches (Caligola et al., 2022). Secondly, multi-omics data integration is a promising field in immune profiling. This entails the merging of genomic, transcriptomic, proteomic, and metabolomic data to provide an integrated picture of immune system behavior. By comparing different layers of biology, researchers can spot interdependencies and regulation mechanisms that govern immune responses. For instance, coupling transcriptomic information with proteomic profiles can show how gene expression leads to functional outcomes in immunology. Such integrated research is critical to the development of effective immunotherapeutic strategies, as it identifies predictive biomarkers that may be at the forefront of patient stratification. Future optimization of immune profiling techniques will depend on the collaboration of wet-lab platforms and computational resources (Wang & Sarwal, 2015) (Figure 13.3).

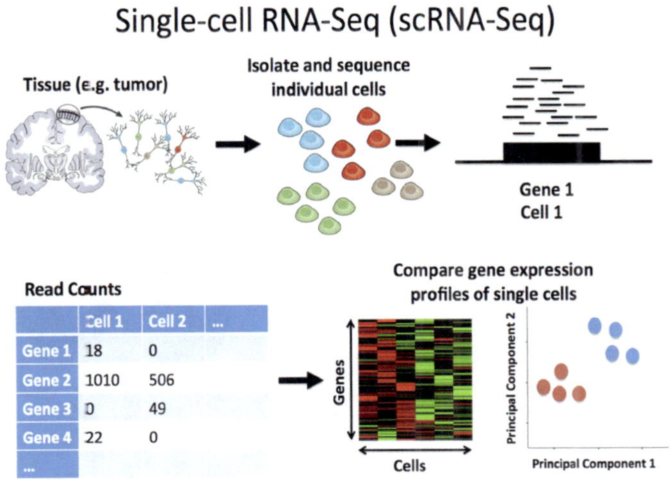

Figure 13.3. Single-cell RNA sequencing (scRNA-seq).

Source: https://learn.gencore.bio.nyu.edu/wp-content/uploads/2018/01/scRNA-overview.jpg.

13.1.2. Types of Immune Cells Analyzed

Immunological characterization of immune cells is central to appreciating the complexities of immune reactions and their implications in health and disease, particularly within the context of immune profiling and omics technologies. Immune cells like lymphocytes, monocytes, and dendritic cells are meticulously profiled to enumerate their specific functionalities and regulation. T cells, for instance, are split into subsets such as CD4+ helper T cells and CD8+ cytotoxic T cells, both of which play vital roles in orchestrating immune response against pathogens. The role of B cells in making antibodies is another determinant of their contribution to humoral immunity. This comprehensive examination of immune cell types not only underscores the intricacy of their diverse functions but also underpins the planning of therapy-based manipulation of immune responses in disease. Monocytes and macrophages represent yet another important group of immune cells. Monocytes are derived from precursors within bone marrow, and they differentiate into macrophages following migration into tissues. Macrophages play initiating and resolving roles in immune responses, as they can present antigens as professional antigen-presenting cells, secrete pro-inflammatory cytokines, and kill pathogens through phagocytosis. Macrophage plasticity allows them to accommodate different microenvironments necessary to maintain homeostasis and fight infections. Clarification of the functional phenotypes of the cells employing techniques like flow cytometry and transcriptomic profiling defines the nuanced interactions of different types of immune cells and may uncover novel targets for the therapy of inflammatory disorders or cancer. Finally, combining the omics approaches provides unprecedented information on the functional dynamics of immune cells.

Techniques such as transcriptomics and metabolomics allow profound insight into cellular signaling cascades, reprogramming of metabolism, and gene expression patterns. For instance, the application of metabolomics to investigate the metabolism of immune cells has provided insights into vital biochemical signatures linked with disease, such as psoriasis and related comorbidities. Connecting these metabolic shifts to the function of the immune cells allows researchers to read the driving mechanisms of the disease pathology. These advances, apart from furthering our understanding of immune networks, also provide a way forward for designing targeted therapies, as evidenced by the need for improved methods to combat powerful diseases as evoked by the emergence of drug-resistant pathogens (Swann et al., 2015). In brief, the complex repertoire of immune cells and conjunction of omics approaches complement each other to better elucidate immune reactions and how they impact health and disease (Yan et al., 2017) (Figure 13.4).

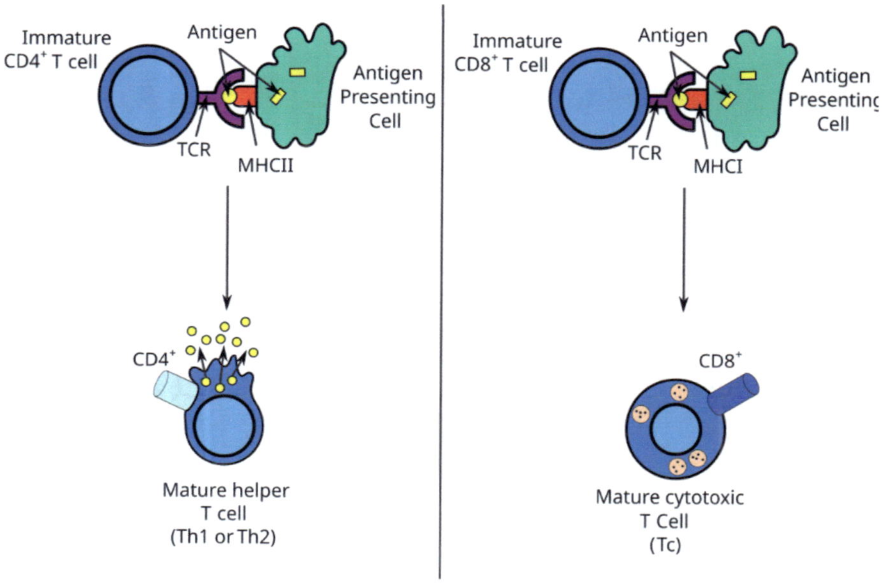

Figure 13.4. Antigen presentation stimulates naïve CD8+ and CD4+ T cells to become mature "cytotoxic" $CD8^+$ cells and "helper" $CD4^+$ cells, respectively.

Source: https://upload.wikimedia.org/wikipedia/commons/thumb/4/4d/Antigen_presentation.svg/1280px-Antigen_presentation.svg.png.

13.1.3. Applications in Disease Diagnosis

Advances in omics technologies have transformed the landscape of disease diagnosis by enabling a more precise and personalized assessment of a patient's condition. Among the key applications is the integration of multi-omics data, including genomics, transcriptomics, proteomics, and metabolomics. By combining knowledge from these different sciences, researchers are able to shed new light on the complex biological networks that operate in various diseases, such as cardiometabolic disease and inflammatory bowel disease. Not only does this integrative approach facilitate the identification of biomarkers, but it also enhances the understanding of disease processes, enabling better diagnostics by physicians and enabling personalized therapeutic strategies. The culmination of such endeavors underscores the potential of optimizing diagnostic approaches to result in improved patient outcomes as well as drive precision medicine in clinical settings. In the context of inflammatory bowel disease (IBD), the integration of immune profiling with omics analyses has outlined the intricate interplay of genetic, epigenetic, and environmental determinants driving pathogenesis of the disease. Recent evidence highlights the implication of heterogeneous cell types, i.e., immune and epithelial cells, in IBD through complex mechanisms of interaction with the microbiome. Using systems biology methods, researchers can investigate high-throughput molecular information to characterize the IBD interactome, which may identify central hubs that regulate disease progression. These advances are crucial for the delineation of novel therapeutic strategies capable of modulating these central regulators to treat the underlying causes of IBD. The incorporation of these advanced diagnostics not only further elucidates IBD but also provides a platform for the creation of personalized therapeutics aimed at the individual molecular alterations present in specific patients, thereby improving the efficacy of treatment. Immune profiling and omics technologies are also critical in the preclinical diagnosis and monitoring of disease, exemplified by their application in cardiometabolic disease. A large range of disease pathway-associated biomarkers serves as potential surrogates for accurate diagnosis and prediction. However, addressing the complexity of the diseases involves incorporating multi-omics data to obtain a broad picture of the molecular scenario. While researchers emphasize the applicability of gender medicine, they can also ensure that biomarkers are appropriately delegated and used in accordance with individual variation in the manifestation of disease. The combination of these methodological breakthroughs and advanced appreciations offers a promising way to the creation of novel diagnostic paradigms that may enhance early detection and increase options for managing cardiometabolic diseases, as well as other chronic conditions that remain difficult to diagnose with precision (Polytarchou et al., 2014; Scola et al., 2019) (Figure 13.5).

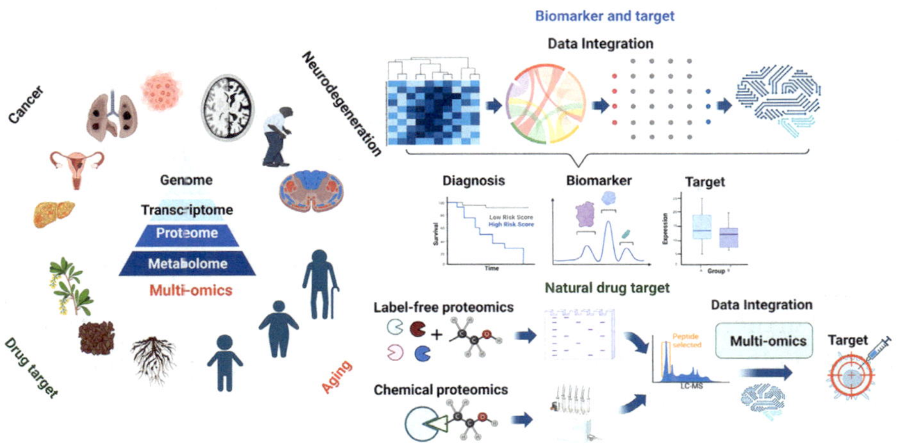

Figure 13.5. The application of multi-omics in disease, aging, and natural drug target identification.

Source: https://www.researchgate.net/publication/372882956/figure/fig5/AS:11431281181870088@1692211641189/The-application-of-multi-omics-in-disease-aging-and-natural-drug-target-identification.png.

13.2. Overview of Omics Technologies

Omics technologies have emerged to become wonderful tools enabling the global analysis of biological systems at the molecular level, such as genomics, transcriptomics, proteomics, and metabolomics. Genomics explores the complete set of an organism's DNA, finding genetic variations that underlie disease and immune responses. Transcriptomics explores RNA transcripts and provides data on patterns of gene expression in different physiological or disease states. These studies are instrumental in immune profiling, where the knowledge of gene expression can be employed to devise targeted therapies and immunotherapies. The intersection of these omics investigations enables researchers to develop multi-dimensional datasets that reflect cellular responses to stimuli and provide the gateway to a holistic understanding of immune function and disease pathogenesis. Proteomics, the study of the proteome, includes an additional layer of complexity by focusing on the vast number of resulting proteins from gene expression. With techniques such as mass spectrometry, proteomics allows researchers to determine protein abundance, modifications, and interactions within many immune environments. This is particularly relevant when considering immune profiling; shifting properties of protein expression can shed light on mechanisms governing immune response as well as disease biomarkers. Furthermore, advances in high-throughput proteomic technologies are sharpening our ability to quickly and accurately identify protein signatures associated with pathological conditions. Such developments are important since they make it possible to identify new drug targets and facilitate personalized medicine approaches based on individual protein profiles. Metabolomics, the study of small molecule metabolites, provides a dynamic snapshot of cellular metabolism and its regulation with respect to disease states or treatment. The method complements genomics and proteomics by illustrating how genomic and proteomic changes manifest through changes in metabolism. During immune profiling, metabolomic analysis can identify metabolic pathways that are individually activated during immune responses, which can have therapeutic implications. For instance, the discovery of metabolic signatures with specific immune cell types may indicate dysfunctions in the immune system. The integration of omics technologies, including metabolomics, also holds tremendous potential for accelerating the translation of fundamental research into clinical utility, particularly in disease diagnosis and treatment involving immune system dysfunction (Sánchez-Vidaña et al., 2017; Consortium OPATHY & Gabaldón, 2019).

13.2.1. Definition and Types of Omics (Genomics, Proteomics, and Metabolomics)

Omics is an umbrella term for a collection of life sciences exploring the complex relationships that underpin life at the molecular level. The best-understood types of omics are genomics, proteomics, and metabolomics, which provide different information important for the understanding of biological function. Genomics deals with the whole DNA set of an organism, examining gene sequence and structure and regulation. Such examination is vital for identifying genetic causes of susceptibility to disease and to therapy. Therefore, genomics is the basis for precision medicine through the revelation of individual genomic profiles, which can be utilized to direct individualized therapy strategies, especially in immunological disorders. Proteomics complements genomics by analyzing the complete set of proteins produced in a cell, tissue, or organism reflecting the dynamicity of biological systems when exposed to various stimuli. By applying high-throughput approaches, researchers can quantify proteins, define their functions, and determine how they function together in signaling pathways. This multiplex approach contributes to our understanding of immune responses as proteins are at the center of cell signaling, enzyme activity, and control of immune processes. Proteomic integration with genomic data is crucial in advancing immune profiling since protein expression tends to provide a functional readout of the genomic landscape and allows for enhanced insight into immune dysfunctions. Metabolomics, or the study of metabolic profiles of biological systems, introduces yet another level of complexity to comprehending organismal responses to environmental perturbations and disease states. Through quantification of small molecules such as metabolites, this omic process provides a measure of cellular function and metabolic pathways that are frequently targeted by disease. Coupled with genomics and proteomics, metabolomics contributes to giving an integrated view of biological organization. Together, these three omics provide an integrated system for immune mechanism dissection, especially host-pathogen interactions and the metabolic requirements of immune cells in an immune response. As highlighted in recent research, multi-omics integration is not only essential to the comprehension of genetic and molecular networks but also is a prospective research avenue for targeted drug generation in immunology (Swann et al., 2015; Scola et al., 2019) (Figure 13.6).

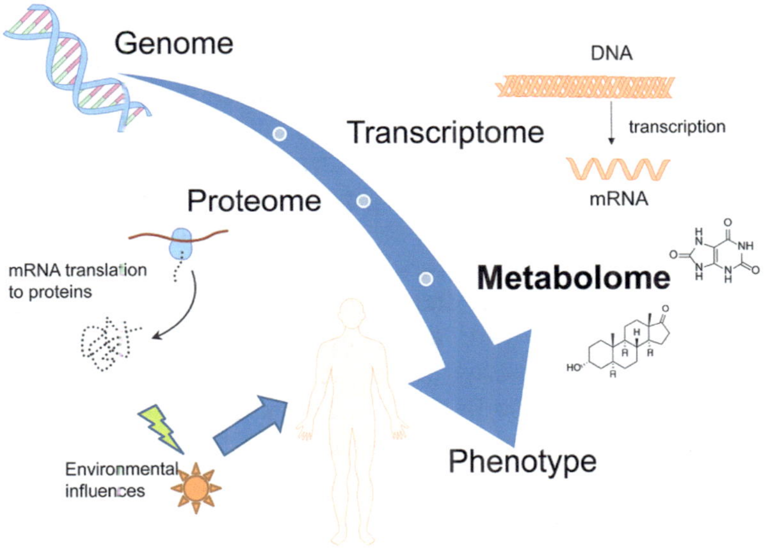

Figure 13.6. Overview of different omics-sciences such as genomics, transcriptomics, and proteomics. Metabolomics represents the downstream output of the genome but also the upstream input from the environment and is therefore positioned at the bottom of the "omics" cascade.

Source: https://www.researchgate.net/publication/333003279/figure/fig1/AS:11431281242988783@1715638694151/Overview-of-different-omics-sciences-such-as-genomics-transcriptomics-and-proteomics.tif.

13.2.2. Role of High-Throughput Technologies

High-throughput technologies have taken a pivotal role in investigating immune profiling and omics approaches, revolutionizing our understanding of complex biological systems. These technologies enable researchers to quantify the expression level of thousands of genes, proteins, and metabolites within a single biological sample at a time. Scientists can exhaustively interrogate TiME and shed light on intricate pathways that modulate immune responses against cancer therapy by employing such technologies. For instance, high-throughput sequencing technologies facilitate wide-ranging analysis of gene expression patterns, enabling identification of novel biomarkers with predictive value for therapeutic response. As such, the use of high-throughput assays enhances our molecular understanding of disease as well as enhances the evolution of precision medicine strategies toward fine-tuning therapies according to individual patient profiles. Application of some high-throughput technologies, such as spatial transcriptomics and multiplex immunofluorescence (mIF), also illustrates their role in progressing immune profiling. By using tools like Vizgens MERSCOPE® and in conjunction with ISP assays, scientists can spatially unscramble the complex molecular interactions between tumors and their microenvironments. By doing so, it is possible to distinguish how local microenvironments influence gene expression as well as immune cell function. In cancer biology, it is especially critical when studying these spatial interactions to understand tumor formation as well as immune evasion mechanisms. The synergy of strong immune profiling and high-resolution spatial analysis allows researchers to draw a more refined picture of the TiME, which is critical to successful immunotherapy design. Hence, high-throughput technologies do not just provide useful information but also provide synergistic opportunities to bridge molecular data to clinical use. Last but not least, high-throughput technologies, particularly single-cell omics, are opening the door to groundbreaking findings in immune profiling. These technologies circumvent the limitations of traditional bulk methods that smokescreen average cell populations, concealing the necessary cellular heterogeneity. By investigating gene expression at the single-cell level, researchers can uncover heterogeneous cellular populations, their various states, and how they participate in immune responses. Such granularity enables the identification of rare cell types potentially decisive in modulating immune responses, hence expanding the scope of potential therapeutic targets. Besides, the integration of multimodal approaches complements a holistic understanding of cellular interactions and regulatory networks. In this case, the high-throughput tools are the building blocks for understanding the complexities of immune profiling and extrapolating our knowledge of pathogenic processes, with the potential to enhance the precision of medicine for immunotherapy and cancer treatment.

13.2.3. Data Analysis Challenges in Omics

The increasing reliance on omics technologies for immune profiling has unfolded a galaxy of data analysis problems that researchers must navigate through. One of the most prominent issues is the sheer and heterogeneous nature of data generated across levels of omics, like genomics, transcriptomics, and proteomics. All of them generate different datasets reflecting biological processes at varied levels of molecules, rendering it challenging to aggregate information to create useful conclusions. In addition, the vast amount of information tends to lead to computational constraints, making sophisticated bioinformatics algorithms and tools a prerequisite for effective analysis. Here, researchers not only must contend with the complexity of single data sets but must also devise integration strategies for these, which defines the relevance and quality of the identified biomarkers in a clinic, as was highlighted in discourses surrounding the interface of multi-omics approaches of disease modeling and biomarker discovery (Scola et al., 2019). In addition, the inherent variability and noise of omics data are key challenges to reproducibility and interpretation. Sample preparation, measurement procedure, and biological variability can all create inconsistencies that render data from different studies problematic to compare. For instance, different sequencing technologies will yield differing outcomes even when used to analyze the same sample, which makes data alignment challenging and determining valid biomarkers difficult. This issue is particularly pertinent to immunology, where patient-specific variables such as age and sex can influence immune responses significantly. As has been stressed recently in research, for example, that on inflammatory bowel disease (Polytarchou et al., 2014), the integration of heterotypic data types is the key to deciphering the multifactorial pathogenesis of immunologic diseases. Therefore, computational tools must account for these variabilities to advance the field and enhance diagnostic accuracy. Lastly, integration of the omics data needs a systems biology strategy to overcome the analytical hurdles. Unraveling the intricacy of interactions in biological systems entails more than mere statistical and computational abilities and requires an intrinsic understanding of the underlying biological mechanisms. As researchers try to associate molecular changes with disease states, the challenge lies in accurately charting such networks. Systems biology approaches can be used to foretell regulatory nodes in biological pathways, and therapeutic targets and disease pathogenesis can be derived from this. Such methods are increasingly applied in conditions like cardiometabolic disease and inflammatory bowel disease, in which multi-omics integration is essential for deciphering mechanisms of disease (Polytarchou et al., 2014; Scola et al., 2019). Overcoming these analytical challenges will finally enhance our understanding of immune profiling and its role in precision medicine (Figure 13.7).

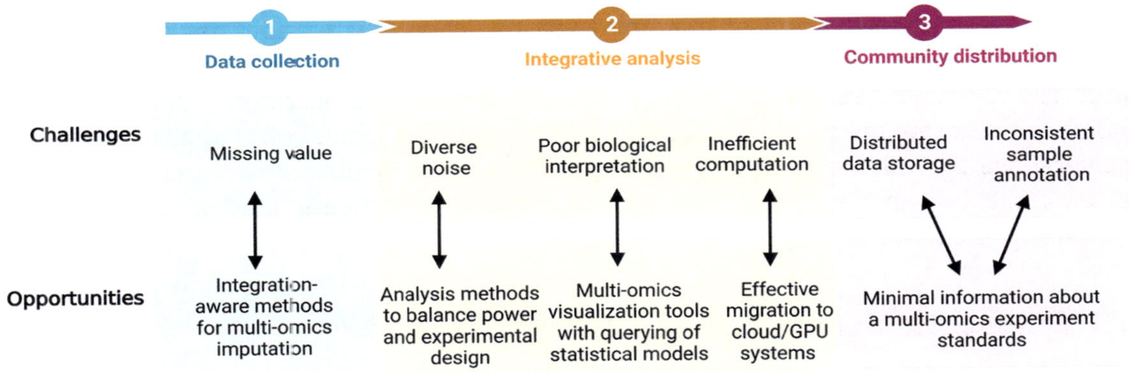

Figure 13.7. Challenges and opportunities for data integration of multi-omics. The analysis challenges together with possible solutions are presented for three different levels, such as data collection, integrative analysis, and community distribution.

Source: https://www.researchgate.net/publication/372882956/figure/fig7/AS:11431281181886513@1692211641574/Challenges-and-opportunities-for-data-integration-of-multi-omics-The-analysis-challenges.png.

13.3. Integration of Immune Profiling and Omics

The integration of immune profiling and omics approaches is a paradigm shift in our comprehension of the intricate immune response and its role in the pathology of disease. By leveraging progress in genomic, transcriptomic, proteomic, and metabolomic technology, researchers can assess the immune landscape across a large number of conditions, including autoimmune diseases and cancer. By combining these, it is possible to find typical biomarker signatures that would be capable of predicting disease progression and treatment response. For instance, the application of computational methods based on mathematical theories enables effective biomarker selection from high-dimensional omics data and thus enhances these clinical tests in terms of reliability. As stressed, the correct use of these computational tools matters when building clinically reasonable biomarker systems, thereby bridging basic research with clinical practice (Wang & Sarwal, 2015). In addition, the interaction between genetic, epigenetic, and immune factors plays a crucial role in multifactorial diseases such as IBD. Current evidence indicates that IBD pathogenesis is the result of intricate interactions among a variety of cellular components, including fibroblasts, immune cells, and the microbiome. A systems biology approach, employing a broad set of omics information, can be employed in the discovery of critical regulatory nodes within the IBD interactome and thereby, in all likelihood, the revelation of novel therapeutic targets. Incorporating molecular data across several levels, from genetic to metabolomic, scientists can deconvolute the intricate signaling cascades involved in IBD and other immune dysfunctions. This in-depth understanding could lead to personalized treatment methods, thus bridging the essential void for more effective therapies for immune-mediated diseases (Polytarchou et al., 2014). Furthermore, the integration of immune profiling with omics technologies is another step closer to dismantling the immune response in real time, enabling dynamic monitoring of patient health. With increasing high-throughput technologies, one can now evaluate multiple layers of biology in parallel, providing an n-dimensional representation of immune function. This holistic view not only elucidates the cooperation of immune components but also illuminates biochemical mechanisms of disease, such as cancer. The continuous refinement of computational models combing these scattered datasets has the ability to accelerate the translation of omics findings into useful clinical applications. Therefore, the convergence of immune profiling and omics transcends academic research to make a direct impact on clinical decision-making, thereby transforming therapeutic models in immunology and beyond (Wang & Sarwal, 2015).

13.3.1. Synergistic Benefits of Combining Approaches

The integration of multiple omics platforms provides a robust platform for comprehensive immune response profiling, with significant synergistic benefits. By integrating immunomics, transcriptomics, metabolomics, proteomics, and microbiomics, researchers are able to provide an unprecedented level of insight into complex biological system interactions. For instance, a recent multiomics pregnancy study found that simultaneous measurement of many biological pathways could be applied to enhance gestational age prediction. This approach not only improved predictive power but also showed new unmasked interactions between different biological modalities, thus providing an indication of clinical utility in the monitoring of pregnancy-associated pathologies such as preterm birth and preeclampsia (Ghaemi et al., 2019). These findings show that the use of multiple data types is capable of creating an integrated view of immune-related processes, paving the way for targeted interventions. Similarly, in the case of ulcerative colitis, synergy derived through the combination of transcriptomics and metabolomics has been a key breakthrough in disease mechanisms as well as patient diagnosis. With an integrated approach, several distinct biomarker panels were discovered that can differentiate between quiescent and active disease states. Through the application of complex analytical procedures, such as lasso regression and orthogonal-projection to latent structure-discriminant analysis, researchers established that the integration of these datasets would significantly improve the predictive potential more than the utilization of smaller, independent biomarker panels (Bjerrum et al., 2013). Not only does this improve the diagnostic precision, but it also facilitates molecular phenotyping of patients, therefore allowing for more personalized treatment regimens. Such successful applications underscore the significance of a multidisciplinary approach to surmounting complex biological challenges. Synergistic benefit in the concatenation of various omics strategies goes beyond diagnostics and catalyzes enhancements in personalized therapy and medicine. Through the integration of disparate biological data, researchers can successfully discover and validate new therapeutic targets, thus enhancing the precision of intervention designs. The information obtained through the use of multiomics analysis can propel the creation of immune-modulating therapies that are personalized to the patient profile, particularly in complex diseases where conventional methods might be lacking. With understanding coming to light regarding the intricacies of diseases, adopting this complete perspective calls for a paradigm shift in addressing diseases with comprehensive treatment strategies that cater to the individualized biological interaction inherent in every patient. The continuously evolving study and refinement of these combined methods in the context of immune profiling, therefore, has the potential to revolutionize patient care by personalizing therapies to the intricate biological landscape of diseases (Figure 13.8).

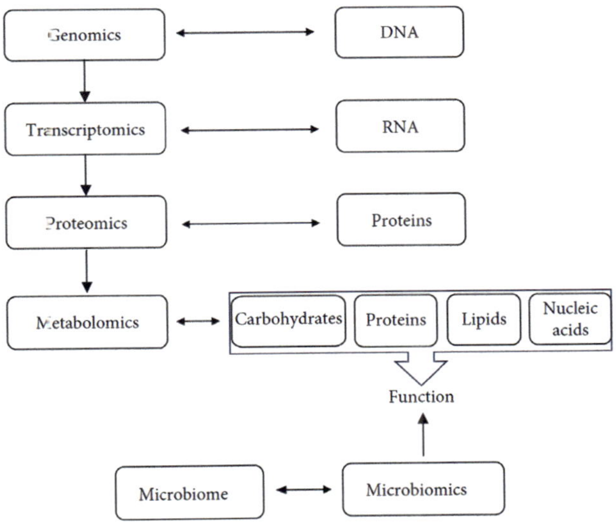

Figure 13.8. The relationship between genomics, transcriptomics, proteomics, metabolomics, and microbiomics.

Source: https://www.researchgate.net/publication/337746774/figure/fig1/AS:1086065838424066@1635949682140/The-relationship-between-genomics-transcriptomics-proteomics-metabolomics-and.jpg.

13.3.2. Case Studies Demonstrating Integration

In the domain of immune profiling and omics approaches, integration of multimodal data has made great strides towards unveiling our understanding of immune responses. A case study is incorporating single-cell omics technologies, which have transformed heterogeneity analysis of immune cells. Scientists have been able to dissect the complex cellular makeup of immune responses at unprecedented resolution with these technologies. The integration of transcriptomics and proteomics at the single-cell level allows for improved assessment of immune cell interaction dynamics, revealing previously obscured cell types and states. Eventually, such a comprehensive approach facilitates better insight into immune cell adaptation during infections and in disease, and the significance of integrating multiple distinct omics technologies in immune profiling has been emphasized (Lim et al., 2024).

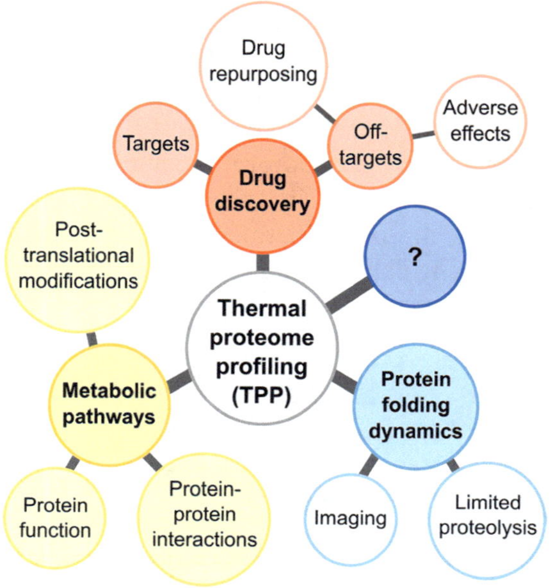

Figure 13.9. Examples of applications of thermal proteome profiling (TPP). In drug discovery, TPP can identify targets and off-targets. The latter can explain adverse effects or allow drug repurposing.

Source: https://www.researchgate.net/publication/317955415/figure/fig3/AS:963510376857640@1606730183567/Examples-of-applications-of-thermal-proteome-profiling-TPP-In-drug-discovery-TPP-can.gif.

Yet another fascinating case study demonstrates the strength in the integration of Thermal Proteome Profiling (TPP) with phosphoproteomics and transcriptomics in cancer studies, namely on Poly (ADP-ribose) polymerase (PARP) inhibition in ovarian cancer cells. COSMOS, an integrated multi-omics platform, makes this integration possible to discern the functional consequences of pharmacological treatments at different levels of biology. TPP provides insights into functional protein changes derived from thermal stability analysis, supplemented by information derived from transcriptomics and phosphoproteomics. This enabled scientists to map out the critical signaling pathways involved in cell cycle control and DNA damage response, thereby illuminating the subtle mechanisms through which PARP inhibition affects ovarian cancer cells. These findings highlight the utility of the integrative strategy, demonstrating how several omics modalities combined can collectively better clarify complex biological processes (Burtscher et al., 2024). Together, integrated insights obtained through combined omics strategies also have the potential to significantly aid precision medicine by tailoring treatment strategies based on one's molecular profile. A case in point, albeit high-profile, is immune response studies during chronic infection, where integration of multi-omics has discovered biomarkers for treatment response to be patient-specific. By using comparative transcriptomics, proteomics, and metabolomics analysis of immune cells, researchers have discovered certain molecular signatures that predict a successful therapeutic outcome. This multi-ancestry strategy not only illuminates more about the differences in immune response among individuals but also helps in the rational design of targeted intervention. Integrative case studies like these demonstrate the transformative potential of combining multiple omics technologies, a route to more effective, more personalized treatment regimens in immunology and other areas (Lim et al., 2024) (Figure 13.9).

13.3.3. Future Directions for Research

As researchers probe deeper into the intricate interface between immune profiling and omics technologies, the destiny of this area will more than likely lie with integrative systems biology approaches. These approaches have the potential to uncover greater understanding of the dynamics of complex diseases like IBD by explaining the interplay among genetic, epigenetic, and microbiomic factors. With the use of a holistic systems biology approach, researchers can identify regulatory centers in the intricate networks that direct disease pathogenesis and hence initiate the production of targeted therapies. This is particularly significant since evidence keeps demonstrating that various types of cells, such as fibroblasts and immune cells, dynamically interact in disease environments. Hence, integration of omics data from various platforms could significantly boost existing treatment strategies and reveal new facts and concepts in the immune dysregulation mechanisms governing IBD and other conditions (Polytarchou et al., 2014). Refining immunomonitoring research needs to move towards multi-omics integration that gives a multi-dimensional view of disease mechanisms. Through the integration of data from genomics, transcriptomics, proteomics, and metabolomics, researchers are now capable of constructing an integrative understanding of disease mechanisms, especially in cardiometabolic disorders (CMD). Future studies need to work on gathering and examining multidimensional data, recognizing that the study of each omics separately gives only a partial image of disease processes. The potential to decide reasonably well-fitted biomarkers relies on the integrative examination of these interconnected networks. Moreover, incorporating gender medicine into future studies could facilitate the identification of biomarkers specific to various populations, with consideration of the complex roles that biological and cultural determinants play in disease management (Scola et al., 2019). Furthermore, new technologies in bioinformatics and computational biology will be the focal point in determining the direction of future studies in immune profiling and omics approaches. The business of developing machine learning software and artificial intelligence techniques will assist in adding capabilities to manage and interpret the complex data generated by multi-omics studies. By facilitating recognition of patterns and correlation across big data, this technology can potentially improve predictive disease risk and response modeling. Furthermore, as databases grow bigger at public repositories, institutional knowledge interchange will be essential to integrate knowledge and tools. This collaboration will ensure that future research work is poised, permitting researchers to identify as-yet-unknown interactions within biological systems and enhance therapeutic interventions in various disease contexts. Interfacing sophisticated technologies is a significant milestone toward personalized medicine in immune profiling and omics research.

13.4. Immune Profiling in Cancer Research

The intricate interaction of the immune response with cancer has been an area of increasing interest during the past decade or so, particularly in the context of immune profiling. Such an analysis enables researchers to truly marvel at the nuanced interactions of tumor and immune effector cells, which are pertinent to the development of targeted therapies. Immune profiling employs advanced techniques such as flow cytometry and mass cytometry to profile immune cell populations within the tumor microenvironment. These approaches uncover the composition and functional characteristics of immune cells and facilitate unraveling tumor immune evasion mechanisms. Insights gained from immune profiling can aid in the discovery of biomarkers to predict patient response to immunotherapies, which subsequently contribute to better therapeutic regimens. In addition, integration of immune profiling with other omics technologies significantly enhances the understanding of cancer biology. For instance, genomics and transcriptomics can discover changes in the genes and patterns of expression within tumors that are capable of regulating the behavior of immune cells. By applying a systems biology approach, researchers can dissect complicated networks consisting of immune cells, tumor cells, and tumor stroma. Knowledge of these complicated networks allows researchers to uncover regulatory nodes of vital significance—hubs within the interactome that could prove valuable as therapeutic targets. Consistent with this, the combination of immune profiling and metabolomics, as was recently highlighted, can illuminate metabolic pathways responsible for immune dysregulation in cancer, and thus provide novel biomarkers to use in the clinic (Yan et al., 2017). Further augmenting such combined analyses, immune profiling with patient-derived samples can lead to revolutionary breakthroughs for personalized medicine. By characterizing the immune landscape inside tumors in patients with different genetic backgrounds and disease histories, researchers can determine differences that influence the reaction to cancer treatment. This tailoring can also enhance the categorization of cancer so that the treatment is accurately matched to a patient's unique immune signature. Immune profiling data can also inform inflammatory response research, for instance, in inflammatory bowel diseases, where there are cancer risk considerations (Polytarchou et al., 2014). Thus, the convergence of immune profiling and personalized omics technologies forms a sound platform to build on our understanding of cancer immunology and maximize patients' outcomes.

13.4.1. Role of Immune Profiling in Tumor Microenvironment

Immune profiling has more recently emerged as a key component in the elucidation of the complexity of the tumor microenvironment (TME). TME represents an evolving heterogeneous system composed of cancer cells, immune cells, stromal components, and extracellular matrix, all which interact with each other to shape the tumor behavior and patient prognosis. Immune profiling is used to identify immune cell subsets and their states of activation within tumors and offers useful information regarding the mechanisms by which tumors evade immune surveillance and react to therapeutic stress. Scientists are able to define the genomic, transcriptomic, and proteomic alterations occurring in immune cells from various cancers through the application of high-dimensional omics technologies. This global understanding facilitates the design of customized treatment plans that might maximize the patient's response to immunotherapies and other promising therapies for the immune system, thereby projecting the intrinsic role of immune profiling in the TME and its implied uses in clinics (Hu., 2017). Immune profiling also facilitates patient stratification based on the unique characteristics of their immune microenvironment. This stratification is particularly critical in those cancers with high immune response heterogeneity, e.g., mantle cell lymphoma (MCL), where traditional approaches might overlook subtle but significant differences in immune cell populations. Immune profiling has been proven to result in the identification of prognostic biomarkers that inform decision-making on treatment. For instance, the development of the minimal residual disease (MRD) monitoring strategies relies on the understanding of immune cell dynamics and their correlation with the drug response. By correlating the incidence of certain immune signatures with clinical responses, such as overall survival, researchers can potentially enhance risk stratification that guides therapeutic interventions based on individual patients.

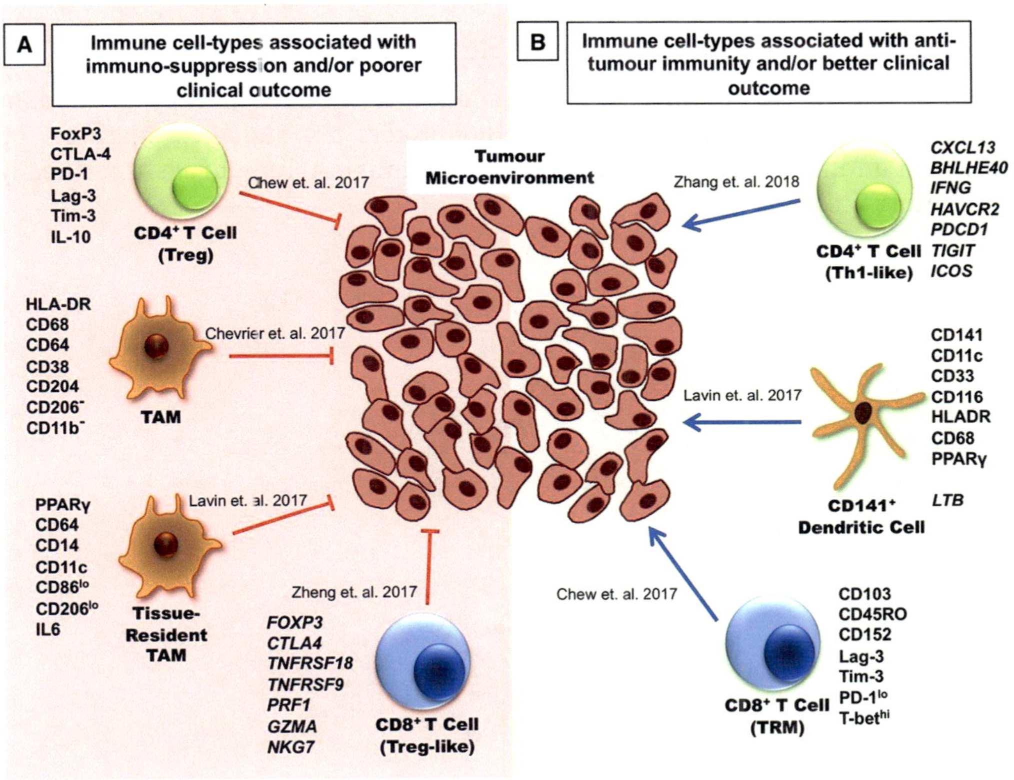

Figure 13.10. Characteristics of selective immune subsets important for antitumor immune activity as revealed by multidimensional immunoprofiling. (A) Immune cell-types correlated with immunosuppressive characteristics in the TME and poorer clinical outcomes in patients with cancer. (B) Immune cell types correlated with antitumor immunity and better clinical outcomes in patients with cancer. TAM, tumor-associated macrophage; Th1, T-helper type 1 cells; TME, tumor microenvironment; Treg, regulatory T cells; TRM, tissue-resident memory cells.

Source: https://jitc.bmj.com/content/jitc/8/1/e000363/F2.medium.gif.

Thus, immune profiling not only enhances the accuracy of cancer diagnosis but also plays a critical role in therapeutic stratification (Lokhande, 2023). Moreover, integrating immune profiling data with other omics approaches, such as genomics and transcriptomics, is an opportunity for synergism to unscramble the complex interactions in the TME. By examining the interaction between genetic changes in tumor cells and resulting immune responses, researchers can better understand mechanisms of tumor progression and resistance. For example, studies on the inflammatory landscape and infiltration of immune cells surrounding tumors reveal important correlations with several molecular signatures that inform the development of combination therapies aimed at resistant tumor phenotypes. Increased understanding of these interactions further supports the hypothesis that therapeutic efficacy can be significantly enhanced by leveraging knowledge from immune profiling coupled with genomic and proteomic data. In this regard, this multi-dimensional strategy emphasizes the central role immune profiling must play as a cornerstone in studies of the TME and the development of novel therapeutic paradigms aimed at maximizing cancer patient outcomes (Hu, 2017) (Figure 13.10).

13.4.2. Biomarkers for Immunotherapy Response

Comprehension of the role of biomarkers in response to immunotherapy is fundamental for maximizing treatment effectiveness in oncology. Biomarkers are biological markers that predict the extent to which an individual will react to certain immunotherapy drugs, specifically immune checkpoint inhibitors (ICIs).

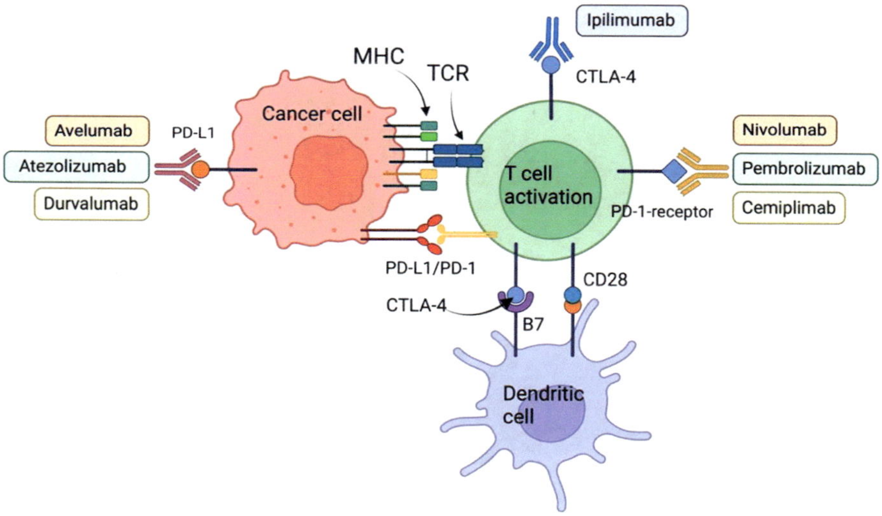

Figure 13.11. Illustration of immune checkpoint inhibitors (ICIs).

Source: https://www.researchgate.net/profile/Richard-Bauer-3/publication/364344739/figure/fig1/AS:11431281090201719@1666002986926/mmune-checkpoint-inhibitors-ICIs-with-FDA-approval-The-scheme-shows-pembrolizumab.png.

The detection of these biomarkers can greatly improve patient stratification, enabling personalized treatment strategies that maximize effectiveness and minimize side effects. With the emergence of immune profiling, researchers are able to measure tumor characteristics as well as the microenvironment and hence identify particular biomarkers associated with patient outcomes. Thus, their integration into the clinical environment has the capacity to assist in the selection of patients most likely to benefit from immunotherapy, literally changing the future of cancer treatment.

Recent advances in omics technologies, including genomics, proteomics, and metabolomics, have greatly enabled the identification and validation of response biomarkers of immunotherapy. These high-throughput profiling technologies allow for the full understanding of molecular interactions involved in tumorigenesis and immune response. For instance, genomic data can determine mutation or gene expression linked with the response to treatment, and proteomic research can determine protein expression profile alterations that influence immune activation. Furthermore, omics technologies enable the identification of tumor-infiltrating lymphocytes and cytokine profiles as predictors of immune response to therapy. However, despite all these advances, there remain issues in translating omics data to clinically useful biomarkers that are actionable in everyday practice, so it is crucial to pursue research on the subject (Nuti et al., 2018; Limeta et al., 2023). The use of artificial intelligence and machine learning for the interpretation of omics data holds great potential for enhancing the predictive power of biomarker profiles. By capitalizing on large amounts of data generated from diverse patient populations and treatment responses, such computational methods can discern subtle patterns that may not be accessible to traditional statistical methods. AI-driven models can integrate different types of omic data and deliver insights into the cause of treatment response. Thus, these models not only have the potential to augment the choice of the patients for immunotherapy but also help find novel therapeutic targets and biomarkers yet to be discovered. This novel data analysis process proves to be a reflection of the power of computational approaches and machine learning in revolutionizing cancer therapy, making the path smoother to a more tailored and efficient cure for the patients (Nuti et al., 2018; Limeta et al., 2023) (Figure 13.11).

13.4.3. Challenges in Translating Findings to Clinical Practice

Translation of immune profiling and omics approaches to clinical practice encompasses a variety of challenges that might impede the effective use of new therapeutic strategies. One primary challenge includes the complexity of biological systems, which usually leads to issues of correlating the omics data with clinical endpoints. For instance, identification of single biomarkers using high-throughput technologies may not detect the IgA nephropathy (IgAN), the most prevalent primary glomerulopathy globally, multifactorial etiology of diseases. Although novel studies have utilized integrative analysis of urinary proteome data to identify promising IgAN biomarkers, the underlying biology and therapeutic targets are partially understood, creating a gap between discovery and utility for clinical use (Diao et al., 2017). This highlights the requirement for a more comprehensive understanding of disease mechanisms to facilitate fruitful research-to-clinics translation. In addition, the need to validate and reproduce omics findings makes them more difficult to utilize in the clinic. Results based on omics analyses are often context-dependent, conditional on patient heterogeneity and variations in sample handling. Thus, findings that seem solid in one population may not be replicated in larger and more diverse patient populations. The example of yeast infection is a case in point, where advancement in high-throughput technologies has significantly changed the identification of pathogens; yet, many methods still need solid assessment for their sensitivity and specificity. Antifungal drug resistance serves to highlight the validation of such methods and bring them into usable clinical diagnostics (Consortium OPATHY & Gabaldón, 2019). Therefore, it is essential for researchers to build sound validation frameworks and standard protocols that will validate findings to be reliable and generalizable across various clinical settings. Lastly, yet another major challenge is incorporating omics data into clinical workflows and decision-making. The complexity of the analysis of omics data is such that it may not readily be available within the clinical setting, hence suboptimal for utilization by clinicians. Additionally, efficient communication of omics findings to clinical teams is crucial to overcome the disconnect in the translation of these results into patient care. For example, as demonstrated by the identification of new molecular signatures in IgAN, without a clearly defined way of incorporating such results into prevailing clinical paradigms, important information is not released. Eliminating such barriers entails transdisciplinary synergy between domains such as bioinformatics, clinical medicine, and health policy, providing room where omics approaches can be readily embedded into routine clinical practice and end up leading to improved outcomes for patients.

13.5. Immune Profiling in Infectious Diseases

The emergence of immune profiling as a core ability to unravel infectious diseases has transformed the pursuit of diagnostics and therapies. By leveraging advanced omics sciences, researchers can map the complex interactions between immune cells and how they respond to pathogens. Such mapping allows for comprehensive insight into the immune environment in infections, making it possible to identify selective biomarkers that signal the disease to be ongoing or resolving. The integration of heterologous molecular information, such as genomic and immunological profiles, allows for improved disease mechanism understanding and the development of personalized therapeutic interventions. Immune profiling, for instance, can explain heterogeneity in immune responses among disparate populations, ultimately to be followed by improved disease management strategies. The relevance of these profiling approaches is most striking in personalized medicine, whereby personalized strategies can lead to superior interventions, especially in composite infectious diseases characterized by heterogeneous responses among patients. In recent years, publicly accessible repositories with extensive 'omics data have also emerged as valuable sources for investigators who conduct studies on immune profiling in the context of infectious diseases. March of Dimes Database for Preterm Birth Research is a classic example of such a movement, offering a comprehensive database that integrates multiple molecular studies into large datasets. This database has various data types, including genomic and transcriptomic data to immunology and microbiome measurements. By making such vast amounts of information accessible, these repositories enable collaborative research projects, enhance discovery velocity, and enable researchers to make connections between independent omics datasets. Access to these open data ultimately results in enhanced knowledge about immune responses against different pathogens and guides the search for novel diagnostic and therapeutic modalities based on patient-specific information. The intersection of these databases and immune profiling is central to the appreciation of the intricate nature of infectious diseases. Systems biology plays a central role in enabling the application of immune profiling in infectious diseases. Embracing an entire system perspective, systems biology goes beyond discrete components to appreciate the intricate relationships that inform biological systems, particularly in the immune response. With the advent of advanced computational and modeling tools, researchers can now delve into massive datasets that are the outcome of immune profiling investigations, leading to comprehension of dynamic interactions of the immune system during infections. Systems biology also enables one to extract predictive models that can offer insight into clinical practice and guide the discovery of novel therapeutics. As highlighted in recent research, such integrative approaches have proven effective in human medicine and animal sciences, too, symbolizing the cross-disciplinary applicability of systems biology. The ongoing evolution of omics technologies along with systems biology concepts is likely to provide increased understanding of immune profiling, thus rewarding approaches in combating infectious diseases successfully (Woelders et al., 2011; Sirota et al., 2018).

13.5.1. Understanding Host-Pathogen Interactions

Host-pathogen interactions are crucial in dissecting the complex biological processes underlying infectious diseases. Omics technologies, such as genomics and proteomics, have now revolutionized the way scientists research host-pathogen interactions. By generating vast amounts of data that provide clarity on the molecular signatures of hosts and pathogens, scientists can identify the key biological pathways and immune reactions that have central roles in fighting infections. This combined strategy is used to provide a clearer image of the manner in which pathogens take over host cellular machinery to develop and propagate infection. These dynamics need to be understood in a bid to generate focused therapies and preventive measures. This is especially crucial because standard treatment strategies are threatened by the rapid emergence of drug-resistant pathogens, and as a result, what is gleaned through these analyses has never been more important (Swann et al., 2015). In order to unleash the full potential of omics technologies, systems biology must be incorporated. This interdisciplinary field aims to understand biological systems as a whole, not focusing on separate parts. Through the integration of high-throughput omic data with bioinformatics and computational modeling, researchers can unravel the complex interactions that drive host-pathogen dynamics. These methods enable the understanding of how pathogens employ various strategies, such as immune evasion and manipulation of host pathways, to survive. Notably, systems biology makes it possible to identify biomarkers that can indicate susceptibility or resistance to infection and thereby enhance the likelihood of forecasting disease outcomes and individually tailored therapy (Woelders et al., 2011). Therefore, this integration makes it possible for scientists to make significant progress in understanding the multifaceted nature of host-pathogen interactions (Woelders et al., 2011). Furthermore, the importance of host-pathogen interactions goes beyond basic research and extends to public health programs as well as to drug development.

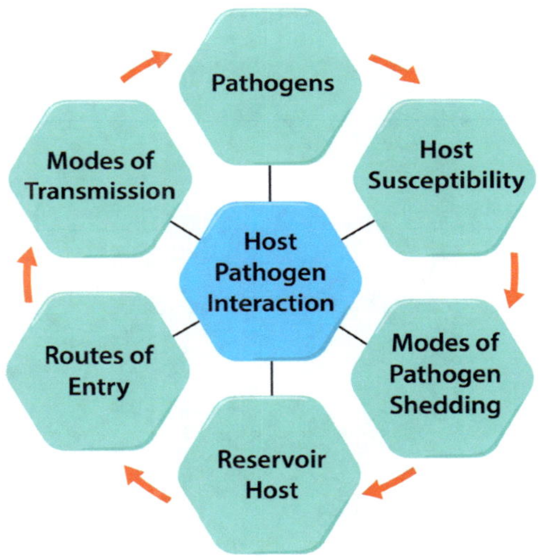

Figure 13.12. The study of host-pathogen interactions is critical in deciphering the complex biological processes that underlie infectious diseases.

Source: https://open.oregonstate.education/app/uploads/sites/54/2019/08/Host-pathogen-interaction-e1497296935850-1024x1018.png.

The information obtained through omics research paves the way for the development of novel vaccines and therapeutics targeted towards selected locations along these interactions. For instance, the discovery of important immune evasion strategies adopted by pathogens offers vital information needed for vaccine development. In addition, an understanding of variability in host responses can be applied to guide personalized medicine approaches, with treatment being tailored based on individual genetic histories and immune responses. As the technology continues to advance, researchers need to continue to push the limits of these technologies and collaborations to fully map host-pathogen interactions. In this way, we can encourage the development of more effective treatments and prevention to counter infectious diseases that mainly present themselves in global populations (Swann et al., 2015) (Figure 13.12).

13.5.2. Applications in Vaccine Development

In vaccine research and development, the application of immune profiling and omics technology has revolutionary potential. Immune profiling allows researchers to deconstruct immunological complexity in responding to pathogens and vaccines and to determine candidate targets for vaccines. Using advanced technologies such as transcriptomics and proteomics, researchers are able to define molecular signatures associated with effective immunity. These signatures also help identify the characteristics of robust immune responses so that one can develop targeted vaccines that create the desired protective effects.

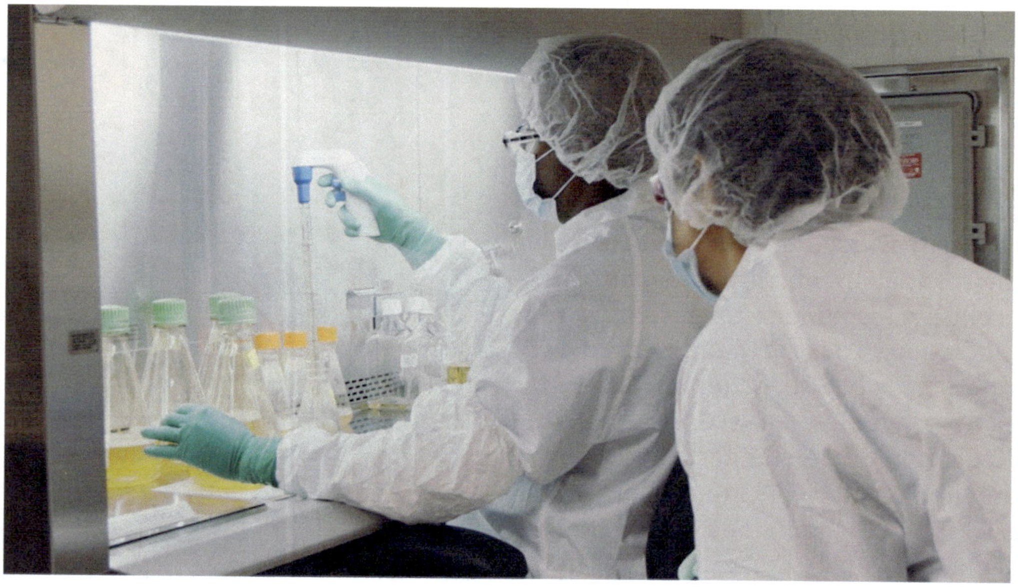

Figure 13.13. Integration of immune profiling in the realm of vaccine development.

Source: https://m.wsj.net/video/20200717/072020elilillyv8/072020elilillyv8_1920x1080.jpg.

Thus, the prospect of tailoring vaccines to fight immunogenicity in a way optimized through immune profiling is becoming more and more feasible, hence providing a new future of personalized vaccine strategies that address infectious diseases and autoimmune disorders. New omics technologies have also accelerated vaccine research and development. For instance, proteomics demonstrates how mass-scale protein profiling can contribute to the discovery of specific antigens required for vaccine construction. Scientists can achieve a general map of the proteome through the use of state-of-the-art proteomics platforms, and it becomes simpler to find novel biomarkers and drug targets. This capability is important in understanding the interaction between diverse pathogens and host systems, which is crucial in developing vaccines capable of withstanding constantly evolving viral and bacterial onslaughts. At the center of this is creating formidable bioinformatics tools that enhance high-throughput data analysis, leading to timely insights into antigenic variation and immune response critical in designing effective vaccines (da Costa et al., 2015). The uses of omics methods and immune profiling go well beyond vaccine development; they also yield critical data that can help address public health challenges. The ongoing malaria war is an example of the uses these methodologies have. Utilization of genomic tools has significantly enhanced our understanding of the Plasmodium species responsible for malaria. These technologies have made it possible to identify genes under selective pressure, which has given insights into drug resistance mechanisms, critical for formulating new drugs. Also, these findings can be used to guide vaccine design by indicating retention and variation in immune responses across different populations, which may lead to better and universally effective vaccines. This intersection of vaccine development and omics research portends an era in which vaccines will not only be more potent but tailored to tackle specific public health challenges in diverse demographic contexts (Kirchner et al., 2016) (Figure 13.13).

13.5.3. Case Studies of Successful Immune Profiling in Infections

The study of immune profiling by the omics approaches has made tremendous contributions towards control of infectious diseases, particularly in the understanding of individualized immune response. The case studies of successful application of immune profiling have explained many infectious agents and their corresponding host immune interactions. For instance, systematic studies by genomics and proteomics have enabled the characterization of specific biomarkers implicated in various infections. These biomarkers hold potential for early diagnosis, enabling the tailoring of therapeutic approaches to optimize patient prognosis. By employing high-dimensional data analysis, scientists are optimizing predictive models connecting immune profiles to infection severity and thus optimizing treatment regimens for subjects predisposed to severe complications of immune failure. Porting computational algorithms to such biological data sets is critical, as it allows for the effective selection of relevant biomarkers, which translates to more precise clinical applications for the infectious disease field (Wang & Sarwal, 2015). Illuminating the dynamic interactions of the host microbiome and its impact on the pathogens, immune profiling has contributed significantly to our understanding of opportunistic infections, such as those caused by yeast species. As these infections become increasingly complex and resistant to old therapies, antiquated diagnostic tests are often insensitive and nonspecific. Novel case reports that integrate next-generation sequencing and proteomic profiling suggest that omics technology can rapidly identify both the causative pathogen and the resistance pattern. With these advanced techniques, researchers can speed up diagnosis, which significantly reduces the delay from conventional culture techniques. The effectiveness of these approaches indicates the potential for not only identifying pathogen diversity, but also identifying effective antifungal treatments based on particular resistance profiles observed (Consortium OPATHY & Gabaldón, 2019). Thus, this development indicates the need for continued development and translation of omics technologies in the clinic. Furthermore, the coming together of immune profiling and omics has provided insights into how to move forward towards effective therapeutic interventions. Case studies suggest that employment of multi-omics data—coalescing genomic, transcriptomic, and proteomic data—enables the interpretation of host-pathogen interactions in more depth. An integrative strategy unravels new therapeutic targets and unearths mechanisms of immune response during infection. Sustained progress in computing algorithms enables this shift through enhanced analysis and interpretation of complex biological data. Significant advances in prediction models and biomarkers from immune profiling lay the groundwork for personalized medicine strategies, encouraging patient-focused management of infectious diseases. This remarkable synergy of immune profiling and omics technologies is essential, providing the basic information required to develop next-generation therapeutics and diagnostics with the potential to cure infections in a growing, challenging clinical setting (Wang & Sarwal, 2015; Consortium OPATHY & Gabaldón, 2019).

13.6. Ethical Considerations in Omics Research

With the advent of omics technologies, biology and medicine have been revolutionized, and scientists can now disentangle intricate biological mechanisms at an unprecedented magnitude. However, this advance is made in concert with a set of ethical challenges that must be addressed. Among the significant challenges is informed consent; subjects must be adequately informed as to how their genetic and microbiomic information will be utilized. In contrast to traditional research methods, omics studies more often utilize large data sets, which can be tricky to interpret concerning future implications for subjects or their family members. Moreover, the potential for secondary findings, revealing unsuspected health risks, makes it crucial to have robust ethical standards for deciding how such information is made available to the research study participants to maintain their autonomy and promote ethical transparency during research. Respect for privacy is also a key ethical consideration in omics studies. With the increasing ability to analyze personal biological data through high-throughput technologies increasing, rigorous data handling practices must be established to ensure the protection of participants' data. As noted, microbes and their interactions within the human microbiome underpin the foundation for a person's well-being, thereby invoking concern over genetic privacy in immune profiling and omics technologies. The effects of data misuse or breaches are profound, not just on the participants but also on their families and communities. Researchers should ensure anonymity and exercise caution to safeguard data, particularly in research that involves sensitive health information.

This action not only builds trust but also ensures the integrity of scientific inquiry in the broader public sphere. Furthermore, the implications of omics research findings extend beyond the laboratory into socio-economic domains. Identification of some biomarkers related to diseases could advance personalized medicine, but also produce inequalities in the provision of healthcare. Ethical concerns are induced by the fact that only particular populations are favored over others through improvement in immune profiling as a result of omics research, potentially amplifying health inequities. The scientific community in general has a responsibility to advocate for equitable access to the benefits of omics research and promote inclusive study designs to ensure representative participation. Thus, addressing such ethical concerns is not merely compliance; it is required to make sure that stakeholders benefit from omics research and make the healthcare system fairer and more equitable, according to the inherent complexity of the microbiome and its implications for human health as described in Rivera & Izard (2015) and Mikaeloff (2023).

13.6.1. Privacy Concerns Related to Genetic Data

The development of novel genetic technologies, such as next-generation sequencing, has revolutionized molecular biology with the ability to obtain highly detailed genetic information that can be used to guide immune profiling and omics approaches. However, this unprecedented ability to obtain and process personal genetic information poses serious issues of privacy. Individuals can inadvertently provide information that could reveal sensitive information about their health predispositions or genetic threats, which would be exploited by third parties like employers and insurance companies. The threat of exploitation of genetic information justifies robust data protection measures, as individuals have limited awareness of how their genetic information will be stored, transmitted, or utilized in the future.

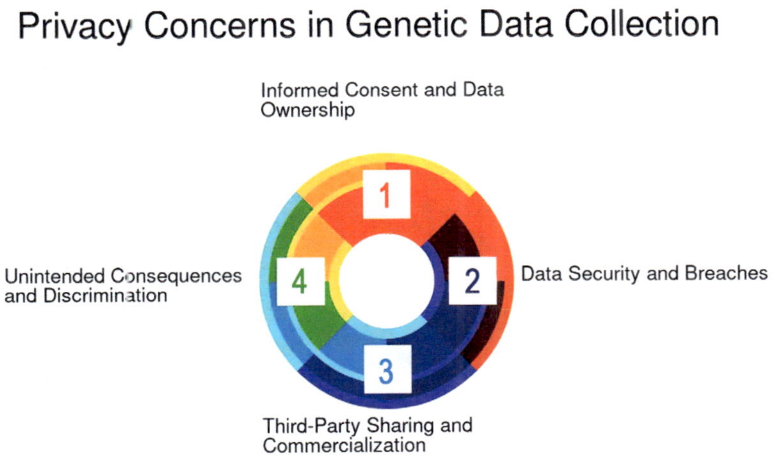

Figure 13.14. Privacy concerns in genetic data collection.

Source: https://fastercapital.co/i/Genetic-Fingerprinting-Risk-and-Liability-Navigating-Genetic-Privacy--Risks-and-Opportunities-for-Entrepreneurs--Privacy-Concerns-in-Genetic-Data-Collection.webp.

The solutions to these privacy concerns are important not only to safeguard individuals but also to maintain public trust in genetic research and its uses. As more genetic data is introduced into healthcare systems, issues of ownership and consent arise. The ethic of informed consent with genetic testing requires individuals to be informed of the ramifications of relinquishing their genetic material, such as potential future analysis that may become an outcome of their data. With the ability to generate massive datasets, researchers must maneuver the prickly problems of privacy and consent. Sharing of genetic data is not generally restricted to immediate use in research, but may include secondary analysis by database sharing. This opens the issue of who actually owns genetic data and under what conditions it can be shared. In addition, provisions must be made to allow people to maintain control of their genetic information so that it is not accessed or divulged without authority and that their health-related privacy is not violated (Gomes et al., 2017). The ethical considerations of genetic data privacy also cover the consequences of data breaches and the growing incidence of cybersecurity threats. As personal health information becomes a cybercrime target, the risks to keeping confidential genetic data in electronic formats grow. Leaking genetic information may lead to identity theft, discrimination, or stigmatization, with a chilling effect discouraging individuals from having genetic studies or even genetic testing per se. It is crucial for the stakeholders within the genomics industry to create comprehensive regulatory processes that emphasize data protection and ethical use of genetic data. Strengthening legal protection surrounding genetic data can empower individuals by protecting their privacy while facilitating groundbreaking immune profiling and omics approach research, thereby propelling health science responsibly and ethically (Rivera & Izard, 2015) (Figure 13.14).

13.6.2. Implications of Personalized Medicine

The age of personalized medicine is transforming healthcare by facilitating tailored therapeutic approaches in response to unique patient profiles. Immune profiling and omics technologies lie at the core of this revolution, offering vast amounts of data regarding a person's genetic, molecular, and immunological background. Utilizing multi-omics approaches, healthcare professionals are capable of identifying individualized biomarkers indicative of disease susceptibility and progression. This convergence of data types—genomic, transcriptomic, proteomic, and metabolomic—is what enables a multi-dimensional view of disease mechanisms, which in turn enables the ability to formulate targeted treatments. This way, personalized medicine not only offers the promise of improved therapeutic responses but also surmounts the limitations of a one-size-fits-all approach that can overlook significant patient-specific characteristics. Moreover, the import of personalized medicine extends beyond therapeutic efficacy to encompass the prevention and management of diseases. Personalized biomarker identification would facilitate early detection and monitoring of diseases, and thus, timely interventions that can prevent conditions such as cardiometabolic diseases from progressing. Revolutionary breakthroughs in the area of metabolomics, as well as other omics disciplines, provide information on metabolic pathways that potentially alter disease trajectories. For instance, studies have proven that the integration of information from different omics types can reveal complex interactions between biological systems, allowing researchers and clinicians to gain a clearer view of the mechanisms behind diseases, and therefore allow them to make more educated clinical decisions (Scola et al., 2019).

Such integrated information underscores the potential of personalized medicine in shaping new paradigms of healthcare through more forward-looking management strategies. Furthermore, the integration of gender medicine into personalized medicine highlights another critical point that must be addressed in personalized treatment planning. Gender differences can potentially have a profound effect on disease pathophysiology and the response to therapeutic intervention. Identification of these differences through the use of personalized biomarkers is critical to optimize patient outcomes. For example, research has shown that gender variation in the expression of some biomarkers can be used for more accurate diagnosis and treatment planning in conditions such as cardiometabolic disease (Scola et al., 2019). By incorporating macro-founders such as gender into omics-driven platforms for personalized medicine, not only can health be made more effective but also fairer, allowing populations to benefit from advances in metabolic research and immunoprofiling. This approach will be instrumental in the improvement of treatment modalities that are in harmony with the dynamic interaction of biological and environmental determinants of health.

13.6.3. Regulatory Frameworks Governing Omics Research

There is a need for regulatory systems for omics research to guarantee the ethical use of technologies being developed exponentially within the biomedical realm. Since scientists increasingly apply immunological data based on omics sciences, it is essential that there are integrated guidelines that deal with various issues related to confidentiality of data, informed consent, and genetic discrimination.

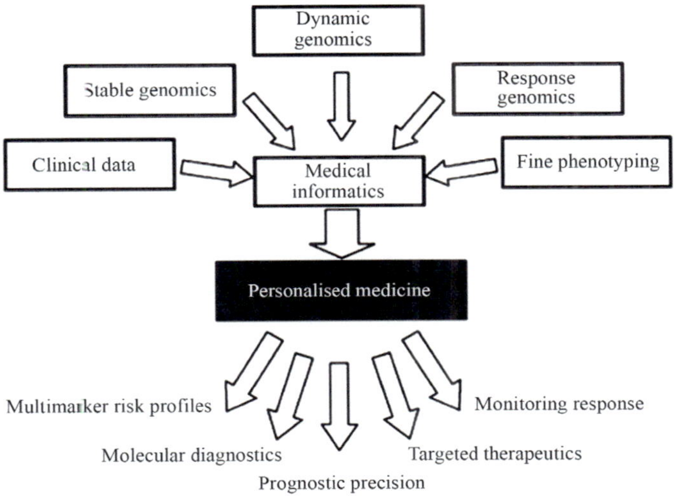

Figure 13.15. The scheme depicts the underpinnings of personalized medicine and principal approaches to be included in the PPPM protocols.

Source: https://www.scirp.org/html/htmlimages/6-2100852x/d142138c-6435-4689-a478-89874f3f5e8a.png.

An example of a PPPM application in cancer treatment has been utilized to identify the need for harmonization across medical disciplines. In reality, its seamless integration among healthcare professionals is necessitated by the complexity of omics data, which requires precisely defined competencies and harmonized guidance to ensure that the researchers and the patients reap beneficial outcomes from technological advances without compromising ethical principles. In such a situation, aging regulations are likely to hamper innovation and collaboration and hence render dynamic regulatory strategies most vital. Additionally, the establishment of effective regulatory frameworks is paramount not just for safeguarding patient rights but also for safe and responsible development of novel technologies, such as nanomaterials (NMs) commonly exploited in omics analyses. Such materials introduce unique functionalities, which can be made specific to certain applications, thus giving rise to a vast array of NM forms. In order to better control such complexity, the deployment of New Approach Methodologies (NAMs) becomes indispensable. These methodologies allow scientists to classify similar NMs and perform read-across assessments, hence filling gaps in data without undermining safety. Such regulatory clarity is not only inevitable but also vital because it provokes innovation alongside ensuring that physicochemical characteristics and potential hazards of NMs are well understood and justified. Thus, integrating NAMs into regulatory frameworks can render risk assessment processes more efficient, such that the research-to-clinics route is rendered robust and secure. In addition, omics studies and regulatory advice must be combined with respect to emerging technologies influencing our understanding of biological processes on a molecular basis. The combination of machine learning (ML) and bioinformatics in omics approaches can revolutionize the manner in which hazards of NMs are correlated to their physicochemical attributes. With the use of large datasets, ML is able to recognize patterns and properties of interest to toxicity, allowing for more mechanistic risk assessment. As is apparent with current research, these sophisticated methods offer a hopeful means by which hypotheses can be developed in terms of groupings of NMs, and that will reduce regulatory processes. Management of such intricate interactions with regulatory frameworks not only facilitates innovation but also maximizes the safety profile of emerging technologies in immune profiling and omics modalities, thereby maximizing returns in personalized medicine (Figure 13.15).

SUMMARY

The integration of immune profiling with omics technologies has the potential to revolutionize the understanding of complex diseases and their biomarkers. As observed, multi-omics analysis that includes genomics, proteomics, and metabolomics provides a holistic view of the biological basis of diseases such as CMD. Integration of multiple omics data allows researchers to identify novel pathways and biomarkers, enabling more precise diagnoses and treatment suggestions. Generally, this multi-dimensional data strategy makes it possible to disentangle the intricate mechanisms of disease and highlight the significance of biomarkers with the possibility of serving as surrogates for CMD and other conditions. Not only does this consolidation strengthen enhanced risk assessment but also opens the door for personalized therapeutic interventions that are consideration of patient profiles, thus addressing the modern paradigm of personalized medicine. Furthermore, the application of gender-specific analysis in biomarker discovery work gives a key dimension to the current efforts. Gender medicine that considers biological and psychosocial heterogeneity between the sexes allows for a subtle appreciation of how CMD manifests differently in women and men. The findings indicate that disease pathway-specific biomarkers may vary with gender, which would demand differential treatment approaches. By understanding gender interaction with disease mechanisms, researchers can make biomarkers more gender-specific and relevant, which will lead to prevention and treatment modalities. As explained, even proven biomarkers require validation and gender-specific modulation based on gender differences to maximize clinical outcomes as well as fair healthcare practices. Finally, the quest for novel biomarkers, most notably in conditions like IgAN, further underscores the necessity of integrating -omics data for comprehensive analysis. The recent studies delve into the urinary proteomics that correlate to IgAN have also underscored the identification of novel molecular signatures and biological pathways, which may have otherwise been missed. By combining different datasets, scientists discovered proteins of interest to the disease, which would be potential targets for future therapeutic targets. The combined strategy not only offers insights into IgAN, but its application can also be extended to other glomerular diseases. Thus, applying multi-omics approaches can bring revolutionary outcomes in the identification of diseases at the molecular level, and, in doing so, open the door to revolutionary advancement in diagnostic as well as therapeutic approaches in all fields of medicine.

The research into immune profiling and the omics techniques has transformed our understanding of complex diseases, most notably autoimmune diseases and IBD. The latest evidence emphasizes the interaction between genetic, epigenetic, and microbiomic determinants of IBD pathogenesis to affect the therapeutic strategy for conditions like ulcerative colitis and Crohn's disease. Systems biology is a method that uses several omics data and hypothesizes potential for the identification of central regulating hubs in the IBD network, enhancing comprehension of its molecular mechanisms. Researchers may create targeted therapeutics that address the root causes of IBD, and not only provide symptom relief. This paradigm shift ushers in an exciting era for precision medicine, where therapies are tailored to individual molecular profiles, dramatically improving patient outcomes and quality of life (Polytarchou et al., 2014). Furthermore, integrating multiomics into clinical studies demonstrates the sophistication and interconnectedness of biological systems. By examining the immunome, transcriptome, proteome, and metabolome in tandem, researchers can better understand important adaptations in physiological function, such as pregnancy. Emerging advances show how these biological clocks create key immunologic and metabolomic responses that are essential to healthy term delivery. For instance, modeling such interactions generates predictive models shedding light on deviations in relation to pregnancy pathology, such as preterm birth. Multivariate predictive modeling, for instance, the Elastic Net algorithm, in research has identified that the integration of several omics datasets can lead to enhanced predictive power, unraveling novel interactions that could inform upcoming therapeutic interventions (Ghaemi et al., 2019). This represents an expanding extent of understanding across various fields of medicine, informing novel treatments for complex diseases. In short, the combination of immune profiling and omics approaches greatly enhances our ability to examine intricate biological systems and their pathologic states. Through the adoption of advanced computational methodologies and the integration of high-throughput molecular data, researchers are at the very edge of personalized medicine. The prospect of ascertaining regulatory nodes of paramount importance allows the potential redirection of therapeutic intervention towards the most potent targets. Moreover, the synergy of multiomics analysis gives clinicians very nuanced information regarding diseases that have to be addressed in a complex manner, such as IBD and pregnancy pathologies. Generally speaking, the transition towards a systems biology view integrates a total understanding of health and disease, which finally results in the development of novel, improved clinical interventions that are sensitive to patient profiles (Polytarchou et al., 2014; Ghaemi et al., 2019).

A CLOSER LOOK

ANTIGEN-PRESENTING CELLS (APCS)

APCs are a vital part of the immune system that is responsible for capturing, processing, and presenting antigens to T cells, thereby leading to adaptive immune responses. APCs are predominantly classified as professional and non-professional APCs, with professional APCs like dendritic cells, macrophages, and B cells playing a primary role in T cell activation (Figure 13.16).

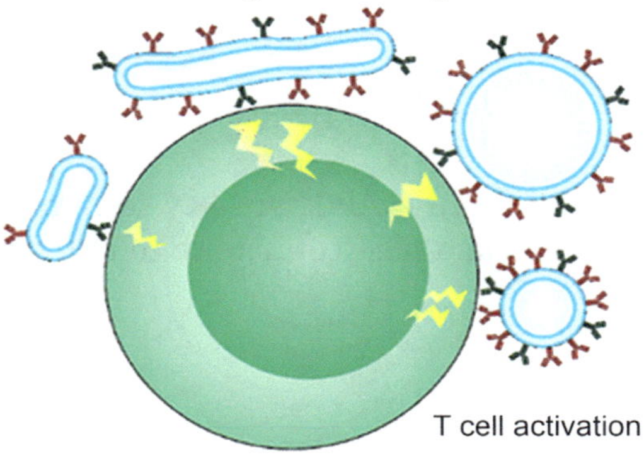

Figure 13.16. Illustration of artificial antigen-presenting cell T.

Source: https://pubs.acs.org/cms/10.1021/acsnano.2c06211/asset/images/medium/nn2c06211_0008.gif.

Key functions of APCs:

a. **Antigen Uptake:** APCs engulf pathogens or foreign substances through phagocytosis or receptor-mediated endocytosis.
b. **Antigen Processing:** The ingested material is broken down into smaller peptide fragments.
c. **Antigen Presentation:** The peptide fragments are presented on the cell surface in association with MHC molecules (Major Histocompatibility Complex).
d. **T Cell Activation:** APCs present these antigen-MHC complexes to T cells, which results in an adaptive immune response.

Types of APCs:

a. **Professional APCs:**These are professional cells that can efficiently present antigens and provide co-stimulatory signals to T cells.
   (i) **Dendritic cells:** Highly efficient in activating naive T cells and inducing immunity.
   (ii) **Macrophages:** Found in tissue and can phagocytose pathogens and present them as antigens.
   (iii) **B Cells:** Can engulf antigens via their B cell receptors and present them to T cells to generate antibodies.

b. **Non-professional APCs:** Although not professional antigen-presenting cells, these cells are capable of presenting antigens under certain conditions. These include:
   (i) Thymic epithelial cells.
   (ii) Vascular endothelial cells.
   (iii) Fibroblasts.
   (iv) Lymph node stromal cells.

Role of APCs

a. **Trigger Adaptive Immunity:** APCs are required to activate both helper T cells (which coordinate immune responses) and cytotoxic T cells (which kill infected or tumor cells).
b. **Regulate Immune Response:** APCs can decide whether an immune response or immune tolerance is initiated.
c. **Pathogen and Tumor Immunity:** APCs are key to immunity against both intracellular and extracellular pathogens and also contribute to anti-tumor immunity.

REFERENCES

1. Moreira, M., Schrama, D., Soares, F., Wulff, T., Pousão-Ferreira, P., & Rodrigues, P. (2017). Physiological responses of reared sea bream (Sparus aurata Linnaeus, 1758) to an Amyloodinium ocellatum outbreak. *Journal of fish diseases*, *40*(11), 1545–1560. https://doi.org/10.1111/jfd.12623(accessed on 27th June 2025).
2. Yan, D., Afifi, L., Jeon, C., Trivedi, M., Chang, H. W., Lee, K., & Liao, W. (2017). The metabolomics of psoriatic disease. *Psoriasis (Auckland, N.Z.)*, *7*, 1–15. https://doi.org/10.2147/PTT.S118348(accessed on 27th June 2025).
3. Ghaemi, M. S., DiGiulio, D. B., Contrepois, K., Callahan, B., Ngo, T. T. M., Lee-McMullen, B., Lehallier, B., Robaczewska, A., Mcilwain, D., Rosenberg-Hasson, Y., Wong, R. J., Quaintance, C., Culos, A., Stanley, N., Tanada, A., Tsai, A., Gaudilliere, D., Ganio, E., Han, X., Ando, K., ... Aghaeepour, N. (2019). Multiomics modeling of the immunome, transcriptome, microbiome, proteome and metabolome adaptations during human pregnancy. *Bioinformatics (Oxford, England)*, *35*(1), 95–103. https://doi.org/10.1093/bioinformatics/bty537(accessed on 27th June 2025).
4. Lin A, Torres CM, Hobbs EC, et al. Computational and Systems Biology Advances to Enable Bioagent Agnostic Signatures. *Health Secur*. 2024;22(2):130-139. doi:10.1089/hs.2023.0076 (accessed on 27th June 2025).
5. da Costa, J. P., Carvalhais, V., Ferreira, R., Amado, F., Vilanova, M., Cerca, N., & Vitorino, R. (2015). Proteome signatures--how are they obtained and what do they teach us?. *Applied microbiology and biotechnology*, *99*(18), 7417–7431. https://doi.org/10.1007/s00253-015-6795-7 (accessed on 27th June 2025).
6. Sirota, M., Thomas, C. G., Liu, R., Zuhl, M., Banerjee, P., Wong, R. J., Quaintance, C. C., Leite, R., Chubiz, J., Anderson, R., Chappell, J., Kim, M., Grobman, W., Zhang, G., Rokas, A., England, S. K., Parry, S., Shaw, G. M., Simpson, J. L., Thomson, E., ... March of Dimes Prematurity Research Centers (2018). Enabling precision medicine in neonatology, an integrated repository for preterm birth research. *Scientific data*, *5*, 180219. https://doi.org/10.1038/sdata.2018.219(accessed on 27th June 2025).
7. Consortium OPATHY, Gabaldón T. Recent trends in molecular diagnostics of yeast infections: from PCR to NGS. *FEMS Microbiol Rev*. 2019;43(5):517-547. doi:10.1093/femsre/fuz015(accessed on 27th June 2025).
8. Scola, L., Giarratana, R. M., Torre, S., Argano, V., Lio, D., & Balistreri, C. R. (2019). On the Road to Accurate Biomarkers for Cardiometabolic Diseases by Integrating Precision and Gender Medicine Approaches. *International journal of molecular sciences*, *20*(23), 6015. https://doi.org/10.3390/ijms20236015(accessed on 27th June 2025).
9. Bahl, A., Haase, A., Halappanavar, S., Kohonen, P., et al. (2024). Bioinformatics and machine learning to support nanomaterial grouping. https://core.ac.uk/download/621473291.pdf (accessed on 27th June 2025).
10. Woelders, H., Te Pas, M. F., Bannink, A., Veerkamp, R. F., & Smits, M. A. (2011). Systems biology in animal sciences. *Animal : an international journal of animal bioscience*, *5*(7), 1036–1047. https://doi.org/10.1017/S1751731111000036(accessed on 27th June 2025).

11. Bjerrum, J. T., Olsen, J., Rantalainen, M., Nielsen, O. H., & Wang, Y. (2013). Integration of transcriptomics and metabonomic: Improving diagnostics, biomarker identification and phenotyping in ulcerative colitis. https://core.ac.uk/download/pdf/81636872.pdf (accessed on 27th June 2025).

12. Nuti M, Zizzari IG, Botticelli A, Putignani L, Marchetti P. The microbiota impact: bacteria shaping immunity, disease and response to therapy. Transl Cancer Res 2018;7(Suppl 5):S616-S619. doi: 10.21037/tcr.2018.05.25 (accessed on 27th June 2025).

13. Labuda, Ján, Bowater, Richard P., Fojta, Miroslav, Gauglitz, Günter, Glatz, Zdeněk, Hapala, Ivan, Havliš, Jan, Kilar, Ferenc, Kilar, Aniko, Malinovská, Lenka, Sirén, Heli M. M., Skládal, Petr, Torta, Federico, Valachovič, Martin, Wimmerová, Michaela, Zdráhal, Zbyněk and Hibbert, David Brynn. "Terminology of bioanalytical methods (IUPAC Recommendations 2018)" Pure and Applied Chemistry, vol. 90, no. 7, 2018, pp. 1121-1198. https://doi.org/10.1515/pac-2016-1120

14. Bubnov, R., Danesi, R., Desiderio, D. M., Grech, G., et al. (2015). EPMA position paper in cancer: Current overview and future perspectives. https://core.ac.uk/download/293881196.pdf (accessed on 27th June 2025).

15. Burtscher, M., Gade, S., Garrido-Rodriguez, M., Rutkowska, A., Werner, T., Eberl, C., Petretich, M., et al. (2024). Network integration of thermal proteome profiling with multi-omics data decodes PARP inhibition. *Molecular Systems Biology, 20*, 458–474. https://www.semanticscholar.org/paper/70735d91f2a3e16ff2ede26515d830de166e3072 (accessed on 27th June 2025).

16. Caligola, S., Canè, S., De Sanctis, F., Ugel, S., et al. (2022). Breaking the immune complexity of the tumor microenvironment using single-cell technologies. https://core.ac.uk/download/596751594.pdf (accessed on 27th June 2025).

17. Diao M, Wu Y, Yang J, et al. Identification of Novel Key Molecular Signatures in the Pathogenesis of Experimental Diabetic Kidney Disease. *Front Endocrinol (Lausanne)*. 2022;13:843721. Published 2022 Mar 30. doi:10.3389/fendo.2022.843721(accessed on 27th June 2025).

18. Dorrestein, P. C., Knight, R., & Mazmanian, S. K. (2014). Finding the missing links among metabolites, microbes, and the host. https://core.ac.uk/download/33113984.pdf (accessed on 27th June 2025).

19. Fels, U., Gevaert, K., & Van Damme, P. (2017). Proteogenomic in aid of host-pathogen interaction studies: A bacterial perspective. https://core.ac.uk/download/153398357.pdf (accessed on 27th June 2025).

20. Frei, A. L. (2024). Tumor and immune profiling by image analysis and digital pathology. https://core.ac.uk/download/621172205.pdf (accessed on 27th June 2025).

21. Limeta A, Gatto F, Herrgård MJ, Ji B, Nielsen J. Leveraging high-resolution omics data for predicting responses and adverse events to immune checkpoint inhibitors. *Comput Struct Biotechnol J*. 2023;21:3912-3919. Published 2023 Jul 24. doi:10.1016/j.csbj.2023.07.032 (accessed on 27th June 2025).

22. Gomes, A. Q., & Soares, H. (2017). Metodologias emergentes de larga escala na era pós-genómica: benefícios e questões éticas. https://core.ac.uk/download/94085599.pdf (accessed on 27th June 2025).

23. Hu, X. (2017). Integrative analysis of omics data in adult glioma and other TCGA cancers to guide precision medicine. https://core.ac.uk/download/80296563.pdf (accessed on 27th June 2025).

24. Polytarchou, C., Koukos, G., & Iliopoulos, D. (2014). Systems biology in inflammatory bowel diseases: ready for prime time. *Current opinion in gastroenterology, 30*(4), 339–346. https://doi.org/10.1097/MOG.0000000000000081(accessed on 27th June 2025).
25. Rivera, Maria C. and Izard, Jacques, "Promises and Prospects of Microbiome Studies" (2015). Department of Food Science and Technology: Faculty Publications. 332. https://digitalcommons.unl.edu/foodsciefacpub/332 (accessed on 27th June 2025).
26. Swann, J., Jamshidi, N., Lewis, N. E., & Winzeler, E. A. (2015). Systems analysis of host-parasite interactions. *Wiley interdisciplinary reviews. Systems biology and medicine, 7*(6), 381–400. https://doi.org/10.1002/wsbm.1311(accessed on 27th June 2025).
27. Kirchner, S., Power, B. J., & Waters, A. P. (2016). Recent advances in malaria genomics and epigenomics. https://core.ac.uk/download/46580201.pdf (accessed on 27th June 2025).
28. Lim, J., Park, C., Kim, M., Kim, H., Kim, J., & Lee, D. S. (2024). Advances in single-cell omics and multimers for high-resolution molecular profiling. *Experimental & Molecular Medicine, 56*, 515–526. https://www.semanticscholar.org/paper/44d251020aad0d8e1ce473dd0b188538bde342ab (accessed on 27th June 2025).
29. Lokhande, L. (2023). The immune microenvironment in mantle cell lymphoma: Targeted liquid and spatial proteomic analyses. https://core.ac.uk/download/553782687.pdf (accessed on 27th June 2025).
30. Mikaeloff, F. (2023). An integrative systems biology study to understand immune aging in people living with HIV. https://core.ac.uk/download/570950700.pdf (accessed on 27th June 2025).
31. Sánchez-Vidaña DI, Rajwani R, Wong MS. The Use of Omic Technologies Applied to Traditional Chinese Medicine Research. *Evid Based Complement Alternat Med.* 2017;2017:6359730. doi:10.1155/2017/6359730(accessed on 27th June 2025).
32. Wang, A., & Sarwal, M. M. (2015). Computational Models for Transplant Biomarker Discovery. *Frontiers in immunology, 6*, 458. https://doi.org/10.3389/fimmu.2015.00458(accessed on 27th June 2025).
33. Vasaturo, A., Kysilovsky, C., Duro, L., Tattikota, S., Chen, R., He, J., Ray, M., et al. (2025). Abstract 2075: Combining Vizgen's MERSCOPE spatial transcriptomics profiling and InSituPlex (ISP) multiplex immunofluorescence (mIF) to unravel the complexity of the tumor-immune microenvironment (TiME). *Cancer Research.* https://www.semanticscholar.org/paper/2f1c5b61915bb42d8ac0674ffd7a657285c0c6e2 (accessed on 27th June 2025).

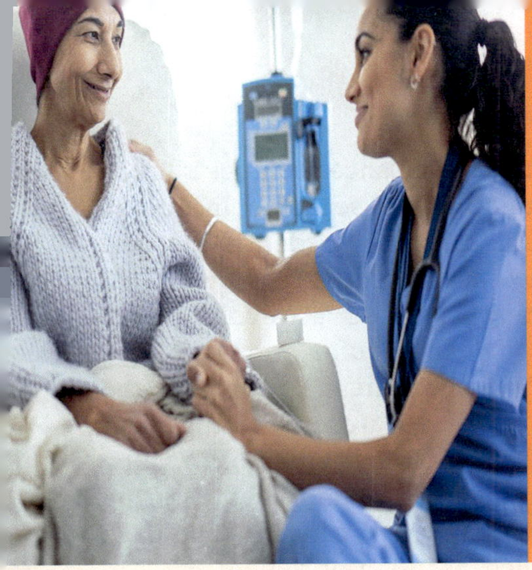

Chapter 14

IMMUNOTHERAPY AND CAR-T TECHNOLOGY

Contents

Introduction

The past decade has seen a revolution in molecular immunology, particularly with the advent of immunotherapy and some of the technologies, such as Chimeric Antigen Receptor T-cell (CAR-T) therapy. This new form of treatment utilizes the body's immune system to identify and kill the cancer cells and has resulted in a revolution among the therapeutic approaches that have delivered remarkable outcomes, particularly in hematological malignancies. Yet, this innovation is not without its challenges; the use of CAR-T technology in solid tumors has been frustrated by concerns, including immune evasion and tumor heterogeneity. To address these complexities, ongoing research aims to refine CAR-T therapies so that they are more specifically targeted and limit potential off-target effects, lending credibility to an urgent need for ongoing innovation in the field of immunotherapy, as has been demonstrated in recent reviews and studies (Shirzadian et al., 2025). The combination of the advances of CAR-T technology with novel mechanisms is a significant area of focus in modern immunological research. These include the integration of synthetic Notch (synNotch) systems, molecular logic gates that control the T-cell response. By facilitating the specific control of gene expression and T-cell activation, synNotch receptors can facilitate targeted responses to many antigens simultaneously, thereby enhancing the therapeutic potential of CAR-T therapies. Such convergence not only addresses the specificity and safety concerns that are specific to traditional CAR-T approaches but also signals the advent of more adaptive treatment protocols that can dynamically respond to the evolving context of tumor biology. This synergy between CAR-T technology and synthetic biology stands at the vanguard of personalized medicine (Shirzadian et al., 2025). Another crucial aspect of CAR-T therapy advancement is to advance tracking technologies, which are critical for uncovering the mechanism of CAR-T cell dynamics in the TME. Traditional technologies have limitations in real-time tracking, thus novel platforms such as gas vesicle (GV)-labeled CAR-T cells have emerged. This novel technology enables stable ultrasound imaging, which provides crucial information on CAR-T cell migration, infiltration, and persistence in tumors. Research has confirmed that such GVs are not at the expense of CAR-T cell anti-tumor activity, thereby granting researchers assurance of their translational potential. The ability to track CAR-T cell migration provides a valuable tool for maximizing treatment protocols and ultimately improving patient outcomes, demonstrating the synergy between technological progress and therapeutic development within the field.

Definition of Immunotherapy

Immunotherapy, a new mode of treatment, utilizes the body's own immune system to fight off diseases, most notably cancer. Immunotherapy applies various drugs that are intended to trigger or inhibit the immune system in order to successfully target cancer cells. Unlike chemotherapy and radiation therapy, which execute cancer cell destruction directly, immunotherapy seeks to make the immune system capable of identifying and eliminating the cancer cells on its own. This shift in therapy signifies a revolutionary advancement in molecular immunology, ushering in more awareness of the immune system's potential. As researchers become adept at understanding the complexities of immune response, immunotherapy improves, offering hope for individuals with cancers that have long been recalcitrant. One of the advances in immunotherapy is CAR-T technology. Chimeric Antigen Receptor T-cell therapy involves gene modification of a patient's T cells to enhance their ability to identify and destroy cancer cells. It involves T cell collection, modification to enable them to express CARs that can identify specific cancer antigens, and reinfusion into the patient. The therapeutic promise of CAR-T therapies has offered excellent results for selected hematologic cancers, with the ability to initiate remission and enhanced survival. The implications show the significance of personalized immunotherapeutic intervention, where the deciphering of individual patient tumor biology must occur in order to optimize treatment effectiveness and reduce off-target effects. Furthermore, the development and enhancement of immunotherapeutic methods necessitate extensive insight into immune system dynamics at the cellular level. Selective differentiation of naive T cells plays a pivotal role in enhancing immunotherapeutic efficiency, particularly in the generation of cell-based therapeutics. As evident through recent literature, naive T cell differentiation to multipotent T cells forms the cornerstone of advancement in cancer immunotherapies. Cellular coordination of differentiation through division state and time is critical in the generation of potent immune responses. Utilizing sophisticated methods, such as time-tracking assays alongside mass cytometry, researchers try to decipher the complexity of T-cell activation and expansion to attain optimal clinical applications (Good et al., 2019). These results not only expand our knowledge of immunotherapy but also provide an entry into new gene therapy approaches, establishing the potential for an era of precision medicine in cancer treatment (Khan et al., 2013) (Figure 14.1).

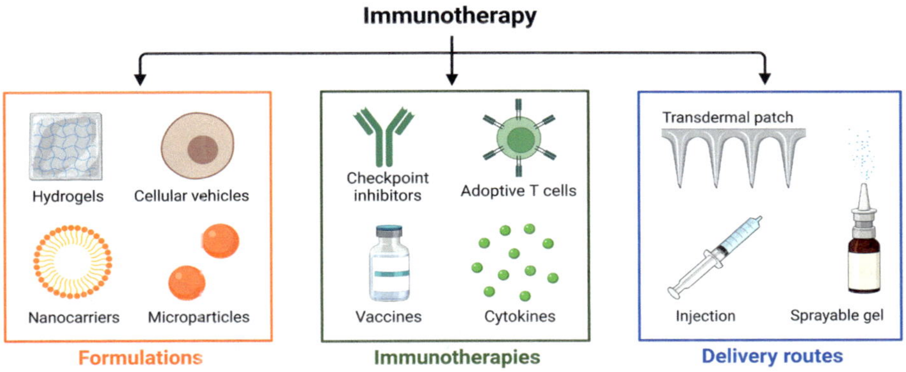

Figure 14.1. Recent advances in local delivery systems for cancer immunotherapy.

Source: https://www.frontiersin.org/files/Articles/1258786/fimmu-14-1258786-HTML/image_m/fimmu-14-1258786-g001.jpg.

Overview of Chimeric Antigen Receptor T-cell (CAR-T) Technology

CAR-T technology represents a revolutionary leap in the science of immunotherapy, particularly in the case of treating hematological malignancies. This new approach includes genetic modification of a patient's T cells to have them produce CARs, which enable the recognition and targeting of specific tumor-associated antigens. It begins with the collection of T cells from the patient, which are then genetically modified in a laboratory to enhance their ability to recognize and kill cancer cells. CAR-T therapy has demonstrated its highest power in certain blood cancers, such as acute lymphoblastic leukemia (ALL) and large B-cell lymphoma, where it has achieved unprecedented remission rates in previously intractable cases. But the transition from success in the laboratory to the clinic is a testament to the potential and challenge of this revolutionary technology. Despite being promising, CAR-T technology use in solid tumors has also experienced significant challenges. For instance, the uniqueness of the tumor microenvironment has the potential to inhibit T-cell activity, as illustrated in malignant gliomas. Standard treatments like chemotherapy and radiation possess relatively low potency and carry undesirable side effects; hence, scientists have been probing CAR-T therapy as a means of obtaining a more targeted immune response. However, the complexity of the glioma tumor microenvironment—beyond what is present in challenges to antigen presentation and T-cell homing—has complicated clinical trials. Investigations have shown that overcoming such hurdles can optimize CAR-T cell potency, as shown by studies on increasing targeting of cardiac or antigen heterogeneity in solid tumors that remain an active area of investigation with immunotherapy. New technologies such as Vapor Nanobubble (VNB) photoporation are providing new means of enhancing CAR-T cell engineering, opening up the landscape in the field even more. VNB photoporation utilizes gold nanoparticles to facilitate T cell macromolecule internalization in a non-toxic way, making it possible for effective CD4+ T cell modification for therapy. Compared to older methods such as viral transduction or electroporation, there are cytotoxicity risks involved. VNB photoporation, however, offers comparable efficacy in terms of a reduced toxicity profile. Such a development is promising not just to facilitate the production of CAR-T cells but to expand their usefulness to even more research and therapeutic applications. As researchers push forward on these developments, the potential for the development of CAR-T technology in molecular immunology is high for bridging some of the gaps it faces today in cancer therapy against solid tumors and enhancing patient outcomes for numerous cancers (Figure 14.2).

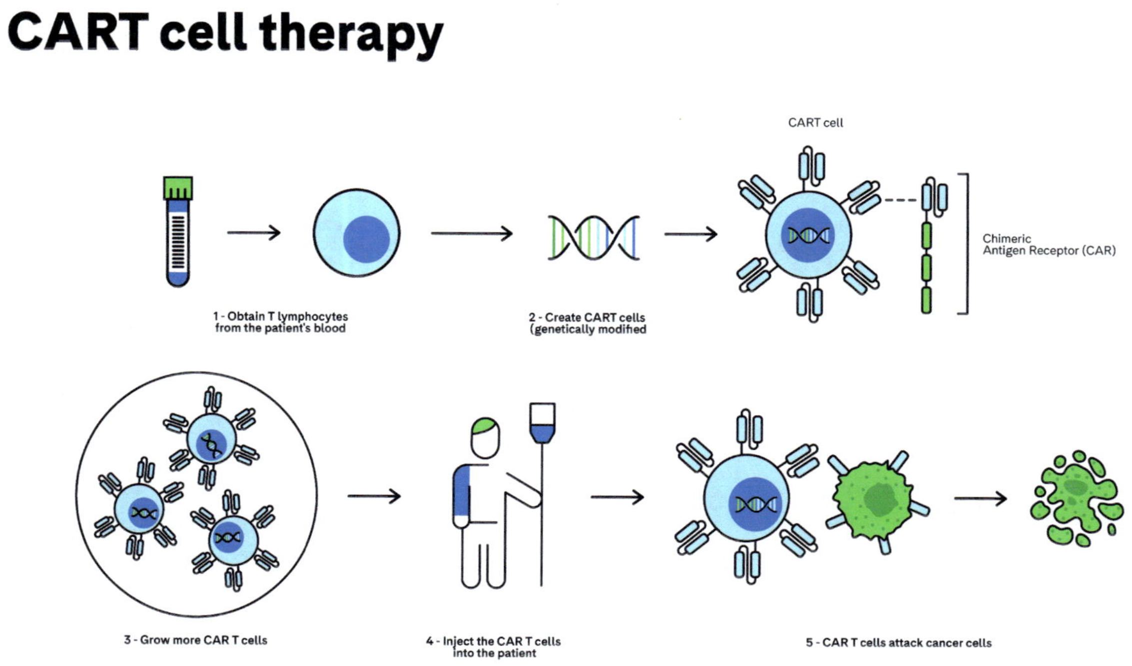

Figure 14.2. Illustration of chimeric antigen receptor T-cell (CAR-T) cell therapy.

Source: https://www.clinicbarcelona.org/uploads/media/default/0011/28/4668e6867b2cb87d2ca2f33b12e3c62865821881.png.

Importance of Molecular Immunology in Cancer Treatment

The applicability of molecular immunology in cancer treatment is underscored by its ability it holds to understand and regulate the interaction of the immune system with cancer cells. By elucidating how tumors evade immune surveillance, researchers have been able to enhance therapeutic modalities like immunotherapy and CAR-T technology. These advancements are founded on a complete understanding of tumor microenvironments (TMEs), which have a propensity to be immunosuppressive that discourages efficient anti-tumor immune responses. The facts gained through molecular immunology research allow precise adaptation of treatment techniques to overcome these challenges, with the ultimate aim of restoring the immune system against tumor cells. As successive research uncovers more about tumor-specific antigens and immune checkpoint mechanisms, the stage is set for more tailored and efficient treatment protocols that tap into the body's own mechanisms for cancer protection. CAR-T technology development and its deployment are some of the exemplary applications of the life-altering potential of molecular immunology in cancer medicine. Chimeric antigen receptors engineered to target specific tumor antigens leverage the inherent cytotoxic capability of T cells, therefore orchestrating an anticancer immunity. The powerful mechanism has been enormously effective in hematopoietic malignancies and points to the central role of molecular insights in the development of effective immunotherapies. However, the intricacies of solid tumors present unique challenges that require new strategies to overcome. For instance, the anatomical barriers of certain cancers may prevent T cell infiltration, and antigen heterogeneity in tumors may result in targeted therapy escape. In accordance with reports, overcoming difficulty in antigen presentation, T-cell homing, and immunosuppression within glioma microenvironments is significant for enhancing CAR-T therapy efficiency (Chuntova et al., 2018). Work on the advancement of these technologies is a major area of interest in current research, with the contribution of molecular immunology at its base. In addition, challenges associated with T-cell dysfunction within the tumor microenvironment reveal other major insights that molecular immunology has in cancer treatment. Immunosuppression is a prevalent issue that typically results in CD8+ T cell dysfunction, as communicated by tolerance and exhaustion, thereby limiting the efficacy of immunotherapy. The senescence of CD8+ T cells is especially worrying because the expanding populations of such cells within the TME can subvert the anti-tumor immune response. Elucidating the complex signals in the process of T cell activation, as well as the several mechanisms that underlie senescence, is crucial for enhancing immunotherapeutic benefits (Huff et al., 2019). By illuminating issues with modulation of the TME and optimizing the activity of T cells, molecular immunology has the potential to lead to novel treatments. Ultimately, the integration of molecular information into treatment protocols has the potential to revolutionize the art of cancer treatment, making immunotherapy a more viable treatment option for patients.

14.1. Historical Background of Immunotherapy

The evolution of immunotherapy in the past offers an indication of a paradigm in cancer treatment, moving away from traditional approaches such as surgery and radiotherapy. It is possible to trace its beginnings back to the late 19th century, when trailblazers William Coley conducted tests involving bacterial toxins to trigger immune reactions against cancerous tumors. Coley's work laid the groundwork for further research on the immune system's function against malignancies. Over the course of the decades, immunological advances catalyzed the discovery of monoclonal antibodies and checkpoint inhibitors, leading to the establishment of immunotherapy as a treatment modality. These discoveries have underscored the enormous potential in utilizing the body's immune system in specifically targeting and killing cancer cells, representing a fundamental revolution in onco-immunology strategies. When the field entered the late 20th century, immunological understanding gained from molecular biology provided a more advanced view of the immune system and enabled the development of targeted immunotherapies. The emergence of vaccine-related treatments, such as the HPV vaccine, illustrated how the immune mechanisms could be utilized to prevent, rather than treat, disease. In addition, human genome sequencing and exploration of tumor microenvironments have enhanced researchers' capacity to design therapies that optimize immune response with minimal side effects. Importantly, the discovery of immune checkpoints, the controllers of immune activation, allowed the development of checkpoint inhibitors that restore functional T cells. This deliberate stimulation of the immune system is a new era of cancer therapy, as combination treatments become the new standard, a reflection of the innovative spirit of modern medicine. The development of chimeric antigen receptor T-cell (CAR-T) technology is proof of the culmination of decades of scientific inquiry into immunotherapy as a testament to remarkable advancements in engineering and clinical applications. From the fundamental concept of T-cell activation and specificity, CAR-T therapy was developed to optimize the ability of T cells to recognize and kill cancer cells. This new method involves genetically modified T cells to produce specific receptors targeting tumor-associated antigens. As demonstrated in the cases of hematologic malignancies, CAR-T therapy has achieved miraculous clinical success, particularly in the case of relapsed or refractory disease. However, a consideration has to be made. There are complexities entailed in CAR-T therapy, including safety and efficacy. The interplay between genetic manipulation and immunotherapy is a promise of constant research and innovation, which will pave the way for future developments in the management paradigm of cancers as researchers unveil the immunological underpinnings of immune dysregulation, such as in disease affecting RAS guanyl-releasing protein 1 (Nashrudin et al., 2025) and sex-dependent immune responses (Feng et al., 2024).

14.1.1. Early Developments in Immunotherapy

The early developments in immunotherapy offered a groundbreaking era in the treatment of numerous cancers, making the preoccupation against traditional chemotherapeutic agents towards the manipulation of the body's own immune system reasonable. The early 20th-century discoveries laid the foundation for the design of the manipulation of immune responses against tumors. The creation of interleukins and interferons as biological response modifiers was representative of initial efforts, demonstrating these cytokines possess the capacity to enhance the immune response to cancer. Researchers highlighted that the activation of immune cells not only bore the possibility of potentiating anti-tumor effectiveness but also extended the survival of patients. These findings provided a proof of principle that reconstitution of a patient's immune system might constitute a new type of cancer treatment, paving the path for more sophisticated technologies, such as monoclonal antibodies and cell-based modalities, which emerged in subsequent decades and further defined the immunotherapeutic canvas. One of the earliest breakthroughs in early immunotherapy was the generation of monoclonal antibodies, which allowed for targeted therapeutic interventions against single antigens expressed by cancer cells. Monoclonal antibodies transformed the care of hematologic malignancies, particularly with the introduction of rituximab in the 1990s for the treatment of non-Hodgkin lymphoma. This achievement demonstrated that targeting cell surface antigens could effectively induce tumor lysis through various mechanisms, including direct cytotoxicity and immune-mediated lysis. Significantly, monoclonal antibodies such as trastuzumab in breast cancer highlighted the promise of personalized therapy given individual tumor biology. It was such groundbreaking work that paved the way for further research into chimeric antigen receptor (CAR) T-cell technology, as it became clear that exploiting the selectivity of antibodies could be successfully applied to cellular therapies and hence expand the cancer therapeutic toolkit. In the context of CAR-T technology, early immunotherapeutic advances enabled an understanding of how modified immune cells could be programmed against cancer. Early research in T-cell therapy efforts attempted to enhance the natural capacity of T cells to recognize and destroy cancer cells, drawing lessons from past studies that highlighted immune modulation. The theoretical leap to design CARs—man-made receptors that enable T cells to identify specific tumor antigens—was a direct outcome of these efforts. Developments in gene engineering and molecular biology continued to spur the design of CAR T-cells, which have gone on to be hugely successful in hematologic malignancies. Meanwhile, as researchers worked towards defining the functional imperfections of solid tumors, the field of immunotherapy only continued to evolve further. The successful application of CAR technology in clinical settings heralded a new era in cancer treatment, thereby highlighting the significance of previous immunotherapeutic advancements in shaping current and future strategies in molecular immunology (Figure 14.3).

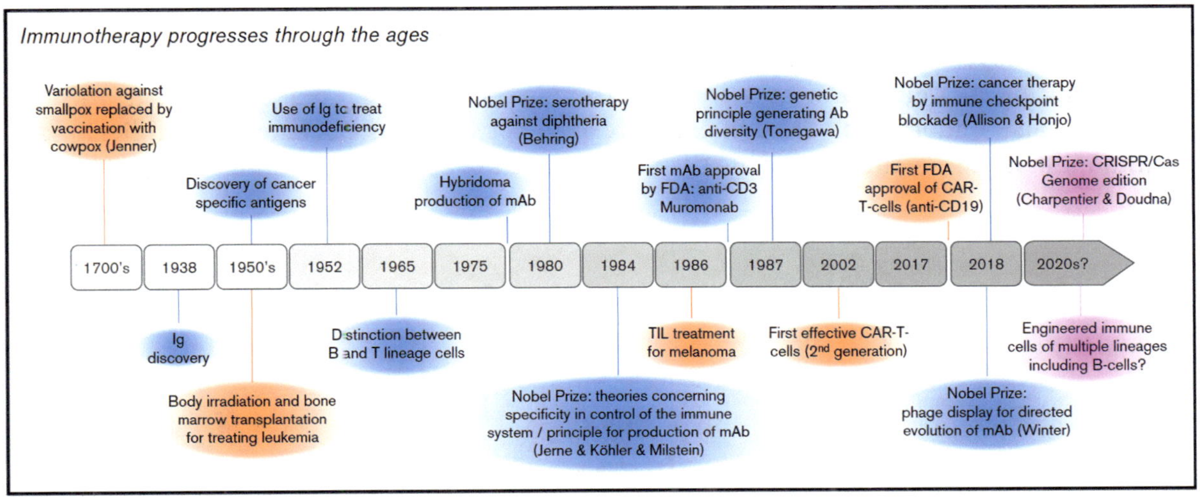

Figure 14.3. A timeline of the history of immunotherapy.

Source: https://www.researchgate.net/profile/Jerome-Moreaux/publication/350329540/figure/fig1/AS:1006550839750657@1616991829280/A-timeline-of-the-history-of-immunotherapy-Although-based-on-old-medical-practices-such.png.

14.1.2. Milestones in Cancer Treatment

As cancer treatment evolved, major milestones have laid the foundation for major breakthroughs in the area. The beginning of chemotherapy in the mid-20th century was a landmark event, bringing with it systemic therapy that greatly enhanced patient survival. With this method came brutal side effects and unpredictable effectiveness against different types of cancer. The advent in the late 1990s of targeted therapies brought new promise, as these drugs specifically targeted cancer cell pathways with minimal harm to normal tissues. As researchers began to better comprehend the molecular basis of cancer, focus shifted to taking advantage of the body's own immune system's natural ability to combat malignancies and birthed immunotherapy—a modality that has grown exponentially in prominence in recent years. Immune checkpoint inhibitors radically transformed cancer treatment by releasing the body's immune attack against tumors. These drugs, such as the PD-1 and CTLA-4 pathway-targeting drugs, have demonstrated phenomenal strength against numerous cancers, including melanoma and lung cancer. However, the creation of immune-related side effects served as an eye-opener on the complexities of immunomodulation. This paved the way for further innovations, particularly CAR-T cell therapy, through which a patient's T cells can be genetically engineered to target and eliminate tumor cells with enhanced efficiency. The advances that have been made in hematological malignancies have instilled hope for applications to solid tumors, underscoring the necessity of continued research toward expanding CAR-T technology's therapeutic potential. At the same time, patient-derived xenograft (PDX) models have developed as a valuable tool for cancer research, continuing to hone treatment paradigms. Through the transplantation of patient tumor tissues into immunocompromised or humanized mice, researchers can replicate the complexity of human tumors, their heterogeneity and three-dimensional structure, which is key to understanding the mechanisms of resistance to treatment. The model's ability to preserve genomic features across various stages and subtypes provides precious insight into drug sensitivity and mechanisms of resistance. By adding cutting-edge technologies such as multi-omics and deep learning, PDX models increase the scope of preclinical trials, ultimately guiding the development of novel therapies like immunotherapies and targeted medicines. This convergence of next-generation modeling and new treatment modalities not only marks milestones in cancer treatment but also underscores the dynamic interface between basic science and clinical practice, propelling momentum in the war against cancer (Hu et al., 2023; Liu et al., 2023) (Figure 14.4).

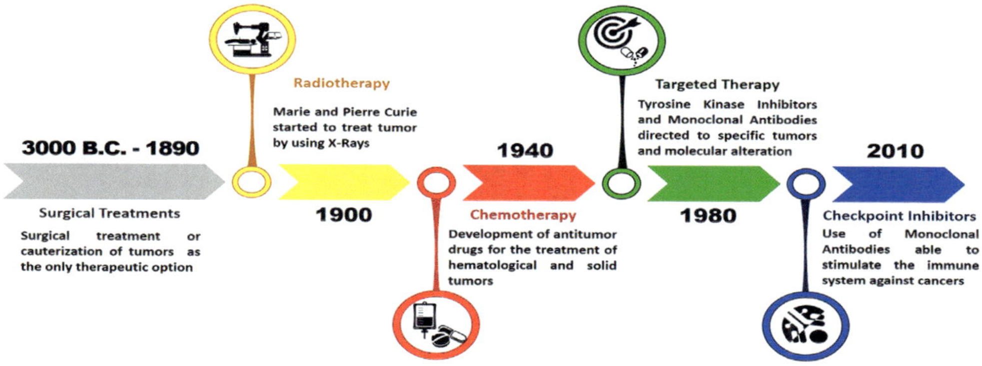

Figure 14.4. Timeline of epochal turning points in modern oncology.

Source: https://www.researchgate.net/publication/328915358/figure/fig2/AS:11431281251405504@1718211413732/Timeline-of-epochal-turning-points-in-modern-oncology-After-the-development-of.tif.

14.1.3. Evolution of Chimeric Antigen Receptor T-cell (CAR-T) cell therapy

Development of CAR-T cell therapy is a landmark event in the history of immunotherapy, marked by its groundbreaking role in controlling certain cancers. In the late 1980s, it was first conceptualized as a CAR-T technology wherein T cells would be engineered by genetics to express CARs that bind to tumor-associated antigens. This milestone opened the door to even more sophisticated ways of taking advantage of the body's immune system against cancer. Decades have elapsed since gene editing tools have been revolutionized by innovations in gene editing tools, particularly with the use of CRISPR and lentiviral vectors, to make T cell modifications more accurate and efficient. It is now possible to engineer CAR-T cells to counter the immunosuppressive tumor microenvironment that typically compromises their effectiveness, a consideration that is most important in the ongoing development of this therapeutic approach to treating hematological malignancies and other diseases. Furthermore, the inclusion of robust preclinical and clinical trial data has played a key role in CAR-T cell therapy. Initial clinical data from trials started to indicate encouraging potential for engineered cells to induce profound remission in patients with refractory disease of leukemia and lymphoma. However, inherent problems, including the resulting toxicities and variable rates of response, spurred subsequent refinements to the CAR design and treatment regimens. It has increasingly become clear that the clarification of T cell dysfunction mechanisms, such as senescence, can be utilized to inform CAR-T therapy optimization. It is, for instance, noted that senescence of T cells induced by tumors contributes to inhibiting durable response induction in cancer therapy and therefore calls for ongoing research into CAR-T cell subsets and their behavior within the tumor microenvironment, which remains a determinant of patient outcome improvement (Huff et al., 2019).

With the field advancing, the prospects for CAR-T cell therapy are optimistic, and several new directions are being explored. New strategies, such as dual-targeting CARs and the use of combination therapies with immune checkpoint inhibitors, are creating opportunities to move beyond hematological malignancies into solid tumors. These similarities between oral canine malignant melanoma (CMM) and human melanoma have also encouraged comparative oncology interest, highlighting the potential to capitalize on findings in veterinary medicine in order to advance human therapies (Atherton et al., 2016). The translational potential of CAR-T therapies, fueled by progress in the knowledge of how cancer cells evade the immune system, puts this technology at the forefront of modern cancer treatment. Lastly, the continuous evolution of CAR-T cell therapy will revolutionize therapeutic practices, enhancing the efficacy of immunotherapeutic strategies against a wide range of cancers (Figure 14.5).

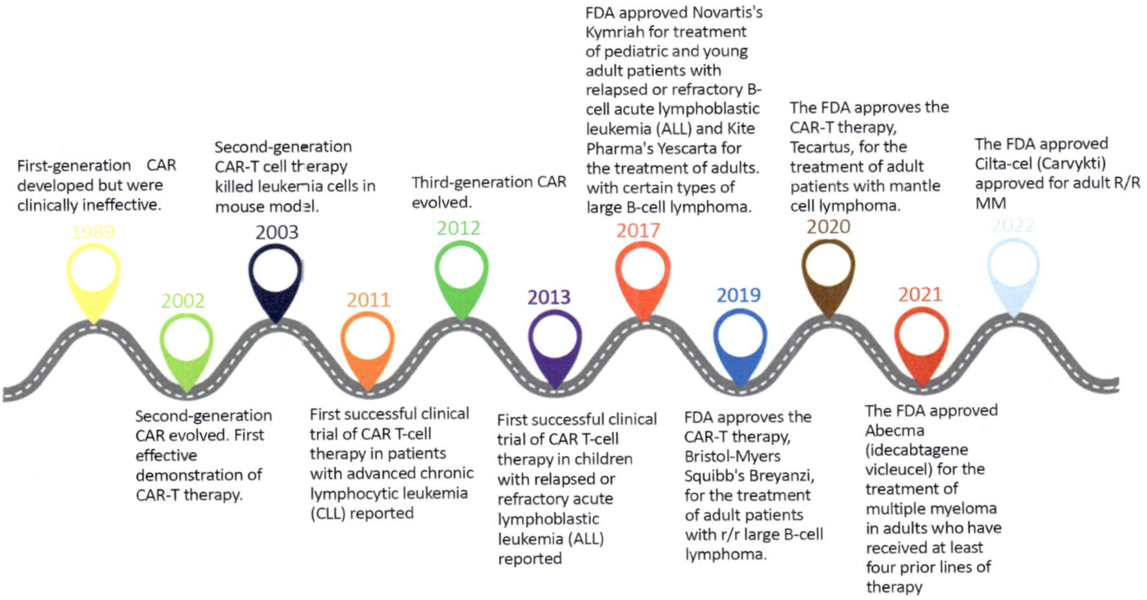

Figure 14.5. History and timeline of chimeric antigen receptor T-cell (CAR-T) therapy development.

Source: https://www.researchgate.net/publication/373297256/figure/fig3/AS:11431281185071611@1693537631782/History-and-timeline-of-CAR-T-therapy-development.png.

14.2. Mechanisms of Action in Immunotherapy

The intricate mechanisms behind immunotherapy are crucial for effective cancer treatments to be formulated. Among the notable features is the modulation of natural killer (NK) cells, significant components of the innate immune system. NK cells execute their cytotoxic function primarily by an equilibrated balance of activating and inhibitory receptors. For instance, ligands such as Necl-5 and Nectin-2, which are usually expressed on tumor cells, bind to receptors such as DNAM-1 and TIGIT. Activation by DNAM-1 leads to enhanced cytotoxicity, while binding to TIGIT leads to inhibition, significantly affecting NK cell activity. Such regulation of NK cell activity highlights the significance of understanding such mechanisms, given that they hold promise for therapeutic intervention through checkpoint blockade maneuvers aimed at boosting or reviving the anti-tumor immune response capable of opposing immune suppression caused by tumors in most cancer types (Sanchez-Correa et al., 2019). Aside from the modulation of NK cells, advances in the development of novel molecules to maximize CAR-T cell therapy are also in the pipeline, particularly as researchers investigate the role of bryostatin analogs. Bryostatin 1 has been very promising in most applications, including enhancing immunotherapeutic activity through the control of the activity of protein kinase C (PKC). The development of bryostatin analogs with preserved PKC affinity and maximized for other biological activities demonstrates a focused method of improving CAR-T cell performance. Interestingly, the analogs can result in enhanced expression of surface antigens like CD22 on CAR-T cells, suggesting their ability to enhance the effectiveness of targeted therapies against malignancies such as leukemia. Through function-oriented synthesis techniques, researchers are studying these derivatives to establish their specific actions and potentially expand the therapeutic armamentarium against drug-resistant malignancies (Hardman et al., 2020). Integration of such molecular mechanisms into immunotherapy strategies offers a comprehensive option for drug development. Elucidation of the inhibitory mechanisms exerted by mechanisms such as TIGIT/PVRIG is essential, with such modulatory activities significantly contributing to the efficacy of immunotherapeutic interventions. Through the application of targeted strategies such as checkpoint inhibitors in conjunction with powerful CAR-T technologies or bryostatin analogs, the aim is twofold: to restore vigorous immune function and to equip immune cells with the armamentarium they require to dismantle tumor defenses. This multi-faceted approach underscores the ever-changing paradigm of cancer immunology, in which emerging findings frequently revise our strategies. In general, an evident understanding of these mechanisms not only clarifies how immune cells can recognize tumors but also provides the foundation for new therapeutic approaches that have the promise to optimize patient outcomes in the ever-evolving cancer therapy landscape (Sanchez-Correa et al., 2019; Hardman et al., 2020).

14.2.1. Immune System Activation

Activation of the immune system is an important aspect to achieve effective therapeutic outcomes in immunotherapy, particularly through CAR-T technology. Immune system activation is founded on the ability of immune cells to identify foreign antigens, and subsequently, a cascade of signals initiates various immune mechanisms to kill abnormal cells. The mechanism is typically hampered by the TME, which may evade immune surveillance and enhance tumor growth. Tumors are capable of creating an immunosuppressive environment by the secretion of cytokines and the attraction of regulatory immune cells, further making the activation of T cells a complicated process. For example, in mechanisms of T cell activation in solid tumors, immune activation and suppression dynamics play a key role in the effectiveness of CAR-T therapies, necessitating the understanding of the mechanisms in place that control the immune system's activation to improve therapeutic procedures. Studies in the tumor microenvironment are revealing how certain factors may be used to amplify immune activation. As an example, fibroblast activation protein (FAP) has proven to be a key biomarker and therapeutic target in sarcomas, which has been described in studies of dog soft tissue sarcomas. Based on these studies, FAP+ cancer-associated fibroblasts within the TME seem to dynamically regulate immunity, effectively leading to T cell exclusion and dysfunction.

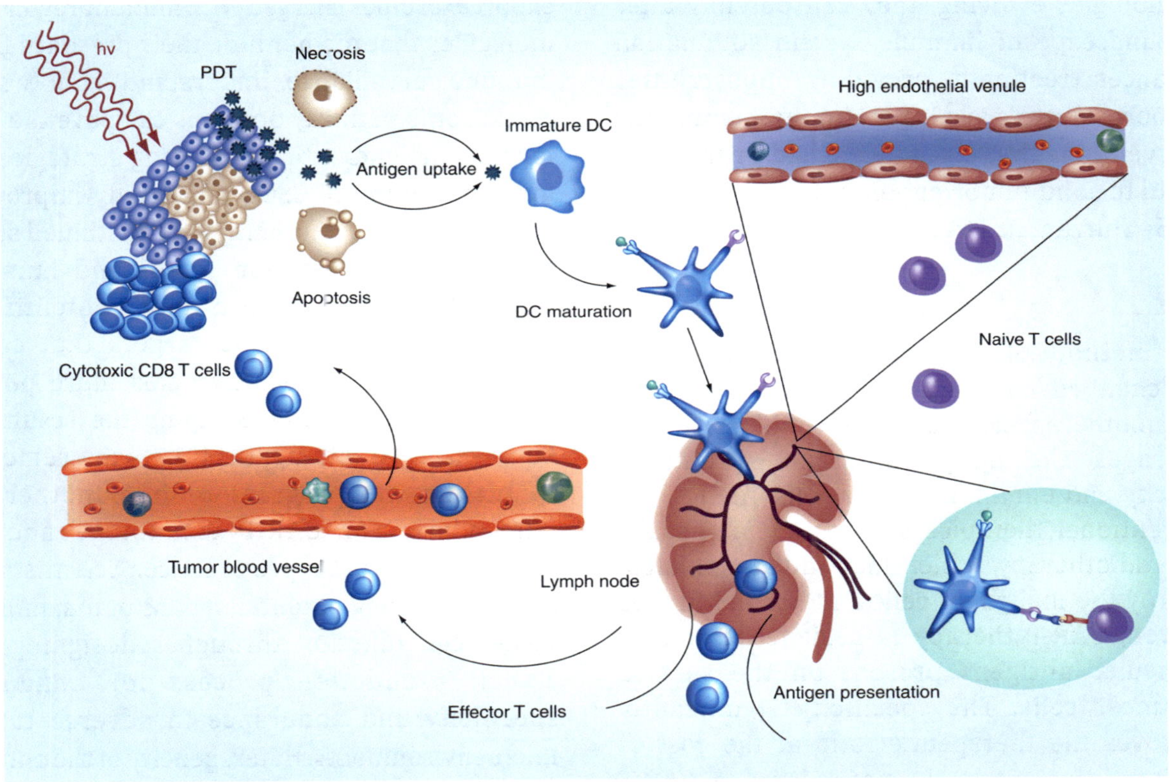

Figure 14.6. Local activation of the innate immune system can be strongly potentiated by strategies that facilitate better activation of dendritic cells, macrophages or neutrophils.

Source: https://www.researchgate.net/profile/Michael-Hamblin/publication/49687617/figure/fig5/AS:394226270523395@1471002275363/Local-activation-of-the-innate-immune-system-can-be-strongly-potentiated-by-strategies.png.

The dual function of FAP as a prognostic factor and CAR-T cell therapeutic target reflects the necessity to enhance immune activation and surmount the inherent hurdle of TME. By targeting immune-dysfunction-facilitating factors, new immunotherapeutic approaches, including FAP-targeting therapy, are being developed to boost T cell infiltration and activity to combat cancer more effectively. Moreover, developments in synthetic biology, such as the development of synthetic Notch (synNotch) receptors, represent a novel approach to enhancing the specificity and activation of anticancer immune responses to cancer treatment. By creating signaling pathways that can be very tightly controlled, synNotch systems can redefine T cell activation in the context of tumor antigens. This technology allows CAR-T cells to gain more regulation of their activation and function, reducing off-target effects but keeping robust anti-tumor potency. Recent studies indicate that synNotch receptors can have the potential to discriminate between cancer and normal cells, improving the therapeutic index of CAR-T therapies. With these technologies evolving, they can possibly alter the landscape of immune system stimulation in cancer treatment, providing opportunities for more effective and safer immunotherapeutic interventions that ultimately could prove to be useful to solid tumor patients (Klosowski et al., 2025; Shirzadian et al., 2025) (Figure 14.6).

14.2.2. Targeting Cancer Cells

The method of targeting the cancer cells has changed completely with the advent of immunotherapy and CAR-T technology, which leverages the body's immune system to identify and eliminate cancer cells. Along with conventional therapies such as chemotherapy and radiotherapy, which may indiscriminately destroy the malignant cells and normal tissues as well, CAR-T therapy is designed to target particular antigens present on the surface of cancer cells. The specificity significantly improves the therapeutic ratio at the cost of collateral damage to the normal tissue. CAR-T cell therapy has, in particular, been shown to have high potential against hematological malignancies, leading to complete remission in several patients.

However, the challenges faced with solid tumors such as gliomas point towards the complexity faced in effectively engineering T cell immunity against heterogeneous antigenic landscapes and tumor microenvironments, which will prove to be critical in the direction of improving patient outcomes in the future (Chuntova et al., 2018). One of the greatest challenges in the case of cancer cell targeting is addressing mechanisms through which tumors manage to evade immunosurveillance, particularly in solid tumors. Cancer stem cells (CSCs), which have been implicated in tumor recurrence and drug resistance, possess unique immunosuppressive properties that allow them to evade recognition and killing by the immune system. Recent evidence suggests that CSCs can export exosomes charged with immunoregulatory molecules that further hide their presence from immune surveillance. Understanding how such an exosome pathway operates can pave the way for new insights into pathfinding strategies for direct targeting of CSCs, potentially improving outcomes in immunotherapy. As continued study of interactions between tumor and immune cells takes place, there is more potential to identify novel druggable targets that could render existing CAR-T therapies more potent (Clayton et al., 2020). Bringing the results of basic research into application is instrumental in fueling the progress of immunotherapy, particularly for CAR-T technology and its application across types of cancer. Scientists are also considering potential means of maximizing CAR-T cell function through redesigning the T cell production process for enhanced specificity and endurance in adverse tumor microenvironments. Heterogeneity of the antigen and the immunosuppressive glioma environment presents a challenge and necessitates new approaches that could include combination strategies or engineered cells that can break through them. Besides, efforts to personalize CAR-T cell design, aiming at every patient's unique tumor pattern, remain a crucial cancer therapy frontier. By systematically addressing such hurdles, researchers could develop a new standard in treating cancer cells, ultimately improving survival rates and patients' quality of life combating malignancies (Chuntova et al., 2018) (Figure 14.7).

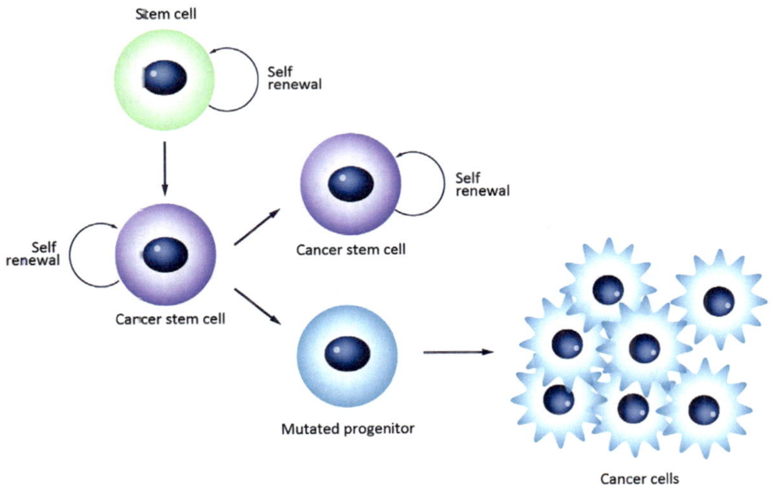

Figure 14.7. Cancer stem cells (CSCs).

Source: https://www.genetex.com/upload/media/research/Cancer/Cancer_Stem_Cells/cancer%20 stem%20cell-header_%E5%E7%A5%E4%BD%9C%E5%8D%80%E5%9F%9F%201.jpg.

14.2.3. Role of Cytokines in Therapy

Cytokines play a pivotal role in enhancing the therapeutic effect of immunotherapies, particularly in CAR-T cell therapies. The tiny signaling proteins facilitate cell-to-cell communication between immune cells and are vital for the control of the immune system. In CAR-T therapy, the incorporation of cytokine genes in the gene-modified T cells has been seen to yield promising results, facilitating increased proliferation, persistence, and anti-tumor activity. For instance, cytokine induction of cytokines such as interleukin-2 (IL-2) and interleukin-15 (IL-15) is likely to enhance CAR-T cell survival and expansion in the tumor microenvironment. In addition, bidirectional crosstalk between immune cells and cytokines not only influences the efficacy of CAR-T treatments but also helps overcome immunosuppressive states characteristic of tumor milieus, promoting a more cancer-targeting environment for eradication. The therapeutic use of cytokines is also beyond CAR-T cell therapy and paves the way for further applications in molecular immunology. In particular, analysis of cytokine profiles in the tumor environment can be a very useful contribution to understanding the pathophysiology of the tumor and the immune reactions induced by the tumor. For example, cytokines such as tumor necrosis factor-alpha (TNF-α) and interferon-gamma (IFN-γ) have been reported to be involved in the activation of both innate and adaptive immune mechanisms against tumors. Nevertheless, some cytokines could inadvertently increase tumor progression or produce undesirable side effects if uncontrolled. Therefore, the optimization of cytokine delivery—through nanoparticle technology or combination therapy—is set to maximize therapeutic benefit with diminished systemic toxicity. Balanced cytokine therapy is a hopeful route to maximizing immune activation against cancer. In addition, research on cytokine-targeted therapies, particularly in combination with existing immunotherapeutic approaches, is necessary for cancer therapy model progression. Recent evidence demonstrates that cytokine modification has the potential to significantly improve when combined with checkpoint inhibitors or other agents. For instance, cytokines facilitating T-cell activation and function can synergize with immune checkpoint inhibitors to significantly amplify the anti-tumor immune response. Similarly, investigation of CAR-T cells engineered to secrete a single cytokine is gaining significance, as this may preserve their therapeutic effect within the cancer microenvironment. Through investigation of the dual role of cytokines—as therapeutic agents and controllers of immune responses—scientists expect to develop more effective and customized anticancer treatments. Furthermore, the deductions drawn from the cytokine interactions on oncology will likely direct simultaneous developments in related sciences such as immuno-cardiology and other long-term inflammatory diseases, eventually broadening therapeutic boundaries (Biondi-Zoccai et al., 2025; Klosowski et al., 2025) (Figure 14.8).

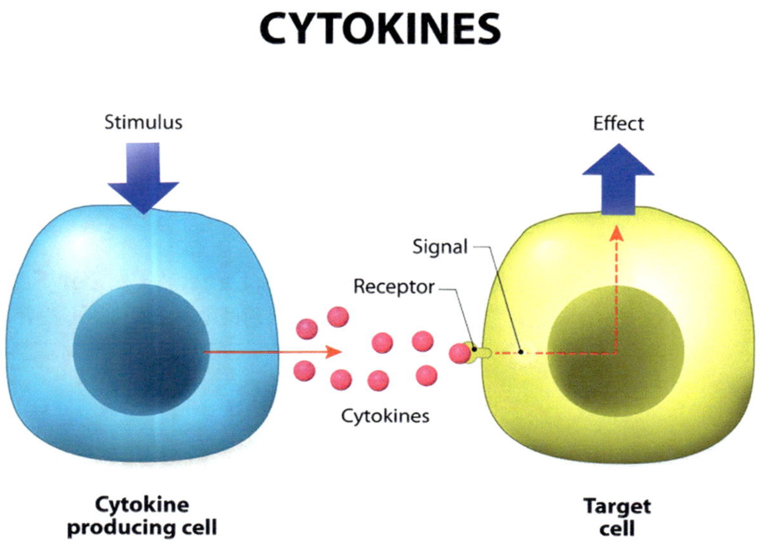

Figure 14.8. Cytokines play a pivotal role in enhancing the therapeutic efficacy of immunotherapies.

Source: https://lifeclinic.com.hk/wp-content/uploads/2021/06/Cytokines-Graphic-August-2017.jpeg.

14.3. Chimeric Antigen Receptor T-cell (CAR-T) Cell Therapy: Process and Development

CAR-T cell therapy is an innovative approach in the area of cancer therapy with its innovative method of accessing the body's immune system. CAR-T cell therapy is founded on the gene editing of T cells to enable them to manufacture CARs, which bind specific tumor antigens. The process begins with harvesting peripheral blood T cells from the patient and stimulating them, prior to transducing them using a viral vector that carries the CAR gene. The modified T cells are then expanded in the laboratory and re-infused into the patient, where they hunt and destroy cancer cells that have the antigens of interest. This personalized therapeutic strategy has been remarkably effective, particularly against hematological malignancies such as acute lymphoblastic leukemia, but the challenge is encountered in transferring its efficacy to solid tumors due to the quirkiness of the tumor microenvironment. Whereas CAR-T cell treatment has demonstrated spectacular success in a few types of cancer, the potential of this modality of treatment is usually dashed by a number of immunologic barriers existing in the TME.

The most striking among them is the state of T cell dysfunction, particularly in combination with the coexistence of regulatory T cells, which generate an immunosuppressive environment. Notably, CD8+ T cell dysfunction has been driven by several factors, some of which are exhaustion and senescence caused by chronic antigen exposure in the TME. Downregulation of costimulatory molecules such as CD28 on T cells brings about defective functionality, leading to diminished anti-tumor responses. As such mechanisms can limit CAR-T efficacy, research efforts should be focused on ways to modulate the TME to enhance CAR-T cell activity and survival in order to improve patient outcomes for solid tumor patients (Huff et al., 2019).

In addition, CAR-T cell therapy engineering should handle the intricacies involved in antigen heterogeneity and the potential for off-tumor toxicity. Because tumors express different antigens and become less targetable in their characteristics over time, the identification of a stable and tumor-specific target is a major problem. The problem is compounded by safety concerns resulting from the risk of damaging normal tissues with the same antigens, which places a premium on achieving greater precision in targeting. Recent studies are directed towards addressing these problems using innovative engineering approaches that optimize the specificity and safety profiles of CAR-T cells. Ongoing studies entail the use of dual CARs to recognize two or more antigens and improved safety switches that are capable of deactivating CAR-T cells upon the occurrence of serious adverse effects. Lastly, by overcoming these limitations in a systematic way, the future of CAR-T cell therapy is very bright in expanding its application in the field of molecular immunology (Chuntova et al., 2018).

14.3.1. Design And Engineering Of Chimeric Antigen Receptor T-cell (CAR-T) Cells

CAR-T cell design and engineering are a significant advancement in the field of cancer immunotherapy. At the heart of this innovation is a synthetic receptor design that possesses the capacity to bind and target tumor-specific antigens on cancer cells specifically. This specificity becomes a critical aspect in differentiating between cancer and non-cancer cells, thereby minimizing potential off-target effects, which remain a problem for conventional cancer treatment. The latest developments have used state-of-the-art techniques, including CRISPR-Cas9 gene editing, to allow researchers to tune into the functional characteristics of CAR-T cells. By enhancing the signaling pathways for T-cell activation upon being presented with the target antigen, researchers aim to increase the persistence, potency, and safety of such engineered cells to combat various malignancies, including solid tumors and hematologic malignancies (Meng et al., 2025). In order to maximize CAR-T cell activity, recent advances have started introducing novel technologies like mRNA and lipid nanoparticles (LNPs) into the design platform. These technologies enable rapid and precise engineering of CAR-T cells such that scientists can react to emerging issues in the tumor microenvironment. Perhaps most importantly, mRNA-based approaches enable the transient expression of CAR constructs, reducing the risk of long-term side effects associated with stably integrated CAR genes. This flexibility is opening up new prospects for active therapeutic reactions to the unique characteristics of particular tumors (Meng et al., 2025). By applying these new methods, scientists can optimize not only the accuracy of targeting by CAR-T cells but also their ability to penetrate and respond to the immunosuppressive factors in solid tumor microenvironments. In addition, the incorporation of synthetic biology principles into CAR-T fabrication is transforming cancer therapy into a new era. SynNotch receptors are the most promising developments, in which molecular logic gates are formed. SynNotch receptors provide a method for selective T cell response to multiple antigens, which can lead to a more nuanced attack on tumors with heterogeneous antigen expression. By linking T-cell activation to combinations of antigens, synNotch systems enhance CAR-T therapies' specificity and control, which guards against on-target, but off-tumor toxicity (Shirzadian et al., 2025). The ability to engineer CAR-T cells with multi-antigen targeting capability is a promising advantage that can transform the therapy of solid tumors and further enable CAR-T technologies to be applied in molecular immunology (Figure 14.9).

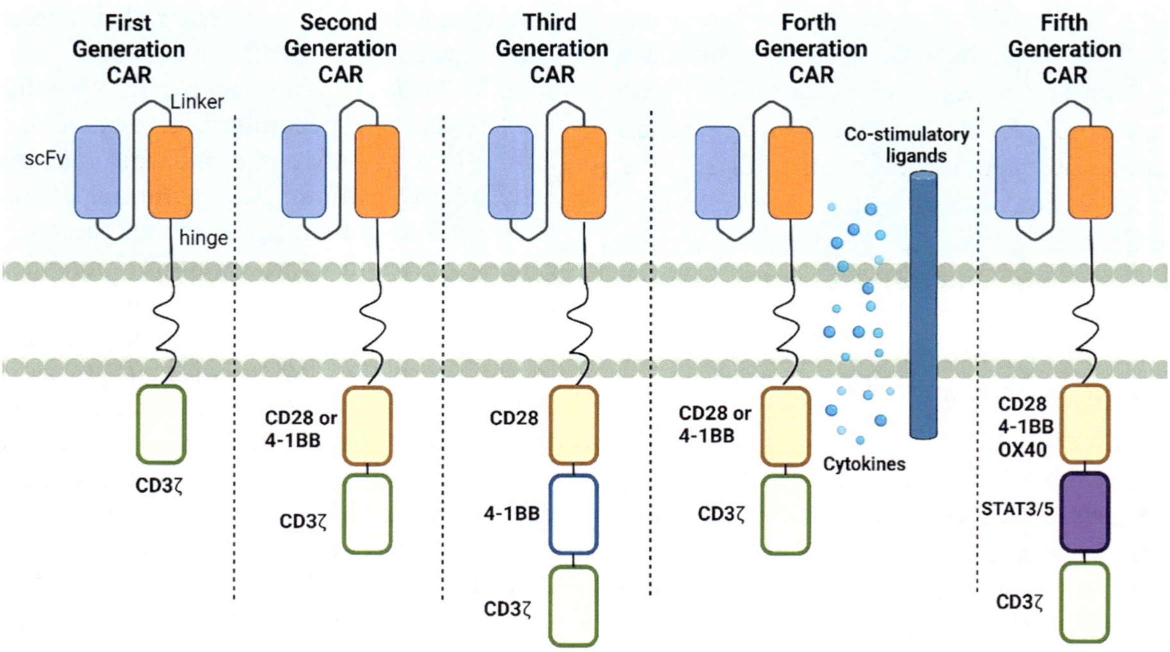

Figure 14.9. The development of the CAR-T cell design, showing changes in structures.

Source: https://www.researchgate.net/publication/381395464/figure/fig3/AS:11431281255833516@1719436239868/The-development-of-the-CAR-T-cell-design-showing-changes-in-structures.tif.

14.3.2. Patient Selection Criteria

Appropriate patient selection for immunotherapy, and in this case CAR-T cell therapy, is important to maximizing the therapeutic benefit and preventing the risk of toxicities. The method of patient selection entails a multi-parameter evaluation of patient characteristics such as age, performance status, and treatment history. Specifically, patients must demonstrate a sufficient level of physical health to endure immunotherapeutic treatment and bear tumor structures expressing similar antigens targeted by CAR-T cells. Malignant gliomas, for example, present special difficulty, as they can be heterogeneous in antigen expression and contain an immunosuppressive environment, thus complicating treatment (Chuntova et al., 2018). Hence, careful assessment of tumor biology in conjunction with the patient's health status is essential in determining the most likely candidates for effective immunotherapy, thus ensuring individualized treatment models. Also, an important aspect of patient selection is an understanding of the intricacies of the tumor microenvironment and how the same plays a role in treatment response. For instance, glioma patients may face antigen presentation and T-cell homing challenges, resulting in lower therapeutic response where these are neglected (Chuntova et al., 2018). This highlights the importance of clinical trials where not only the overall condition of the patient is considered, but also extensive research of the biological profile of the tumor. Patient stratification for tumors with benign immune profiles can significantly enhance the likelihood of a successful outcome to CAR-T therapy. The interactive nature of tumor biology and immune response also identifies the imperative of multidisciplinary care in the identification of candidates as well as the development of specific therapies directed against the patient's unique individual tumor profile. Here, in addition to biological factors, there are also significant logistical factors inherent in choosing patients for immunotherapy. Due to the intricacies of CAR-T cell preparation and delivery, proximity to treatment centers specialized in providing this procedure is frequently the deciding factor in patient qualification. Timing is also crucial since the lag time between developing innovative therapies and bringing them into clinical trials may delay access to potentially life-saving therapy. Groups such as the World Immunotherapy Council call for the primacy of streamlining such processes to eliminate obstacles to the timely enrollment of patients. By addressing both the scientific and the logistical issues of patient selection, the healthcare community can maximize the efficacy of immunotherapies and ensure that the best candidates receive these new medicines promptly (Figure 14.10).

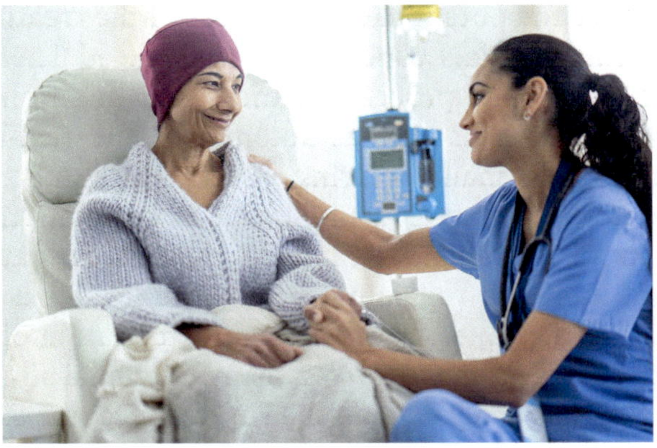

Figure 14.10. Selection of appropriate patients for immunotherapy.

Source: https://www.lungcancercenter.com/app/uploads/2023/10/Immunotherapy-vs.-Chemotherapy.jpg.

14.3.3. Manufacturing and Quality Control Processes

The generation of CAR-T cells is a complex and multifaceted process that involves stringent quality control procedures to ensure safety and efficacy. It begins with patient T cell isolation, which is then genetically modified to express a chimeric antigen receptor to target specific cancer cells. During this complex process, various factors, including cell viability and transduction efficiency, must be closely monitored. Quality control measures take precedence at each step to prevent contamination and ensure reproducibility in the final product. With the advancement of the discipline of molecular immunology, there lies a critical necessity for standardized methods that can streamline the manufacturing process, thereby enabling easier access by patients and better outcomes in immunotherapy. With the rapid advancement in biomanufacturing technology, there is considerable heterogeneity in the practices adopted across labs. Contemporary manufacturing practices in immune cell therapies lean towards being based on outdated practices, which are destined to induce inconsistency and reduce the potential effectiveness of the treatments. Pörtner et al. (2017) identify that the majority of clinical trials conducted on Advanced Therapy Medicinal Products (ATMP) face the variability of quality and process for the generation of immune cells. In this regard, the application of state-of-the-art tools such as automation and real-time monitoring platforms can greatly contribute to improving manufacturing effectiveness and reproducibility. These advancements would lead to better-characterized immune cell populations, in which more accurate therapeutic predictions can be made, and ultimately, the success rates of immunotherapies increase. Quality control is not merely a regulatory requirement; it is a fundamental element that is central to the trust in CAR-T therapies. Complete characterization of *ex vivo* expanded immune cells is essential because it provides information on their functional abilities. Pörtner et al. (2017) emphasize the importance of deeper analysis than the surface receptor expression, e.g., the identification of secreted effectors and their dynamics in time. Such precise quality determinations have the capacity to provide important information concerning the products of immune cells and improve their therapeutic potency. As demand for personalized medicine and targeted therapies continues to grow, stringent quality control during production will be central to the advancement of CA technology in molecular immunology (Figure 14.11).

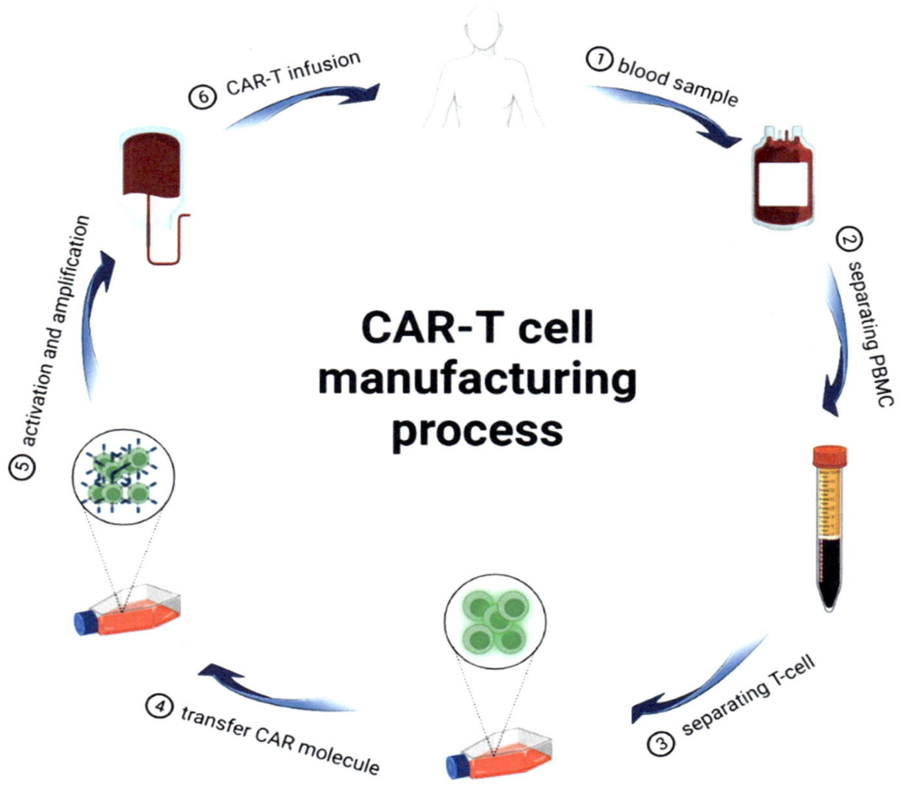

Figure 14.11. The chimeric antigen receptor T-cell (CAR-T) cell manufacturing process.

Source: https://www.researchgate.net/publication/370114028/figure/fig1/AS:114312812105773 96@1702054677682/The-CAR-T-cell-manufacturing-process.tif.

14.4. Clinical Applications of Chimeric Antigen Receptor T-cell (CAR-T) Technology

The clinical applications of CAR-T technology have unmistakably transformed the landscape of cancer treatment, with remarkable efficacy, particularly in hematological malignancies. Initially designed to treat blood cancers such as ALL and non-Hodgkin lymphoma, CAR-T therapies have recorded phenomenal success rates, where some patients record complete remission. This new technique takes advantage of patients' T-cells, which are modified to produce receptors that bind tumor-associated antigens specifically and hence, mediate a specific immune response. The treatment procedure, however, is not complication-free. Complications such as cytokine release syndrome and neurotoxicity, which have been implicated to result from the intense immune activation, underscore the necessity for maximizing treatment protocols for enhanced safety and effectiveness. Moreover, the tractability of CAR-T technology continues to enhance with new antigen targets and better T-cell designs that enter clinical trials, providing hope to patients afflicted with previously untreatable diseases. Despite the promising advances in CAR-T therapy, several significant obstacles still remain, particularly in solid tumors, as the tissue-specific microenvironment presents multi-faceted challenges to effective treatment. Unlike hematologic malignancies, however, solid tumors such as gliomas possess complex architectures and immunosuppressive microenvironments that can dampen T-cell infiltration and function. CAR-T cells, while engineered to be specific, are typically beset by the problems of antigen heterogeneity within the tumor, with ensuing less-than-complete responses. Clinical trials for CAR-T therapy in gliomas are underway to be initiated; nonetheless, it is essential to appreciate the complexity of the immune landscape of the brain. Recent studies have also outlined suggestions of how to enhance CAR-T effectiveness in this application, such as overcoming antigen presentation and homing of T-cells in the brain. Resolving these problems should maximize the therapeutic value of CAR-T technology in recurrent solid tumors and extend its clinical use (Chuntova et al., 2018). Gains in T-cell differentiation knowledge also further expand the possibilities of optimizing CAR-T therapy outcomes. Recent research has unlocked insight into naive T-cell activation, revealing that specific cellular behavior during signaling and division can contribute significantly to differentiation into functional immune cell types. By knowing how naive T cells convert to multipotent T cells, researchers can streamline CAR-T cell production protocols to generate wanted phenotypes, such as T stem cell memory (TSCM)-like cells, with long-lasting persistence and enhanced anti-tumor activity. This tactic not only highlights the importance of individualized immunological therapy but is also part of an overarching shift toward precision medicine in oncologic treatment. Given the current clinical trials, data from these new methods may be opening the door for more effective and safer CAR-T implementations, solidifying the importance of this technology within the evolving field of cancer immunotherapy (Good et al., 2019).

14.4.1. Successes in Hematological Malignancies

The evolution of immunotherapy, in particular the use of CAR technology, has dramatically changed the management of hematologic malignancies. CAR-T cell therapy has been a revolutionary treatment with unprecedented efficacy in the case of relapsed or refractory B-cell malignancies. Patients with ALL and certain other non-Hodgkin lymphomas have shown remarkable responses, with high proportions of complete remission. These therapeutic successes are due to the ability of the CAR-T cells to target specifically CD19, a protein often expressed on the surface of B-cell cancers. Shortcomings still remain, however, such as antigen escape, where cancer cells adapt to shut off CD19 expression, hindering treatment. Resolution of these matters is critical in maintaining progress towards improving patient survival rates for those afflicted with hematological cancers and overall the success of CAR-T treatments (Lühle et al., 2025). Ongoing progress has been made through the development of bifunctional CAR-T cells, created to overcome issues related to antigen escape. With CAR-T cell engineering to target other targets that identify malignant growth, researchers have expanded the application of CAR technology. In particular, through the use of cysteine-mutated CAR variants, targeting and killing CD19 non-reacting B-cell lymphomas is possible. This novel approach provides a two-faceted attack on CD19-positive and CD19-negative malignant cells. These advancements are set to dramatically enhance patient response rates, as attested in preclinical models that show strong cytotoxicity against a range of hematological malignancies. This advancement is a testament to the dedication towards optimizing CAR-T therapy, which eventually resulted in increased efficacy and better patient survival rates in what were once difficult clinical situations (Lühle et al., 2025).

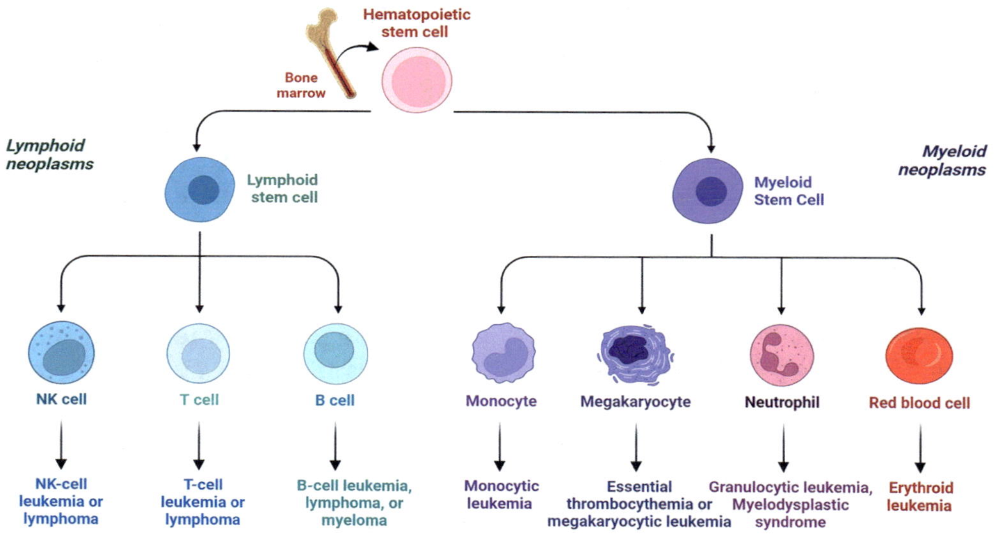

Figure 14.12. The main subtypes of hematological malignancies.

Source: https://www.researchgate.net/publication/371808997/figure/fig1/AS:11431281170009800@1687573157019/The-main-subtypes-of-hematological-malignancies.png.

In addition to CAR-T cells, new strategies such as CAR-macrophage (CAR-M) treatments have also come under the spotlight due to their potential to revolutionize therapy in hematological malignancies and overcome some of the shortcomings of CAR-T strategies. Macrophages possess inherent characteristics that enable them to migrate through complex tumor microenvironments, making them ideal candidates for the therapy of solid tumors and certain hematological conditions. Preclinical studies indicate CAR-Ms' dual function—exerting direct cytotoxic activity while enhancing the infiltration of other immune cells to the tumor. This action has the potential to be a more advantageous alternative to the traditional CAR-T therapy and may provide patients with improved safety and durability. As CAR-M technology advances through research, the integration of these innovative therapies into clinical settings holds the potential to improve current treatment protocols for hematological malignancies, ultimately transforming the landscape of cellular immunotherapy (Figure 14.12).

14.4.2. Challenges in Solid Tumors

The evolution of solid tumors generates inherent issues that together greatly impede the functionality of immunotherapy and CAR-T cell technologies. Unlike hematological tumors, solid tumors possess a complex tumor microenvironment that is characterized by unique anatomical and physiological barriers, which hinder effective immune cell infiltration and functioning. For instance, the excessive extracellular matrix composition in tumors has physical limitations that limit T cell migration and function. Further, the immunosuppressive factors present in the tumor microenvironment can create a harmful environment for T cells and lead to their dysfunction.

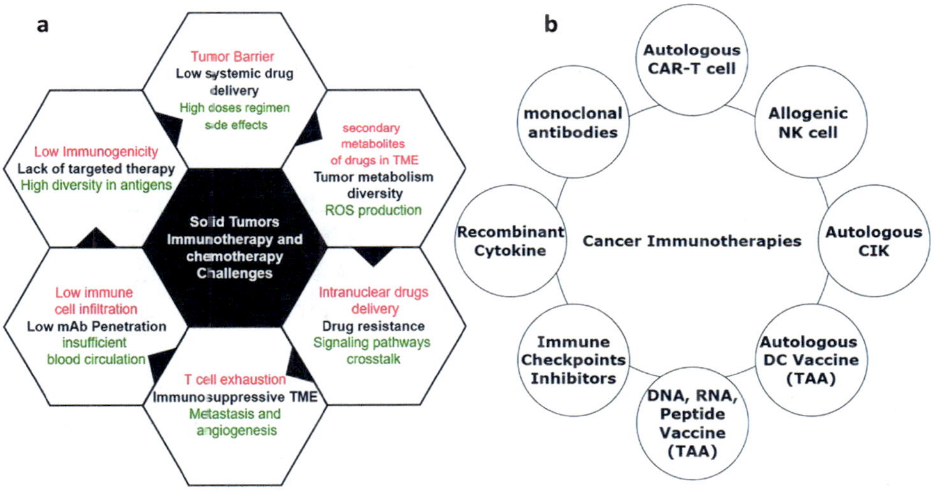

Figure 14.13. a) Immunotherapy and Chemotherapy challenges in solid tumors: The main challenges are the bold font, direct causes are pink, and passive feedback is green. b) General classification of cancer immunotherapy approaches in solid tumors.

Source:

These barriers necessitate a novel means of increasing localization and residence of T cells in solid tumors, particularly with the application of engineered T-cells immune to such obstacles and capable of an effective immune response. Additionally, antigen heterogeneity of solid tumors complicates CAR-T therapy, as antigen variations can lead to asymmetrical targeting by the responsive immune cells. This heterogeneity is generally the result of tumor evolution through clonal selection and mutation, rendering a subgroup of tumor cells resistant to treatment. Hence, the treatment directed against a single antigen will result in the inability to kill the tumor outright since cells lacking that target remain alive and proliferate. Added to this, off-tumor toxicity whereby the CAR-T cells kill normal tissues with identical antigens also generates additional safety concerns. As discussed, rigorous clinical trials need to be conducted to maximize CAR T-cell constructs with improved specificity and fewer potential side effects and in overcoming the heterogeneity and plasticity of solid tumors so as to facilitate enhanced patient outcomes in immunotherapy strategies (Chuntova et al., 2018). T cell senescence within the tumor microenvironment also exacerbates the issues faced by immunotherapy. Naïve CD8+ T cells that are critical for the best anti-tumor responses can become senescent as a result of one of a number of factors, potentially the tumor-related stressors or actions of regulatory T (Treg) cells. Senescent T cells also demonstrate a reduction of co-stimulatory molecules like CD28, which contributes significantly to their activation and proliferation. This dysfunction keeps T cells from effectively launching a proper attack on solid tumors because they are typically stuck in tolerance or anergy. Thus, there is a need for a profound comprehension of senescence pathways in T cells, as discussed in recent publications, to develop targeted strategies that would restore T cell function and increase the effectiveness of immunotherapy in the context of different tumors (Huff et al., 2019) (Figure 14.13).

14.4.3. Ongoing Clinical Trials and Research

The landscape of ongoing clinical trials and studies in immunotherapy, particularly in CAR-T technology, remains dynamic and holds immense hope for oncology treatment methodology enhancement. Ongoing research is focused primarily on addressing the problems related to the successful application of CAR-T cell therapies, particularly in multicystic tumor conditions such as gliomas. These tumors are notoriously resistant to standard therapy, and most standard therapies, like chemotherapy and radiation, yield meager results. The potential of CAR-T cells to bind to tumor antigens selectively is a revolutionary approach, albeit recent clinical trial data give rise to an imperative need for sustained innovation to overcome the challenges intrinsic to glioma therapy, including antigen heterogeneity and immunosuppressive tumor microenvironment, as described in current research initiatives (Chuntova et al., 2018). Planning and execution of clinical trials of CAR-T therapies are aimed at maximizing the therapeutic modality by various means. Investigators remain engaged in exploring modifications in CAR constructs, which are capable of enhancing T-cell survival and intratumoral homing properties. Newer generations of CAR-T therapies have emerged as a result of recent breakthroughs that are intended to circumvent the specific mechanisms of immune escape exhibited by gliomas. Second, upcoming trials are examining combinations of CAR-T therapies with immune checkpoint proteins to enhance the net efficacy. Learning about the complexities of the glioma microenvironment, these new-generation clinical trials aim to derive information that potentially can be translated into meaningful patient improvement and become a model for future immunotherapeutic trials (Chuntova et al., 2018). Further, the data obtained from such continuous trials holds the promise of revolutionary innovations in molecular immunology. While bearing particular challenges in CAR-T execution in mind, scientists can use this data to create innovative treatment strategies. For instance, an understanding of the brain's unique anatomical and biological attributes could lead to more effective means of T-cell delivery as well as minimal off-tumor toxicity. Furthermore, lessons learned from ongoing trials provide valuable feedback loops to refine protocol designs and choose patients better, resulting in more targeted and effective interventions. Scientific investigation into these treatments not only enhances the understanding of immunological responses in gliomas but also contributes to building a larger framework of research into CAR-T technology applicability in other forms of cancer (Chuntova et al., 2018).

14.5. Side Effects and Risks of Chimeric Antigen Receptor T-cell (CAR-T) Therapy

CAR-T therapy has been a significant achievement in the evolution of immunotherapy, particularly in the treatment of hematological malignancies. CAR-T therapy, with its potential for therapeutic benefit, also has a broad range of side effects that have the potential to impact patient outcomes. The most dramatic of these is cytokine release syndrome (CRS), an often lethal disease characterized by a massive inflammatory response upon reintroduction of the engineered T cells into the patient's system. Symptoms of CRS can range from mild flu-like symptoms to severe neurological complications, especially requiring intensive care and treatment. These unanticipated responses highlight the necessity of close monitoring and preparedness for immediate therapeutic interventions both during and after CAR-T cell infusion, in order to offer maximum patient protection with simultaneous exploitation of this new treatment modality. Besides CRS, neurotoxicity has also emerged as a concerning side effect of CAR-T therapy. These patients may manifest a range of neurological toxicities, including encephalopathy, confusion, and seizures, that complicate their cancer clinical management. The underlying pathophysiology of these neurotoxicities is unclear, but they are thought to be a result of central nervous system activation and proliferation of CAR-T cells or systemic inflammation secondary to CRS. This nuance calls for well-conducted clinical trials and long-term studies to define the risk factors of neurotoxicity and establish measures to mitigate such risks. An understanding of the whole spectrum of neurological complications is vital to improve patient outcomes and maximize CAR-T therapy applications in clinical oncology practice. Furthermore, beyond the transient side effects, CAR-T therapy also has long-term risks that should be factored into judging its clinical application. Long-term engraftment of CAR-T cells in the body also poses a risk to off-tumor toxicity, where the engineered cells might end up attacking normal cells that carry the same antigens as tumor cells. This may cause catastrophic damage to healthy tissues and lead to negative implications in otherwise healthy organs. Recent clinical trials have shown such risks, particularly when targeting multi-specific antigens in various tumors. With therapies showing constant advancements, improved CAR constructs must be found in a bid to reduce the rate of off-target effects with higher efficacy towards tumors to a maximum degree, such that CAR-T therapy does justice as a revolutionary treatment within the field of molecular immunology (Chuntova et al., 2018; Krmpotić, 2018).

14.5.1. Cytokine Release Syndrome (CRS)

CRS is one of the most serious side effects of CAR-T cell therapy, with a significant impact on the safety profile of these revolutionary treatments. CRS is a hyper-inflammatory syndrome caused by the extreme activation and proliferation of CAR-T cells, which translates to the overabundance of cytokine release. It exhibits signs ranging from mild flu-like illness to high-grade complications like acute respiratory distress syndrome and multi-organ failure. The clinical presentation of CRS is widely variable depending on CAR-T product and underlying disease, thus making vigilant monitoring of treated patients a must. Early detection and diagnosis of CRS are of utmost importance, as prompt treatment can significantly impact patient outcomes, allowing for the preservation of potentially curative therapy while regulating unwanted consequences of inflammation and cytokine overflow (Huang, 2025). Advances in the knowledge of molecular pathophysiology of CRS have contributed to the discovery of targeted therapies to mitigate its severity.

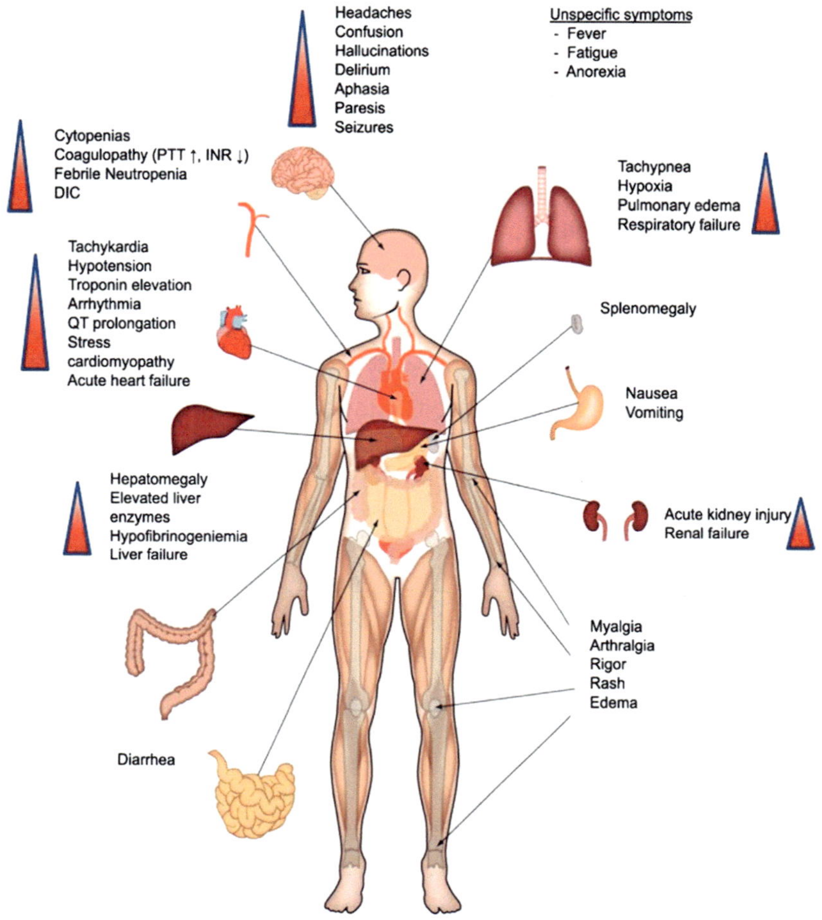

Figure 14.14. Clinical presentation of cytokine release syndrome (CRS).

Source: https://cdn.ncbi.nlm.nih.gov/pmc/blobs/9a26/6003181/f47ac37cdb44/40425_2018_343_Fig1_HTML.jpg.

Tocilizumab, an IL-6 receptor antagonist, has been extensively given to control the inflammatory process of CRS. By inhibiting the IL-6 signaling pathway, tocilizumab suppresses the cytokine storm, thus decreasing symptoms and recovering the compromised patient. Other approaches with potential include the employment of kinase inhibitors, potentially modulating downstream signaling to suppress cytokine production and T-cell hyperactivation. In addition, technologies such as CAR-NK (Natural Killer) cells represent a further avenue of investigation, attempting to utilize the efficacy of CAR technology while minimizing CRS risk. Continuing research will be required to advance these treatment regimens and integrate them best into the clinical management of CAR-T-treated patients (Teibo et al., 2025). CRS worries have driven ongoing debate about the future of immunotherapy of the CAR-T technology, and fascinating developments in the field have ensued. Technologies such as reversible CAR switches attempt to provide clinicians with greater control over T-cell activation and dissociate CRS events. Such groundbreaking technologies are engineered to toggle CAR-T cell function on and off, allowing for tailored immune responses that are tailored to the unique needs of individual patients. Furthermore, understanding the proteomic composition of CAR-T cells has unveiled critical effector molecules implicated in CRS, holding the potential to bring personalized prevention and management strategies into being. The need for in-depth studies in this area remains acute in view of the fact that the therapeutic benefit of CAR-T cell therapy has been balanced with safety issues. Resolution of CRS not only will enhance patient outcomes but also solidify CAR-T position in the evolving landscape of cancer immunotherapy (Huang, 2025; Teibo et al., 2025) (Figure 14.14).

14.5.2. Neurological Toxicities

With the introduction of immunotherapy and CAR-T therapy, cancer therapy has been revolutionized, but at a cost of grave risk, most notably neurological toxicities. These toxicities, which range from mild to severe, can occur because the engineered T-cells target tumor cells but also normal neural cells. Neurological toxicities are typically manifested as confusion, agitation, seizures, or even confusional encephalopathy. It is valuable to know these side effects, especially since the brain's unique environment complicates the therapeutic process. For instance, though CAR-T cells may easily penetrate the tumor microenvironment, they might inadvertently cause inflammation or damage to the adjacent neural tissues, leading to a variety of neurological adverse effects that should be monitored and controlled carefully within clinical settings. The growing body of evidence points us toward the need to develop strategies that mitigate such toxicities without giving up therapeutic efficacy. Additionally, the abundance of neurological toxicities has encouraged rigorous explorations into the mechanisms behind the toxicities. In view of the anatomical dissimilarities of the brains, researchers are forced to investigate how CAR-T cells communicate with neural cells and whether there is an off-target activity. Clinical trials have shown that the immune response within the central nervous system is not always identical to that in peripheral tissues and that this can cause unexpected side effects when using these treatments. In addition, CAR-T cells can cause overstimulation of the immune system or cytokine release, which can increase neurological toxicity. Experience in several clinical trials emphasizes the need for increasing understanding of such complications. Resolution of the antigen specificity issue and T-cell optimization can decrease the safety profile of CAR-T therapies while avoiding neurological side effects, thus improving patient outcomes in oncology treatment. Clinical trials with CAR-T technology indicate that while the therapeutic impacts are most striking, the accompanying neurological toxicities must be avoided. For instance, findings of primary research on CAR-T therapy for gliomas reveal an intricate association between tumor invasion and neuroinflammatory responses. As discussed in the literature, these responses have been shown to maximize the toxicities within the central nervous system and impact patient quality of life. Improved, safer, and more specific immunotherapies rely on demystifying these toxicities. Future advancements in CAR-T technology must focus on minimizing neurological toxicities using sophisticated designs involving engineered safety switches or dual-targeting mechanisms. Through the development of a more advanced method of CAR-T therapy, practitioners can increase therapeutic potential while protecting against the neurologic effects that at present restrict broader use of these novel treatments in molecular immunology, specifically for brain malignancies and lymphomas, as highlighted in research (Koduri et al., 2017; Chuntova et al., 2018) (Figure 14.15).

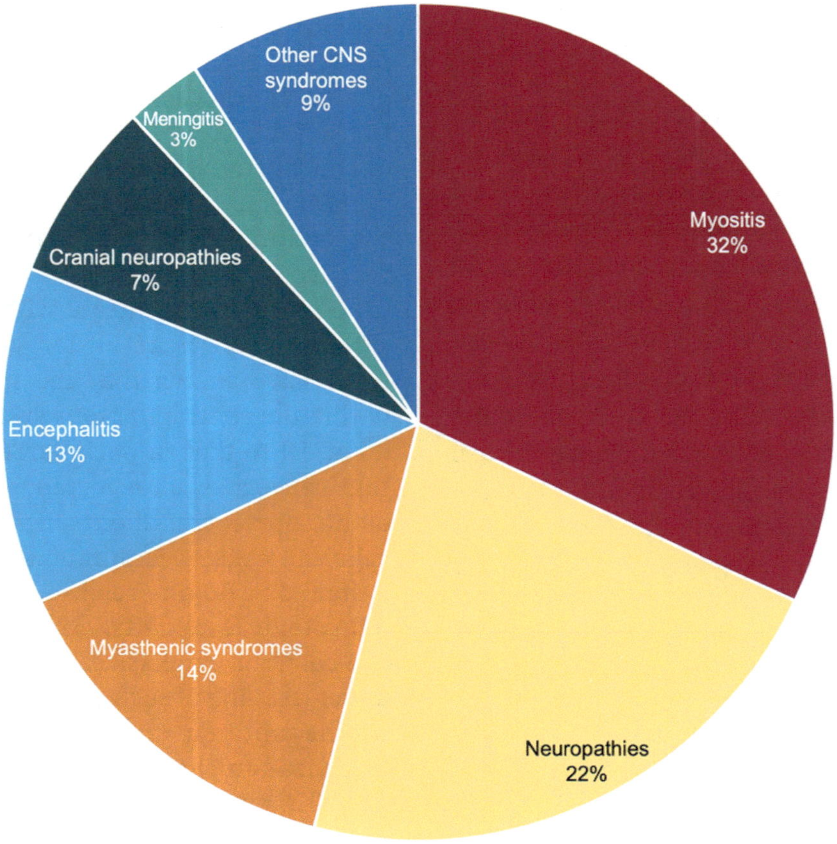

Figure 14.15. Relative frequency of the different neurological toxicities of immune checkpoint inhibitors.

Source: https://www.researchgate.net/profile/Alberto-Vogrig/publication/355686216/figure/fig2/AS:1125024438190082@1645238136771/Relative-frequency-of-the-different-neurological-toxicities-of-immune-checkpoint.png.

14.5.3. Long-Term Effects and Monitoring

The long-term implications of immunotherapy, in particular CAR-T cell therapy, are a focus of research in molecular immunology. With these treatments having positive outcomes in many cancers, their long-term implications gain significance. Particular attention is given to the response duration, which may be influenced by such factors as the durability of CAR-T cells, the tumor microenvironment, and CSCs. Research indicates that treatment may be intense at first, but the patients normally experience relapses, which are normally due to the potency of CSCs that are quite resistant to drugs. Therefore, ongoing assessment of these patients is required to determine the efficacy and duration of the response over time, with specific focus on the kinetics of CSC populations and correlation with recurrence of cancer, as indicated in studies with a focus on CSC immunosuppressive properties (Stroncek et al., 2012). Follow-up of patients after immunotherapy is an essential component of ensuring maximum outcomes, as it enables early action upon relapse or failure of treatment. Imaging techniques and laboratory tests, every now and then, can assist in the detection of the recurrence of cancer cells and determine the persistence of CAR-T cells. Furthermore, medical teams must implement intensive monitoring for possible adverse effects of CAR-T therapy, such as cytokine release syndrome and neurotoxicity, which have been found to manifest far beyond after treatment. These are the aspects of such a multidisciplinary team, ensuring not just that survivors are immediately treated but are also educated on what the possible long-term effects of their treatment will be. Best post-treatment practices can enhance the quality of life for patients and promote early control of any undesirable consequences, thereby maximizing the effectiveness of CAR-T technologies (Stroncek et al., 2012). The evolving landscape of immunotherapy requires continuous study of long-term consequences to optimize measures that counter the new hurdles offered by cancer. Investigating the cross-talk between different adoptive cell therapies, including CAR-T cells, and cancer stem cells has the potential to unveil novel therapeutic targets that can counteract recurrence risk. Studies have demonstrated that CSCs are highly skilled at evading immunotherapy and consequently promoting tumor recurrence. Therefore, further research into CSC-mediated mechanisms of immunorecurrence and the potential for immunoregulatory activity of exosomes derived from such cells is necessary. This line of research holds the promise to deliver essential insights into novel druggable targets and enhance the effectiveness of existing treatments. With the continuous refinement of monitoring and treatment regimes, the field of molecular immunology can ensure that patients are being treated with the most effective cancer therapies available now and optimizing their survival and remission chances in the long run (Clayton et al., 2020).

14.6. Future Directions in Immunotherapy

The future developments in immunotherapy will be dictated by a greater understanding of the tumor microenvironment and the complex interactions between cancer cells and the immune systems. New studies have concentrated on how diverse immunological responses are modulated by various biomolecular factors. Recent progress in precision medicine is aimed at tailoring immunotherapy approaches through informing treatment regimens based on the individual's genomic and immunologic signatures. With molecular biomarkers, physicians can select the best therapies, optimizing treatment while minimizing side effects. Of special interest is the work on combined therapies with CAR-T technology applied in combination with immune checkpoint inhibitors, an extremely promising field for investigation and to facilitate synergistic action against neoplasms. This venture is crucial because there is an intrinsic challenge to properly treating heterogeneously occurring tumors that are variably responsive to monotherapies, generating a need for multi-faceted interventions grounded in early scientific evidence (Garg et al., 2024). Further, the development of next-generation CAR-T cell therapy is promising advancements in immunotherapy science. The evolution of these treatments is marked by efforts to maximize them for effectiveness against solid tumors, where indigenous CAR-T applications have fared poorly. Current research is focused on CAR-T cell engineering for the expression of additional receptors or cytokines in the hope of maximizing their effectiveness and duration of stay in the tumor microenvironment. Techniques such as

CRISPR gene editing are also being explored to improve the efficacy and safety of CAR-T therapies, reducing the possibility of on-target, off-tumor toxicity. As clinical trials expand, the application of artificial intelligence and machine learning to analyze patient data and predictive modeling will be the revolutionary force in the optimization of CAR-T therapy protocols. This combination of technology and immunological progress will likely set new standards in treatment success and patient survivorship (Mutebi, 2024). The future of immunotherapy is also moving toward the application of novel agents such as oncolytic viruses and tumor-infiltrating lymphocytes (TILs), which provide alternative modalities to augment immune responses against cancer. Translation of these therapies requires an integrative approach that not only addresses the intrinsic immune-evasion capacity employed by cancers but also brings more comprehensive therapy to the masses across geographic or socioeconomic boundaries. Some new research underlines the importance of multidisciplinary approaches with an emphasis on cooperation among specialties such as genetics, bioengineering, and public health to accelerate the pace of innovation. Also, increasingly expensive costs of advanced immunotherapies necessitate a call to discussions for equitable access to healthcare and sustainable approaches in cancer therapy. As these promising avenues in immunotherapy develop, they also present a path towards not only enhanced therapeutic results but also enhanced quality of care for cancer patients globally (Garg et al., 2024; Mutebi, 2024).

14.6.1. Combination Therapies with Chimeric Antigen Receptor T-cell (CAR-T)

Combination therapies with CAR-T cell therapy represent a new avenue of research in cancer therapy, particularly for those who are not optimally responsive to single-agent therapies. By combining CAR-T therapy with other treatment modalities, including immune checkpoint inhibitors or targeted therapies, the aim is to optimize treatment regimens. This approach overcomes the issue of immune evasion and tumor heterogeneity that would otherwise compromise the effectiveness of CAR-T therapies when used alone. For instance, when CAR-T cells are used in combination with checkpoint inhibitors, they may reinvigorate exhausted T cells, thereby increasing their proliferation and survival in the tumor microenvironment. Such an intervention would change the treatment paradigm fundamentally, for which reason synergistic effects must be investigated and maximized in clinical trials. Clarifying how these therapies interact will be important to maximizing patient outcomes and the evolution of immunotherapy as a whole. Further, the inclusion of novel technologies such as CRISPR/Cas9 in CAR-T cell therapy is opening new avenues for combination regimens. This revolutionary gene-editing strategy allows for the targeted manipulation of CAR-T cells, enhancing their function while reducing apprehension about off-target effects. For example, CRISPR can be employed to knock out inhibitory receptors on CAR-T cells to effectively eliminate checkpoints that limit their activity against tumors. Concurrently, using CRISPR in combination with CAR-T therapy and nanomedicine may result in transformative synergies that attempt to deliver targeted therapeutics within tumor cells while circumventing systemic toxicity. With the potential of gene editing to tailor changes, researchers can come up with more potent and specific CAR-T therapies that will also reduce the costs of production and improve access to treatments, thereby addressing the bigger problem of current cancer treatments, which include their very high economic expense and variable patient response. Furthermore, the evolving landscape of combination therapies highlights the potential of multifunctional strategies that combine disparate treatment modalities to bypass the drawbacks inherent in traditional cancer treatments. Nanomedicine revolutionizes the delivery and efficacy of therapeutic agents at the site of cancer, complementing CAR-T technology. Multifunctional nanomaterials can be engineered to concomitantly deliver CAR-T cells and chemotherapy drugs with modulation of the tumor microenvironment to augment an immune response against cancers.

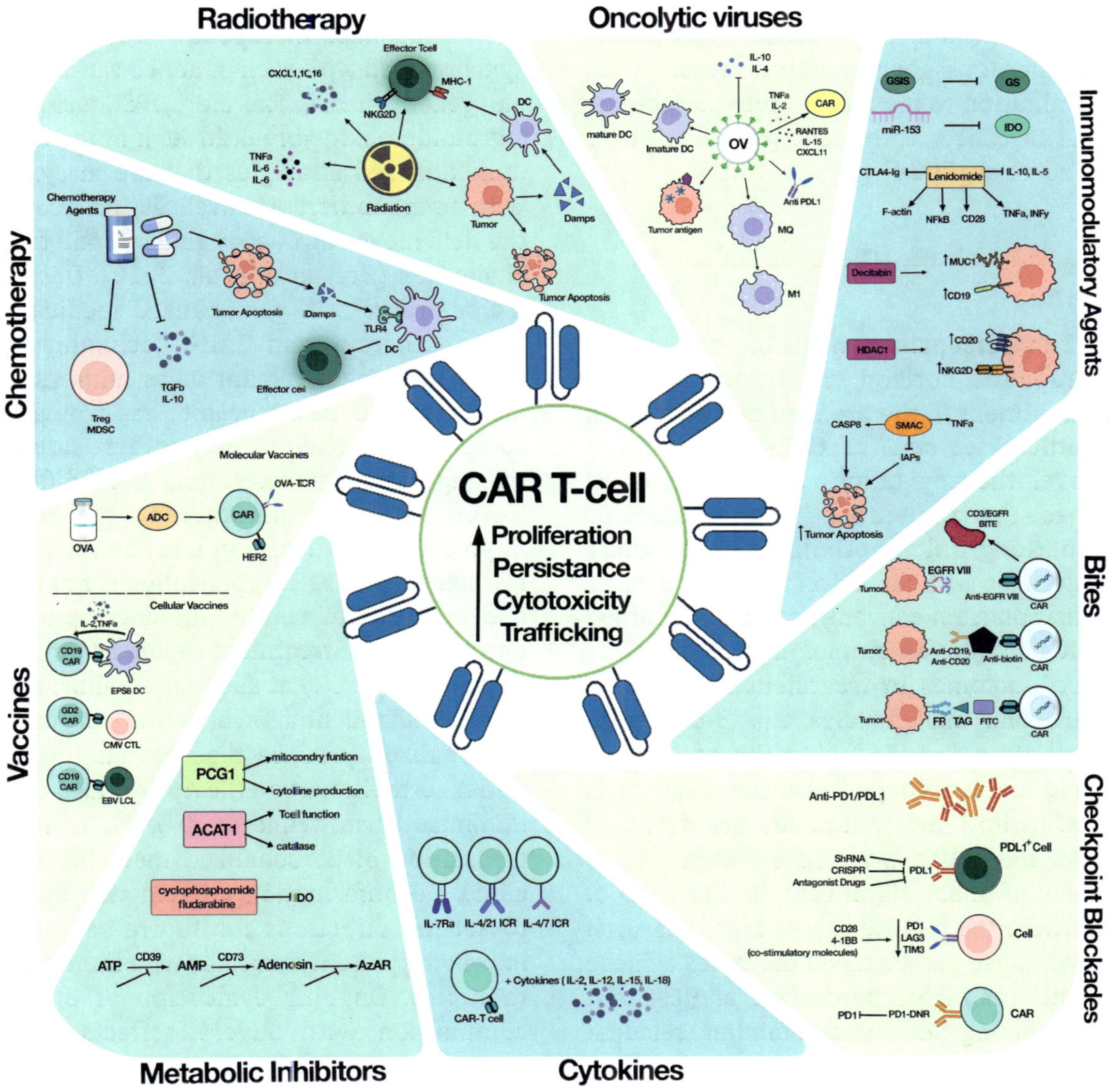

Figure 14.16. Chimeric antigen receptor T-cell (CAR-T) cell combination therapy with other cancer therapeutic approaches.

Source: https://www.researchgate.net/publication/365713911/figure/fig1/AS:1143128110033958 9@1669346429894/CAR-T-cell-combination-therapy-with-other-cancer-therapeutic-approaches.png.

As is clear from recent advances, these novel approaches not only augment the therapeutic index of immunotherapies but also leverage the enhanced permeability and retention effect for enhanced drug consolidation in tumors. The therapeutic potential of future combination therapies with CAR-T cells will, however, hinge on these integration approaches, highlighting the necessity for rigorous clinical investigation and examination to maximize their therapeutic potential in cancer treatment (do Rêgo et al., 2024; Tao et al., 2024) (Figure 14.16).

14.6.2. Advances in Personalized Medicine

Progress in personalized medicine has altered the therapeutic horizon, most specifically in cancer treatment in the arena of oncology, with immunotherapies such as CAR-T cell therapy. This novel therapy tailors the treatment of cancer to the individual's own molecular and genetic profile, optimizing therapeutic responsiveness with few adverse consequences. The transition from conventional chemotherapy to targeted immunotherapies has significantly improved outcomes in treatment for patients with particular malignancies, e.g., B-cell acute lymphoblastic leukemia (B-ALL). One of the most noticeable successes of personalized medicine is observed in how the treatments are designed to engage the patient's immune system better, a fact that is most significant in the case of B-ALL, where the relapse rate is high. Research has shown these personalized therapies achieve remission in as high a percentage as 90%, but reveal continuing challenges in minimal residual disease that require research and development using molecular immunology. The integration of induced pluripotent stem cells (iPSCs) into personalized medicine has further expanded the potential for customized therapies. Through its provision of the capacity to generate pluripotent stem cells from somatic cells of adults, iPSC technology offers scientists the capacity to model disease processes with unprecedented accuracy. These cells provide a system for examining the specific molecular mechanisms of various diseases, including cancer and genetic disorders, and offer a source for cell-based therapeutics. The ability to create patient-specific iPSCs has the priceless potential not only in the understanding of disease pathology but also in the creation of individualized therapeutic strategies that are synchronized with each patient's variant cellular and genetic profile. Therefore, iPSC technology is a groundbreaking breakthrough in the quest for individualized strategies that are in synchrony with immunotherapy advances, particularly as the field moves through regulatory and technical challenges (Bragança et al., 2019). Despite the major progress in personalized medicine with immunotherapy and CAR-T technology, many major challenges remain to be addressed. The introduction of new therapies has brought along complexities, including new adverse side effects, making patient management more difficult. In B-ALL, while immunotherapy has achieved unprecedented success in treating relapsed and refractory disease, its application is not risk-free and necessitates continuous development and optimization of treatment regimens for patients (Besada, 2018). That such an equilibrium must be maintained underscores the very spirit of personalized practice that not only strives to optimize therapeutic efficacy but also seeks to minimize harm. While more work explores the translation of personalized medicine into the clinic, the information created will be crucial to setting directions for future research and improving patient outcomes with immunological therapies. Ongoing evaluation of efficacy in comparison with adverse effects will give motivation for continued evolution of the field and greater safety and efficacy of new therapies in molecular immunology.

14.6.3. Potential for Treating Other Diseases

The hope of immunotherapy, particularly CAR-T technology, extends beyond hematological neoplasms and is increasingly being explored for the management of solid tumors and other disorders. Recent advances demonstrate that CAR-T cell manipulation can enhance their efficacy against solid tumors through evasion of the immunosuppressive environment within the tumor microenvironment. For instance, CAR-T cells armored to secrete interleukin-12 (IL-12) have been promising for treating ovarian cancer models by increasing T-cell function and regulating the tumor microenvironment in a favorable manner. This groundbreaking modality illustrates how CAR-T technology can be modified not only for oncology but also for treating autoimmune diseases and perhaps chronic infections, in which augmentation of local immune responses might contribute to more effective management and resolution of disease. As more research is conducted, the promise of CAR-T use expands beyond cancer treatment, with new treatments for many health ailments waiting in the wings. In addition to solid tumor management, CAR-T technology holds out the promise of treating mechanisms of disease in autoimmune illnesses. By developing T-cells to detect and control specific autoimmune antigens, researchers envision developing targeted therapies that will suppress disease manifestations but preserve overall immune function. This approach holds particular potential for conditions like rheumatoid arthritis and multiple sclerosis, where immune response dysregulation is pathogenic. The ability to engineer T-cells able to selectively delete pathologic immune cells provides a novel route to restore immune homeostasis without generalized immunosuppression, thereby curtailing side effects and optimizing therapeutic index. As the field explores this intersection of autoimmunity and immunotherapy, the likelihood of CAR-T therapy becoming an effective treatment for such recurrent debilitating illnesses becomes clearer. Moreover, exploring the possibility of applications of immunotherapy outside of oncology into the infectious disease field is a significant step forward in the field of molecular immunology. CAR-T technology and other modalities of immunotherapy can possibly be applied to the treatment of chronic viral infections, such as HIV and hepatitis. These infections generally counter immune response by utilizing various mechanisms including latency and immune suppression. By engineering T-cells to kill certain viral antigens, researchers are seeking to introduce functional cures and even eradicate these hard-to-treat infections. In addition, what has been learned from CAR-T therapy development in cancer can be applied to strategies for optimizing immune responses against pathogens. Such cross-disciplinary applications highlight the revolutionizing potential of immunotherapy, i.e., with every advancing insight, the scope of treating a wide variety of diseases expands exponentially, reshaping clinical practice in the future.

SUMMARY

Research on immunotherapy, and particularly through the novel paradigms of CAR-T technology, has transformed cancer treatment dramatically. Evolution in this field has elucidated the potential of harnessing the immune system in order to specifically attack and kill cancer cells. CAR-T cells, especially in hematological malignancies, have yielded exceptional clinical outcomes and demonstrated the efficiency of the approach. However, as more and more immunotherapy is being introduced into conventional cancer treatment, issues are still evident. These include the drawbacks of single-antigen-targeted CAR-T treatments, where antigen mutation or loss would constrain treatment effectiveness. Solving these issues is essential as researchers continue to work on dual and multi-antigen targeted CAR-T treatments, which represent promising directions for achieving optimum therapy effectiveness and reducing tumor recurrence, paving the way for improved therapeutic strategies (Wang et al., 2025). Furthermore, the intersection of cancer immunotherapy and synthetic biology provides a hopeful new horizon in overcoming the deficiencies of CAR-T therapies presently. The evolution of synthetic Notch (synNotch) receptors represents a significant breakthrough that allows for the precise regulation of T-cell activation upon tumor-specific antigens. This new technique not only enhances the specificity of CAR-T cells but also offers an extremely sophisticated approach towards tackling the intricacies entailed in tumor heterogeneity and immune evasion. By acting as molecular logic gates, synNotch systems are able to distinguish between cancer cells and normal cells, enhancing safety in treatment while maximizing target specificity. The union of synNotch and CAR-T technology holds the promise for a new era where T cells can be engineered for greater responsiveness and efficiency, especially in the challenging field of solid tumors (Shirzadian et al., 2025).

Overall, the current research and development involving CAR-T technology and immunotherapy suggest an epochal shift in the approach to cancer treatment and management. The overall progress in therapeutic modalities, driven by advances like dual-antigen targeting and synNotch systems, provides a firm foundation for the resolution of the limitations existing in practice today. With continuous advancement in knowledge about the tumor microenvironment and mechanisms of the immune response, hopes for more effective, targeted, and personalized therapy draw steadily nearer. The promise of such innovations is not only in the advantage of patients with malignancies but also represents a significant leap in the study of molecular immunology, with the burden of incessant discovery and partnership in this rapidly growing discipline. Immunotherapy has achieved much in the recent past, especially in the realization of cancer cures like multiple myeloma (MM). The multi-drug combination has been impressively effective, with hope for patients with this formerly recalcitrant disease. Most notable is the combination with standard treatment of monoclonal antibodies, e.g., daratumumab, and the resulting improved progression-free survival (PFS) and overall survival (OS) outcomes. For newly diagnosed multiple myeloma patients, these new treatment approaches utilize very sensitive molecular assays to quantify minimal residual disease (MRD) status, thereby making follow-up therapies more efficacious with reduced toxicity. Furthermore, the introduction of CAR-T cell therapies for relapse and refractory disease shows a striking response in those populations that previously had few alternatives, pointing to the importance of additional research and trial innovation in this area (Morè et al., 2023). Immune system-tumor biology interaction will be a key factor in advancing treatment and disease outcomes. With the development of immunotherapy modalities, understanding cancer cell evasion of immune surveillance is increasingly relevant. The research on noncoding RNAs (ncRNAs) has been a promising front, revealing their promise in modulating immunity and tumor microenvironment dynamics. Through governing key biological pathways, ncRNAs are involved in processes such as angiogenesis and immune evasion. As these insights evolve, ncRNAs have the potential to act as key biomarkers for the monitoring of treatment responses and prognostic outcomes. Furthermore, combining ncRNA-targeting therapies with traditional modalities like immune checkpoint inhibitors and CAR-T technology may yield new mechanisms to enhance patient responses and bypass mechanisms of resistance to therapy (Martino et al., 2021). The future of molecular immunology depends upon the potential to innovate and reshape treatment paradigms. As progressive trials test new drugs and combinations, cancer treatment continues to move towards targeted and personalized treatments. The incorporation of CAR-T technology with standard treatments has particular potential to radically alter the treatment of drug-refractory tumors. With mounting evidence of the success of these multimodal therapies, clinicians are urged to consider patient-level parameters, including genetic risk stratification and immune status, when devising treatment. Ultimately, where intersecting findings between immunology, molecular biology, and clinical science will lead to effective therapy for increasing survival rates and quality of life among malignancy patients, such as multiple myeloma (Morè et al., 2023).

A CLOSER LOOK

CANCER STEM CELLS (CSCS)

CSCs are a minor subpopulation of cells within a tumor that possess stem cell-like properties, including self-renewal and the ability to differentiate into a wide range of cancer cell phenotypes. These cells are believed to play a crucial role in tumor initiation, growth, metastasis, and chemoresistance (Figure 14.17).

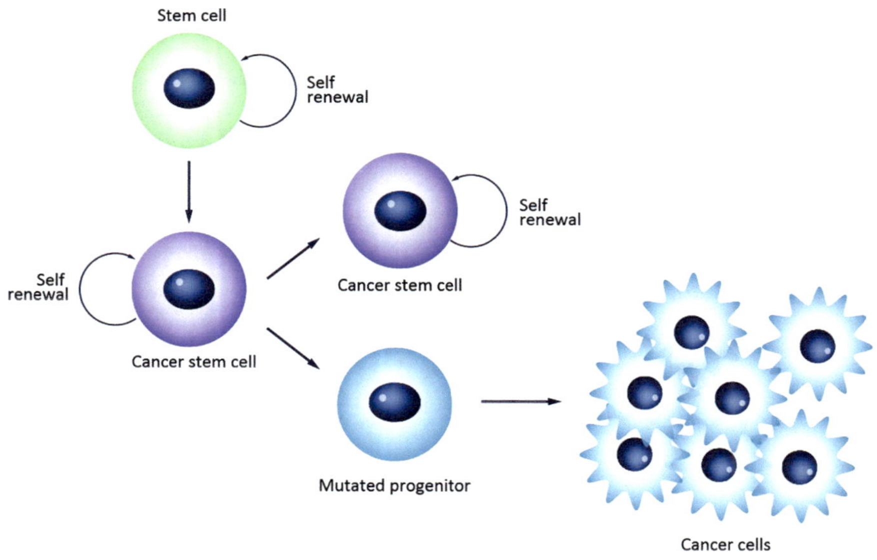

Figure 14.17. Cancer Stem Cells (CSCs).

Source: https://www.genetex.com/upload/media/research/Cancer/Cancer_Stem_Cells/cancer%20stem%20cell-header_%E5%B7%A5%E4%BD%9C%E5%8D%80%E5%9F%9F%201.jpg.

Key Features of CSCs:

- **Self-renewal:** CSCs can divide and produce more CSCs, self-renewing the tumor-initiating population.
- **Cellular Differentiation:** CSCs can differentiate into various other cancer cell types, resulting in tumor heterogeneity.
- **Tumorigenicity:** CSCs can produce tumors upon implantation in animal models.
- **Therapy Resistance:** CSCs are more resistant to conventional chemotherapy and radiation therapy.
- **Quiescence:** CSCs can be quiescent, which would make them resistant to therapy directed against proliferating cells.

- **Implications for Cancer Treatment:** The CSC model also has significant implications for cancer therapy. If CSCs are the cause of tumor recurrence and metastasis, specifically targeting CSCs would lead to more successful and sustained cancer therapies.

Obstacles and Directions:

- **Identification of CSCs:** Precise isolation and identification of CSCs may be challenging as CSCs are heterogeneous and have varying markers in various tumors.
- **Targeting CSCs:** Developing therapies that target CSCs alone without interfering with normal stem cells is one of the major areas of research.
- **Unraveling CSC Origins:** Further studies are needed to identify the origins of CSCs and the mechanisms that lead to their self-renewal and differentiation.

REFERENCES

1. Fox, B. A., Schendel, D. J., Butterfield, L. H., Aamdal, S., Allison, J. P., Ascierto, P. A., Atkins, M. B., Bartunkova, J., Bergmann, L., Berinstein, N., Bonorino, C. C., Borden, E., Bramson, J. L., Britten, C. M., Cao, X., Carson, W. E., Chang, A. E., Characiejus, D., Choudhury, A. R., Coukos, G., ... Disis, M. L. (2011). Defining the critical hurdles in cancer immunotherapy. *Journal of translational medicine*, *9*, 214. https://doi.org/10.1186/1479-5876-9-214 (accessed on 27th June 2025).

2. Clayton SM, Archard JA, Wagner J, et al. Immunoregulatory Potential of Exosomes Derived from Cancer Stem Cells. *Stem Cells Dev*. 2020;29(6):327-335. doi:10.1089/scd.2019.0197(accessed on 27th June 2025).

3. Chuntova, P., Downey, K. M., Hegde, B., Almeida, N. D., & Okada, H. (2019). Genetically Engineered T-Cells for Malignant Glioma: Overcoming the Barriers to Effective Immunotherapy. *Frontiers in immunology*, *9*, 3062. https://doi.org/10.3389/fimmu.2018.03062(accessed on 27th June 2025).

4. Sanchez-Correa, B., Valhondo, I., Hassouneh, F., Lopez-Sejas, N., Pera, A., Bergua, J. M., Arcos, M. J., Bañas, H., Casas-Avilés, I., Durán, E., Alonso, C., Solana, R., & Tarazona, R. (2019). DNAM-1 and the TIGIT/PVRIG/TACTILE Axis: Novel Immune Checkpoints for Natural Killer Cell-Based Cancer Immunotherapy. *Cancers*, *11*(6), 877. https://doi.org/10.3390/cancers11060877(accessed on 27th June 2025).

5. Ascierto, P., Agarwala, S., Botti, G., Cesano, A., Ciliberto, G., Davies, M., Demaria, S., et al. (2016). Future perspectives in melanoma research. *Journal of Translational Medicine, 14*. https://www.semanticscholar.org/paper/3574f966364f29823214dae013cb8086b32882f0 (accessed on 27th June 2025).

6. Atherton, M. J., Morris, J. S., McDermott, M. R., & Lichty, B. D. (2016). Cancer immunology and canine malignant melanoma: A comparative review. *Veterinary immunology and immunopathology*, *169*, 15–26. https://doi.org/10.1016/j.vetimm.2015.11.003(accessed on 27th June 2025).

7. Good, Z., Borges, L., Vivanco Gonzalez, N., Sahaf, B., Samusik, N., Tibshirani, R., Nolan, G. P., & Bendall, S. C. (2019). Proliferation tracing with single-cell mass cytometry optimizes generation of stem cell memory-like T cells. *Nature biotechnology*, *37*(3), 259–266. https://doi.org/10.1038/s41587-019-0033-2(accessed on 27th June 2025).

8. Besada, R. H. (2018). Immunotherapy in childhood B-cell acute lymphoblastic leukemia. https://core.ac.uk/download/158415235.pdf (accessed on 27th June 2025).

9. Biondi-Zoccai, G., Weber, B. N., Abbate, A., & Booz, G. (2025). Cardiac immunotherapy, immuno-cardiology and the future of cardiovascular pharmacology. *Journal of Cardiovascular Pharmacology*. https://www.semanticscholar.org/paper/890b853c1544f289f5589f4fe69c6f65d7410735 (accessed on 27th June 2025).

10. Braeckmans, K., Brans, T., De Smedt, S., Fraire, J., et al. (2019). Gold nanoparticle-mediated photoporation enables delivery of macromolecules over a wide range of molecular weights in human CD4+ T cells. https://core.ac.uk/download/237011703.pdf (accessed on 27th June 2025).

11. Bragança, J., Lopes, J. A. P., Santos, J., Silva, D., et al. (2019). Induced pluripotent stem cells, a giant leap for mankind therapeutic applications. https://core.ac.uk/download/227081218.pdf (accessed on 27th June 2025).

12. Khan, G., E., S., Denniss, F., Sigurdardottir, D., & Gui, B. (2013). Identification and Validation of Targets for Cancer Immunotherapy: From the Bench-to-Bedside. InTech. doi: 10.5772/54698(accessed on 27th June 2025).

13. Huff, W. X., Kwon, J. H., Henriquez, M., Fetcko, K., & Dey, M. (2019). The Evolving Role of $CD8^{+}CD28^{-}$ Immunosenescent T Cells in Cancer Immunology. *International journal of molecular sciences, 20*(11), 2810. https://doi.org/10.3390/ijms20112810(accessed on 27th June 2025).

14. Di Martino, M. T., Riillo, C., Scionti, F., Grillone, K., Polerà, N., Caracciolo, D., Arbitrio, M., et al. (2021). miRNAs and lncRNAs as novel therapeutic targets to improve cancer immunotherapy. *Cancers, 13.* https://www.semanticscholar.org/paper/12dc934175563d5c0bc399058a0876643f921b53 (accessed on 27th June 2025).

15. Feng, Z., Liao, M., & Zhang, L. (2024). Sex differences in disease: Sex chromosome and immunity. *Journal of Translational Medicine, 22.* https://doi.org/10.1186/s12967-024-05990-2 (accessed on 27th June 2025).

16. Garg, P., Singhal, S., Kulkarni, P., Horne, D., Malhotra, J., Salgia, R., & Singhal, S. S. (2024). Advances in non-small cell lung cancer: Current insights and future directions. *Journal of Clinical Medicine, 13.* https://www.semanticscholar.org/paper/16dbd889459b540e198c5fb7e3c31462d24ed1f7 (accessed on 27th June 2025).

17. Hardman, C., Ho, S., Luu-Nguyen, Q., Marsden, R., et al. (2020). Synthesis and evaluation of designed PKC modulators for enhanced cancer immunotherapy. https://core.ac.uk/download/323075886.pdf (accessed on 27th June 2025).

18. Pörtner, R., Parida, S. K., Schaffer, C., & Hoffmeister, H. (2018). Landscape of Manufacturing Process of ATMP Cell Therapy Products for Unmet Clinical Needs. InTech. doi: 10.5772/intechopen.69335(accessed on 27th June 2025).

19. Hu, Y., Hu, Q., Li, Y., Lu, L., Xiang, Z., Yin, Z., Kabelitz, D., et al. (2023). γδ T cells: Origin and fate, subsets, diseases and immunotherapy. *Signal Transduction and Targeted Therapy, 8.* https://doi.org/10.1038/s41392-023-01653-8 (accessed on 27th June 2025).

20. Huang, H. (2025). Challenges and innovations in managing cytokine release syndrome in CAR-T therapy: Mechanisms, clinical impact, and future directions. *Theoretical and Natural Science.* https://www.semanticscholar.org/paper/e49f1ae03d507e186099e8c72636e577be82159c (accessed on 27th June 2025).

21. Huang, T., Bei, C., Hu, Z., & Li, Y. (2024). CAR-macrophage: Breaking new ground in cellular immunotherapy. *Frontiers in Cell and Developmental Biology, 12.* https://www.semanticscholar.org/paper/de4c3f56b666bdf3c4e6461d76d8a9eb8a94da65 (accessed on 27th June 2025).

22. Huang, Y., Yin, Z., Xu, R., Zheng, W., Zhang, Q., Zhou, M., Xu, Z., et al. (2025). Gas vesicle-assisted ultrasound imaging for effective anti-tumor CAR-T cell immunotherapy efficacy in mice model. *International Journal of Nanomedicine, 20,* 4849–4862. https://www.semanticscholar.org/paper/ff24216275c73bc864422daa0b7d5f947dd30029 (accessed on 27th June 2025).

23. Klosowski, M. L., McMellen, A., Burton, J., Cronise, K. E., Leibowitz, M. S., & Regan, D. P. (2025). Abstract A028: Assessing fibroblast activation protein as an immunotherapy biomarker and

CAR T cell therapeutic target in the tumor microenvironment of canine sarcomas. *Cancer Immunology Research.* https://www.semanticscholar.org/paper/3fb8c5b1bb96edb5da80c7b4956618913a78c236 (accessed on 27th June 2025).

24. Koduri, M. P. (2017). The curative potential of chimeric antigen receptor T-cell therapy for B-cell malignancies. https://open.bu.edu/bitstream/2144/23818/5/Koduri_bu_0017N_12719.pdf (accessed on 27th June 2025).

25. Krmpotić, K. (2018). Application of CAR-T cells in cancer gene therapy. https://core.ac.uk/download/162616157.pdf (accessed on 27th June 2025).

26. Liu, Y., Wu, W., Cai, C., Zhang, H., Shen, H., & Han, Y. (2023). Patient-derived xenograft models in cancer therapy: Technologies and applications. *Signal Transduction and Targeted Therapy, 8.* https://doi.org/10.1038/s41392-023-01419-2 (accessed on 27th June 2025).

27. Lühle, J., Krost, S., Goerdeler, F., Seitz, C., Seeberger, P. H., & Moscovitz, O. (2025). Abstract A017: Cysteine-engineered CAR-T cells to counter antigen escape in B cell lymphoma. *Cancer Immunology Research.* https://www.semanticscholar.org/paper/327bbf0f4baecb9bd81367766fdfaf04221d680f (accessed on 27th June 2025).

28. Stroncek, D. F., Berger, C., Cheever, M. A., Childs, R. W., Dudley, M. E., Flynn, P., Gattinoni, L., Heath, J. R., Kalos, M., Marincola, F. M., Miller, J. S., Mostoslavsky, G., Powell, D. J., Jr, Rao, M., Restifo, N. P., Rosenberg, S. A., O'Shea, J., & Melief, C. J. (2012). New directions in cellular therapy of cancer: a summary of the summit on cellular therapy for cancer. *Journal of translational medicine, 10,* 48. https://doi.org/10.1186/1479-5876-10-48(accessed on 27th June 2025).

29. Meneses do Rêgo, A. C., & Araújo Filho, I. (2024). Nanomedicine-driven advances: Enhancing checkpoint inhibition and CAR-T therapies in cancer immunotherapy. *International Journal of Current Microbiology and Applied Sciences.* https://www.semanticscholar.org/paper/d64deaaa9e09e4a47d9c80bb7dbcf0d55d2f07e6 (accessed on 27th June 2025).

30. Meng, S., Hara, T., Miura, Y., Arao, Y., Saito, Y., Inoue, K., Hirotsu, T., et al. (2025). *In vivo* engineered CAR-T cell therapy: Lessons built from COVID-19 mRNA vaccines. *International Journal of Molecular Sciences, 26.* https://www.semanticscholar.org/paper/ff18b1e53fad1ace1dac5bac559c5e159b35b78e (accessed on 27th June 2025).

31. Mohamed Nashrudin, K. N., Zainal Abidin, M. A., Ng, S., Razali, H., Jawin, V., Zakaria, A. F., Mohd Ali, R., et al. (2025). RASGRP1 deficiency associated with diffuse mesangial sclerosis infantile nephrotic syndrome and Epstein–Barr virus-induced Hodgkin's lymphoma. *Pediatric Allergy Immunology and Pulmonology.* https://doi.org/10.1089/ped.2024.0062 (accessed on 27th June 2025).

32. Morè, S., Corvatta, L., Manieri, V. M., Olivieri, A., & Offidani, M. (2023). Current main topics in multiple myeloma. *Cancers, 15.* https://www.semanticscholar.org/paper/0008986315aa19868c7ac820b61ba972c78ebf1f (accessed on 27th June 2025).

33. Mutebi, I. (2024). Renewed insight into cancer mechanism and therapy: Advances, challenges, and future directions. *Research Output Journal of Public Health and Medicine.* https://www.semanticscholar.org/paper/11cf101d6a87067f2d7e82f37ab467d2fdac9e9e (accessed on 27th June 2025).

34. Richon, V., Fisher, D., Letai, A., Haber, D., Bardia, A., Stott, S. L., Yeku, O., et al. (2018). Channer Colloquium: Answering the big questions in cancer research & 2018 STO

Annual Meeting. *The Oncologist, 23,* S1–S6. https://www.semanticscholar.org/paper/eb847663ef2b837396b41996129cb1b2442e446f (accessed on 27th June 2025).

35. Shirzadian, M., Moori, S., Rabbani, R., & Rahbarizadeh, F. (2025). SynNotch CAR-T cell, when synthetic biology and immunology meet again. *Frontiers in Immunology, 16.* https://www.semanticscholar.org/paper/0ffe29e9c077f78f6d2044f31796b6d977f54bc9 (accessed on 27th June 2025).

36. Tao, R., Han, X., Bai, X., Yu, J., Ma, Y., Chen, W., Zhang, D., et al. (2024). Revolutionizing cancer treatment: Enhancing CAR-T cell therapy with CRISPR/Cas9 gene editing technology. *Frontiers in Immunology, 15.* https://www.semanticscholar.org/paper/2ec33a956fd6f8ee3ef3be4e3324da62b5e00375 (accessed on 27th June 2025).

37. Teibo, J., Picanço-Castro, V., de Souza, L. E. B., & Faça, V. (2025). A proteomics outlook on the molecular effectors of CART cell therapy in cancer management. *Journal of Proteome Research, 24,* 2571–2583. https://www.semanticscholar.org/paper/46ffef79f012ac5f4f60c63f6df3887ec8c0ad56 (accessed on 27th June 2025).

38. Wang, Z., Wang, M., Wang, M., Zhou, R., Deng, X., Xin, O., Chu, M., et al. (2025). From molecular design to clinical translation: Dual-targeted CAR-T strategies in cancer immunotherapy. *International Journal of Biological Sciences, 21,* 2676–2691. https://www.semanticscholar.org/paper/6c3cfaee0fc161a4b72c5afe7b7222c21d764a1a (accessed on 27th June 2025).

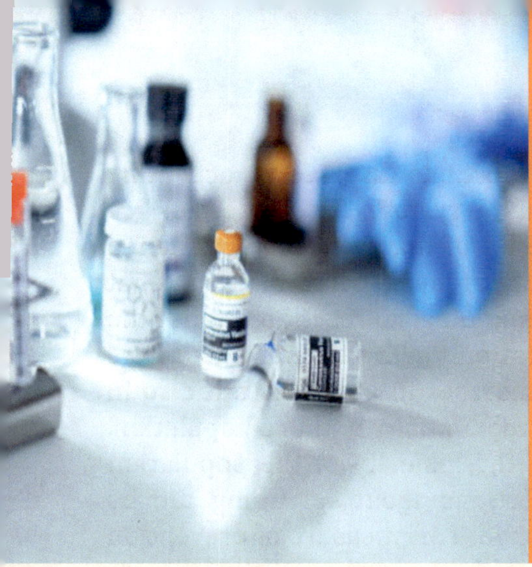

Chapter 15

ADVANCEMENTS IN VACCINE DEVELOPMENT TECHNIQUES

Contents

Introduction

The public health scenario has been revolutionized by advancements in methods of vaccine development, particularly to treat global public health crises such as the COVID-19 pandemic. Not only are these innovations focused on quick and efficient manufacturing of vaccines, but they also focus on addressing the need for diversity in the delivery mechanisms that have the potential to address various logistical challenges. Traditional vaccine delivery methods, though effective, have been hampered by issues such as needle phobia, access, and cold chain preservation of vaccines. Thus, the search for novel delivery systems has emerged as a significant field of interest in developing modern vaccines. Advances in needle-less technology, coupled with the inclusion of biotechnological approaches, are paving the way towards more patient-friendly products—ultimately leading to enhanced vaccination coverage in diverse groups and environments. Among the many emerging technologies, 3D-printed microneedle technology stands out due to its precision and applicability. 3D-printed microneedle technology offers a pioneering strategy over conventional injection techniques through offering painless, efficient, and convenient vaccine delivery. The microneedle patches consist of extremely fine needles that melt upon skin contact, facilitating transdermal delivery directly. Through customized shape, size, and density via 3D printing, scientists can customize the vaccine pharmacokinetics and immunogenicity, hence its overall efficacy. Studies identify that this new method improves antigen delivery and causes robust immune responses by targeting the skin's immunocompetent layers. Microneedle technology not only simplifies the process of immunization but also makes it more accessible, particularly in resource-limited regions, which is crucial in guaranteeing global health equity. Among such innovations, besides microneedle technology, are new vaccine development platforms like new adjuvants, messenger RNA (mRNA) platforms, and viral vector approaches. These revolutions are transforming vaccine development and facilitating faster responses to emerging pathogens, as well as enhancing the potency of current vaccines. For instance, mRNA vaccines, which stepped into the spotlight during the COVID-19 pandemic, demonstrate the capability of new technologies to expedite the development process while maintaining efficacy and safety. Moreover, the use of such strategies not only promotes the fast prototyping of therapeutics but also allows the healthcare system to respond promptly to public health emergencies. Overall, the coming together of all these advancements is bringing about a paradigm shift in vaccine creation, which ultimately results in an accelerated, more efficient, and more equitable global vaccination strategy that is optimally poised to meet the evolving challenges of infectious diseases.

Definition of Vaccines and Their Importance

Vaccines can be defined as biological preparations intended to provide immunity against some infectious diseases by activating the body's immune system. These vaccines are typically made up of inactivated or weakened microorganisms, or even parts of them, that provoke an immunological reaction but not the illness itself. Not only will vaccines play a role in preventing diseases in a person, but also in establishing herd immunity within a population. By vaccinating the majority of the population effectively, infectious agent spreading can be greatly diminished. This measure of prevention not only safeguards the unvaccinatable due to medical reasons but also results in eventual disease eradication, as has been observed in the past with smallpox. Therefore, the continuing emergence of innovative vaccine development methods is essential, which calls for improving efficacy, safety, and access to strengthen global health impact. The role of vaccines transcends human health, having a substantial impact on animal agriculture as well. Advances in vaccine production techniques are revolutionizing how vaccines are manufactured and administered to animals. Advances in the field of biotechnology have enabled the production of more effective vaccines that eliminate the need for antibiotics. Such vaccines help manage animal infectious diseases, and this is significant given the increasing concerns about antibiotic resistance in agriculture. The second International Symposium on Alternatives to Antibiotics highlighted the position of vaccines as driving forces behind this initiative, calling for increased cooperation among partners, including researchers, producers, and policymakers (Hoelzer et al., 2018). New vaccine technologies, including new delivery methods and multi-pathogen protection, are emerging as critical solutions to meet the complex threats facing animal health and agricultural productivity. In developing countries, vaccine efforts are not only key in combating infectious diseases but also in addressing agriculture-related challenges through innovative technologies such as nanotechnology. The addition of advanced technologies to vaccine designs is capable of making them more efficient and potent in delivery, especially in resource-poor settings where traditional methods may be insufficient. For example, new research and development priorities in vaccine science can enable farmers at the local level, enabling them to adopt forward-looking farming techniques while ensuring public and animal health (Gruère et al., 2011). As research in vaccine development progresses, its importance in ensuring both animal and human populations cannot be overstated. Granting equitable access to these innovations will be crucial in attaining world health equity, promoting resilience to emerging health threats, and facilitating global food security (Figure 15.1).

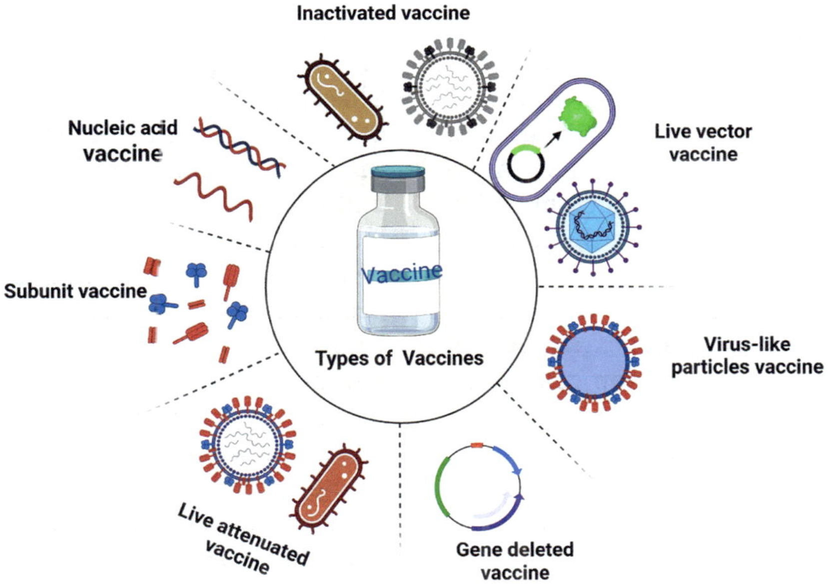

Figure 15.1. Types of vaccines.

Source: https://images-provider.frontiersin.org/api/ipx/w=1200&f=png/https://www.frontiersin.org/files/Articles/1243835/fvets-10-1243835-HTML/image_m/fvets-10-1243835-g001.jpg.

Overview of Traditional Vaccine Development Methods

The foundation of traditional vaccine development strategies lies in using inactivated or weakened pathogens to induce an immune response. This approach has been successfully employed in vaccine development for polio, measles, and hepatitis diseases. Using these attenuated or killed pathogens, researchers are hoping to stimulate the body's immune system to recognize and fight the actual disease-causing agents when exposed. While these methods have proved successful in rescuing thousands of lives, development cycles for these can be long due to the wide range of testing required for proof of efficacy as well as safety. As well, the need for special handling and storage conditions means that distribution within resource-poor settings poses problems. All these call for ongoing demands for new vaccine development methods that can potentially enhance rapid deployment without sacrificing effectiveness in the combat against infectious disease. Another very well-known ancient vaccine development strategy involves the use of subunit vaccines, which contain isolated portions of pathogens like proteins or carbohydrates that trigger a body response without the threat of making one ill. The technique presents a greater level of safety over whole-organism vaccines, particularly in those with impaired immune systems. An example is the human papillomavirus (HPV) vaccine, which works against particular virus proteins to trigger immunity. However, a significant drawback of subunit vaccines is that they can trigger a weaker immune response in comparison to live attenuated and inactivated vaccines. Adjuvants are thus typically added to improve efficiency. This requirement of employing adjuvants demonstrates the fine balance between efficacy and safety that exists in traditional vaccine development methods once more, keeping constant the necessity for innovation that could enhance and maximize the immune response elicited by such vaccines (Saranya et al., 2025). Further, traditional vaccine methods have also used infectious agents extensively in recombinant technology to develop genetically altered organisms for the purpose of creating antigens. Vaccines like the hepatitis B vaccine serve as an example of such a method, where the virus surface antigen is produced in yeast and subsequently utilized to create immunity. Although successful in producing protective reactions, this process is time-consuming and time and resource-intensive. Such inefficiencies in the old approach are areas where newer methods intend to improve. Advancements in computational approaches and deep learning technology, for instance, hold the potential to transform the process of vaccine development through the provision of predictive models that can potentially decrease the amount of time it takes to design and test vaccines, ultimately translating to quicker reactions to the shifting health issues (Yao et al., 2025).

Purpose and Significance of Advancements in Vaccine Techniques

Vaccine development technology is at the core of reviving public health and fighting infectious illnesses. Producing vaccines has been a protracted and complex process that has achieved limited success in safety and effectiveness. That is no longer the case since the invention of biotechnology. Biotechnology has provided new technologies, such as recombinant DNA technology and genetic engineering, that enable scientists to design vaccines that are safer and more effective. For instance, the biotechnological use of immunity enables it to create vaccines with the capacity to provoke greater immune responses against pathogens. This shift towards new techniques is indicative of the necessity to modernize techniques applied in vaccine production to tackle both current and future health needs, enabling populations worldwide to be better shielded from infectious diseases with the potential to impact social and economic stability, particularly for vulnerable communities (Bruce, 1989). Furthermore, the advances in vaccine technique hold significant promise to overcome the challenges in parasitic diseases heretofore largely neglected in vaccine design efforts. No matter how heavily viral vaccines have traditionally drawn interest, the new focus on developing vaccines against parasitic infection is a significant shift in public health policy. With much attention focused on malaria and schistosomiasis, scientists are employing the technique of biotechnology to dissect the complex life cycles of such parasites, as well as finding good vaccine targets. This research not only constitutes a step forward in vaccine technology but also reflects an emerging appreciation for the need to address the global burden of the neglected tropical diseases. And while these advancements are yet to be seen, they provide opportunities for novel solutions to traditional health problems that promote better chances at global health equity (Saxena, 2022). Lastly, the significance and purpose of advances in vaccine methodology extend beyond tech advancements themselves; they represent an entire paradigm shift in disease prevention and public health thought in society. Through the integration of traditional immunological principles and cutting-edge biotechnological methods, researchers are now capable of formulating vaccines that can keep pace with the dynamic needs of an ever-changing world. This development re-emphasizes the need for sustained investment in vaccine R&D, which is essential in preparing against emergent infectious diseases. The potential dividends of these profits are not only improved health outcomes, but economic and social resilience in populations as well. In light of the shifting landscape of infectious diseases, the integration of advanced methods in vaccine development will be critical to safeguarding public health and enabling global communities to thrive amidst health crises (Bruce, 1989).

15.1. Historical Context of Vaccine Development

The historical evidence for vaccine development portrays a past of scientific research driven by the need to combat infectious diseases. The origins of today's vaccine practice can be traced back to Edward Jenner's initial innovation in 1796, when he created the smallpox vaccine from cowpox. This method was revolutionary because it was the beginning of immunology and provided a new tool to combat the devastating effects of smallpox, which had devastated mankind for centuries. Jenner's success was a milestone in public health, which paved the way for future vaccines. As human society faced more and more problematic viral issues, including polio and measles in the 20th century, vaccinology evolved with tremendous momentum from progress in microbiology and immunology that has continued to shape vaccine strategies (Alowais et al., 2023). Early 20th-century technological advancements drove the development of more sophisticated vaccines. The application of inactivated and live attenuated virus vaccines offered more effective immunization protocols, particularly against diseases like tetanus and diphtheria. These protocols availed themselves of information regarding pathogen biology as well as host immunity to devise vaccination systems that substantially reduced the occurrence of disease. Besides, the establishment of global health organizations at this period pointed to the importance of vaccinations as a public health measure, which saw mass immunization programs implemented. It was instrumental in demonstrating the efficacy of vaccines as a preventative, significantly impacting global health outcomes and disease prevention public policy (Ji et al., 2022). The second half of the 20th and the early 21st centuries have seen an unprecedented acceleration in the rate of vaccine development processes, using novel technology and techniques. The advent of recombinant DNA technology and advances in genomics allowed for the rapid development of vaccines for a variety of pathogens, enhancing safety and efficacy. Vaccines for human papillomavirus (HPV) and hepatitis B are reported examples of the impact of these advances, illustrating how genetic manipulation has come to dominate vaccine manufacture. Moreover, the uncovering of adjuvants and delivery systems further improved immune responses, optimizing vaccinations. This ongoing innovation in vaccine technology demonstrates the significance of experience gained previously, since current practices make use of the principles established by the pioneers themselves, tending to accelerate the field towards new solutions for challenges that confront current public health (Alowais et al., 2023).

15.1.1. Early Vaccine Development and Key Milestones

The history of vaccine development begins with Edward Jenner's pioneering work in the late 18th century. Jenner's historic experiment in 1796 included inoculating a boy with cowpox virus to give him immunity against smallpox, and this was the beginning of vaccination. This strategy demonstrated that a less virulent pathogen exposure could confer immunity against more severe disease, a principle that is the foundation of immunization today. Afterwards, the successful eradication of smallpox during the late 20th century is a testament to the efficacy of vaccines. Technological advancements and improved methods of research have supported this practice, providing opportunities for further progress in vaccine science. The early milestones solidified vaccination as a critical tool in preventing infectious diseases, leading to further innovations that harnessed emerging scientific knowledge to enhance public health globally. Further milestones in vaccine development can be traced through the late 19th and early 20th centuries, with the advent of immunological research that introduced the concepts of attenuation and inactivation of pathogens. Louis Pasteur's success of the rabies vaccine in 1885 was the pinnacle of these techniques, which were able to trigger protective immunity without causing disease, employing weakened or inactivated viruses. This era also witnessed the emergence of serological techniques, which further elucidated the functioning of the immune system and enabled the identification of isolating antigens. These developments created a new era in which vaccines were created against life-threatening diseases such as tetanus and diphtheria. These early improvements laid critical groundwork for modern vaccine strategies, demonstrating the power of concentrated scientific investigation to create life-saving measures against disease causatives. The latter half of the 20th century introduced accelerating vaccine development through notable technological progress. The development of tissue culture techniques enabled the production of vaccines in aseptic systems, highly enhancing safety and efficacy. The development of recombinant DNA technology also provided new avenues for the construction of vaccines, such as the manipulation of genetic codes to design more effective immunogens. Vaccines such as hepatitis B, developed through these advances, continued to signal a transition towards safer and more precise immunization techniques. In addition, the role of international collaborative work within vaccine production came to the fore during this time, characterized by activities like the Expanded Programme on Immunization (EPI). This collaborative work provided not just improved access to vaccination, but it also activated research drives to conquer upcoming infectious challenges, an investment in public health that continues to be felt today (Figure 15.2).

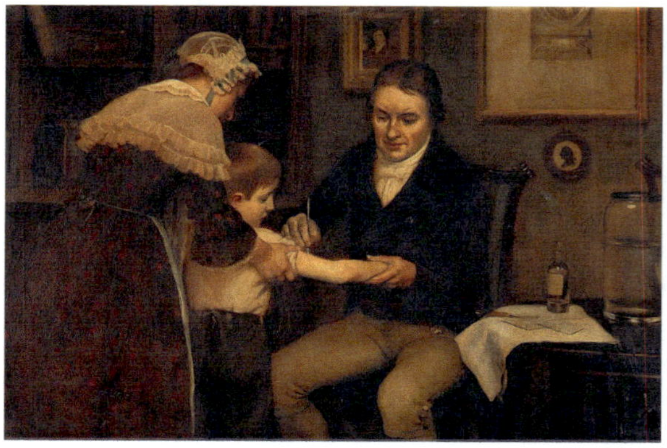

Figure 15.2. Jenner performing his first vaccination on James Phipps, a boy of age 8, on 14 May 1796.

Source: https://upload.wikimedia.org/wikipedia/commons/thumb/1/1a/Jenner_phipps_01_%28cropped%29.jpg/1280px-Jenner_phipps_01_%28cropped%29.jpg.

15.1.2. The Role of the Scientific Community in Vaccine Innovation

The scientific community is leading the way with vaccine innovation as the driving force behind research and development. This kind of community is made up of a pool of experts, including immunologists, virologists, and biostatisticians, who have a collective skill that is needed to address new and re-emerging infectious diseases. The recent technological advancements in vaccination, especially during the COVID-19 pandemic, reflect the collaborative nature of scientific endeavor. Scientists utilized multiple methodologies, including mRNA technology, which facilitated prototyping and widespread distribution of vaccines. Such technological advancement indicates how the scientific community leverages available knowledge and expertise to challenge, adapt, and react to global health emergencies. Importantly, this interaction extends beyond the lab, to public health professionals and policy-makers who synthesize scientific evidence into comprehensive health policy. To summarize, interdisciplinary synergy among scientific disciplines and public health administration optimizes the effectiveness of vaccine deployment. Moreover, the use of advanced technology has been crucial in streamlining vaccine development. The utilization of artificial intelligence (AI) and machine learning algorithms is a leap in the direction of enhanced research effectiveness. AI interventions propel medical research through the acceleration of drug discovery and the identification of potential vaccine candidates more quickly than traditional methods. For instance, algorithms analyzing big data are capable of finding links between viral genomes and host immunity at a quicker rate, making successful vaccine targets faster to identify (Al Kuwaiti et al., 2023). Furthermore, AI's role in data management has proven invaluable, enabling researchers to simulate vaccine responses and optimize formulations before clinical trials commence. These technological advancements not only enhance innovation but also ensure that vaccines can be developed and deployed on time, which is crucial during public health emergencies. Additionally, the scientific community is increasingly recognizing the importance of ethical considerations and public engagement in vaccine innovation. With the advancements in new technologies, such as synthetic biology, their implications on ethics need to be addressed. Safety, efficacy, and equity in vaccine access are concerns that demand open communication and community participation in vaccination (Uddin et al., 2021). There is a call for scientists and public health officials to collaborate in coming up with guidelines to govern the utilization of emerging vaccine technologies ethically. Engaging with the people not only fosters trust but also ensures increased vaccination participation, which is necessary to achieve herd immunity. Therefore, the role of the scientific community extends beyond mere innovation, involving a responsibility of upholding ethical standards and generating public awareness and acceptability towards vaccines (Figure 15.3).

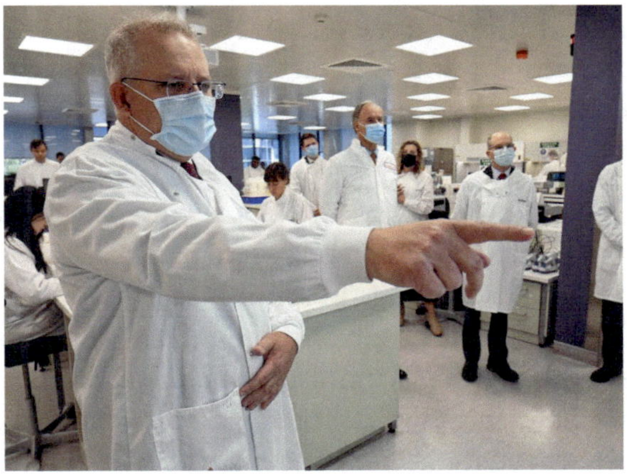

Figure 15.3. The scientific community plays a pivotal role in the innovation of vaccines.

Source: https://content.api.news/v3/images/bin/a8188bf32640ea44a24daefa8e465976.

15.1.3. Impact of Historical Pandemics on Vaccine Research

The past history of pandemics has had a significant impact in charting the path of vaccine research in shaping milestone advances that redefined public health responses. The early outbreaks, such as smallpox, fueled efforts towards vaccine formulation, leading to Edward Jenner's seminal contribution in the late 18th century. This groundbreaking approach paved the way for immunization through the use of a cousin virus to grant protection against smallpox. Releasing this innovation brings out the extent to which serious health crises propel societies towards concern for the prevention of infectious diseases, ultimately accelerating research and technological advances in vaccine strategies. Every emerging pandemic, like the 1918 flu and recent ones like SARS and the H1N1 virus, has kept fueling the quest for even improved vaccines. This has unraveled the continuing cycle of medical progress and disease epidemic. The response to recent pandemics, particularly the COVID-19 pandemic, demonstrates this reciprocal relationship between historical challenges and current vaccine development strategies. The urgency of the situation necessitated unmatched collaborations between governments, pharma companies, and research institutions and therefore hastened improvements in vaccine technology.

As an instance, mRNA vaccine platforms were leveraged at an increased pace, being very effective in treating the viral disease agent for COVID-19. These advancements are noted to be a departure from traditional methods in vaccine discovery, exhibiting a new significant breakthrough in response strategies to new contagious diseases. The experiences gained from previous pandemics have allowed health authorities to optimize the regulatory processes, leading to the rapid rollout of vaccines that can be modified for new strains, eventually making the whole world better prepared for emerging health crises. In addition to the direct influence on vaccine research during the immediacy of a pandemic, pandemics have far-reaching effects on the ethical and functional guidelines governing vaccine development. Application of AI in healthcare is a quintessential example of such transformation, allowing advanced tools to support vaccine discovery and delivery, as has been exemplified by the COVID-19 response. Application of AI has revolutionized medical imaging, diagnosis, and patient communication, with significant contributions to vaccine research and distribution planning. This tech-led change spotlights the challenge and potential for historical pandemics, challenging effective governance to respond to the regulatory, ethical, and trust issues surrounding the deployment of vaccines. While societies around the world reflect on the consequences of past health crises, it is more important than ever that innovation in methods of making vaccines does not simply look to effectiveness but also to their ethical consequences, both ensuring public understandability and fair access during subsequent epidemics (Miethke et al., 2021; Al Kuwaiti et al., 2023) (Figure 15.4).

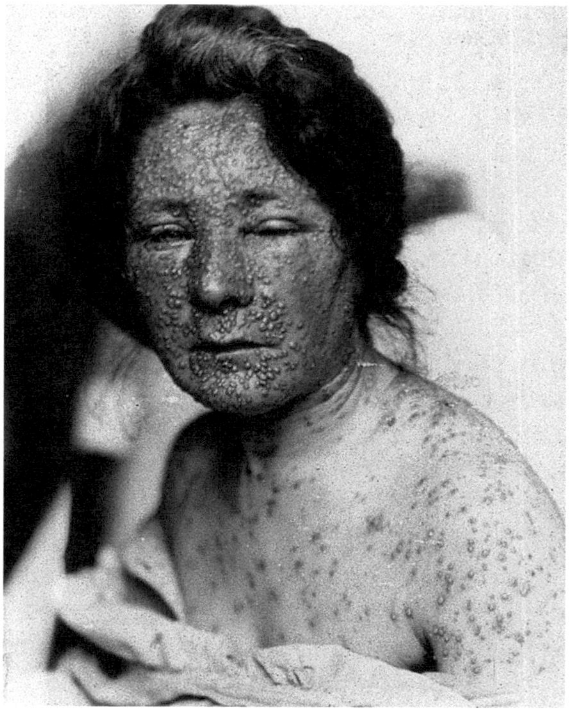

Figure 15.4. Female smallpox patient in London, c. 1890.

Source: https://upload.wikimedia.org/wikipedia/commons/thumb/3/3a/Friern_Hospital%2C_London%3B_a_young_girl%2C_head_and_shoulders%2C_w_Wellcome_V0029631.jpg/800px-Friern_Hospital%2C_London%3B_a_young_girl%2C_head_and_shoulders%2C_w_Wellcome_V0029631.jpg.

15.2. Novel Vaccine Platforms

The landscape of vaccine development is being revolutionized in a dramatic way with the emergence of new vaccine platforms. These platforms include an extensive range of new technologies, from mRNA-based vaccines, viral vector systems, to protein subunit formulations. All of these approaches have their own special advantages, including the potential to enhance immunogenicity, support rapid production, and allow for targeted action against specific pathogens. Particularly, mRNA vaccines have been in the limelight due to their ability to rapidly transfer genetic codes for antigen production, thus enabling immediate immune reactions. This rapid adaptability is extremely crucial in the wake of rising and re-emerging infectious diseases, marking a milestone achievement in the manner in which vaccines can be produced and deployed. This technology not only enhances effectiveness but also demonstrates the versatility of modern vaccine strategies in addressing global health challenges. Blending novel vaccine platforms with advanced immunological techniques is equally critical to the achievement of such vaccines. Techniques such as immunoblotting are critical to the determination of the immune response elicited by such vaccines. It is through immunoblotting that it becomes achievable for researchers to identify and quantify unique proteins that indicate an immune response, hence playing a significant role in the validation of vaccine candidates. Contemporary advancements have enhanced the sensitivity and specificity of this technique, allowing for high-throughput screenings and productive workflows. As complexity in vaccine formulations has increased, understanding antigen-antibody interactions becomes imperative to maximize vaccine efficacy. The synergy between new immunological technologies and novel vaccine platforms displays an integrated approach to developing vaccines. Such synergy is essential in vaccine provision, not only to provoke robust immune reactions but also to attain high safety and efficacy levels. AI is emerging as a powerful collaborator in the design of new vaccine platforms, revolutionizing how scientists identify viral threats and craft appropriate responses. Through the use of machine learning and predictive modeling, AI reduces the process of discovering new vaccine targets to a breeze, shortening the time it takes to identify vaccine candidates by roughly half. Furthermore, AI can also make clinical trial designs more streamlined and make regulatory processes more efficient, so it is easier to cope with mutating viral strains. This is particularly valid in the case of continuously evolving viral pathogens, where traditional approaches may falter. Moreover, AI's capacity to facilitate personalized medicine approaches could help tailor vaccines to individual responses, enhancing their effectiveness. As the synergy of AI and novel vaccine platforms continues to unfold, it holds significant promise for reshaping our capability to respond to viral outbreaks and ultimately preserving global health (Malpani & Telrandhe, 2024).

15.2.1. mRNA Vaccine Technology and Its Applications

The development of mRNA vaccine technology is a fundamental advance in vaccine technology, particularly as an answer to acute public health demands. Unlike traditional vaccines that are often developed using attenuated or inactivated pathogens, mRNA vaccines employ synthetic genetic material to instruct cells to make a non-harmful piece of the target virus. This novel technology not only speeds up vaccine development but also boosts the immune response through the natural processes of the body. The case of COVID-19 vaccines, which utilized mRNA technology, exemplifies the response speed provided by the platform, ultimately changing vaccine deployment strategies during emergencies. Apart from that, the versatility of mRNA technology can also be applied to combat not only viral diseases but also cancer and other infectious diseases, which would allow for the creation of tailored vaccines according to the patient's profile. When researchers are looking at the potential of mRNA technology, scientists are particularly looking at its efficiency and versatility. The mRNA technology facilitates quick changes based on evolving pathogen genomes, thereby allowing for instant adaptations in vaccine formulations, such as with circulating forms of COVID-19. This adaptability constitutes a shift in paradigms in vaccine development with the potential for quick clinical trials and regulatory approvals compared to conventional approaches. In addition, the incorporation of advanced delivery mechanisms such as lipid nanoparticles facilitates the stability and efficacy of mRNA vaccines for long-term immune responses. Such technological advancement is crucial in an increasingly faced world of newly emerging pathogens, and therefore, the pertinence of mRNA vaccines as a key tool in upcoming public health interventions. While the potential of mRNA vaccines is great, their utilization is not trouble-free, particularly with respect to access equity and health systems. The fast-tracking of vaccine science enabled by the COVID-19 pandemic groundwork underscored these challenges and highlighted the need for interconnected public health strategies. The effective deployment of mRNA vaccines involves technological progress as much as socio-political confidence factors, regulatory harmonization, and resource equitability among global health systems. According to recent studies, such advancements' translation into real applications is still vulnerable to structural gaps and health capacity differences in geopolitics (Mafuts, 2025). Providing free access to mRNA vaccines is of top priority in achieving widespread immunization, especially among low- and middle-income countries, thereby reaffirming the need for unified global efforts in filling such gaps (Johansen et al., 2024) (Figure 15.5).

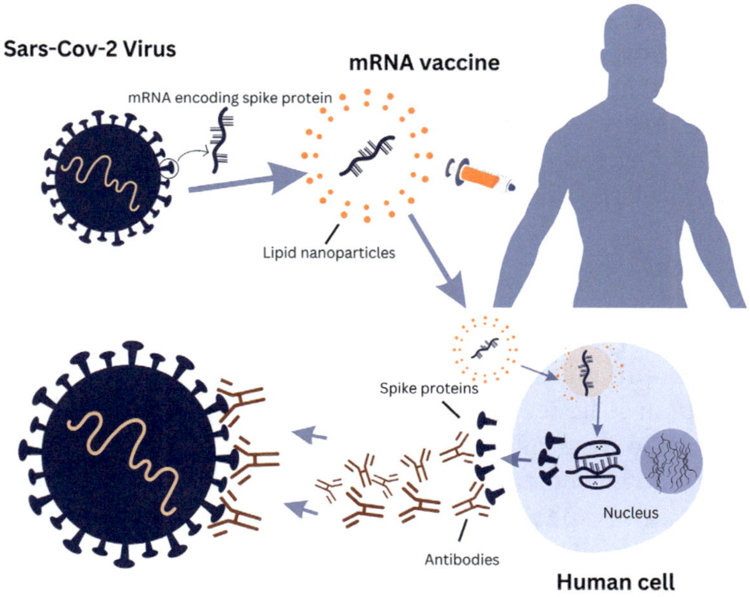

Figure 15.5. Schematic representation of the mechanism of action of mRNA vaccines.

Source: https://www.researchgate.net/profile/Ilkin-Aygun/publication/374848083/figure/fig1/AS:11431281200133102@1697792121531/Schematic-representation-of-the-mechanism-of-action-of-mRNA-vaccines-This-figure.png.

15.2.2. Viral Vector Vaccines and Their Mechanisms

Viral vector vaccines are one of the advancements in vaccine development strategies, where viruses are utilized as delivery systems by genetically modifying them to trigger immune responses against a specific pathogen. By taking advantage of the natural ability of viruses to infect host cells, these vaccines are capable of presenting antigens efficiently and triggering humoral and cellular immunity. The mechanisms of viral vector vaccines are diverse but generally involve the incorporation of a gene encoding for a target antigen of a disease-causing agent in a non-pathogenic viral vector. Once injected, the vector infects cells of the host, which then respond by producing the antigen. This mechanism not only provokes the immune system to recognize and attack the foreign antigen but also the formation of immunological memory to ensure long-term immunity against future infection. This new mechanism also facilitates rapid adaptation to new infectious disease threats, exhibiting its adaptability in a dynamic environment of public health pathogens. Additionally, viral vector vaccines have also been very flexible in their applications, particularly in the event of various viral epidemics. For instance, the successful application of viral vectors during the COVID-19 pandemic illustrated the capability of such vectors to rapidly develop effective immunizations. Adenoviruses and vesicular stomatitis viruses are some of the vector systems that were used to produce the SARS-CoV-2 spike protein and induce neutralizing antibodies and produce robust T-cell responses successfully.

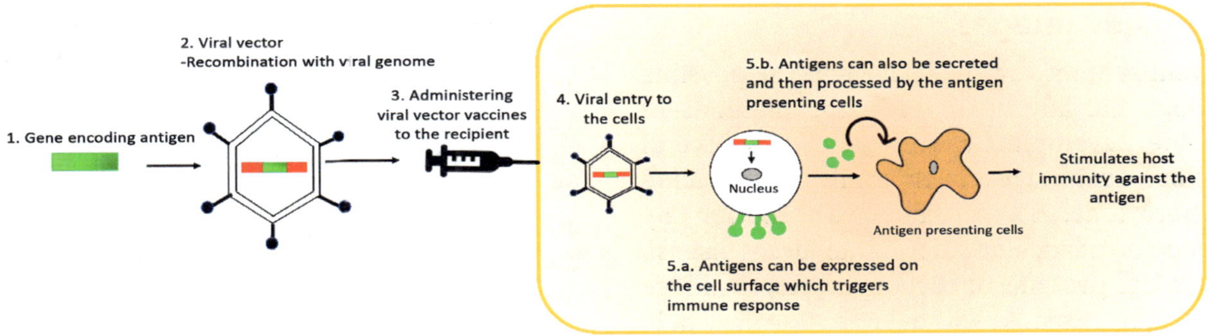

Figure 15.6. Illustration of viral vector vaccine delivery method.

Source: https://www.researchgate.net/publication/328974465/figure/fig4/AS:11431281212002487@1702513604920/Illustration-of-viral-vector-vaccine-delivery-method-The-gene-encoding-the-antigen-of.tif.

The rapid development and deployment of these vaccines underscore the utility of viral vectors in compact timelines, underlining their significance in modern vaccine strategies. Not only do they offer the promise of rapid response to public health crises, but they also potential for application against a wide range of pathogens, including cancers, where novel tumor-specific antigens can be addressed by therapy, enhancing their usefulness and worth within the context of preventing and controlling infectious disease. Though they have so many advantages, the application of viral vector vaccines also has its problems and issues. The biggest among these is pre-existing immunity to the viral vectors, which may reduce the effectiveness of the vaccines if the population is already exposed to the vector. This can lead to a poorer immune response, hence the need for different vector platforms to overcome this drawback. Further, utmost care should be taken to prevent the risk of insertional mutagenesis, wherein the viral vector DNA gets inserted into the host genome, which has the potential to initiate oncogenic pathways. Overcoming these challenges is essential to the safe and effective use of viral vector vaccines. Recent studies still pursue new ways of bolstering vector construction and reducing the risks associated with their use, thereby solidifying their position as a cornerstone of future vaccine construction methods as attested by recent advances in the field of immunotherapy and biotherapeutics, especially in oncology and aggressive infectious diseases like those outlined in Uddin et al. (2021) and Lahiri et al. (2023) (Figure 15.6).

15.2.3. Protein Subunit Vaccines and Their Advantages

Protein subunit vaccines have become possible through the advancement in the methods of vaccine development, and they have several distinct advantages over traditional vaccine preparations. These vaccines function by employing particular parts of the target disease agent, e.g., proteins or carbohydrates, to induce an immune response without releasing the whole pathogen. Thus, protein subunit vaccines are inherently safer, with less likelihood of causing adverse effects associated with live attenuated or inactivated vaccines. Their potential to trigger a specific immune response can also lead to greater efficacy against the pathogen in question. Moreover, advancements in biotechnology have facilitated mass production of such vaccines with ease and speed, so that it is now possible to respond more readily to fresh infectious dangers unfolding before us, thereby enhancing public health preparedness. Thus, protein subunit vaccines represent a significant development in vaccine technology that harmonizes safety with efficacy against infectious pathogens. Beyond their safety record, protein subunit vaccines offer scalability and ease of manufacture, rendering them attractive for large-scale use. The recombinant DNA method employed in their production enables quick and efficient generation of the target immune components. As opposed to traditional methods that rely on the culture growth of entire pathogens, the production of subunits is often possible in mature laboratory systems like yeast or bacterial cultures. Besides lowering development-to-market times, this versatility also allows for adaptation to vaccines for new pathogens because scientists can simply modify the protein constituents based on genomic information. Furthermore, the stability of protein subunit vaccines makes their shelf-life better, which is priceless in areas with limited accessibility to cold storage for more fragile vaccines. These production efficiencies are an argument for protein subunit vaccines as a viable alternative in vaccine programs worldwide. The application of protein subunit vaccines extends beyond human medicine to animal health, providing a significant benefit in disease management in animal populations. Vaccination programs for livestock and poultry have the capacity to slow down the transmission of infectious disease, thus improving food security and minimizing financial losses in agriculture. The establishment of vaccines for preventing the likes of coccidiosis in poultry is a case example of the effectiveness of protein subunits in lowering the dependence on antibiotics and meeting drug-resistant challenges in bacterial infections among animals (Hoelzer et al., 2018). By inducing targeted immunity through the application of selected antigens, the vaccines become capable of controlling disease transmission among dense animal populations. With an increasing awareness among veterinarians and agricultural stakeholders about the importance of vaccination in sustainable agriculture, protein subunit vaccines are poised to reshape animal health protection and productivity maintenance in agricultural systems (Fernández et al., 2012) (Figure 15.7).

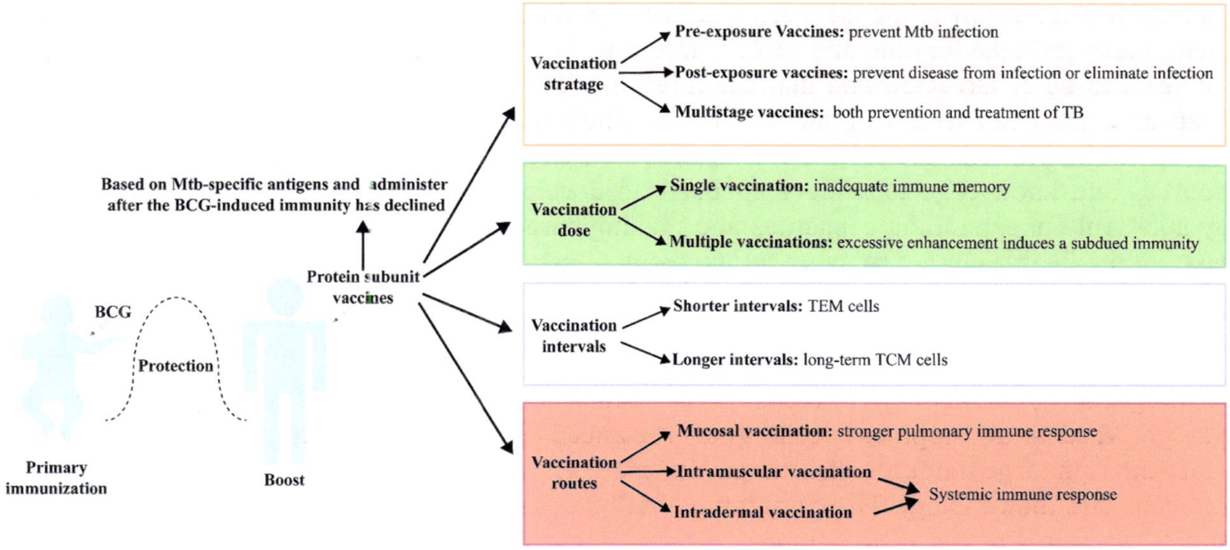

Figure 15.7. Vaccination strategies of protein subunit vaccines.

Source: https://www.researchgate.net/publication/373581121/figure/fig2/AS:11431281254749931@1719300208882/Vaccination-strategies-of-protein-subunit-vaccines.tif.

15.3. Speeding Up Vaccine Development

The attempt to speed up vaccine development is increasingly important in meeting public health crises, an activity significantly accelerated by recent technological advancements. The utilization of AI in vaccine research has shown promising potential in streamlining processes from the identification of vaccine candidate choices to the optimization of clinical trial design. AI enables researchers to screen massive data sets rapidly, enabling them to identify functional antigens and streamline the process of vaccine design. Additionally, AI-driven predictive models can complement decision-making through simulated results, improving the overall efficiency and responsiveness of vaccine development processes. This technological shift highlights a revolutionary phase in the healthcare sector, forcing stakeholders to embrace innovative methods that not only accelerate vaccine production but also enable agile adaptability in crisis phases, thus securing populations well against newly emerging pathogens (Varnosfaderani & Forouzanfar, 2024). In addition to AI development, the concept of digital twins is likely to revolutionize vaccine production processes. Application of digital twin technology in healthcare, also known as digital twin for health (DT4H), supports personalized vaccine regimens that adapt based on individual health patterns. Through the creation of virtual replicas of biological systems, researchers can simulate vaccine interactions, predict immunity, and optimize formulations without expensive physical trials. This method accelerates the process of research, particularly in understanding how different populations will respond to vaccines. The intersection of big data, data science, and DT4H promises doors to groundbreaking innovations in vaccine development, manufacturing, and delivery, ultimately boosting the speed at which safe and effective vaccines hit the market (Katsoulakis et al., 2024). Moreover, advancements in manufacturing technologies such as mRNA and viral vector platforms have drastically changed the field of vaccine manufacturing. Such platforms carry the specific advantage of high scalability, which allows for rapid response during times of public health emergencies. Traditional vaccine development can take months and be resource-intensive; however, newer methods, such as mRNA vaccines, can be constructed and manufactured in weeks and not months, with the same efficacy. Moreover, as has been seen with the rapid development of COVID-19 vaccines, collaboration between government institutions, the private sector, and research institutions plays a critical role in managing resources and knowledge to achieve speeded-up development timelines. Strategic collaborations play a key role in expanding capacities and making sure that technologies of development lead to actual public health impact to avert future pandemics.

15.3.1. The Role of Technology in Accelerating Research

The integration of technology in research has transformed many fields of work, particularly with regard to vaccine development techniques. Advanced computer applications enable researchers to sort through large amounts of data, paving the way for comprehensive knowledge of infectious pathogens and immunology. The combining of efforts through technology can be seen through the rapid development of vaccines for emerging pathogens, where bioinformatics and machine learning are involved when modeling the efficacy of vaccines.

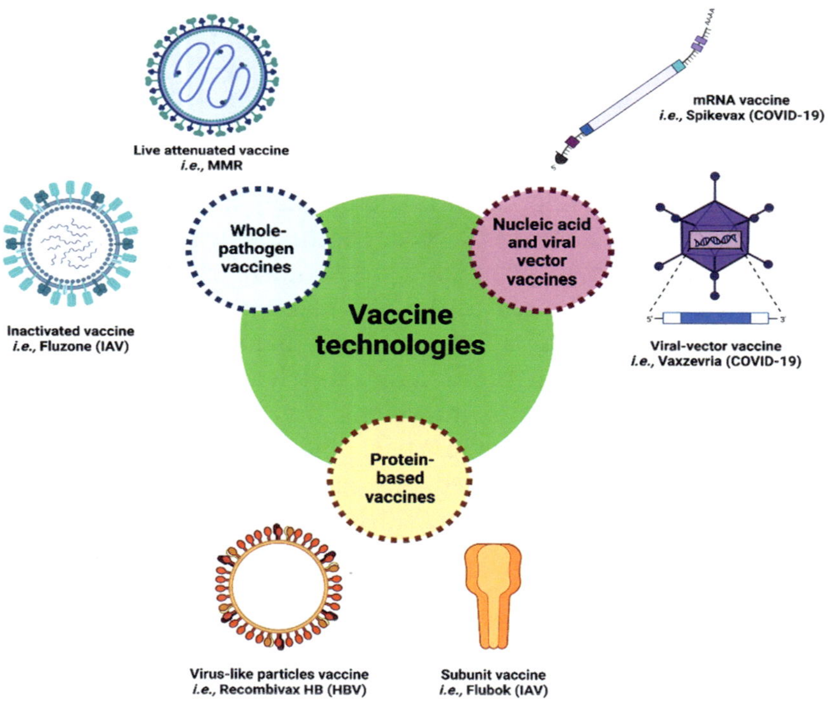

Figure 15.8. Schematic representation of vaccine technologies.

Source: https://www.researchgate.net/publication/365394324/figure/fig2/AS:11431281217222739@1705042417788/Schematic-representation-of-vaccine-technologies-and-examples-of-commercialized-vaccines.tif.

By simulating immune responses and forecasting potential antigens based on genomic information, researchers can significantly shorten the design process, reducing the time traditionally linked to traditional vaccine manufacturing methods. Such speed is of paramount importance when responding to newly arising health threats, highlighting the way that technology not only maximizes research efficiency but may even save lives. Also, the emergence of single-cell sequencing technologies is revolutionizing our vaccine research strategy. These approaches allow for detailed analysis of the immune cell populations at the single-cell level, which informs cellular heterogeneity and function. For instance, scRNA-seq is important in vaccine-induced immunity, where it is possible to recognize the cell types that contribute most toward protection against infection. These data are important for optimizing vaccine design because they identify specific immune pathways whose modulation can be addressed for enhanced efficacy. With advanced analytical tools, this approach guides decision-making processes in vaccine research, emphasizing the value of using the most up-to-date technology in study designs for quick and efficient intervention in worldwide diseases (de Sande et al., 2023). In addition to improving vaccine design and evaluation, technology takes a central role in making manufacturing and delivery processes simpler. Biomanufacturing technologies' recent advancements, such as the use of cell-free protein synthesis systems and continuous manufacturing platforms, enable efficient and high-speed development of vaccine candidates. Not only are they cost-efficient but also easily scalable, making it possible to produce them in mass instantly should a public health outbreak occur. Furthermore, digital monitoring and tracking ensure that the vaccines are stored and transported in perfect conditions until reach end-consumers. Therefore, the convergence of various technological innovations throughout the vaccine development life cycle is one of the best examples of how research can be leveraged and accelerated, and communities can obtain safe and effective vaccines in a more complicated world (Figure 15.8).

15.3.2. Regulatory Changes And Emergency Use Authorizations

Regulatory procedures that govern vaccine production have fundamentally transformed to stay current with the urgencies of the COVID-19 pandemic. Traditional procedures for vaccine approval, typically featuring comprehensive safety testing and long clinical trials, were modified to advance access to lifesaving vaccines. The issuance of Emergency Use Authorizations (EUAs) was the pinnacle of such a shift, which facilitated accelerated deployment of vaccines that had early evidence of safety and efficacy in diverse populations. That was particularly important to combat the emergent public health emergency due to COVID-19 by facilitating rapid access to vaccines that would otherwise require years of regulatory approval. Thus, the agility of adjusting to emerging health needs through regulatory adjustment underscores the dialogue between scientific breakthrough and effective navigation of bureaucratic barriers amidst crisis. Furthermore, the use of EUAs has also been an impetus for important dialogue between regulatory agencies, healthcare facilities, and biotech firms to make sure that vaccines not only come out quickly but also meet stringent safety standards. Regulatory agencies, like the Food and Drug Administration (FDA), have played a significant role in streamlining data submission protocols and refining assessment standards to keep pace with rapid advances in vaccine technology, including mRNA platforms and novel adjuvants. This collaborative strategy has made remarkable strides in vaccine development technology by fostering shared knowledge and expertise. An example of such a collaborative strategy is the NIH's RADx-UP initiative, which aims to enhance diagnostics in under-resourced populations and thereby bridge gaps in healthcare access and equity (Narayanasamy et al., 2023). Such partnerships effectively improve the impact and coverage of vaccination campaigns and thereby enhance public health resilience. While the triumph associated with EUAs cannot be doubted, criticism of the resulting regulatory changes identifies the risk of compromising safety levels in the name of expediency. Guarding against the risk that the rapid response to vaccine development does not compromise the public's confidence or the integrity of the approval process is crucial. As put forth in available literature, the relationship between technological innovation and equitable public health implementation remains an essential challenge, necessitating ongoing debate surrounding regulatory processes (Mafuts, 2025).

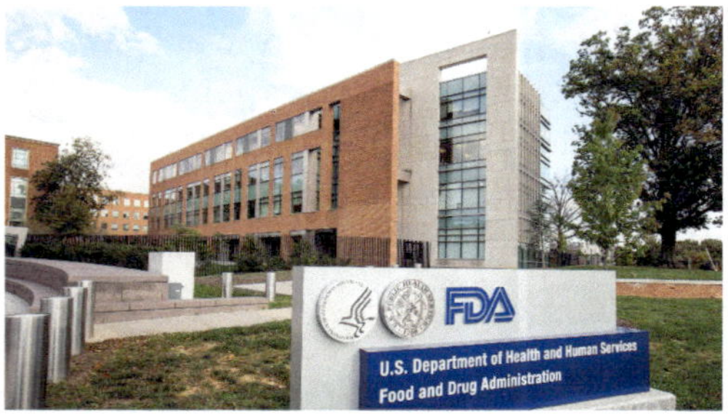

Figure 15.9. The Food and Drug Administration (FDA) played a pivotal role in streamlining data submission processes and revising evaluative criteria to keep pace with rapid advancements in vaccine technologies.

Source: https://media.wired.com/photos/67c1f9f43b2d5224177a3108/16:9/w_2000,h_1125,c_limit/FDA-Chaos-Business-AP23124686409590.jpg.

There is a necessity for frameworks that ensure swift response against health emergencies while ensuring strict safety and efficacy standards. This balance will play an important role in informing future responses to emerging infectious disease outbreaks, such as ensuring that the COVID-19 pandemic experience provides lessons for more effective public health response and regulation strategies in the future (Figure 15.9).

15.3.3. Collaborative Efforts in Global Vaccine Development

Joint efforts in international vaccine research and development have been essential in combating the increasing plague of contagious diseases that do not discriminate where they occur. The partnership among governments, international organizations, drug companies, and research institutions facilitates the pooling of resources and technical expertise, which accelerates the innovation process. For example, collaborations made via organizations such as the Coalition for Epidemic Preparedness Innovations (CEPI) are aimed at advancing vaccine development against epidemics, prioritizing quick response mechanisms. This can mean quicker regulatory approvals and clinical trials, thereby getting vaccines to populations in need in a timely manner. This element of collaboration not only reduces the economic burden on solitary entities but also engenders the shared feeling of fate towards international health security, which proves that when organizations collaborate, the efficiency and effectiveness of vaccine development are considerably enhanced. Integrating diverse scientific knowledge through collaborative efforts has also been fundamental in enhancing vaccine technologies. By integrating information from various fields—such as mRNA technology, nanotechnology, and traditional immunology—researchers are able to design more sophisticated and effective vaccine candidates. The multidisciplinary strategy allows researchers to find novel adjuvants, delivery systems, and production procedures that perhaps would not have been discovered in single research departments. For instance, CGIAR's collaboration with other agri- and health bodies underscores the significance of combining agricultural science with information on health needs, thereby strengthening the vaccine pipeline with fresh uses of biotechnology (Gruère et al., 2011). Such collaborative research processes have been pivotal in establishing novel methods of disease prevention that disproportionately benefit poor communities while ensuring equitable access to vaccine technologies. Moreover, the public-private partnerships' impact on global vaccine programs highlights the game-changing potential of partnership models. Governments provide the necessary finance and infrastructure, while corporations contribute cutting-edge research and development capabilities. The best example of such synergy lies in the partnerships formed during the COVID-19 pandemic, where companies such as Pfizer and BioNTech collaborated with government agencies in an effort to accelerate the manufacture and delivery of vaccines. These collaborations allow for both private innovation and public investment to be utilized, closely bridging the timeline between deployment and research.

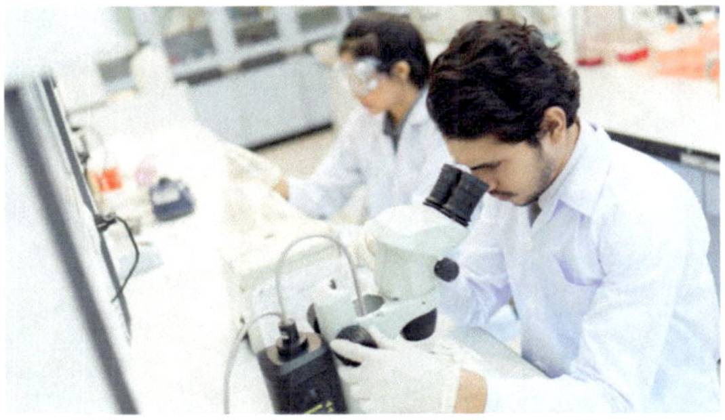

Figure 15.10. Coalition for Epidemic Preparedness Innovations (CEPI) focuses on enhancing vaccine development for epidemics.

Source: https://static.cepi.net/images/3840x2160/2024-01/Web-Image-Institut-Pasteur-and-Themis.webp.

Further, collaborative action also involves international agencies that allow for global coordination and financing, as seen in initiatives led by CEPI and the World Health Organization. Through these collaborative efforts, global response to pandemics has demonstrated that collaborative vaccine development is not only helpful; it is indispensable to the advancement of public health programs that traverse international borders (Figure 15.10).

15.4. Enhancements in Vaccine Efficacy

The formulation of vaccines has been one of the most influential factors for enhancing vaccine efficacy and the center of new advancements in vaccine development techniques in recent years. New theories, such as the incorporation of adjuvants and enhanced delivery systems, have optimized immune responses by making antigens more accessible to the immune system. This tactical enhancement is designed to induce a stronger and more enduring immune response, a prerequisite for effective vaccination. For instance, newer adjuvants can induce recruitment and activation of dendritic cells, which are instrumental in inducing adaptive immunity. This augmented activation has been converted into improved immunogenicity and defense against infectious diseases, ushering in the prospect for more effective vaccines to counter new emerging pathogens and reassortant viral strains. Beyond traditional improvements, use of genetically altered viruses, such as oncolytic measles virus (MV), represents a revolutionary step forward in vaccine effectiveness, particularly in cancer immunotherapy. The Edmonston MV strain, as reported, has a good safety profile and has been modified at the genomic level to become increasingly selective for cancer cells with minimal damage to normal tissue. These optimizations not only enhance therapy but also enable activation of the immune system against cancer. The therapeutic value of viral vector adaptations underscores their position in breaking the dichotomy between vaccine technology and therapy. This move not only enhances performance but also represents a paradigm shift in the use of vaccines beyond prevention, extending to cancer therapy, and therefore expanding the scope of vaccine development approaches. Moreover, advances in formulation science are essential in addressing the complexity of delivering therapeutic vaccines efficiently. Formulation scientists face the task of achieving maximum bioavailability and therapeutic response with chemotherapeutic agents and vaccines. Due to the increasing incidence of cancer-related diagnoses, new systems for cancer vaccine delivery are becoming increasingly important. Modulating vaccine formulations to elicit robust protective immunity to cancer presents unique opportunities for redefining immunotherapy. As the investigations continue in pursuit of developing better designs and preparations of such vaccines, interaction with cutting-edge technologies has not only the potential for increased vaccine performance but also for extending the boundaries of vaccine applications towards better patient outcomes (Chablani, 2016). This multi-disciplinary approach is a critical move in the evolution of vaccine production techniques, with a keen emphasis on the potential of therapeutic vaccines for cancer treatment.

15.4.1. Adjuvants and Their Role in Immune Response

The contribution of adjuvants towards enhancing immune response is a critical feature in the evolution of vaccine production techniques. Adjuvants are additives in vaccines that help amplify the immune response of the body against the presented antigen. This increase has the potential to produce more vigorous and sustained immunity, of importance in the current era when emergent pathogens pose significant public health risks. Through the activation of innate immune responses, adjuvants enable more intense stimulation of adaptive immunity, producing increased antibody and enhanced T cell responses (Figure 15.11).

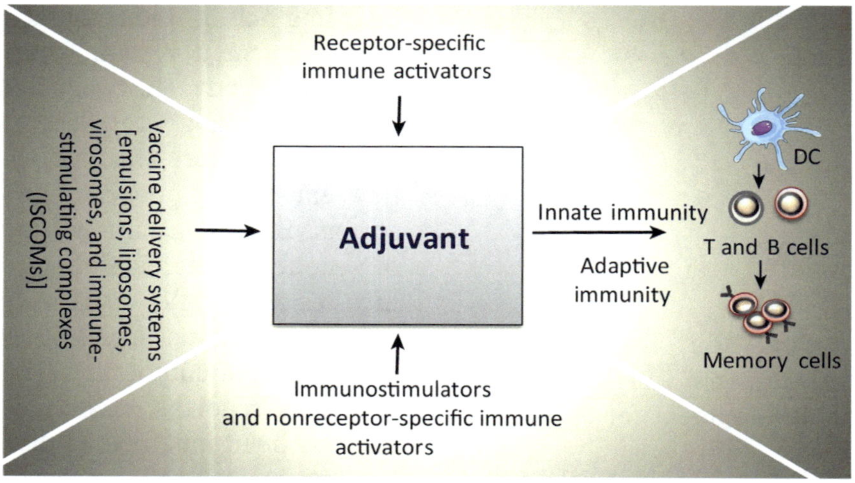

Figure 15.11. Adjuvants.

Source: https://www.cell.com/cms/10.1016/j.tips.2017.06.002/asset/e190d098-71ae-4d4e-822a-69fa76589a1a/main.assets/gr3_lrg.jpg.

Various adjuvant forms, such as the traditional aluminum salts and new contenders such as toll-like receptor agonists, have been comprehensively studied with a view to understanding their mechanisms of action. E.g., aluminum salts induce a local inflammatory response that attracts immune cells to the injection site, enhancing the visibility of antigens to the immune system. Also, it has recently been found that certain adjuvants also play a role in immunotype modulation, i.e., influencing the type of immune response induced, basically channeling it into an optimal route most appropriate for combating certain pathogens. Interestingly, the use of adjuvants is increasingly recognized as a strategic step in preventive and therapeutic vaccine production with promise for the treatment of a variety of conditions from infectious diseases to malignancies, calling for continued research into their optimal use. The study of adjuvants is not just at the core of enhancing traditional vaccines but also in new therapeutic strategies, most notably to cancer immunotherapy.

Research illustrates how adjuvants increase the therapeutic vaccine efficacy by inducing an immune state that promotes identification and death of cancer cells. Macrophages as critical immune system actors are regulated by adjuvants that lead to their repolarization to an immunogenic phenotype capable of further targeting the tumors (Chen et al., 2023). Application of adjuvants in combination treatments, including checkpoint inhibitor therapies, has also been promising in augmenting overall therapeutic outcomes in cancer treatment, such as inducing synergy that could unlock potential in immunotherapy approaches (Lahiri et al., 2023). Despite advancements in vaccine research, understanding and leveraging the potential of adjuvants remain the pivotal elements (Figure 15.12).

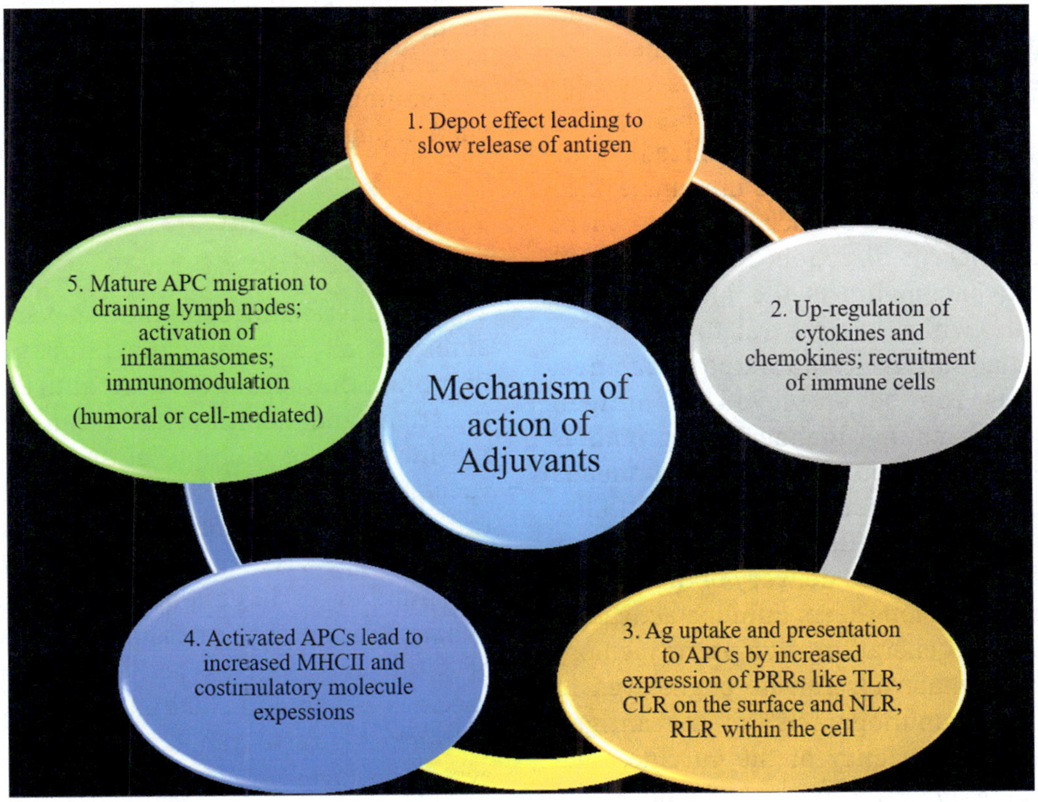

Figure 15.12. Mechanism of action of adjuvants.

Source: https://www.researchgate.net/profile/Kuldeep-Dhama-2/publication/346945608/figure/fig1/AS:967520559308803@1607686285675/Mechanism-of-action-of-adjuvants.png.

15.4.2. Personalized Vaccines and Tailored Approaches

The concept of personalized vaccines is a significant improvement in immunization technologies from the generic one-size-fits-all solutions to more tailored, patient-specific interventions. Personalized vaccines are designed to generate maximal immune responses, taking into account individual patient parameters such as genetic makeup and personal disease profiles. This individualization is extremely relevant in cancer treatment, where tumor antigens can be discovered and targeted, maximizing vaccine efficacy and reducing unpredictable side effects. Application of this form of individualization has the ability to maximize therapeutic benefit, particularly for cancer with definable molecular signatures, through triggering the immune system specifically against cancer cells. Along with continuing research, the nexus of genomics and vaccine technology is opening doors to unprecedented possibilities for the development of vaccines as customized as the individuals they are intended to immunize, thus transforming methods of vaccine development towards a different direction. At the forefront of these advancements is the integration of biomaterials, which are central to enhancing the efficacy of individualized vaccines. Biomaterials can be employed as antigen delivery platforms in a manner that promotes targeted immune responses with simultaneous removal of challenges such as biocompatibility and biodegradability. Biomaterials allow for controlled and sustained delivery of the vaccine components, with long-term immune activation being vital in the generation of long-term memory responses. Biomaterials can be engineered to increase the immunogenicity of the antigen with enhanced efficiency of the vaccine. This novel use of biomaterials not only enhances the therapeutic potential but also underlines the utility of personalized approaches in tailoring vaccinations to each patient's needs, once more bridging the distance between technology and patient care (Trucillo, 2024). Moreover, in the discipline of neuro-oncology, personalized immunotherapy, such as personalized vaccines, is fighting back against malignant brain tumors such as glioblastoma. Due to the sheer difficulty of glioma treatment—i.e., the tumor's immunosuppressive environment and the blood-brain barrier—personalized vaccines are a promising solution. Targeting specific antigens that are characteristic of certain tumors, these vaccines are capable of initiating a stronger immune response better designed to penetrate the gliomas' special defenses. Immunotherapies, including individualized vaccines, are becoming key components of a multitask treatment strategy for glioblastoma, with the promising results of clinical trials having been observed. With an ever-growing body of knowledge regarding glioma biology, relentless efforts to develop individualized immunotherapies, including individualized vaccines, may lead to astounding developments in treating this challenging malignancy (Yasinjan et al., 2023).

15.4.3. Combination Vaccines and Their Potential Benefits

The production of combination vaccines has emerged as a significant improvement in immunization practice that addresses both logistical and health-related concerns. With the inclusion of multiple antigens in a single vaccine product, these vaccines consolidate the vaccination process for patients and for healthcare professionals as well. This minimizes the number of injections greatly, which can enhance compliance rates and reduce the effect of multiple visits. In addition, combination vaccines are able to elicit more robust immune responses due to the fact that the immune system is presented with multiple antigens simultaneously, even with the highest level of immunological synergy. This way, such vaccines can potentially simplify healthcare programs while also ensuring greater population immunity levels can be achieved with ease. One of the most significant developments among combination vaccines is the five-in-one vaccine microneedle patch, which has antigens for Pertussis, Tetanus, Diphtheria, Hepatitis B, and Haemophilus influenzae type b. The groundbreaking delivery system not only enhances the convenience of vaccine availability but also offers greater stability and efficiency with the vaccines. The microneedle patch enables stable antigenicity to be stored at room temperature, something that is especially valuable when resources are limited and refrigeration cannot be relied upon. As demonstrated by the study, combination patch immunogenic responses are the same as with traditional intramuscular injections, but with the advantage of being less invasive and easier to administer. These advancements highlight the potential of combination vaccines to be of immense impact on public health, particularly where healthcare capacity is limited (Choi et al., 2024). Moreover, judicious application of combination vaccines in immunization regimens can produce ample health benefits. Through being able to combat several diseases simultaneously, combination vaccines are capable of alleviating the overall immunization load on patients and the health system. This becomes especially important in controlling diseases with high levels of morbidity and mortality, where coverage for vaccination may be lower because of logistical factors. Additionally, the smaller number of vaccines required can lead to lower healthcare expenditure, and hence, immunization programs become more sustainable and effective in resource-poor settings. With the demand for global health needs to be addressed through innovative solutions on the rise, combination vaccines can emerge as a prominent driver of public health initiatives and patient enhancement (Hussain et al., 2025) (Figure 15.13).

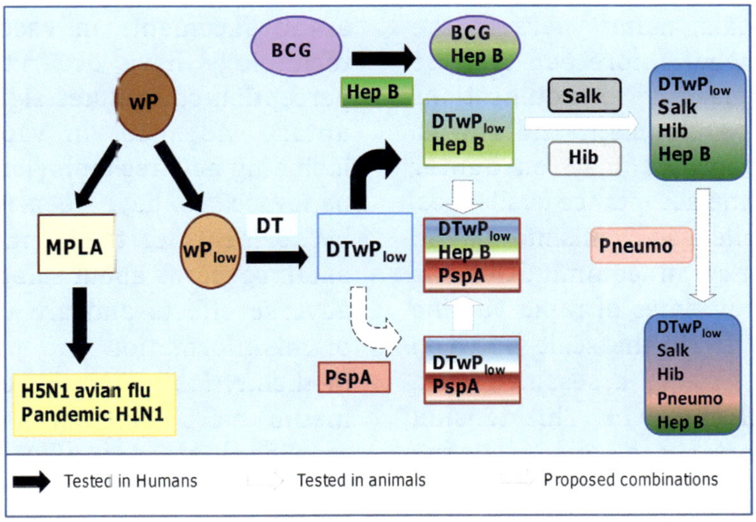

Figure 15.13. Schematic representation of combined vaccines as well as new vaccines.

Source: https://www.researchgate.net/profile/Paulo-Ho/publication/51852712/figure/fig2/AS:292459072110593@1446739084906/Schematic-representation-of-combined-vaccines-as-well-as-new-vaccines-under-development.png.

15.5. Challenges in Vaccine Development

The development of vaccines is plagued with challenges that can stop progress despite monumental advances in technology. Perhaps the biggest challenge is the complexity of the pathogens themselves.

Viruses and bacteria have vast genetic diversity and a high mutation rate, rendering current vaccines increasingly less effective with time. This is perhaps most pronounced in infections like influenza, whose antigenic drift necessitates annual vaccine reformulation. Additionally, vaccines against diseases caused by more complex organisms, such as malaria or HIV, present unique challenges due to their complex life cycles and immune evasion strategies. Thus, vaccine developers must embark on serious study and research in an attempt to engineer immunogens that are capable of initiating strong and long-term immune responses that result in the timeline for a vaccine to reach the public taking significantly longer. Furthermore, safety and effectiveness concerns are formidable barriers in the pipeline for vaccine creation. The need for meticulous examination of potential side effects and desired immune action requires rigorous clinical trials, many years in the making. Along the way, unforeseen adverse reactions may arise, leading to modifications or even complete development shutdowns. Even established vaccines may encounter public trust and vaccine acceptance challenges, particularly when challenged by misinformation and vaccine hesitancy in communities. As illustrated through our times of rapid vaccine deployment for COVID-19, the scale between speed and sufficient safety assessment is a delicate and critical endeavor. This tension underlines the importance of open dialogue and robust regulatory mechanisms to underpin public trust in emerging vaccines and ultimately determine the course of immunization efforts. To address these challenges, new manufacturing techniques are being explored to render vaccine manufacture more efficient and adaptable. Recent developments in plant-based antigen manufacturing technology, for example, have underscored great potential in the manufacture of cost-effective and mass-scalable vaccines. This approach employs genetically engineered plants, such as Nicotiana benthamiana, to produce recombinant proteins that are more immunogenic, with the potential to revolutionize the rate of vaccine development against new infections. The use of techniques like CRISPR/Cas9 offers the potential for ease in the process of editing the genome, with the way open for rapid advances in vaccine design. Nevertheless, reliance on these new technologies still demands an intimate acquaintance with regulatory barriers and long-term efficacy. Though the vaccine development platform continues to expand, classical and modern challenges have to be overcome to advance public health initiatives and safeguard populations from infectious diseases, as pointed out by the critical reviews of new platforms (Hutzen et al., 2015; Evju, 2023).

15.5.1. Addressing Vaccine Hesitancy and Public Perception

It is vital to comprehend vaccine hesitancy, as advancements in vaccine manufacturing technology have occurred, because public perception contributes significantly to vaccine uptake. Advances in vaccine development, including new technologies such as mRNA and nanovaccines, have been met with skepticism by segments of the population. All of these entail concerns about safety, effectiveness, and adverse effects and are commonly products of misinformation and previous distrust in medicine. Moreover, the emergence of social media as a primary information source amplifies these fears, allowing unverified claims to shape public discourse. Addressing these concerns requires a multifaceted approach, emphasizing open communication between healthcare professionals and the community while disseminating evidence-based information to eradicate myths. Moreover, actions taken to enhance public trust, such as community communication, transparency towards clinical trial processes, and highlighting the advancement and success in vaccine technology, could certainly limit resistance and build a more favorable public perception. The convergence of new vaccine technologies is particularly conducive to an overhaul of public opinion. By way of illustration, the demystification of new vaccine modalities is crucial because they leave more favorable efficacy profiles and safety features. Innovations such as nonlipid and lipid nanovaccines are a classic case of this phenomenon, with their enhanced antigen stability and targeted delivery mechanisms unavailable in traditional vaccines. Through the promotion of such innovations, public health initiatives can demonstrate how these surpass previous limitations effectively. The potential for individualized immunization protocols, which adapt vaccinations in accordance with personal needs, also creates the perception of ownership and involvement in the process of making health decisions among the public. As recognized through research into these innovations, addressing both scientific effectiveness and public perception allows for complete comprehension of the role of immunization in the prevention of disease spread, and, when combined with outreach, can enhance overall vaccine acceptance among groups (Gholap et al., 2023). Lessons drawn from avian influenza immunization campaigns provide important lessons regarding public perception and vaccine acceptance within the backdrop of scientific advancement. It was initially opposition from stakeholders like broiler producers due to economic and fear of worthless products reasons. However, with advancements demonstrating the efficiency of the vaccination method, including vector-based and recombinant vaccines, public confidence changed for the better. The change emphasizes the need for education and stakeholder agreement, highlighting that transparency for vaccine development and stringent regulatory processes form acceptance at the community level. In addition, successful narratives surrounding vaccination campaigns can contribute positively to public debate, stressing the relevance of vaccines in safeguarding public health. A holistic approach combining scientific advancement, sustained public discourse, and emphasis on ethical considerations will be instrumental in overcoming resistance and enhancing public attitudes toward vaccination in an era of rapid scientific development (Shehata & Tellez-Isaias, 2023) (Figure 15.14).

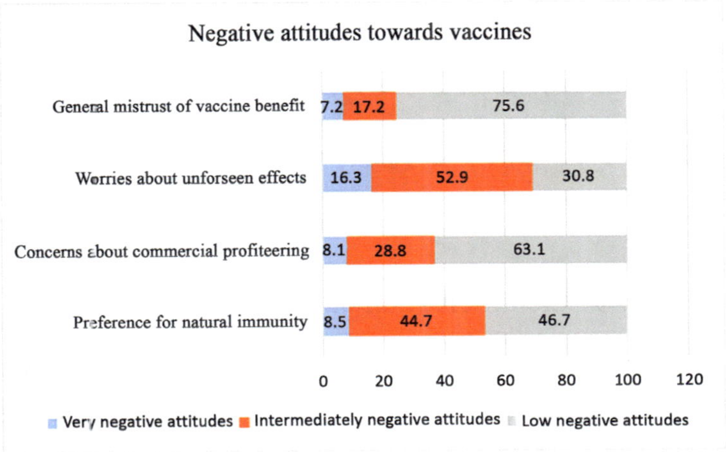

Figure 15.14. Negative attitudes towards vaccines.

Source: https://ars.els-cdn.com/content/image/1-s2.0-S2666776220300120-gr1.jpg.

15.5.2. Overcoming Logistical Challenges in Distribution

As the methods of vaccine production evolve, the distribution of vaccines has also emerged as a main challenge requiring innovative breakthroughs. Logistical hurdles in the distribution of vaccines, which were glaringly highlighted in the midst of the COVID-19 pandemic, are the storage requirements, coordination of transport, and timely delivery to various geographic locations. For instance, the ultra-low storage requirement for certain of the mRNA vaccines complicates the process of distribution, especially in low-resource settings. Ghana and Rwanda, among others, have been successful in employing advanced technologies, such as artificial intelligence, to combat such challenges through demand forecasting and supply chain logistics optimization, where vaccines are made available to even the remotest areas (Addy, 2023). The capacity to incorporate such technologies represents a significant step ahead in breaking the stranglehold of conventional methods, evidence that distribution is heavily reliant on planning and strategic implementation. Moreover, successful vaccine deployment relies on an understanding of local health care infrastructure and population. Using the capability of analytics, countries can identify populations that are most at risk and prioritize them for immunization.

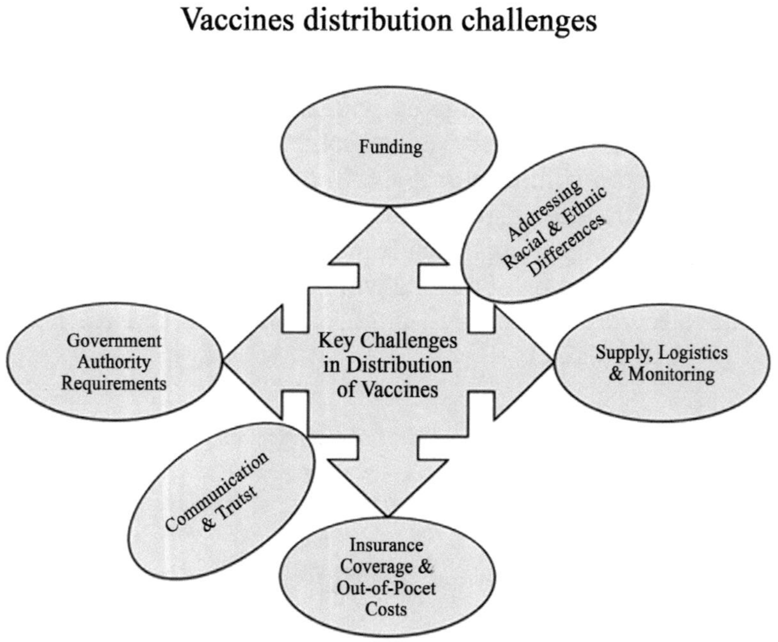

Figure 15.15. Key challenges in the distribution of vaccines.

Source: https://www.researchgate.net/profile/Tauseef-Ahmad-10/publication/355007209/figure/fig2/AS:1076022619451400@1633555192899/Key-challenges-in-the-distribution-of-vaccines.png.

For example, AI-powered models can distribute resources most efficiently and be key to guiding the fair distribution of vaccines, whereby resources are sent to the right location at the right time. In a recent study, an improvement in the fairness of resource distribution was observed, with strong advances in logistical structure assisting sin enhancing higher vaccination among marginalized communities (Sharmin et al., 2025). These analytical methods not only enhance the efficiency of vaccine coverage but also facilitate higher aspects of justice in public health programs, ultimately resulting in higher community acceptance of vaccination efforts. Lastly, while technology advancements have worked significantly to fill gaps in logistics, the complexities of distribution mechanisms cannot be addressed by technology alone. Collective actions by governments, private industry, and international organizations must converge to form strong distribution systems. Developed nations such as the US and UK have utilized collaboration with technology companies to enhance immunization campaigns. However, this needs ongoing investment in health infrastructure by developing nations in a bid to make them capable of joining efforts to outsmart such adversity effectively. An equitable method of vaccine distribution not only serves public health but should also make the whole world prepared to handle subsequent pandemics (Addy, 2023). Lastly, effective vaccine distribution is a multifaceted endeavor with synergy between technology and partnership, highlighting the necessity of overall strategies to enhance public health programs (Figure 15.15).

15.5.3. Ensuring Equitable Access to Vaccines Worldwide

In the context of global health, ensuring equal access to vaccines is an outstanding issue that has become further appreciated with the onset of the COVID-19 pandemic. Technological innovations in vaccine production, particularly mRNA and nanoparticle delivery technology, have enabled the production of vaccines in bulk and at a quicker pace. However, the innovations themselves are not able to guarantee that all populations in low- and middle-income countries receive the necessary immunization coverage. Structural inequalities in terms of insufficient healthcare infrastructure and insufficient funding also further exacerbate the existing inequalities. As cited in new literature, the success of vaccine breakthroughs as robust public health interventions relies on a multifaceted process that considers not only scientific progress but also the social and political determinants that influence access to healthcare resources. Progress in scientific method must therefore be augmented by collective action that demolishes barriers to equitable vaccine distribution in global health rule systems (Mafuts, 2025). Health equity depends on the effective implementation of technological advancements into effective immunization techniques. Above all, countries like Ghana and Rwanda have been examples of effective use of AI in making vaccine distribution smoother, where remote areas also get access to timely vaccinations. Using demand forecasting and supply chain optimization, these nations have demonstrated how technology systems can make a radical difference in access. On the other hand, although more densely populated nations with higher densities, such as India and China, are faced with extraordinary problems in fairly distributing vaccines despite the application of cutting-edge technologies, their enormous populations create mind-boggling distributional challenges that necessitate tailor-made solutions.

The disparate infrastructure preparedness levels and resource availability are themselves pivotal in the effectiveness of vaccine distribution strategies, so a differentiated strategy with sensitivity to local needs and obstacles is required (Addy, 2023). Furthermore, the ethical imperatives of vaccine equity call for increased international cooperation among countries, public health agencies, and the private sector. Next-generation vaccine development approaches, as groundbreaking as they are, must put a priority on access for disadvantaged groups to meet global health goals. It is an urgent need for international cooperation to assist vaccine production capacity in resource-scarce settings and facilitate technology transfer. Such collaborations might allow lower-income countries to develop independent manufacturing capacity of their own, reducing reliance on external resources and enhancing self-sufficiency. By bringing biotechnological innovation together with fair public health benefits, the world can begin to close the gaps in vaccine access laid bare by the pandemic.

Ethical considerations must be employed to inform the policy for vaccine distribution so that innovation gains benefit all individuals and no group is left out (Mafuts, 2025).

15.6. Future Directions in Vaccine Research

With continued research on vaccines, one of many of the most crucial future breakthroughs is the application of oncolytic viruses, namely genetically modified strains of the MV. The new therapies capitalize on the natural ability of certain viruses to home in and destroy cancer cells without damaging normal tissue. The Edmonston strain of MV, which has an established safety profile from earlier vaccinations, was genetically altered to be selective and more effective against cancer cells. Its conversion into an anticancer modality from a preventative vaccine represents a new model in vaccine technology, which holds promise for future applications within the industry. The research into oncolytic viruses not only opens up new avenues for cancer treatment but also offers an added model for traditional vaccination methods, suggesting a confluence of preventative and therapeutic approaches in future vaccine research (Hutzen et al., 2015). Another major area of future vaccine research involves the solution to the universal issue of vaccine misinformation. With increased reliance on digital information, the dissemination of misinformation in assumptions about vaccine safety and effectiveness poses a challenge to public health initiatives. With multiple spheres of decision-making affected by misinformation, an increased interest in the dissemination of misinformation and its impact on vaccination rates is being felt. This necessitates further innovative methods in the battle against misinformation through the integration of technology and social science methods. Through the development of algorithms and applications that are effective in fighting disinformation, the scientific community can assist in building public confidence and acceptance of vaccines. To overcome this barrier is essential to the destiny of vaccine campaigns since it directly influences the success of new vaccine technologies and their acceptance (Fernandez & Alani, 2018). Finally, incorporating novel adjuvants into vaccine formulations is an exhilarating area of research that is conceivable in the future, with a focus on enhancing immune responses more forcefully and broadening the window of vaccine actions. Current adjuvants all have safety liabilities and the inconvenience of causing higher doses, which has prompted researchers to venture toward natural source-derived or engineered immunostimulant entities. The synergy between adjuvants and vaccines can boost both humoral and cellular immunity extremely effectively, especially for those conditions which require to be immunized with vigorous long-term immunity. Additional studies need to determine the mode of action of such novel adjuvants so that further optimized adjuvant vaccine combinations may be produced in vaccines. As this work progresses, it potentially offers breakthroughs that optimize the use of vaccines for new infectious diseases as well as established pathogens, setting an enhanced global health response (Hutzen et al., 2015).

15.6.1. Innovations in Delivery Methods

Breakthroughs in delivery formats have revolutionized vaccine development, optimizing efficacy and availability. The identification of new technologies such as microneedle patches illustrates the shift towards more patient-focused products in immunization. In contrast to traditional injection methods that are anxiogenic and injurious, microneedles facilitate painless delivery by introducing a series of short, thin needles that penetrate only the outer skin layer. These methods not only increase compliance among patients but also allow self-administration, which is particularly worthwhile in remote areas with no health care facilities. Along with this, microneedle technology is also capable of lowering the amount of required dosage, with the delivery system directly targeting the immune system more effectively than is currently practiced. This indicates a broader trend towards decreasing the impediments to vaccination and thus enhancing public health results. Aside from microneedles, the application of nanoparticle-based delivery systems has made a significant progress in vaccine technology. These systems permit protection of antigens, adjuvants, and other essential components from destruction and for delivery via controlled release. Stability and bioavailability of the vaccine components are optimized by nanoparticle systems, which have the potential to induce enhanced immune responses. Such widespread application is the potential of nanotechnology not only in vaccines but also in a majority of therapeutic treatments, foreshadowing a revolutionary shift in methods of medical intervention. As shown in recent research, nanoparticle formulations can also target specific cells, enhancing their immunogenicity and decreasing side effects. Relyance on such sophisticated delivery systems is complementary to the need for more personalized, effective immunization strategies appropriate for heterogeneous populations. In addition, the existing vaccine delivery environment is increasingly being driven by AI and data analytics, which refine and enhance the process. AI can be of tremendous help in simulating and forecasting immune responses, providing insight into the optimal set of antigens and modes of delivery. Such functionalities enable vaccine candidates to be refined iteratively based on real-time information, accelerating the process from development to market. By combining these technologies, scientists can more effectively meet such global challenges as emerging infectious diseases. However, the application of AI in medicine is not without its challenges; i.e., concerns over data privacy and trust involved in algorithmic decision-making, as mentioned in the literature recently (Alowais et al., 2023). As these developments advance, both the benefits and the risks will need to be balanced to get the maximum out of contemporary vaccine delivery systems.

15.6.2. The Potential of Universal Vaccines

The advent of universal vaccines is a revolutionary leap in the area of immunization that holds the potential for more efficiency and wider protection against a variety of pathogens. Conventional vaccines tend to be specific to strains or species, requiring periodic renewal to remain effective, particularly with the changing epidemiology of viruses and bacteria. Universal vaccines, by contrast, aim to elicit a stronger immune response across multiple variants or even different pathogens, thus optimizing their use in different populations and regions. This innovation optimizes the minimization of the logistical challenges of vaccine delivery, ensuring quicker and more efficient response times in public health crises, such as pandemics. Particularly, the innovation of 3D-printed microneedle technology in vaccine delivery contributes to the tractability of the delivery of universal vaccines. The pain-free and user-friendly delivery of microneedle patches can render populations more compliant and accepting, thereby maximizing immunity across groups (Bhadouria et al., 2025). The science of universal vaccine design is progressing at a very fast pace by employing computational science and immunology to identify future candidates. For instance, current research has used reverse vaccinology to screen the core proteome from a series of bacterial pathogens and has found potential universal vaccine candidates that can be administered across the board. Targeting conserved proteins from a series of different species, researchers are in the hope to develop vaccines that induce robust immune responses but are less likely to fail due to mutations in the pathogen. One of the most significant studies unveiled numerous promising proteins through large-scale core proteome analysis, suggesting that vaccines developed from such elements may neutralize the obstacles presented by drug-resistant pathogens. This method is particularly vital in combating infections like endocarditis, wherein traditional treatment avenues are impaired by evolving bacterial defenses, pointing towards a significant breakthrough in vaccine technology that would redefine preventive medicine (Chao et al., 2025). The consequences of universal vaccines extend beyond the patient, with significant public health repercussions. Higher vaccine efficacy would translate into herd immunity levels that constrain transmission of the pathogen, further reducing the healthcare burden of infectious disease. Universal vaccines could also further simplify vaccination schedules, making immunization campaigns more cost-effective and efficient. Their design often incorporates antigenic formulations that induce lasting immunity, and therefore minimize the number of booster doses and related healthcare costs. Against the rising danger posed by re-emerging infectious diseases and antibiotic resistance, the development of universal vaccines may well provide an enduring solution to these issues. And as science continues to develop in this field, so-called "universal vaccines" not only bring human health but also promise to enhance the resilience of global public health infrastructure (Bhadouria et al., 2025; Chao et al., 2025).

15.6.3. Integration of Artificial Intelligence (AI) in Vaccine Design

The application of AI in vaccine design is a great advancement in the methods applied in the field of immunology. Traditionally, vaccine discovery has been a long and slow process, normally plagued by inefficiencies and high failure rates. However, with the advent of AI technologies, researchers can quickly scan through vast amounts of information, identify patterns, and develop insights that were previously impossible. For instance, AI computer programs are able to fine-tune the detection of epitopes, which are crucial entities used to trigger an immune response. By being able to predict exactly which epitopes will elicit the strongest responses, AI enhances the validity of vaccine design and maximizes the potential for success. This innovative impact allows it to accelerate the vaccine development timeline, which is increasingly critical in the context of new emerging infectious diseases. In addition to reducing the design time, AI also plays a significant role in customizing vaccine strategies. Each individual's immune response necessitates the need for adaptable approaches to vaccine design, especially considering genetic variation within populations. AI achieves this adaptability by employing machine learning algorithms utilized in processing patient data, including genomic and immunological information. Personalized medicine aims at optimizing therapeutic response using vaccine design adapted to the individual's own distinct immune profile. Furthermore, AI use in predictive modeling can be capable of facilitate the development of therapeutic cancer vaccines, which have specific requirements as opposed to traditional vaccines, thus driving the advancement in vaccine technologies in a manner that is nearer to the needs of individual patients and hence attaining improved health outcomes (Kumar et al., 2024). Regardless of the advantages introduced by AI incorporation, issues continue to exist in the field of vaccine development. Notably, issues such as tumor heterogeneity and the complexity of immune system interactions can complicate predictions for vaccine effectiveness. Additionally, there are ethical considerations concerning data privacy, algorithmic bias, and AI model integrity used in the context of vaccine design. It is important that the challenges are overcome to guarantee the successful utilization of AI technologies. Again, interdisciplinary collaboration is required to effectively harness the potential of AI in this context. By creating partnerships between computational scientists, immunologists, and ethical researchers, the community of vaccine development can work together toward the eradication of today's challenges, ultimately finding breakthrough, AI-based vaccines that can better meet public health needs (Panchariya et al., 2024) (Figure 15.16).

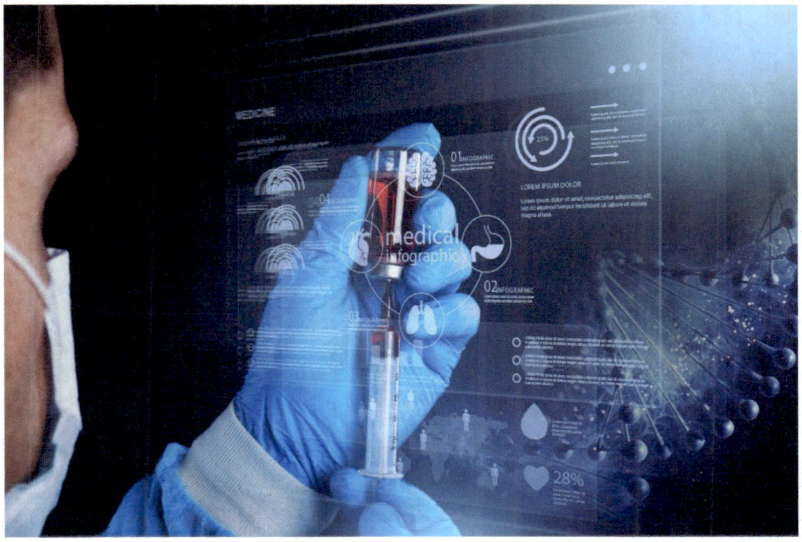

Figure 15.16. The integration of artificial intelligence (AI) in vaccine design marks a significant shift in the methodologies employed in the field of immunology.

Source: https://www.drugtargetreview.com/wp-content/uploads/shutterstock_1718486710-1536x1023.jpg.

SUMMARY

With the emergence of advancements in vaccine development, the innovations that have been made in the methods employed are a huge step toward public health. The innovation of mRNA technology, recombinant proteins, and viral vectors has transformed the landscape of vaccine research, development, and delivery. These innovations not only advance the pace and efficiency of vaccine development but also provide the adaptability needed to respond rapidly to outbreak diseases. The ongoing refinement of these techniques is a methodical effort by the scientific fraternity to employ cutting-edge methods, ultimately leading to more effective vaccine technologies that can tackle worldwide health challenges. The addition of newer techniques like immunoblotting has played a pivotal role in augmenting the information regarding immune responses against vaccines. By enabling precise measurement of antigen expression and protein interaction, techniques such as these permit researchers to more precisely analyze the possible immunogenicity of future vaccine candidates. Sensitive increases and high-throughput formats are only a small example of the advances that have increased the productivity of vaccine research. As identified from the literature, these technologies focus on the importance of sustained investment in methodological advances that are key to establishing immune responses and ensuring novel vaccine platforms are effective and safe in the evolving vaccinology environment (Dubey, 2025). Overall, the future of vaccine development is bright with rapid innovation and increasing capacity to combat infectious diseases. Academic, business, and public health institution collaboration has been a main stimulator for these advances, with conclusive evidence that a multidisciplinary approach is critical for future progress. Additionally, identified knowledge deficits in ongoing research will prove critical for refining existing methodologies and contributing to the bank of available vaccines. As we enter this new era, taking an integral approach that brings together cutting-edge technology and potent epidemiological data will be in a position to enhance our ability to handle public health matters efficiently. This togetherness of the stakeholders will, by extension, seal our preparedness for potential future pandemics and enhance global health outcomes (Mustorpha et al., 2025).

The landscape of vaccine development has evolved revolutionarily and has dramatically transformed the technologies and approaches employed to create successful vaccines. Biomedical sciences, such as the study of virology, immunology, and molecular biology, lay a robust foundation that drives advancements in vaccine formulation and potency. Eminent progress, specifically the development of messenger RNA (mRNA) technology, has revolutionized the field by making it possible to develop and deploy vaccines at a rapid pace during public health emergencies. This approach, especially employed in COVID-19 vaccines, makes it easy to adapt to new pathogens at a fast pace, illustrating the adaptability and responsiveness of modern vaccines. Moreover, with the advent of reverse vaccinology, novel vaccine candidates have been discovered and the vaccine discovery process is being optimized by focusing on specific antigens of the pathogen that elicit high immune responses, as highlighted by the recent reviews of vaccine development trends (Weerarathna et al., 2024). Moreover, the integration of state-of-the-art biotechnological tools has played a key role in optimizing the precision and effectiveness of vaccines. Tools such as CRISPR-Cas9 gene editing, genome sequencing, and computational modeling have enormously increased the ability to study pathogen interaction and optimize vaccine designs tailored to populations. These tools not only provide information on how to maximize the structural integrity of vaccines but also how to understand host-pathogen dynamics, which is central to the development of immunity.

Also, monoclonal antibody development has proved to be a key strategy, which has facilitated the production of highly specific preventive and therapeutic vaccines. The marriage between biotechnology and immunological research is a prime example of how targeted techniques can combat multifaceted infectious diseases as well as challenges associated with vaccine production and hence advance public health on a global level (Weerarathna et al., 2024). Curiously enough, the veterinary vaccine industry also has seen thrilling advances, particularly against diseases such as coccidiosis caused by Eimeria parasites. Though problems like drug resistance and vaccine efficacy continue to crop up, researchers have had to turn to innovative methods based on a greater understanding of parasite biology and host-parasite relationships. Recent studies revealed intricate interactions between Eimeria and host immunity, which are suggestive of the development of more efficient vaccines. Making use of sophisticated approaches, such as genome research and novel immunological techniques, allowed researchers to develop different anticoccidial vaccines that can deal with evolving parasite strains. This interdisciplinary approach points to a key trend in vaccine design: the necessity of bringing advances in biological understanding together with novel approaches to therapy to establish the well-being and productivity of poultry and livestock.

A CLOSER LOOK

VACCINE HESITANCY

Vaccine hesitancy refers to refusal or resistance to vaccination in the context of vaccine availability. It is a complex issue caused by numerous factors, including misinformation, complacency, convenience, and confidence in vaccines. Vaccine hesitancy results in declining vaccination rates, vaccine-preventable disease spread, and public health in general (Figure 15.17).

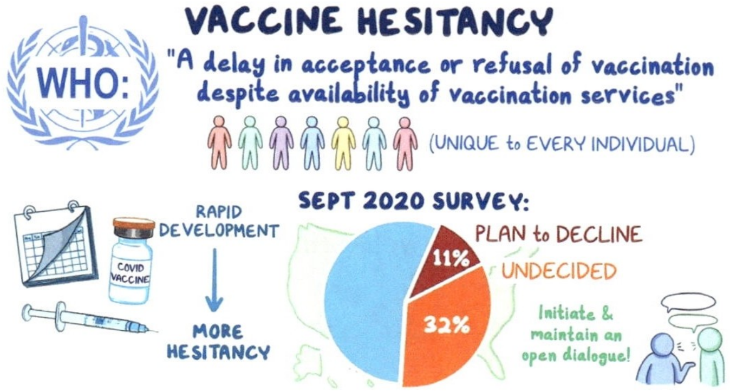

Figure 15.17. Vaccine hesitancy.

Source: https://www.osmosis.org/_next/image?url=https%3A%2F%2Fd16qt3wv6xm098.cloudfront.net%2FtqS6LkOKR_ONSIuwpmRUqDG8Q_KfSGqq%2F_.jpg&w=3840&q=75.

Factors Contributing to Vaccine Hesitancy:

- **Lack of Awareness and Misinformation:** False or misleading information about the vaccine can spread quite rapidly, particularly on social media, and can lead to unjustified fear and uncertainties.
- **Complacency:** When people view a disease to be at low risk or not serious, people become complacent about vaccination despite the fact that the disease may be preventable.
- **Convenience:** Unavailability of access to vaccination services, be it transportation problems, problems in making an appointment, or limited clinic working hours, can lead to hesitancy.
- **Confidence:** Distrust in healthcare professionals, drug companies, or health departments can lower confidence in immunizations.
- **Cultural Beliefs:** Religious and cultural beliefs do play a part now and then in the acceptance and rejection of vaccines.
- **Past Experiences:** Traumatic experiences with vaccines at a personal level or rumors from others may result in hesitancy.
- **Fear of Side Effects:** Fear of potential side effects, although unlikely, can be a compelling disincentive to vaccination.

Tackling Vaccine Hesitancy:

- **Communication and Education:** Providing accurate, fact-based information about vaccines from reliable sources can overcome misinformation and build confidence.
- **Community Mobilization:** Engaging community leaders, health workers, and influential people in pro-vaccination activities and responding to questions can be effective.
- **Removal of Practical Barriers:** Making vaccination services readily accessible, e.g., by extending clinic operating hours or through mobile vaccination clinics, can enhance uptake.
- **Fostering Trust:** Fostering trust in public health agencies and healthcare workers by being transparent in communications and addressing concerns can build vaccine confidence.
- **Tailored Intervention:** Designing interventions tailored to the specific concerns and barriers of specific communities or groups can be more useful.

Consequences of Vaccine Hesitancy:

- **Lower Vaccination Coverage:** Hesitancy can lead to fewer individuals being vaccinated, thereby putting them and their communities at risk for outbreaks of preventable disease.
- **Vaccine-Preventable Disease Outbreaks:** Reduced immunity results in more cases of diseases like measles, whooping cough, and flu, which can lead to severe illness and even death.
- **Higher Healthcare Costs:** Outbreaks can overwhelm healthcare infrastructure and lead to increased costs associated with the treatment of disease.
- **Economic Impacts:** Outbreaks of diseases can destabilize populations, affecting productivity and economic activity.

REFERENCES

1. Gruère, Guillaume P.; Narrod, Clare A.; Abbott, Linda. 2011. Agricultural, food, and water nanotechnologies for the poor: Opportunities, constraints, and role of the Consultative Group on International Agricultural Research. IFPRI Discussion Paper 1064. https://hdl.handle.net/10568/154937(accessed on 27th June 2025).
2. Addy, A. (2023). Comparative analysis: AI-assisted vaccine distribution during COVID-19 pandemic. https://core.ac.uk/download/597470759.pdf (accessed on 27th June 2025).
3. Al Kuwaiti, A., Nazer, K., Alreedy, A. H., AlShehri, S. D., Almuhanna, A., Subbarayalu, A. V., Al Muhanna, D., et al. (2023). A review of the role of artificial intelligence in healthcare. *Journal of Personalized Medicine, 13*, 951–951. https://doi.org/10.3390/jpm13060951 (accessed on 27th June 2025).
4. Miriam Fernandez and Harith Alani. 2018. Online Misinformation: Challenges and Future Directions. In Companion Proceedings of the The Web Conference 2018 (WWW '18). International World Wide Web Conferences Steering Committee, Republic and Canton of Geneva, CHE, 595–602. https://doi.org/10.1145/3184558.3188730(accessed on 27th June 2025).
5. Alowais, S. A., Alghamdi, S. S., Alsuhebany, N., Alqahtani, T., Alshaya, A., Almohareb, S. N., Aldairem, A., et al. (2023). Revolutionizing healthcare: The role of artificial intelligence in clinical practice. *BMC Medical Education, 23.* https://doi.org/10.1186/s12909-023-04698-z (accessed on 27th June 2025).
6. Ananya, Panchariya, D. C., Karthic, A., Singh, S. P., Mani, A., Chawade, A., & Kushwaha, S. (2024). Vaccine design and development: Exploring the interface with computational biology and AI. *International Reviews of Immunology, 43*, 361–380. https://www.semanticscholar.org/paper/1c9123caa6702ec925f4ac25dcf8d43c358e9940 (accessed on 27th June 2025).
7. Fernández, M. L. S., Engels, K. K., Bender, F., Gassel, M., Marhöfer, R. J., Mottram, J. C., & Selzer, P. M. (2012). High-throughput screening with the Eimeria tenella CDC2-related kinase2/cyclin complex EtCRK2/EtCYC3a. *Microbiology (Reading, England), 158*(Pt 9), 2262–2271. https://doi.org/10.1099/mic.0.059428-0(accessed on 27th June 2025).
8. Bekbolatova, M., Mayer, J., Ong, C. W., & Toma, M. (2024). Transformative potential of AI in healthcare: Definitions, applications, and navigating the ethical landscape and public perspectives. *Healthcare, 12*, 125–125. https://doi.org/10.3390/healthcare12020125 (accessed on 27th June 2025).
9. Bhadouria, N., Yadav, S., Naik Bukke, S. P., & Narapureddy, B. (2025). Advancements in vaccine delivery: Harnessing 3D printing for microneedle patch technology. *Annals of Medicine and Surgery, 87*, 2059–2067. https://www.semanticscholar.org/paper/5a0b89cb42fef37d4a3ec32148dafed2af29f3d6 (accessed on 27th June 2025).
10. Hoelzer, K., Bielke, L., Blake, D.P. *et al.* Vaccines as alternatives to antibiotics for food producing animals. Part 2: new approaches and potential solutions. *Vet Res* **49**, 70 (2018). https://doi.org/10.1186/s13567-018-0561-7(accessed on 27th June 2025).
11. Sharmin, S., Biswas, B., Tiwari, A., Kamruzzaman, M., Saleh, M. A., Ferdousmou, J., & Hassan, M. (2025). Artificial Intelligence for Pandemic Preparedness and Response: Lessons Learned and Future Applications. *Journal of Management World, 2025*(2), 18-25. https://doi.org/10.53935/jomw.v2024i4.863 (accessed on 27th June 2025).

12. Bruce, J. I. (1989). *Biotechnology: An Overview.* https://media.neliti.com/media/publications/64026-EN-biotechnology-an-overview.pdf (accessed on 27th June 2025).

13. Narayanasamy, S., Veldman, T. H., Lee, M. J., Glover, W. A., 2nd, Tillekeratne, L. G., Neighbors, C. E., Harper, B., Raghavan, V., Kennedy, S. W., Carper, M., Denny, T., Tsalik, E. L., Reller, M. E., Kibbe, W. A., Corbie, G., Cohen-Wolkowiez, M., Woods, C. W., & Petti, C. A. (2023). RADx-UP Testing Core: Access to COVID-19 Diagnostics in Community-Engaged Research with Underserved Populations. *Journal of clinical microbiology, 61*(8), e0036723. https://doi.org/10.1128/jcm.00367-23 (accessed on 27th June 2025).

14. Chablani, L. (2016). Micro- and nanoparticulate cancer vaccines: A vision for the future. https://core.ac.uk/download/48623203.pdf (accessed on 27th June 2025).

15. Chao, P., Zhang, X., Zhang, L., Ma, W. Y., Wang, D., Yang, A., & Chen, X. (2025). Pan-vaccinomics strategy for developing a universal multi-epitope vaccine against endocarditis-related pathogens. *Frontiers in Immunology, 16.* https://www.semanticscholar.org/paper/4095203e7d6856b12ba547d2f1a2a181c5942730 (accessed on 27th June 2025).

16. Chen, S., Saeed, A. F. U. H., Liu, Q., Jiang, Q., Xu, H., Xiao, G. G., Rao, L., et al. (2023). Macrophages in immunoregulation and therapeutics. *Signal Transduction and Targeted Therapy, 8.* https://doi.org/10.1038/s41392-023-01452-1 (accessed on 27th June 2025).

17. Choi, I. J., Cha, H. R., Kwon, D., Kang, A., Kim, J. S., Kim, J., Choi, J. E., et al. (2024). Development and evaluation of five-in-one vaccine microneedle array patch for diphtheria, tetanus, pertussis, hepatitis B, and *Haemophilus influenzae* type b: Immunological efficacy and long-term stability. *Pharmaceutics, 16.* https://www.semanticscholar.org/paper/3725be3f84c803c773efb224bfc331f1a1b96d1b (accessed on 27th June 2025).

18. Dubey, R. K. (2025). A mini-review on immunoblotting technique in vaccine development: Current innovations. *Zhongguo Ying Yong Sheng Li Xue Za Zhi = Zhongguo Yingyong Shenglixue Zazhi = Chinese Journal of Applied Physiology, 41,* e20250004. https://www.semanticscholar.org/paper/ac33d004fe1d7a63b0db28c4c7250e7a04af0477 (accessed on 27th June 2025).

19. Evju, E. (2023). General aspects and applications of plant genome editing: Advancements in recombinant protein production and viral vaccine efficiency through CRISPR/Cas9-edited *N. benthamiana.* https://core.ac.uk/download/591078709.pdf (accessed on 27th June 2025).

20. Gao, Y., Sun, P., Hu, D., Tang, X., Zhang, S., Shi, F., Yan, X., et al. (2024). Advancements in understanding chicken coccidiosis: From *Eimeria* biology to innovative control strategies. *One Health Advances.* https://www.semanticscholar.org/paper/da7655b2325eee5be0821874d16ada81bd1e8c9b (accessed on 27th June 2025).

21. Gholap, A., Gupta, J., Kamandar, P., Bhowmik, D. D., Rojekar, S., Faiyazuddin, M., Hatvate, N. T., et al. (2023). Harnessing nano vaccines for effective immunization A special concern on COVID-19: Facts, fidelity, and future prospective. *ACS Biomaterials Science & Engineering.* https://www.semanticscholar.org/paper/7fc570b446dedbc9c68a855d864285be97310f87 (accessed on 27th June 2025).

22. Hay, J., Graham, R., Gresham, E., Mullins, M., et al. (2012). Innovative technologies for global space exploration. https://core.ac.uk/download/pdf/10568212.pdf (accessed on 27th June 2025).

23. Hussain, A., Moxley-Wyles, B., Bryan, M., Gordon-Weeks, A., Al-Obaidi, I., Sandhu, C., & Lee, L. (2025). Cancer vaccine trial evaluations: Immunobinding and potential immunological

endpoints. *Immunotherapy Advances, 5.* https://www.semanticscholar.org/paper/cf7d24c33264b6cd617d5fcb4852fd79f6d838e1 (accessed on 27th June 2025).

24. Hutzen, B., Raffel, C., & Studebaker, A. W. (2015). Advances in the design and development of oncolytic measles viruses. *Oncolytic virotherapy, 4,* 109–118. https://doi.org/10.2147/OV.S66078 (accessed on 27th June 2025).

25. Ji, Z., Lee, N., Frieske, R., Yu, T., Su, D., Xu, Y., Ishii, E., et al. (2022). Survey of hallucination in natural language generation. *ACM Computing Surveys, 55,* 1–38. https://doi.org/10.1145/3571730 (accessed on 27th June 2025).

26. Tone Bjordal Johansen, Elisabeth H. Madslien, Mats Forsman, et al (2024). State of the art of synthetic biology—Literature review. https://core.ac.uk/download/653697438.pdf (accessed on 27th June 2025).

27. Katsoulakis, E., Wang, Q., Wu, H., Shahriyari, L., Fletcher, R., Liu, J., Achenie, L. E. K., et al. (2024). Digital twins for health: A scoping review. *npj Digital Medicine, 7.* https://doi.org/10.1038/s41746-024-01073-0 (accessed on 27th June 2025).

28. Kumar, A., Dixit, S., Srinivasan, K., Dinakaran, M., & Vincent, P. M. (2024). Personalized cancer vaccine design using AI-powered technologies. *Frontiers in Immunology, 15.* https://www.semanticscholar.org/paper/a5a7f5de72a051c944f26a61df88c454294fe95c (accessed on 27th June 2025).

29. Kumar, M. A., Baba, S. K., Sadida, H. Q., Al Marzooqi, S., Jerobin, J., Altemani, F. H., Algehainy, N. A., et al. (2024). Extracellular vesicles as tools and targets in therapy for diseases. *Signal Transduction and Targeted Therapy, 9.* https://doi.org/10.1038/s41392-024-01735-1 (accessed on 27th June 2025).

30. Lahiri, A., Maji, A., Potdar, P. D., Singh, N., Parikh, P. M., Bisht, B., Mukherjee, A., et al. (2023). Lung cancer immunotherapy: Progress, pitfalls, and promises. *Molecular Cancer, 22.* https://doi.org/10.1186/s12943-023-01740-y (accessed on 27th June 2025).

31. Levkiv, M., Chorniy, S., Boitsaniuk, S., Chornij, N., Patskan, L., Pohoretska, K., Manashchuk, N., et al. (2025). Advancements in dental materials and modern perspective on dental restoration techniques. *Перспективи та інновації науки.* https://www.semanticscholar.org/paper/bb1c9b96f1688c69686b69a9189a4daf33480a52 (accessed on 27th June 2025).

32. Mafuts, V. (2025). Emerging trends in vaccine development integrating pharmaceutical science with public health. https://core.ac.uk/download/655274906.pdf (accessed on 27th June 2025).

33. Malpani, M., & Telrandhe, U. B. (2024). AI-powered advancements in drug discovery and vaccine development to combat viral threats. *2024 International Conference on Healthcare Innovations, Software and Engineering Technologies (HISET).* https://www.semanticscholar.org/paper/efc5d0646fa0f89b82242f35fd4dbce67cf80a29 (accessed on 27th June 2025).

34. Miethke, M., Pieroni, M., Weber, T., Brönstrup, M., Hammann, P., Halby, L., Arimondo, P. B., et al. (2021). Towards the sustainable discovery and development of new antibiotics. *Nature Reviews Chemistry, 5,* 726–749. https://doi.org/10.1038/s41570-021-00313-1 (accessed on 27th June 2025).

35. Mustorpha, S. I. S., Ahmad, S. W., Kamarudin, M. A. A., Alsakkaf, H. A., & Shafiq, O. (2025). Advancements in earthquake research and seismic risk analysis: An in-depth review centered on Malaysia. *Journal of Advanced Research in Applied Sciences and Engineering Technology.*

https://www.semanticscholar.org/paper/49fb015499a1ebdab9474ef2f66c8189774bb5f3 (accessed on 27th June 2025).

36. K. Saxena, S. (Ed.). (2022). High-Throughput Screening for Drug Discovery. IntechOpen. doi: 10.5772/intechopen.91075(accessed on 27th June 2025).

37. Saranya, K. R., Usha, L. J., Valarmathi, P., & Suganya, Y. (2025). Next-generation vaccines: Leveraging deep learning for predictive immune response and optimal vaccine design. *Journal of Machine and Computing.* https://www.semanticscholar.org/paper/cc65c8681d6fb708b6ced6a5c8c666a5b363e718 (accessed on 27th June 2025).

38. Shehata, A., & Tellez-Isaias, G. (2023). Vaccination against highly pathogenic avian influenza (HPAI): From opposition to acceptance. *The First International Avian Influenza Summit.* The University of Arkansas. October 16–17, 2023. https://www.semanticscholar.org/paper/c91015cacb5c1ab02b585046875a7fdfd2a636a2 (accessed on 27th June 2025).

39. Trucillo, P. (2024). Biomaterials for drug delivery and human applications. *Materials, 17,* 456–456. https://doi.org/10.3390/ma17020456 (accessed on 27th June 2025).

40. Uddin, T. M., Chakraborty, A., Khusro, A., Zidan, B. M. R. M., Mitra, S., Emran, T. B., Dhama, K., et al. (2021). Antibiotic resistance in microbes: History, mechanisms, therapeutic strategies and future prospects. *Journal of Infection and Public Health, 14,* 1750–1766. https://doi.org/10.1016/j.jiph.2021.10.020 (accessed on 27th June 2025).

41. Van de Sande, B., Lee, J. S., Mutasa-Gottgens, E., Naughton, B. J., Bacon, W., Manning, J., Wang, Y., et al. (2023). Applications of single-cell RNA sequencing in drug discovery and development. *Nature Reviews Drug Discovery, 22,* 496–520. https://doi.org/10.1038/s41573-023-00688-4 (accessed on 27th June 2025).

42. Varnosfaderani, S. M., & Forouzanfar, M. (2024). The role of AI in hospitals and clinics: Transforming healthcare in the 21st century. *Bioengineering, 11,* 337–337. https://doi.org/10.3390/bioengineering11040337 (accessed on 27th June 2025).

43. Weerarathna, I. N., Doelakeh, E. S., Kiwanuka, L., Kumar, P., & Arora, S. (2024). Prophylactic and therapeutic vaccine development: Advancements and challenges. *Molecular Biomedicine, 5.* https://www.semanticscholar.org/paper/2be4374c1e888a4593e49c1af26a936d6992d1ca (accessed on 27th June 2025).

44. Yao, X., Yi, Z., Xu, M., & Han, Y. (2025). A review on the extraction, structural characterization, function, and applications of peptidoglycan. *Macromolecular Rapid Communications.* https://www.semanticscholar.org/paper/bc71394978067dd25e2bf95a8f06d0f8a30100f8 (accessed on 27th June 2025).

45. Yasinjan, F., Yang, X., Geng, H., Guo, R., Yang, L., Liu, Z., & Wang, H. (2023). Immunotherapy: A promising approach for glioma treatment. *Frontiers in Immunology, 14.* https://doi.org/10.3389/fimmu.2023.1255611 (accessed on 27th June 2025).

INDEX

D

E

F

G

H

I

J

L

M

Q

R

S

T